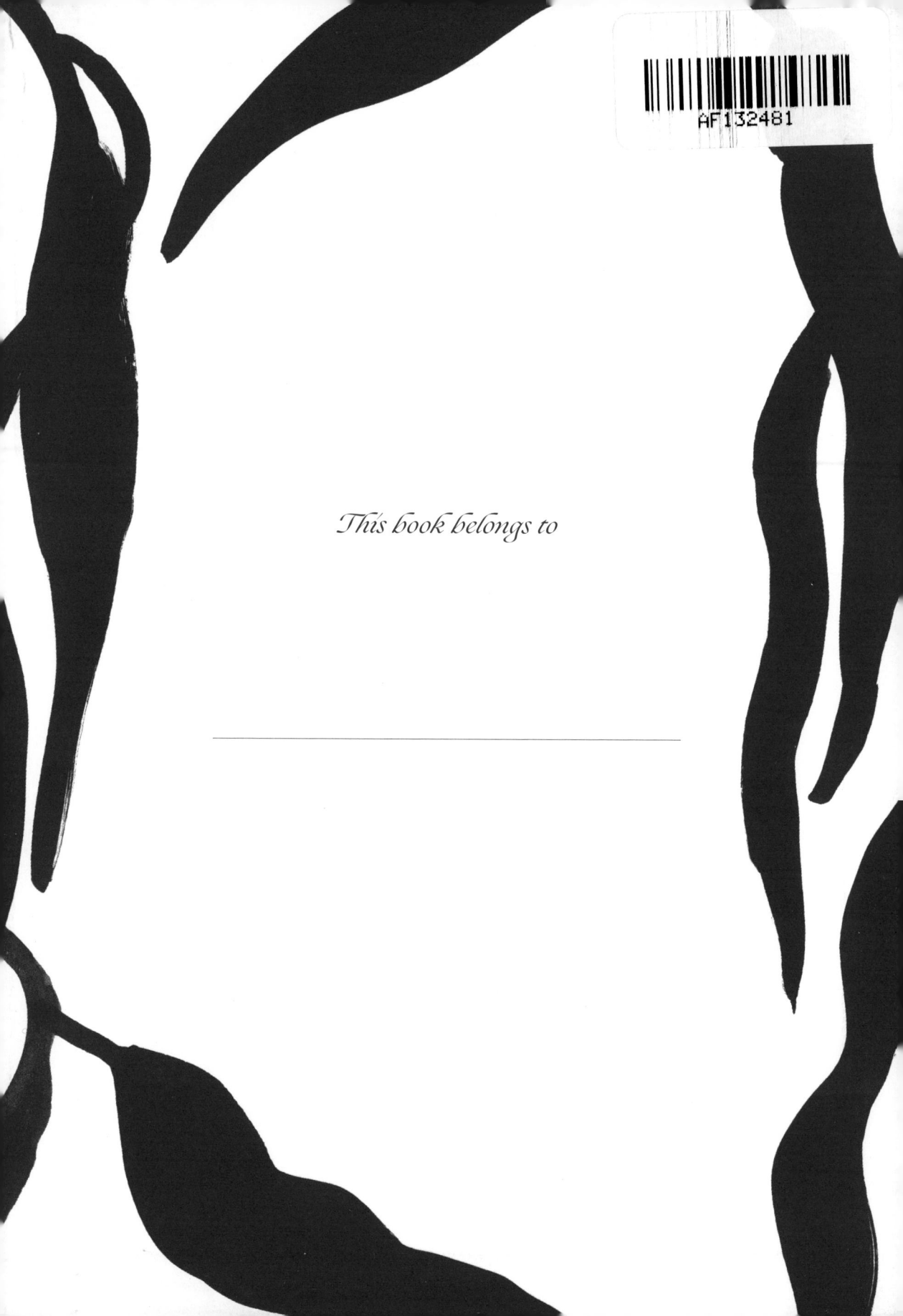

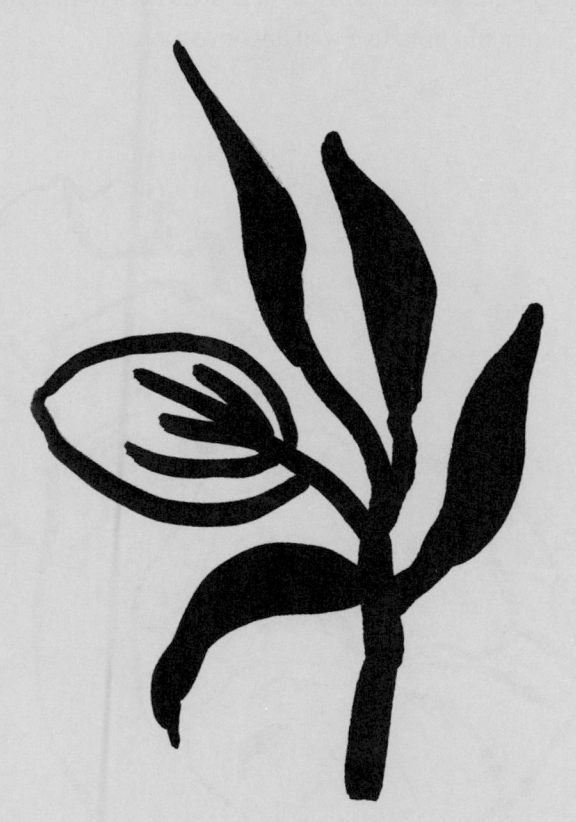

We dedicate this book to the countless women whose honest,
challenging questions inspired us to seek deeper understanding. Your voices guided
our journey. With heartfelt gratitude, we also acknowledge the dedicated scientists
whose research continues to illuminate the path toward greater hormonal health
and empowerment for all women. This book is dedicated to every woman—
remember to live well and love more.

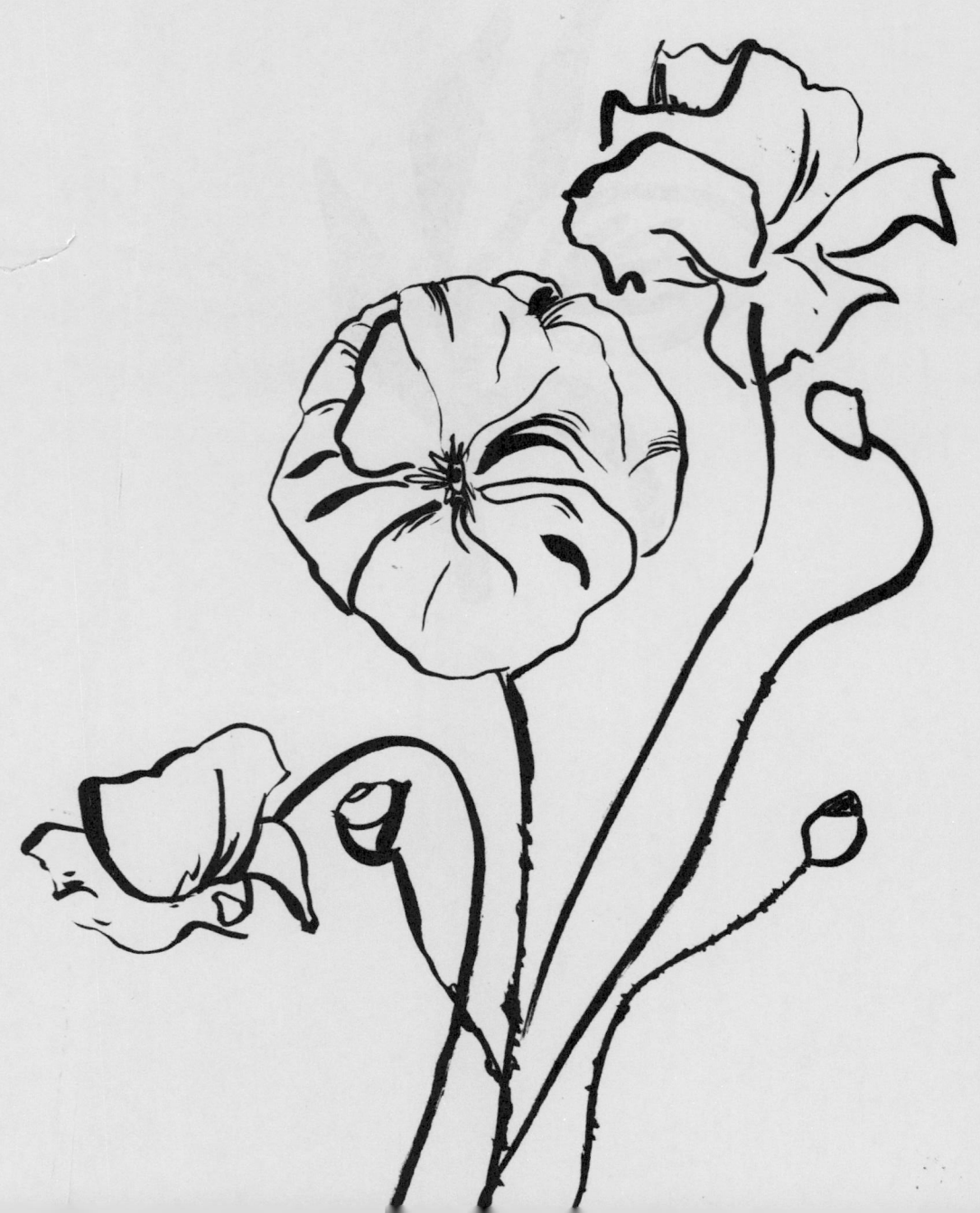

# Hormonal Harmony

## A woman's guide to puberty, fertility, menopause and beyond

DR KAREN COATES & SHARON KOLKKA

A JULIE GIBBS BOOK
for

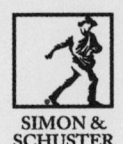

SIMON & SCHUSTER

New York · Amsterdam/Antwerp · London · Toronto · Sydney · New Delhi

# TABLE OF CONTENTS

Welcome 7
About the authors 9
How to use this book for optimal wellness 13

## *Part One*    YOUR HORMONAL JOURNEY            19

| | |
|---|---:|
| **YOUR HORMONES** | 21 |
| **THE FIVE HORMONAL STAGES** | 22 |
| **PUBERTY** | 27 |
| **THE FERTILE YEARS** | 63 |
| **PERIMENOPAUSE** | 119 |
| **MENOPAUSE** | 149 |
| **THE AGE OF WISDOM** | 236 |

## *Part Two*    YOUR HORMONAL HEALTH PILLARS    267

| | |
|---|---:|
| **EPIGENETICS** | 269 |
| **OXIDATIVE STRESS** | 273 |
| **ALCOHOL** | 287 |
| **PSYCHOLOGICAL STRESS** | 290 |
| **ADRENAL GLANDS** | 334 |
| **CORTISOL** | 342 |
| **TULSI HERBAL TEA** | 349 |
| **SLEEP** | 351 |
| **MELATONIN** | 367 |
| **RESTORATIVE PRACTICES** | 372 |
| **NOURISHMENT** | 393 |
| **VITAMINS AND MINERALS** | 443 |
| **MANAGING TOXINS** | 478 |
| **MOVEMENT AND EXERCISE** | 485 |

## Part Three — MASTERING WOMEN'S UNIQUE HEALTH CHALLENGES — 499

| | |
|---|---|
| **PELVIC WELLNESS** | 501 |
| **YOUR CERVIX** | 511 |
| **UTERINE CARE** | 517 |
| **OVARIAN HEALTH** | 524 |
| **BLADDER SUPPORT** | 530 |
| **ENDOMETRIOSIS** | 534 |
| **POLYCYSTIC OVARY SYNDROME (PCOS)** | 546 |
| **INSULIN RESISTANCE** | 564 |
| **BREAST CARE** | 569 |
| **LIVER CARE** | 592 |
| **THYROID** | 599 |
| **BONE CARE** | 612 |
| **BRAIN CARE** | 635 |

## Part Four — MEET YOUR HORMONAL SUPPORT TEAM — 643

| | |
|---|---|
| **YOUR MOOD HORMONES** | 645 |
| **SEROTONIN** | 648 |
| **DOPAMINE** | 658 |
| **GABA FOR RELAXATION** | 667 |
| **TESTOSTERONE** | 673 |
| **OXYTOCIN** | 683 |

Recommended reading 690
Medical references 690
Resources 691
Index 695

If you listen to
your body when it
whispers, you won't
have to hear
it scream.

Planthaya

# Welcome!

You are holding in your hands your passport to a transformative journey through the hormonal landscapes of womanhood. Whether you are reading this for yourself, your daughter, granddaughter or another female in your life, we hope that you consider this your new handbook for your health and hormonal journey.

We write this book with the intention of giving all women a one-stop resource for understanding and navigating the complex hormonal changes that shape our lives. Whether you're approaching puberty, exploring conception and fertility, navigating the sometimes-choppy waters of perimenopause and menopause, or enjoying the freedom from these hormonal disruptors during the Age of Wisdom, you will find information to guide you during this time.

Our intention in writing this book is that as you grow—older and wiser—and your health shifts and changes during your life, you will find the advice and help you seek within these pages.

This handbook has evolved from a profound need: ours and yours. To our knowledge, there is no comprehensive guide that traverses the entire hormonal journey of women in such an inclusive and accessible manner. We have poured our hearts into creating a helpful resource that educates, empowers you to achieve and maintain hormonal balance at every stage of your hormonal life.

We begin with puberty and the often-challenging time this can be, for the teenager, parents or carer. As you move into your Fertile Years, we guide you as you delve into the intricate dance of hormones that can influence everything from mood and metabolism to your fertility and hormonal disruptions. We know this period of your life can be difficult to navigate, and we explore the emotional, mental and physical issues you may encounter during this time. Most importantly, we arm you with the education and solutions that you may not have received from other factions in your life.

The next stage of your life—perimenopause and menopause—can bring with it many changes—both positive and challenging. This time of a woman's life is often poorly explained and can be misunderstood by many practitioners in the medical community, leaving many women feeling alone and invisible. These chapters will provide you with the insights and strategies to help you manage and embrace these significant shifts that occur during this time. With our help you will be steered through these years, with grace, confidence and most of all the knowledge and education needed to help you take control.

Finally, we have rebranded the post-menopause years. No longer the forgotten or twilight years, this is a time we now claim as the Age of Wisdom. Yes, there are challenges physically and mentally during this period, but more importantly this is a time to celebrate the newfound freedom and strength that comes at this stage in life. These pages will offer the guidance to help you maintain optimal health and vitality to enhance your longevity and enjoyment of this time.

What you will find throughout the pages is our collective years of experience within the health and wellness arena. Our advice is evidenced-based, the result of extensive research, learning, and collaboration between two best friends and colleagues who share a passion for women's health. Our first book *How to Be Well* laid the groundwork for women to redress and reclaim their health journey, and we are thrilled to present this comprehensive guide which specifically focuses on hormones. It has been a wonderful project, a true labour of love and we are excited to share our findings, experiences and expertise with you.

Wherever you are in your hormonal journey, *Hormonal Harmony* will provide you with the practical advice and proven strategies all women need to achieve hormonal balance and overcome the many health hurdles that women of all ages can face. With heartfelt gratitude and enthusiasm, we invite you to embark on this adventure with us, towards a beautiful life of balance, wellness, and empowerment.

May the force be with you!

# ABOUT THE AUTHORS

**DR KAREN COATES**

It's a pleasure to share my experiences and insights from over 30 years as a medical doctor and obstetrician—and my personal hormonal journey—with you. Having delivered more than 1000 babies, I've seen almost everything in women's health. Beyond the clinic and delivery room, my own life has been shaped by the hormonal highs and lows we all face.

Let's go back to when I first started in general practice. At the time, women were still celebrating the freedom that the oral contraceptive pill (the Pill) offered—freedom from the fear of an unwanted pregnancy, which, in the 1950s and 60s, often led to immediate dismissal from a government job. In the 1970s, young women tolerated the Pill's side effects because of the career opportunities, financial independence, and control it provided. The trade-off seemed worth it.

Now, decades later, we have more family planning options, but the responsibility for contraception still largely falls on women. Apart from condoms and vasectomy, we're still carrying that load.

Early in my career, I met countless young women suffering from hormonal symptoms—irritability, mood swings, and sore breasts. I knew these symptoms well, both from my patients and my own experience as a newly graduated doctor juggling a stressful career with hormonal chaos. At that time in my life, irritability, fatigue, and breast tenderness were so familiar to me that I reassured women it was all 'normal,' sometimes even joking with their partners to hide the kitchen knives during 'that time of the month.' With limited options, the Pill was often my go-to prescriptive solution.

I faced my own struggles with fertility after four years of trying to conceive my first child, eventually turning to fertility drugs. The stress of delivering babies at all hours of the night had taken its toll on me. But everything changed once I made key lifestyle adjustments.

The second time around I paid attention to the fundamentals of hormonal wellbeing; it took just one cycle to conceive my son. That personal experience ignited my passion for helping women understand their hormones and how profoundly they affect every aspect of life.

In the mid-1990s, a patient gave me a book that changed my perspective on women's hormonal health. *What Your Doctor May Not Tell You About Menopause* by Dr John R Lee was a lightbulb moment. It reconnected me with the biochemistry of the intricate dance of hormones and gave me new tools to help women beyond prescriptions. Interestingly, this same book was pivotal for my co-author, Sharon Kolkka, on her journey in women's health education.

Today, we face a different challenge. Information on health is readily available online but sifting through what's credible and what's cleverly marketed is tricky. I often feel concerned when I see the latest Instagram influencer promoting a 'miracle' hormonal solution. While well-intentioned, hormones are complex. What works for one woman may not work for another because our bodies are influenced by unique genetic, biochemical, and lifestyle factors.

With my foundation in mainstream medicine, I grew as a practitioner, driven to find solutions that conventional medicine did not always provide. I delved into the worlds of nutritional, environmental, and herbal medicine, exploring a rich tapestry of complementary practices.

In addition to my credentials in herbal medicine, I have embarked on postgraduate studies in nutrigenomics—a field that explores the intriguing connection between genetic expression, nutrition, and lifestyle choices, especially in the context of hormonal wellness. Nutrigenomics provides insights into how specific nutrients and lifestyle factors can influence gene activity, allowing us to support hormonal balance and resilience at a cellular level. This personalised approach empowers us to tailor nutrition and lifestyle strategies to our unique genetic makeup, building a strong foundation for optimal hormonal health and overall wellbeing.

Integrating these with conventional medicine has given me a broader toolbox and a fresh perspective, allowing me to offer patients a more holistic and balanced approach to health. It's been both a rewarding and enlightening journey, expanding my understanding of what truly supports wellbeing.

Having worked alongside exceptional naturopaths over my professional life, I have a deep appreciation of their skill and expertise. Many naturopathic principles such as the fundamental importance of food, nutrition, digestion, and the gut microbiome are only recently being appreciated by conventional medicine. These essentials have historically been on the periphery of medical training, yet these pillars of wellness hold profound insights into our overall wellbeing.

Even after decades in integrative medicine, I'm still amazed by how herbs can smooth the bumps on our hormonal journey. The natural world holds firm evidence of how deeply our wellness is connected to it.

While pharmaceutical solutions play a significant role in both prevention and treatment of chronic disease, we need to remember that herbs and natural therapies are powerful allies, especially when combined with the foundations of good health—nourishing food, mindful lifestyle choices, stress management, and gut health. Supporting your body in these ways often leads to more balanced, long-term results. That said, there are times when mainstream medical interventions are the right choice, and that's perfectly fine. But no pharmaceutical option will deliver lasting benefits if you don't address the root causes of hormonal chaos. By blending the best of both worlds, you can navigate hormonal challenges more effectively and enjoy long-term wellbeing.

So, what can you expect from this book? Together, we'll explore the science behind hormonal health, practical steps to support your body, and real-life stories—mine included—that remind you that you're not alone on this journey. From fertility and contraception to perimenopause and menopause, I'll share what I've learned through research, personal experience, and working with women like you.

Ultimately, this book is your guide to making informed choices that support your health and wellbeing. My advice? Always follow the evidence. We've done the research, and we're here to share it with you. Whether you're interested in natural therapies, food as medicine, or mainstream options, this book will give you the tools you need to thrive through every hormonal shift life brings.

Let's get started!
In health,

Dr Karen Coates

## SHARON KOLKKA

In the early 1990s, I worked in the fitness industry as one of the first personal trainers on the Gold Coast, and most of my clients were women. Many younger women were dealing with hormonal imbalances, facing mood swings, heavy periods, and painful breasts, yet had little understanding of why these symptoms occurred or how to manage them. The common solution presented to them was the Pill, but this was not always effective. Many were left wondering how to navigate these uncomfortable symptoms, often being told it was 'normal' and to just 'suck it up, princess.' After all, 'you're a woman!'

Women in their 40s experiencing perimenopause, and those in their mid-50s going through menopause, faced even more complex symptoms. Once again, clear answers were hard to find.

During training sessions, conversations often turned to hormonal symptoms. For younger women, the Pill was a common topic, while for older women, it was hormone replacement therapy (HRT). The decision to take these treatments was frequently debated. At the time, the medical community strongly encouraged the Pill for hormonal balance and HRT for women in perimenopause or post-menopause. However, some women felt uncomfortable with this blanket pharmaceutical approach.

I had no concrete answers either. I knew I couldn't take the Pill, having suffered from migraines during my 20s while on it. My GP insisted it wasn't the Pill, so I tried different brands and even had brain scans to rule out other issues. But no solution emerged. Eventually, I stopped taking the Pill, and like magic, the migraines vanished. This sparked my curiosity. If I couldn't tolerate the Pill in my 20s, how would I handle menopause?

With a background in exercise science, I had always loved researching, so I began focusing on hormones. My flatmate at the time, a general practitioner (GP), was my first source of information. However, despite being an excellent doctor, she didn't have the answers I needed. It turns out that GPs, then and now, often receive limited education on this topic, relying heavily on pharmaceutical representatives to provide guidance. Doctors, strapped for time, rarely have the opportunity to delve deeply into independent research.

Without the convenience of the internet, I turned to books. Two that stood out were *What Your Doctor May Not Tell You About Menopause* by Dr John R Lee MD and *Natural Fertility* by Francesca Naish, a brilliant naturopath and herbalist. These books remain my top recommendations today. (For more, see Recommended reading on page 690.)

Years later, I met Dr Karen Coates, who shared that she, too, had been influenced by Dr Lee's book. His work opened our eyes to the extent of the early use of synthetic hormones, like the Pill, in the 1950s and 60s.

Through ongoing research, I learned to understand my body and its rhythms during my menstrual cycle. I became attuned to the subtle changes in my body each month and learned how to respond to its needs. Understanding how my menstrual cycle worked—and how hormones fluctuated—empowered me to navigate birth control without relying on the Pill. Though it took effort, it was worth it. I felt connected to my body's natural rhythm, and it had little impact on my day-to-day life.

Somehow, almost accidentally, I seemed to have skipped right over the challenges of perimenopause. Reflecting on it now as we write this book, Karen and I can see that my commitment to a healthy lifestyle, stress management, and years spent working within health retreats, surrounded by inspiring naturopathic colleagues, likely paved the way. Some fatigue in my early 40s resolved by tightening up my diet and removing gluten (my magic energy solution). In my late 40s, other symptoms led to removing dairy products (and eventually replacing them with sheep and goat cheese and yoghurt) proved to provide good results. Daily practices like Qigong, regular massage and acupuncture integrated into my self-care plan may have eased my journey through perimenopause, allowing me to arrive at menopause around age 49 with only subtle signs of hormonal shifts. I experienced some sleep disruption and the first interruptions to my once-clockwork menstrual cycle. The year before menopause, I even went 10 months without a period, only for my cycle to start up again before my transition was complete!

By the time I reached menopause, I welcomed it with open arms. At 52, when

Dr Karen, my doctor through these years, confirmed I had officially entered menopause, it felt like I had passed a significant milestone. I've never looked back.

In the late 1990s, while working at a health retreat in Queensland, I began offering a two-hour Women's Health workshop, which soon evolved into three-day retreats. These workshops helped women understand their bodies and explore the natural rhythms of their menstrual cycles and appreciate the influence of the moon and nature on their health. My aim was not to diagnose or offer specific medical advice; instead, simply to educate on the importance of sleep, nutrition, and exercise, as well as inform and celebrate the beauty of femininity.

These workshops offered guidance on what to read and which experts to consult—whether it be a GP, medical specialist, naturopath, or herbalist. When an endocrinologist, who attended a session, complimented me and stated I knew more about hormones than many doctors, my efforts were validated, and I was assured of the path I was on.

Through these workshops, I encountered remarkable women, and together we laughed, cried, and shared wisdom in what felt like sacred women's circles. I was elated by the stories of women who gained a greater sense of control over their hormonal health, and equally horrified by the impact of endocrine disruptors—an issue we discuss further on pages 31, 405 and 478.

Women and their hormonal journeys have remained central to my career, shaping my passion for stress management and life resilience. This journey has led me to work in health retreats for 30 years both as a practitioner and senior leader. Today I work as a strategic wellness advisor for companies keen to include wellness wisdom into their workplaces or design wellness programs for retreats. I also love sharing what I have learned with the corporate world and am often invited to conferences and offsite retreats as a keynote speaker. Regardless of what I do today, I remain passionate about women's health.

I feel incredibly privileged to co-author this book with my dear friend and colleague, Dr Karen Coates. Together, we've poured our combined knowledge about women's hormonal wisdom—from medical, environmental, emotional, and even esoteric perspectives—into these pages. As women, we've lived through every stage of the hormonal journey and now find ourselves in what we call the Age of Wisdom. We believe our role, and that of all women at this stage, is to mentor younger generations, sharing life lessons while empowering each woman to explore her potential.

This book is a celebration of the female journey—its trials, triumphs, and sacredness. It's a guide for you, your daughters, granddaughters, sisters, aunts, and all the women you hold dear. Through it, we aim to support and educate you about your body's wonderful hormonal journey, from the onset of puberty to the Age of Wisdom. Let this book be your companion at every stage, offering support as you navigate the sacred journey of womanhood.

With heartfelt love,

Sharon Kolkka

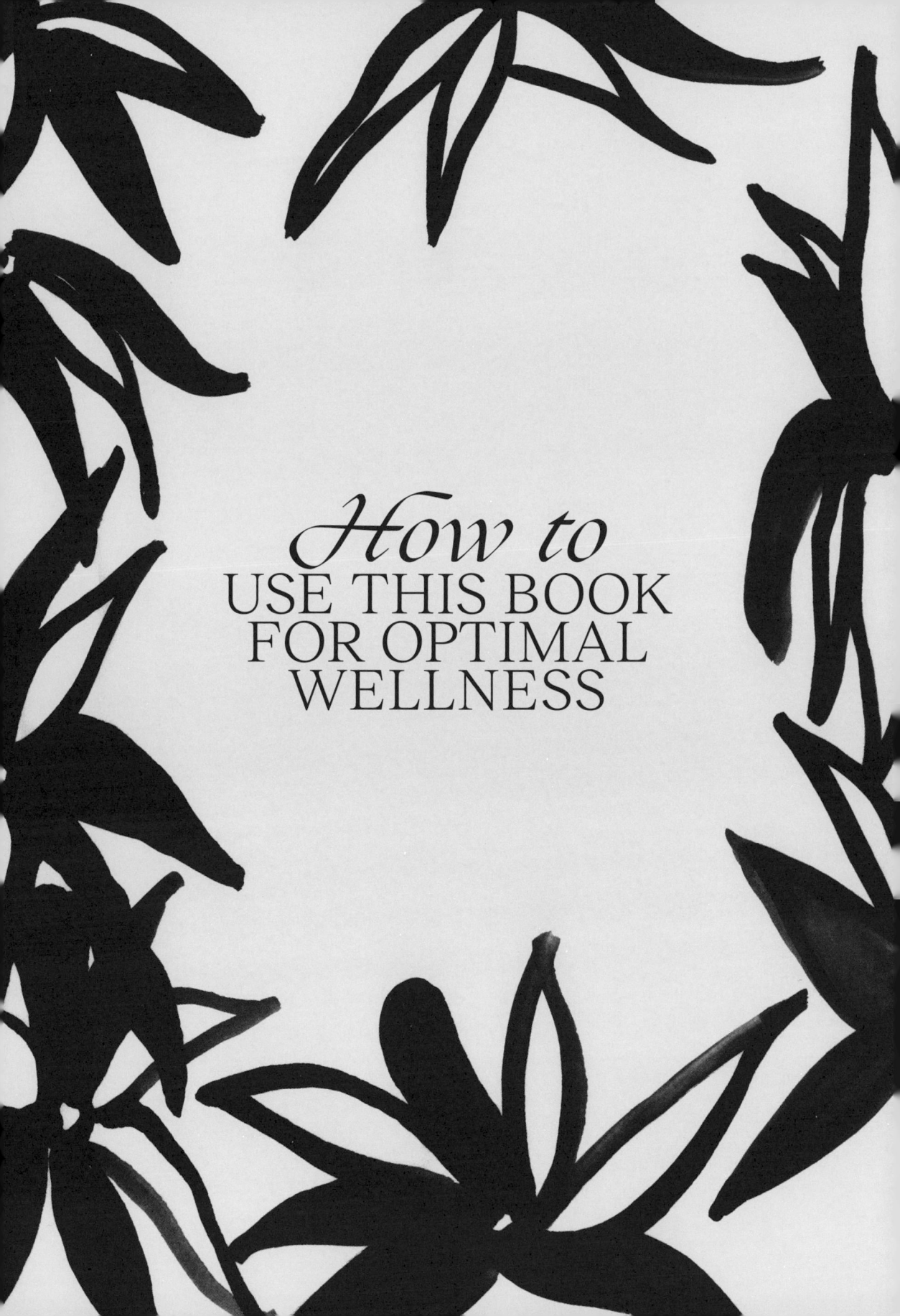

# How to
## USE THIS BOOK FOR OPTIMAL WELLNESS

In *Hormonal Harmony*, we explore every factor that influences hormonal harmony and what disrupts the delicate balance—from sleep and movement to nutrition and lifestyle choices. You'll get to know each of your hormones and how they interact with and influence one another. Our **Spotlight** sections delve deeper into key topics that deserve special attention, while the **Wellness Action Plans** offer practical 'how-to' guides, equipping you with the knowledge needed to make informed decisions about your hormonal health and overall wellbeing.

This book is designed to be a lifelong handbook, a guide to pass down to your daughters or share within your circle of friends. The information here is for all women—to learn, to share, and to empower themselves and others.

**THIS BOOK IS DIVIDED INTO FOUR PARTS**

**Part One:** Your Hormonal Journey
**Part Two:** Your Hormonal Health Pillars
**Part Three:** Mastering Women's Unique Health Challenges
**Part Four:** Meet Your Hormonal Support Team

*Part One*
## YOUR HORMONAL JOURNEY

We delve into the hormonal journey of a woman's life, covering key stages: Puberty, the Fertile Years, Perimenopause, Menopause, and finally, the Age of Wisdom. We invite you to explore these transformative phases, gaining a deeper understanding of how your body evolves over a lifetime.

Even if some sections don't align with your current stage, we encourage you to read—or at least skim—through them. They may offer valuable insights into the paths you've already travelled and the challenges you've faced. These milestones profoundly shape your hormonal and overall health, offering opportunities to make informed changes that support a stronger, healthier future.

By understanding your hormonal landscape and the internal and external factors that influence it, you'll be better prepared to apply the tools and strategies shared in Parts Two, Three, and Four. Let this section empower you to embrace your unique journey and navigate it with clarity and confidence.

*Part Two*
## YOUR HORMONAL HEALTH PILLARS

In this section we invite you to explore the core lifestyle pillars that support hormonal balance, including our Spotlights on stress management, sleep, nutrition, exercise, epigenetics and more. Each topic is presented in a way that's relevant to everyone, with guidance tailored to your age or hormonal stage.

This approach ensures that this handbook becomes a trusted companion throughout your hormonal journey over your lifetime, offering actionable advice and insights to meet your unique needs.

*Part Three*
## MASTERING WOMEN'S UNIQUE HEALTH CHALLENGES

We focus on the health challenges that often arise at different hormonal stages of a woman's life. From menstrual disorders to caring for your female body, this section unpacks the most common concerns women encounter along their hormonal journey.

We explore these challenges and provide practical, evidence-based solutions to help you address them with confidence. Our aim is to empower you with the knowledge and tools to take charge of your health, equipping you to navigate these phases with clarity and resilience.

*Part Four*
## MEET YOUR HORMONAL SUPPORT TEAM

We guide you to understand and nurture the network of supportive hormones that work alongside your primary fertility hormones to maintain balance and overall wellbeing. These often overlooked yet essential hormones play a crucial role in creating hormonal harmony and supporting your health at every stage of life.

We explore practical strategies and insights to help you collaborate effectively with your body—and, if needed, with your fertility team—to optimise these supportive systems. This section is designed to empower you with actionable steps to enhance your hormonal wellness and create a foundation for vitality and balance, no matter where you are on your journey.

**YOUR PERSONAL RESOURCE**

We hope this book becomes a cherished resource for you and the girls and women in your life. We encourage you to keep a highlighter pen handy and mark any text or pieces of advice that resonates with you. As you continue to grow, age and learn, we hope you continue to refer to this book to help you wherever you are in your hormonal journey.

## It's time to take control.
## Let's begin this journey—together.

**A NOTE ON PRONOUNS**

We honour the wide and wonderful spectrum of gender identities and lived experiences with deep respect. To support clarity and ease of reading, we have used she/her pronouns when referring to the reader. However, this book is for everyone. Should you identify with they/them or another pronoun, please know that you are seen, you are welcome, and this book is written with you in mind.

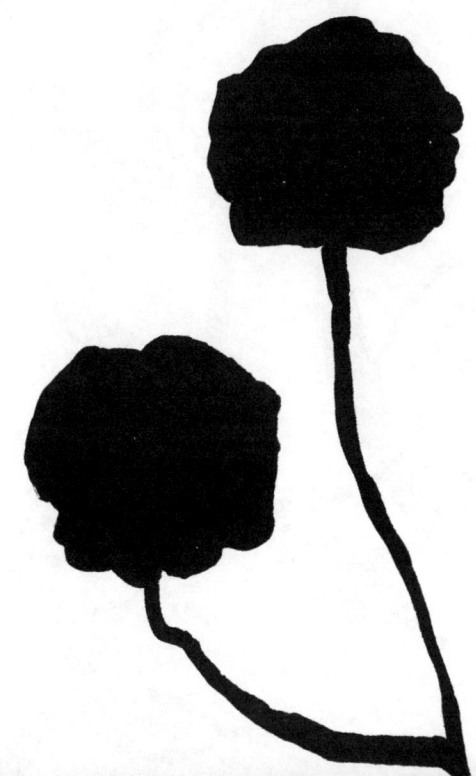

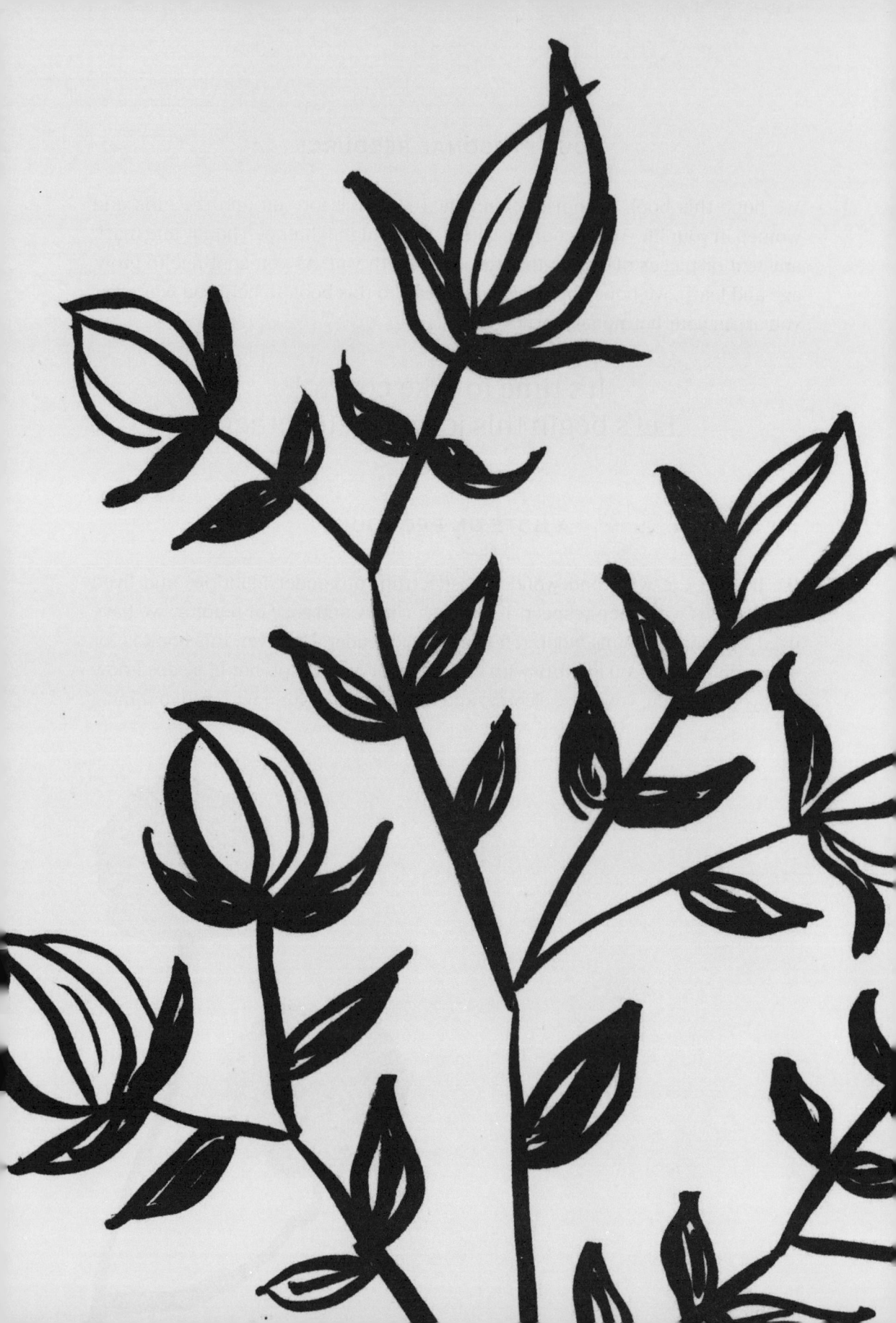

# 1. YOUR HORMONAL JOURNEY

Let's dive into the life stage you're currently experiencing, whether it's Puberty, the Fertile Years, Perimenopause, Menopause or the Age of Wisdom. Our intent is to provide you with practical, tailored strategies to support your health and wellbeing, no matter where you are on the hormonal timeline.

**YOUR HORMONES PAGE 21**

**THE FIVE HORMONAL STAGES PAGE 22**

**PUBERTY PAGE 27**
**THE FERTILE YEARS PAGE 63**
**PERIMENOPAUSE PAGE 119**
**MENOPAUSE PAGE 149**
**THE AGE OF WISDOM PAGE 236**

# Your Hormones

Hormones are the unsung heroes of our bodies, quietly orchestrating nearly every function from our first breath to our final stage of life. As women, our hormonal landscape is a dynamic, ever-changing system that shapes our physical health, emotional wellbeing, and how we experience life. Understanding your hormones isn't just about managing symptoms or conditions — it's about connecting with your body on a deeper level and learning how to nurture it at every stage of your life's journey. Whether you're just beginning your hormonal adventure or navigating your final stages, understanding your hormonal shifts can help you make empowered decisions for your body and mind.

Learning to understand the ebb and flow of hormones, and how to support your body through them, can empower you to take control of your health and wellbeing. By recognising the signs of imbalance, making mindful choices about your diet and lifestyle, and seeking the right support when needed, you can navigate your hormonal journey with greater ease and confidence.

Remember, every woman's hormonal experience is unique. There is no one-size-fits-all approach. Rather, we encourage you to tune into your body and understand its natural rhythms, to be better equipped to face each phase with knowledge, grace, and empowerment.

# The Five Hormonal Stages: From Puberty to the Age of Wisdom

**PUBERTY:
THE SACRED AWAKENING**

Ahh, the teenage years. Who remembers those tumultuous, angst-ridden days? Or perhaps you're dealing with this stage yourself or supporting a beautiful teenage girl. Wherever you are in your hormonal journey now, puberty is where all hormonal stages begin.

Puberty marks the beginning; this is when the pituitary gland signals your ovaries to start producing oestrogen and progesterone—the two key hormones that will define your reproductive years. These hormones regulate the development of your menstrual cycle, breast tissue, and secondary sexual characteristics. Puberty is not just a physical transformation; it's an emotional and psychological one as well. Fluctuating hormone levels can bring mood swings and heightened emotional sensitivity as well as physical changes.

At this stage, it's important to understand the immature body is still fine-tuning itself, and irregular periods, heavy bleeding, and discomfort can all be part of the process. While challenging, this phase is the foundation for reproductive health, and setting healthy habits—like balanced nutrition, adequate sleep, and movement—can help manage symptoms and most essentially, prepare the body for the decades ahead.

**THE PUBERTY CHAPTER BEGINS ON PAGE 27**

## THE FERTILE YEARS

This hormonal stage begins around age 18 and continues to the mid-40s. During this transition into adulthood, your body settles into a regular menstrual cycle, driven by the intricate dance between oestrogen, progesterone, and other hormones. Each month, your ovaries prepare an egg for potential fertilisation, while your uterine lining thickens in anticipation of pregnancy. If the egg isn't fertilised, your hormone levels drop, and your period begins.

During this phase, your hormonal fluctuations are more predictable, yet they can still affect your energy, mood, and physical wellbeing. Fertility is often viewed as the prime function of these hormones, but it's essential to realise they do much more than just regulate reproduction—they impact your bones, muscles, skin, and mental health.

For many women, this stage of life is marked by the use of birth control to regulate periods, prevent pregnancy, or manage hormonal imbalances like Polycystic Ovary Syndrome (PCOS) or endometriosis. Regardless of whether you choose to use contraception, it's important to be aware of how choices like the Pill affect your body's natural hormonal rhythms. Understanding your cycle, tracking your symptoms, and nourishing your body with hormone-supportive foods can help you thrive during these years.

Your fertility levels and the desire to fall pregnant are two connected, yet distinct stages of your hormonal journey. Through this chapter, we explore how to maximise natural fertility through the concept of preconception care. By focusing on this before actively trying to conceive, you can create an ideal environment within your body for a natural pregnancy. This approach not only helps to reduce emotional and financial stress but also harks back to the basics of how our ancestors conceived for thousands of years—basics we often overlook in today's fast-paced world, and we encourage you to revisit them.

We also explore assisted fertility options. Nearly 6% of babies in Australia are born through assisted reproductive technologies like IVF, making it a valuable option for those who need it, whether due to sexual diversity or after extended struggles with conception.

Regardless of the path you choose, preconception care can help prepare your body for a healthy pregnancy, ensuring both you and your baby thrive throughout.

**THE FERTILE YEARS CHAPTER BEGINS ON PAGE 63**

## PERIMENOPAUSE:
## THE THREE PHASES OF TRANSITION

Perimenopause is the natural transition between your reproductive years and menopause, usually beginning in your 40s, sometimes earlier. During the early stage (what we call Phase One) your hormone levels begin to fluctuate more unpredictably as your ovaries produce less progesterone. Subtle at first, you may experience a range of symptoms like erratic or heavy periods, sleep disturbances, and changes in libido. This low progesterone sets the stage for symptoms of oestrogen dominance (Phase Two) to add its flavour to your monthly hormonal rollercoaster. As you move closer to the door of menopause, a fall in oestrogen (Phase Three) adds further layers of symptoms to the mix, with hot flushes, night sweats and missed periods starting to dominate your hormonal landscape.

The three phases of perimenopause can last anywhere from a few months to over a decade, and every woman's experience is unique. This transition is often the most confusing and misunderstood, as women and their doctors may not realise that the symptoms they are experiencing are connected to fluctuating hormones **across the three phases**. It's crucial to listen to your body during this time and, if needed, consult a doctor who specialises in women's hormonal health for tailored support and guidance.

Lifestyle changes, such as stress management, regular movement, and a nutrient-dense diet, can help ease the transition and make perimenopause a more manageable experience.

**THE PERIMENOPAUSE CHAPTER BEGINS ON PAGE 119**

## MENOPAUSE:
## THE END OF REPRODUCTION

Menopause is officially defined as twelve consecutive months without a period. Historically, menopause was identified by the symptoms of oestrogen deficiency, which we now identify as a part of your perimenopausal Phase Three stage. This final transformation, dominated by oestrogen deficiency, can last a couple of years: your ovaries produce less oestrogen, and along with lowered progesterone, bring symptoms such as hot flushes, vaginal dryness and weight gain. It's a sign that your reproductive years have come to an end. Most women reach menopause in their late 40s to mid-50s, but the age can vary widely.

While menopause is often feared for its physical symptoms, it may also be a time of liberation. The end of monthly cycles means freedom from periods, birth control, and the rollercoaster of hormonal fluctuations that have accompanied your reproductive years. For many women, this is a time to focus on their own health, growth, and empowerment.

Hormone replacement therapy (HRT) is one option that can help manage menopausal symptoms, though it's not for everyone. Some women opt for natural alternatives like tailored bioidentical hormones, herbal supplements, or lifestyle interventions to balance their bodies. The key is to find what works for you and remember that menopause is not the end of your hormonal journey—it's simply the beginning of a new and exciting chapter.

**THE MENOPAUSE CHAPTER BEGINS ON PAGE 149**

## THE AGE OF WISDOM

Despite the challenges of declining hormones, we find it more empowering to redefine your post-menopausal time as the 'Age of Wisdom.' This marks the final stage of your hormonal transitions. While your hormone levels have largely stabilised, the long-term effects of lower oestrogen and progesterone can impact your bones, heart, and brain health. This is why it's crucial to focus on preventative care during this period (if not earlier). We encourage you to focus on building strong bones, supporting heart health, and keeping your mind sharp through mental stimulation and stress management.

With the intensity of hormonal fluctuations behind you, many women find this phase of life to be one of clarity, purpose, and self-assurance. Your focus shifts from managing reproductive health to nurturing your body for longevity, with an emphasis on maintaining strength, vitality, and overall wellbeing.

**THE AGE OF WISDOM CHAPTER BEGINS ON PAGE 236**

# Puberty

Let's delve into the fascinating world of puberty with a look at the following topics:
- Understanding the menstrual cycle
- The role of key hormones: oestrogen and progesterone
- The dance of the hormones: how they influence the menstrual cycle
- Is the contraceptive pill a good option?
- Green and Red Flag menstrual cycles: what is normal and when to seek help
- Herbal and lifestyle support
- Skin problems
- The teenage brain: emotional wellbeing and communication
- Sacred celebration: embracing the first menstruation
- Nutritional considerations: what should she eat?
- Movement and exercise: finding the sweet spot

> **Still the same girl with the same name,
> just a different mindset and a new game.**
>
> **NICOLE BROWN**

**CASE STUDY | SHARON**

# My hairy legs, bra straps, and the not-so-comfy 'mattresses'.

I remember the thrill of being the first girl in grade seven to wear a bra—I was about 12. The shopping trip with mum felt like a secret female mission, and I basked in the grown-up glow until the boys discovered flicking my bra straps! As my breasts grew, I had to deal with new body changes: armpit hair (which granted me the privilege of using a razor), pubic hair (which I eventually managed with wax—ouch!), and larger breasts (which were both exciting and inconvenient as a horse rider).

Around 15, I noticed my legs were hairy—how had I never noticed before? My friends shaved but Mum had a firm stance against it. Eventually, peer pressure won out and I secretly shaved my legs. Mum discovered my secret months later and I had to face the consequences.

My period didn't arrive until two years after these changes, which left me feeling concerned and embarrassed. My friends were all at different stages, and I remember feeling confused—didn't puberty have some kind of order? Why did one of my friends not wear a bra but have periods, while I had all the changes but no period? I felt left out and weird at the same time.

When my first period finally arrived, Mum had thankfully prepared me with sanitary napkins, but they were horrendous—it was the early 70s, after all! I wore a belt that connected to a bulky pad, and I remember thinking, 'Why did I want my period so much?' The realisation that this would happen every month hit me hard. Swimming was out and choosing clothes that wouldn't show the bulky 'mattress' between my legs became a challenge.

Then, one day at school, the older girls were discussing tampons. Ignoring Mum's 'nothing enters until marriage' rule, I embraced the freedom of tampons, which allowed me to reclaim my independence without the medieval belt contraption.

Puberty was a wild and scary ride, but looking back, I believe it helped shape me into a resilient and resourceful individual.

# ADVICE FOR MUM, DAD, AND CARERS

*'We thought we were prepared for this time in her life, but OMG, we are not prepared. Who is this person in our house, and what happened to our little girl? The teenage stage is harder than we expected—it makes the toddler years seem easy!'*

If this thought or conversation sounds familiar, take heart—you're not alone. There is so much happening in your girl's body, brain, and emotions, and she is likely just as confused and scared as you are, even if she doesn't admit it.

This chapter is not about parenting —we aren't mental health specialists and, of course, every teenager is different. What we will uncover in this chapter is an exploration of the hormonal changes to expect during puberty, to give you an insight into the physical challenges that can affect behaviour and health. This understanding of the changes that can or may occur during this time can help you support and coach your girl through the transformation from child to young woman with empathy, patience, and love.

Starting conversations about puberty before age 10 can normalise the experience and make it less daunting when it arrives. Something as simple as, 'One day your breasts will develop, and you might see some blood in your pants—that's totally normal. Come talk to me about it anytime,' can make a world of difference.

### YOUR TEENAGER IS NOT AN ADULT

Research shows that a child's environment has a more significant impact on their development than genetics alone. While puberty bombards your child's body with powerful hormones, her brain is still rapidly developing. It's important to adjust your expectations of her emotional intelligence and self-regulation.

The key to navigating this stage is consistency, boundaries, empathy, and reassurance. While this time can be extremely rough, it will pass, and with the right support, an emotionally aware, resilient adult will emerge.

### THE BLOSSOMING OF PUBERTY

Puberty typically begins between the ages of 10 and 14, though timing varies for everyone. Hormonal fluctuations trigger physical, emotional, and psychological changes, marking the transition from childhood to adolescence. This sacred awakening of the feminine spirit is not just a biological process, it's a holistic transformation that encompasses the body, mind, and emotions.

During this time, young girls experience a range of emotions—from excitement and curiosity to uncertainty and vulnerability. It's crucial to provide a supportive environment that encourages open communication. Creating a safe space for discussions about bodily changes and emotional wellbeing can empower girls to navigate puberty with confidence.

### HOW TO EMBRACE THE JOURNEY

Each girl experiences puberty differently, and there is no one-size-fits-all approach. Encouraging self-love and body positivity is crucial, as is creating a supportive environment that fosters open communication.

# Puberty for a girl is like floating down a broadening river into an open sea.

**STANLEY G HALL**

# UNDERSTANDING THE MENSTRUAL CYCLE

As your young girl progresses through puberty, the hormonal interplay between oestrogen and progesterone sets the stage for her menstrual cycle. This intricate dance occurs monthly, with each cycle typically lasting 28 to 30 days. These hormonal shifts influence not just the menstrual cycle but also mood, energy levels, and physical symptoms.

> Some girls begin to show signs of puberty as young as seven or eight years old, a trend that's becoming more common. One significant factor driving early puberty is exposure to endocrine-disrupting chemicals (EDCs)—substances found in plastics, personal care products, and pesticides. These chemicals can mimic or interfere with the body's natural hormones, leading to imbalances that trigger early puberty. (See Spotlight on Managing Toxins page 478.)
> 
> Other factors include rising obesity rates, as higher body fat can affect hormone levels. Understanding these triggers is essential to addressing the physical, emotional, and social impacts of early puberty.

### TRACK AND TAKE CHARGE

Keeping a period diary is a helpful tool for both you and your daughter. If she's too young, disinterested, or has a disability, you can maintain it for her. Tracking her period helps reduce the chances of unexpected surprises during social events or activities, and provides valuable insights into her cycle.

Encourage her to note moods, physical symptoms, and discomfort. This record can be invaluable when consulting healthcare professionals, as it helps them understand her hormonal balance or imbalances. It also guides the timing for hormonal testing, providing a history of symptoms over two to six months. Many young girls and women use period tracking apps such as *Spot On*, *Clue* and *Flow*. Alternatively, we have provided you with a Period Tracking Table on page 33 to be used or referred to as a journal reference to help you keep track of your periods.

> **TIP**
> 
> Keep in mind that during the first 12 months of menstruation, periods are often irregular. It's normal for them to disappear for a few months before returning.

## I remember my friends and I looking forward to puberty because it seemed exciting at first.

**MARA WILSON**

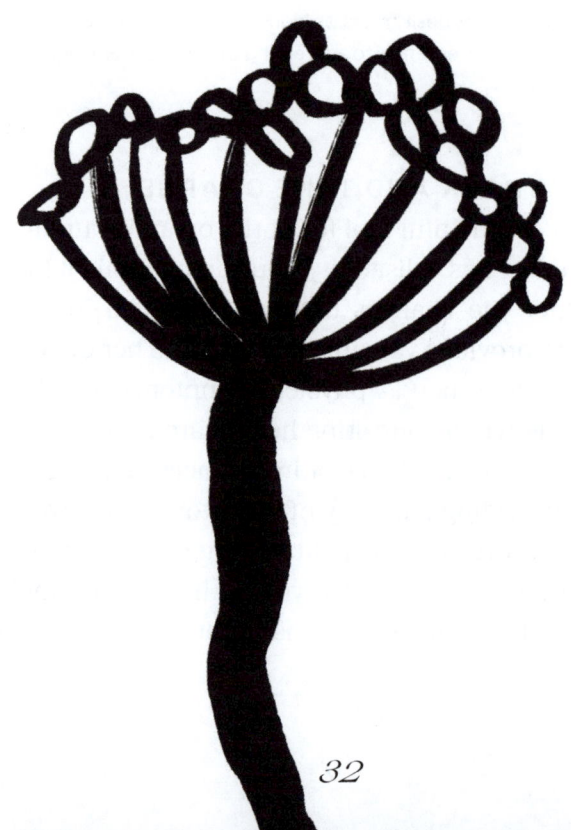

# PERIOD TRACKING TABLE

| DAY | 1 | 2 | 3 | 4 | 5 | 6 | 7 |
|---|---|---|---|---|---|---|---|
| DATE | | | | | | | |
| Period Flow | | | | | | | |
| Cramps | | | | | | | |
| Breast Tenderness | | | | | | | |
| Headaches | | | | | | | |
| Fatigue | | | | | | | |
| Bloating | | | | | | | |
| Acne | | | | | | | |
| Mood | | | | | | | |
| Energy Levels | | | | | | | |
| Sleep Quality | | | | | | | |
| Exercise | | | | | | | |
| Diet Changes | | | | | | | |
| Hydration | | | | | | | |
| Social Activities | | | | | | | |

Use descriptive words such as None/Mild/Moderate/Severe or Poor/Fair/Good.

# OESTROGEN AND PROGESTERONE: THE KEY PLAYERS

The menstrual cycle is orchestrated by two primary hormones: oestrogen and progesterone. These fertility hormones perform a delicate balancing act throughout a woman's life. While their levels fluctuate naturally during the menstrual cycle, their impact on overall health and development is significant, starting from puberty and continuing throughout a woman's reproductive years and beyond.

For young girls, the first appearance of these hormones during puberty marks a pivotal moment in their growth and development. Oestrogen and progesterone influence not only fertility but also bone health, mood, and general wellbeing.

**THE ROLE OF OESTROGEN**

- Retains body fluid
- Thickens the uterine lining for pregnancy
- Supports brain function, especially learning and memory
- Enhances communication skills
- Regulates appetite
- Promotes quality sleep
- Maintains good bone density

**THE ROLE OF PROGESTERONE**

- Balances the effects of oestrogen during the luteal phase (second half) of the menstrual cycle
- Supports pregnancy during the first 12–14 weeks
- Aids thyroid function
- Maintains healthy breast tissue
- Acts as a mood stabiliser and natural antidepressant
- Releases body fluid
- Works with oestrogen to support bone density

## OESTROGEN:
## THE GUARDIAN OF FEMININITY

Oestrogen is one of the primary hormones driving the changes during puberty. It plays a vital role in the development and maintenance of female reproductive organs. In the early stage of puberty, called 'thelarche', oestrogen levels begin to rise. The first visible sign is often changes in the nipples, as breast buds start to form, signalling the start of puberty.

As this process progresses, the ovaries produce more oestrogen, eventually leading to the onset of menstruation—known as 'menarche'—marking the body's potential for conception.

Oestrogen plays a key role in shaping a girl's physical appearance during puberty. It promotes breast growth, widens the hips, and contributes to a more feminine body shape. Additionally, oestrogen stimulates the growth of pubic and underarm hair and the enlargement of the vulva, uterus, and ovaries.

Beyond physical changes, oestrogen affects emotional wellbeing and cognitive development. It influences mood regulation, memory, and cognition, often leading to mood swings, heightened emotions, and changes in thought processes. It's a time where the once innocent child may begin to show the more resistant and stubborn parts of her personality. To be honest, as challenging as this may be, it's quite normal. Sleep patterns may change (see Spotlight on Sleep on page 351), and she may become obsessed with her social circle, often feeling FOMO (fear of missing out). These are typical symptoms of increasing oestrogen and a changing brain.

> **BABY 'MINI-PUBERTY'**
>
> After birth, both testosterone and oestrogen begin to rise, peaking around age 3 months in what scientists' call 'mini-puberty.' In girls, the surge of oestrogen can cause breast bud swelling and vulval fullness, resembling a mini version of puberty. This phase often goes unnoticed by parents and health practitioners.
>
> In rare cases, especially in premature girls, this mini puberty can last longer and may result in vaginal bleeding. While this can be stressful for both parents and doctors, it is a temporary condition that typically resolves without the need for medical intervention.

## PROGESTERONE:
## NURTURING THE PATH TO WOMANHOOD

While oestrogen takes the lead during early puberty, progesterone plays a vital supporting role. Unlike oestrogen, which thickens the uterine lining in preparation for pregnancy, progesterone helps shed the lining if the egg isn't fertilised, leading to menstruation.

Progesterone levels remain relatively low during early puberty, but as a girl nears her first ovulation, her body produces more progesterone to regulate the menstrual cycle and prepare the uterus for potential pregnancy. Initially, erratic bleeding is common as progesterone 'joins the party' to balance the effects of oestrogen. When periods become regular, it signals that progesterone has fully stepped in.

Progesterone acts as a stabiliser, moderating the effects of oestrogen—think of oestrogen as the accelerator and progesterone as the brake. In early puberty, progesterone may be slow to catch up, contributing to oestrogen-dominant symptoms like sore breasts, headaches, mood swings, and cramps. While these echo symptoms of premenstrual syndrome (PMS), it's important to understand that for a young female at this stage in her life these symptoms are not PMS. Rather they are normal developmental symptoms that can often be managed with lifestyle changes. If symptoms persist into later adolescence, an integrative doctor may help to support a normal progesterone surge and prevent potential long-term health issues. (See the Resources section on page 691 for integrative doctors.)

# THE DANCE OF
# THE PUBERTY HORMONES

In early puberty, a girl's body is developing hormonal pathways which take time to fully form. These pathways can be compared to walking through an overgrown forest trail—difficult at first, but over time, it becomes easier to navigate. Eventually, the path widens into a road and finally, a superhighway.

Early puberty is like the barely visible path, and the body is working hard to develop the hormonal 'superhighway' needed for long-term hormonal health. It's normal for periods to be irregular and for hormonal symptoms to fluctuate. While it may be tempting to seek a quick fix, such as the Pill, it's essential to allow the body time to develop these pathways naturally. Intervening too early with synthetic hormones can disrupt the body's ability to regulate itself in the long term.

To support this natural development, focus on a balanced lifestyle: minimal stress, regular movement, nutritious food (covered later in the chapter), sufficient sleep, and emotional support. Herbal remedies like Chaste Tree can also help promote progesterone production and balance oestrogen. (See the herbal remedies recommendations on page 45 or consult a naturopath for more guidance.)

Think of your young girl as embarking on a 28-day adventure every month. Keeping track of her cycle can help you both understand what's going smoothly and what may be out of sync. While the body can be quite precise when hormones are balanced, the timing can vary slightly from person to person. (For example, when we mention Day 14, it may be around Day 12 for some.)

# THE MENSTRUAL CYCLE AS A TEENAGER

Let's begin the cycle at menstruation. During this stage, both oestrogen and progesterone are at very low levels.

## A NORMAL MENSTRUAL CYCLE TABLE

| PHASE | DAYS | DESCRIPTION |
|---|---|---|
| Day 1 | Day 1 | The moment bright red blood appears, count this as Day 1. Ideally, a period should last no longer than five days of bright red blood. Spotting brownish blood is normal for up to two days on either side of the period. |
| Oestrogen Rise | Day 6–14 | Oestrogen increases, enriching the lining of the uterus. |
| Hormonal Surge | Around Day 12–13 | A surge in luteinising hormone (LH) and follicle-stimulating hormone (FSH) occurs, signalling the ovary to release an egg. |
| Ovulation | Day 14 | An egg is released from the ovary. The egg travels through the fallopian tube to the uterus. Oestrogen levels begin to decrease, while progesterone slowly starts to rise above oestrogen levels. |
| Progesterone Surge | Day 18 | Progesterone starts to surge. |
| Progesterone Peak | Day 21 | Progesterone reaches its peak. If fertilisation occurs, ovulation leaves a crater in the ovary called the *corpus luteum*, which becomes a temporary gland, producing a surge in progesterone to support the foetus during early pregnancy. |
| Testing Window | Day 21–22 | Ideal window for hormonal blood tests to observe the progesterone/oestrogen balance. |
| Cycle Restart | Day 28–30 | Menstruation begins, marking the start of a new cycle. A healthy hormonal cycle shows higher oestrogen levels than progesterone in the first two weeks and significantly higher progesterone in the second two weeks of a 28 to 30-day cycle. |

When ovulation doesn't occur there is a hormonal disruption in the second half of the cycle, creating hormonal imbalance.

Before ovulation is fully established in puberty, the hormonal 'dance' is naturally erratic. Oestrogen follows its usual pattern, but progesterone often fails to reach its peak between Days 18 and 25 to counterbalance oestrogen's effects. As a result, oestrogen takes the lead unchecked—not because its levels are unusually high, but because progesterone isn't there to keep it in check. This can trigger symptoms like mood swings, sore breasts or heavier periods. It's all part of the normal hormonal transition during puberty.

### PMS-LIKE SYMPTOMS IN PUBERTY VS PMS IN MATURE WOMEN (18+ YEARS)

During puberty, the balance of hormones is crucial to the overall hormonal system. As the body undergoes significant changes, it's common for girls to experience irritability, mood swings, and discomfort, similar to premenstrual syndrome (PMS). This is largely due to fluctuating progesterone levels as the menstrual cycle begins to regulate.

These symptoms, often resembling PMS, are typically temporary as the body establishes its hormonal pathways. Over time, as the cycle becomes more regular and the progesterone surge stabilises, these symptoms usually lessen by around 18 years of age.

However, if these symptoms persist into the Fertile Years—especially during periods of intense stress—this can be a **Red Flag** (see page 43) and may indicate an underlying issue that needs attention.

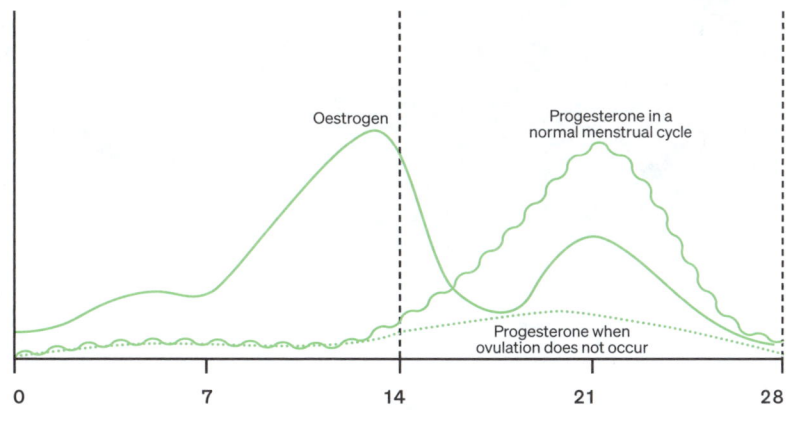

Days of your menstrual cycle

YOUR HORMONAL JOURNEY

# The Menstrual Cycle

**MENSTRUATION**

This is the period when the endometrium or lining of the uterus sheds over 3–7 days if there is no pregnancy.

**LUTEAL PHASE**

This is when the endometrium (the lining of the uterus) is thick and prepared to support a pregnancy or be released in a period.

**FOLLICULAR PHASE**

This is when several eggs mature inside small cysts or follicles within the ovary.

**OVULATION**

This is when an egg is released from the biggest follicle and travels through the fallopian tube, where it can be fertilised. If it is not fertilised, it dissolves in about 24–48 hours.

# THE PILL: YES, OR NO?

Dr Karen says, 'General practitioners, with limited consultation time, often prescribe the Pill for hormonal imbalances in puberty. However, I recommend exploring all natural solutions before turning to pharmaceutical options, unless it's absolutely necessary.

'This can be a tricky path to navigate as a parent or carer, as girls as young as 14 may legally be prescribed the Pill by their doctor without parental consent if they believe them to be "mature minors" and capable of making an informed decision. This is especially true if contraception is the underlying reason for the consultation.

'As a young body matures, it needs time to develop its neural connections and hormonal pathways. The Pill replaces natural hormones with synthetic versions, effectively blocking these pathways by introducing a one-size-fits-all hormonal rhythm. While it may seem like a quick solution, it often contributes to long-term hormonal dysfunction when you stop taking the Pill.

'Before considering the Pill for hormonal imbalances during puberty (or at any age), consult a naturopath or integrative doctor specialising in women's health to explore lifestyle and herbal remedies. Practitioners of Traditional Chinese Medicine or Ayurveda can also help establish balance across the body's systems, which is key to healthy hormones.'

**TIP**
If the Pill is being considered for contraception, ask your doctor to prescribe the lowest dose possible.

# GREEN, ORANGE AND RED FLAGS

The following descriptions of the different menstrual cycles are a guide to help you identify your own menstrual cycle or your daughter's/girl's cycle.

### MENSTRUAL CYCLE: GREEN FLAG

This is an ideal menstrual cycle; this means hormones are likely to be in balance.
- Regular 28 to 30-day cycle
- Light to moderate breast tenderness
- Light to moderate cramping
- No need to change sanitary pads or tampons more than every four hours

### MENSTRUAL CYCLE: ORANGE FLAG

The following symptoms suggest some imbalance.
- Headaches
- Sore breasts
- Dizziness during periods
- Uncomfortable cramping, manageable with basic pain relief (for example, Nurofen or paracetamol)
- Spotting or bright red bleeding before and after the period
- Diarrhoea during periods

**SOLUTIONS**

Respond with lifestyle adjustments—nutrition, exercise, reducing stress. (Read Part Two: Your Hormonal Health Pillars on page 267.)

## MENSTRUAL CYCLE: RED FLAG

These symptoms below represent hormonal imbalance.
- Very heavy or frequent periods.
- Extremely sore or lumpy breasts.
- Severe fatigue.
- Depression or severe mood changes.
- Blood clots and flooding.
- Bright red blood flow lasting longer than six days.
- Severe cramping.

**SOLUTIONS**

First step is to address lifestyle adjustments—nutrition, exercise, reducing stress, adequate sleep etc.

---

Next step is to visit a naturopath for review and herbal support, if there is no improvement over the next 4-6 months, arrange a consultation with an integrative doctor or a GP with a special interest in Women's Health.

---

Review the Your Hormonal Health Pillars in Part Two and Herbal Solutions (page 177). Even when medical intervention is needed, establishing a solid wellness foundation and lifestyle solutions adjustment is crucial for achieving hormonal balance. This approach applies to every stage of a woman's life.

Hormonal balance requires consistent effort from everyone at any age. As challenging as this may be with a tween, the effort is well worth it. Learning to balance hormones early in life will help her understand the importance of healthy habits to support her through every hormonal transition until the Age of Wisdom. For further support, consult a Traditional Chinese Medicine or Ayurvedic practitioner (see our Resources section on page 691 for our recommendations).

CASE STUDY | DR KAREN

# Millie

## Hormonal balance with Chaste Tree

Millie, a first-year journalism student, had recently moved to a new state, living away from home for the first time. She found herself disillusioned by the sensationalism of mainstream journalism and struggled to balance work, studies, and independence.

During a phone call, Millie broke down to her mother, expressing her frustration and emotional stress. Her mother, who had consulted me for hormonal advice, noted that Millie had been experiencing sore breasts, headaches, and severe menstrual cramps, along with emotional ups and downs. The significant lifestyle changes and increased stress were clearly impacting her hormonal balance.

I had worked with Millie during her puberty and transition into her Fertile Years, and I suggested that her mother recommend Chaste Tree as a first step. Additionally, I advised Millie to seek counselling through her university's health services for emotional support.

Months later, her mother shared that her daughter initially ignored the advice. However, after three more months, Millie began taking Chaste Tree daily and noticed a complete resolution of her hormonal symptoms. This experience highlighted the surprising efficacy of herbal remedies like Chaste Tree, which has a 500-year history of use as a natural hormonal support herb.

## RED AND ORANGE FLAG SOLUTIONS: HERBAL AND LIFESTYLE SUPPORT.

| HERB OR INTERVENTION | DOSE | SYMPTOM OF PUBERTY IT ADDRESSES |
|---|---|---|
| Chaste Tree (*Vitex agnus-castus*) | 1000 mg dried herb equivalent | Regulates menstrual cycles, reduces PMS symptoms |
| Cramp Bark | 1–2 ml tincture, 2–3 times daily | Eases menstrual cramps and muscle tension |
| Evening Primrose Oil | 500–1000 mg daily | Reduces breast tenderness and PMS mood swings |
| Magnesium-Rich Foods | Include leafy greens, nuts, seeds | Supports mood stability, reduces muscle cramping |
| Vitamin B6-Rich Foods | Chickpeas, chicken, bananas, potatoes, turkey, tuna, avocados, spinach | Reduces irritability and bloating related to PMS |
| Omega-3 Fatty Acids | 500–1000 mg daily from fish oil | Eases inflammation, stabilises mood |
| Iron-Rich Foods | Red meat, legumes, leafy greens | Supports energy and combats fatigue from menstruation |
| Daily Movement (e.g. walking, yoga) | 30 minutes of light activity | Reduces stress, supports stable mood |
| Hydration | Aim for 6–8 glasses of water daily | Reduces bloating, supports clear skin |
| St John's Wort | Consult your health practitioner | May help with mild mood swings and emotional support; use with caution due to potential medication interactions |

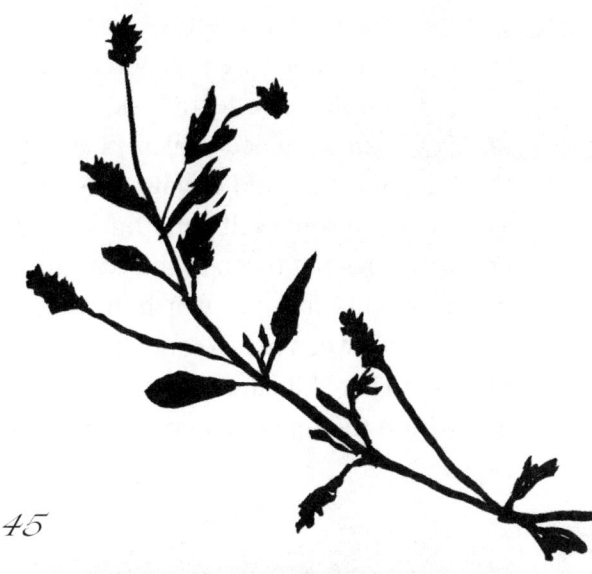

# PUBERTY-RELATED SKIN PROBLEMS

Let's delve into the realm of skincare: this a crucial aspect of puberty. Some of the skin changes during this journey of transformation, can be delightful and others a tad challenging. As hormones kick into gear, the skin becomes a hub of activity, ramping up oil production. Surprisingly, this excess oil may be a bonus to help her skin become supple, maintain hydration and a healthy radiance. However, the flip side is hormonal messages can create too much of a good thing, clogging pores resulting in black heads, white heads, pimples, and acne. This is extremely distressing for anyone, particularly a young girl trying to figure out how to fit into the norm of her tribe.

Prevention is key, so unless acne is severe, a comprehensive skincare routine combined with dietary adjustments targeted to support gut microbiome is recommended. Acne may need the expertise of dermatologists and other health specialists. We advise exploring natural remedies under the guidance of a naturopath or integrative doctor. Educating your tween on how to nourish her body—and gut—with proper nutrition, avoid processed, fatty and sugary foods, getting some regular exercise, and a solid skincare routine can keep her skin in balance, so pimples are less fierce, and hopefully prevent acne.

A simple yet effective skincare routine needs to be introduced to her. Ideally consult a trained clinical beauty therapist, dermatologist, or teach her how to do regular targeted facials (this can be a bonding experience, if you both participate in some self-care time). Find a therapist well-versed in teenage skin, one who does not use a brand with harsh chemicals to get the job done. If you can afford this, it is well worth the investment, as the therapist can instruct and advise your tween not to squeeze spots, and to be consistent every morning and night with her skincare routine. Usually, teenagers respond well and are good at following a therapist's recommendations for skincare between treatments.

> **TIP**
>
> If professional services aren't feasible, opt for gentle, organic skincare products devoid of harmful chemicals. Try Eco Sonya, Phyt's or Subtle Energies available online (see Resources on page 691 for more information).

## PUBERTY SKINCARE: AT A GLANCE

| ROUTINE | FREQUENCY | GUIDANCE AND KEY TIPS |
| --- | --- | --- |
| Cleansing, Toning, Moisturising | Morning and Night | These cornerstone steps help maintain skin's pH balance and vitality. Use gentle products to avoid disrupting the skin's microbiome, which is essential for healthy skin. Over-cleansing or harsh products can worsen pimples. |
| Exfoliation | Once a Week | Use a gentle exfoliant to remove dead skin cells. Avoid over-scrubbing, as it can irritate the skin and disturb its natural balance. |
| Sunscreen | Daily | Apply a lightweight facial sunscreen to protect skin from UV rays without adding excess oil. |
| Pimple Care | As Needed | Discourage squeezing pimples to prevent scarring. Instead, use monthly cleansing masks to unclog pores and maintain skin health. |
| Makeup Selection | Daily | Choose makeup that supports the skin's microbiome, helping prevent blemishes. Organic brands are recommended, as they are free from harmful chemicals and toxins, which can be common even in high-end products. Look for pure, skin-friendly ingredients. |
| Makeup Brush Cleaning | Weekly | Clean makeup brushes with a makeup brush cleanser to prevent bacterial build-up. |
| Investment in Skincare | As Budget Allows | Invest in quality skincare and makeup—it doesn't need to be expensive—prioritising gentle, microbiome-friendly products to promote lasting skin health. |

## ACNE MANAGEMENT

A dermatologist might prescribe oral contraceptives or topical treatments like Roaccutane for acne management. While they're highly skilled in treating skin concerns, they're not as well-versed in the intricate interplay of hormonal and neurological development. So, while it's important to support her skin health, it's equally crucial to weigh the broader impact on her endocrine system before agreeing to the Pill, which warrants careful consideration.

Use this solution only as a last resort. Start with the natural route: focus on clean, nutritious food (a major key factor) and a solid skincare routine. Consult a naturopath to ensure her digestion is working optimally and that her gut microbiome is healthy and balanced. If all of this fails and the acne remains severe, a dermatologist can step in with additional options.

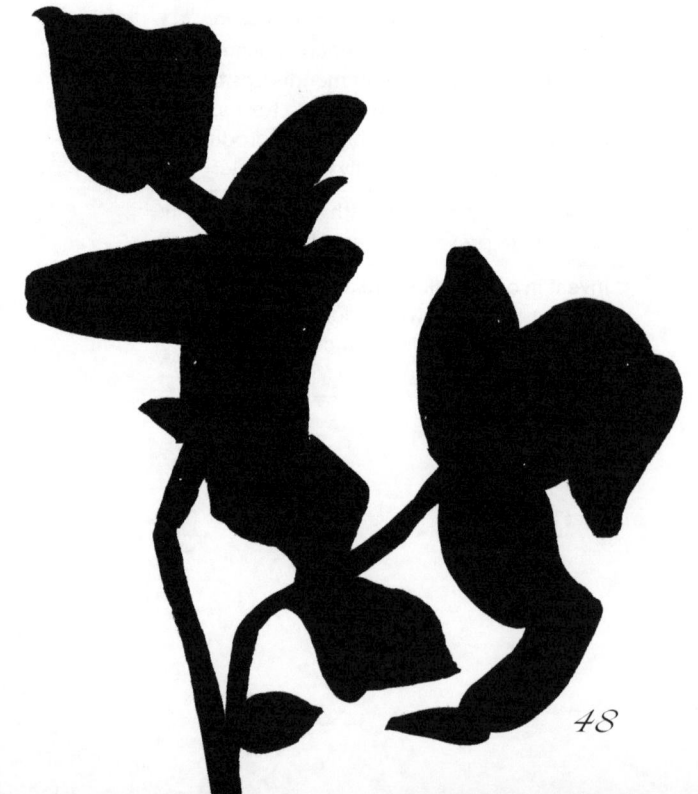

# THE TEENAGE BRAIN

As we discussed earlier in this chapter, your teenager or tween is not an adult. If you've ever wondered what *exactly* is going on inside your teenager's mind, or you wonder why her moods are up and down like a yo-yo, you're not alone. In brief, it's a lot! This is a time of change—in attitude, understanding, acceptance and personal growth.

Studies show that the prefrontal cortex, the area of the brain responsible for complex thought, decision-making, and social behaviour, is still a work in progress during adolescence. It's quite literally under construction. This means that the 'CEO' part of her brain hasn't yet developed all the necessary connections to fully regulate the powerful emotions coming from the amygdala, the brain's emotional centre.

Jay Giedd, a professor of psychiatry at the University of California, San Diego, explains:

> 'I think it's clear that the brain is still undergoing significant development until we are at least 25 years old. Even after the teenage years, the brain is not yet in full possession of all the neurological features critical to processing emotional responses, making decisions, and controlling impulsive behaviour.'

Having empathy and awareness of her brain 'state', may help you understand why your teenager needs to be asked five times to clean up her room, or why she seems over-emotional or extremely forgetful. By understanding a teenager's brain is still developing, you can then approach her emotional swings, impulsivity, and decision-making challenges with empathy and patience.

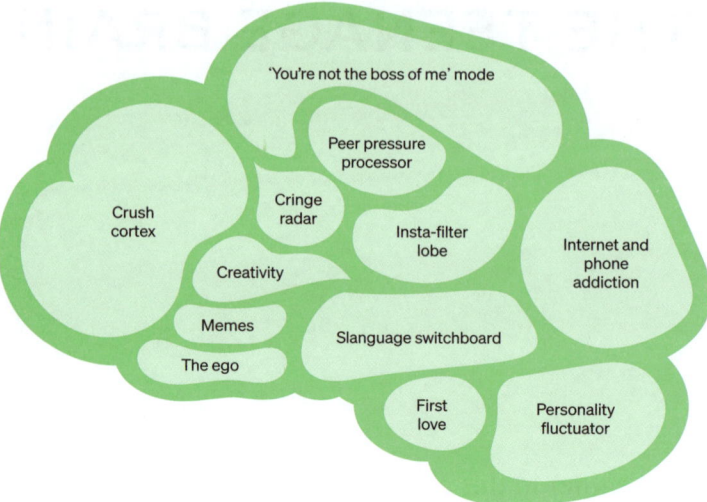

Although this is not an accurate depiction of the teenage brain, we think you get the picture!

Between the ages of 12–24, the brain will change in important, and often maddening ways. It's no wonder many parents approach their child's adolescence with fear and trepidation.

Daniel Siegel, a renowned neuropsychiatrist, helps parents and tweens work together to form a deeper understanding of the brain science behind all the tumult, you can turn conflict into connection and form a deeper understanding of one another. His book *Brainstorm* (see Recommended reading on page 690) illuminates how brain development impacts teenagers' behaviour and relationships. Drawing on important new research in the field of interpersonal neurobiology, it explores exciting ways for you to understand how the teenage brain functions, which helps you to see what is happening to your child. Believe it or not, this time can be an incredibly positive period of growth, change, and experimentation in any child's life. The book helps you to navigate this growth, so your teen is less lonely, and it helps to reduce any distress on both sides of the generational divide. If you're looking for a 'how to' manual for teenagers, *Brainstorm* is your port in a storm!

# EMOTIONAL WELLBEING AND COMMUNICATION

## PUBERTY:
### TIME FOR A SACRED CELEBRATION

Embarking on the journey into womanhood is a sacred passage, one deserving of a cherished celebration that transcends time. Throughout human history, many cultures have woven unique rituals to herald a girl's arrival into womanhood. In ancient civilizations, diverse customs marked this pivotal moment. Some societies embraced the transition as the onset of marriage—though in modern times, this practice has evolved. In other traditions, a girl's first menstrual cycle led to her integration into a women's circle, where her mother, grandmother, sisters, and aunts would offer wisdom and guidance.

Even today, echoes of these ancient customs persist in some cultures, where women gather to honour a young girl's first period. Laughter fills the air as stories are shared, advice is offered, and memories of early womanhood are recalled. While these traditions may no longer be common in many parts of the world, there's something special about acknowledging a girl's first menstruation.

In modern times, however, many significant life events, such as a girl's first period, often go unrecognised. Without traditional rites of passage, younger generations may create their own—sometimes through unhealthy or risky behaviours. Perhaps it's time to return to more meaningful rituals for both young girls and boys, marking these transitions with significance.

For a young girl entering womanhood, the celebration can be simple yet meaningful: a handwritten card, a small token to commemorate the occasion, or a special meal. These small acts create memories that can last a lifetime, and perhaps even be passed on to future generations. By fostering these rituals, we ensure that each new generation feels the significance of their personal milestones.

### BUILDING BRIDGES THROUGH SHARED STORIES

Sharing your own experience of puberty can help build a unique connection with your daughter or young girl. By opening up about your feelings and your own challenges during that time, you create a foundation of trust and mutual understanding. Be honest yet share the positives and humour from your story, weaving in the challenges you faced and how you overcame or approached them. This can help create a strong bond and make her feel more at ease about her own experience.

### RITE OF PASSAGE CONVERSATIONS

Open and supportive questions can guide conversations about puberty, such as:

- 'How are you feeling about the changes happening to your body?'
- 'Is there anything you're worried about or confused by?'
- 'Are there any questions you have about hygiene or how to manage embarrassing situations?'

These discussions help foster understanding and allow your girl to express her concerns in a safe space.

### HOW TO HAVE CONVERSATIONS ABOUT PUBERTY

Families come in all shapes and sizes—whether it's mum, dad, a couple of siblings, a solo parent, separated parents, grandparents, same-sex parents, carers, or foster parents. Each family brings its own unique background, culture, socio-economic status, and religious perspectives. In some homes, discussions about puberty flow freely, with open communication encouraged, and the pubescent child feels comfortable sharing with whoever they trust. In others, these conversations may follow specific guidelines or restrictions based on family values or cultural beliefs.

In more open households, fathers and brothers may be included in conversations about the natural biological changes a young woman is experiencing. This can offer valuable insights for them, helping them understand and navigate the transformation their daughter or sister is going through, as she moves from girlhood to womanhood. It may also provide valuable context for future relationships, such as with a wife or partner.

However, we fully respect that this level of openness may not be the norm for all families. There are many reasons why conversations about puberty may take place privately, behind closed doors—and that's perfectly okay. The most important thing is that every young woman feels supported during this time of transition.

Our goal within this book—and this chapter in particular—is to provide support and ensure a positive, healthy journey for each developing young woman. Regardless of the approach, it's crucial that she has access to a trusted individual or, ideally, a supportive circle of women. This support can help her grow into a confident, healthy adult with emotional resilience.

If conversations about puberty happen in private, it's important to explain why privacy is needed—without framing puberty as something shameful, dirty, or promiscuous. Instead, privacy should be explained as a matter of respecting cultural, religious, or family boundaries surrounding menstruation and women's issues in general.

As their trusted adult, we suggest you gently guide the conversation about what is socially and culturally acceptable both inside and outside the home when it comes to puberty and the menstrual cycle. This includes practical matters such as feminine hygiene, purchasing and disposing of sanitary products, and defining what is appropriate to discuss in public or with others. Having clear boundaries ensures that no one unintentionally crosses any cultural, religious, or family lines—such as a friend accidentally mentioning something that could be seen as inappropriate.

# APPROACHING THE ISSUE OF GENDER IDENTITY

Building a foundation of trust will also help you to have conversations that may be difficult, as sometimes the onset of puberty may reveal gender incongruence. This is not directly related to puberty. It relates to an individual's personal feelings of gender identity. Should questions around gender identity arise with your loved one, as this is not our area of expertise we advise seeking support from health professionals, gender clinics and support groups. Finding right-minded professionals to provide guidance is critical for your loved one; having the resources and support to help navigate very personal and complex feelings, can help provide the smoothest of journeys for all concerned. (See our Resource section for more information.)

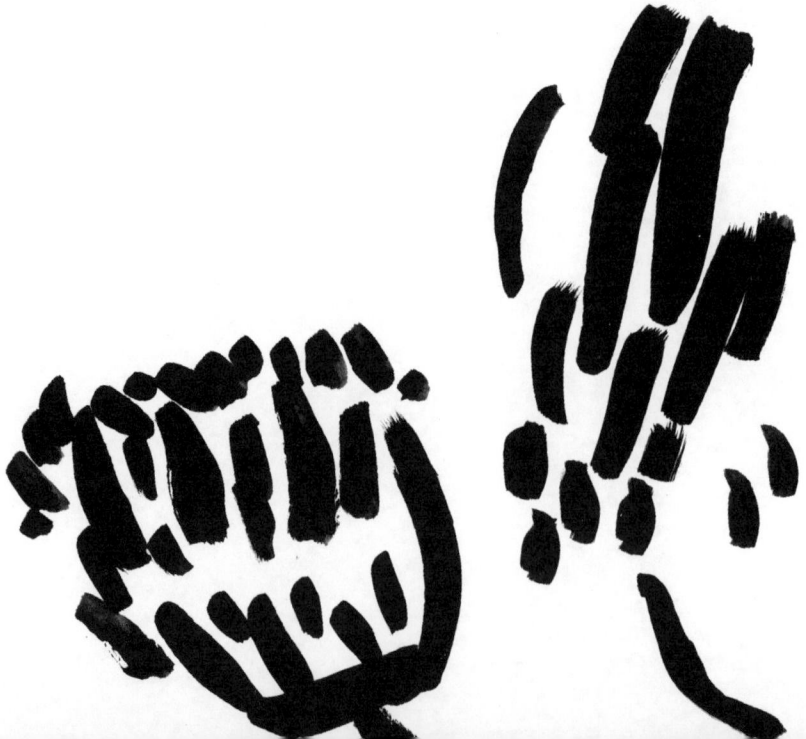

## WELLNESS ACTION PLAN
# PUBERTY

Whether you are working alongside your teenager for solutions to different symptoms or issues in puberty, or you're a teenager reading this for guidance and advice, keep in mind the following. For natural solutions, consult with an experienced naturopath for lifestyle, diet, and herbal options. Your GP or integrative doctor can help with issues such as polycystic ovary syndrome, endometriosis and other medical concerns.

As we explore lifestyle choices it is important to remember what is done most of the time is important—consistency is key.

A young girl moving through puberty requires sufficient sleep as a foundation, as well as a nutrient-rich diet—both promote healthy skin, balanced hormones, and stable moods. (Read our Spotlight on Sleep on page 351 and our Spotlight on Nourishment on page 393.) In the following pages we have included an outline of what a tween needs to eat at least 80% of the time, plus a helpful guide to the essential food groups.

### DAILY NUTRITIONAL PLAN

**Real Food:** Whole, natural foods provide the vitamins and minerals her body needs to grow and thrive. These nutrients support balanced hormones, better sleep, and glowing skin. Real food is nutrient-dense and supports your daughter's growth, hormonal balance, and overall wellbeing as she navigates puberty. Try to encourage her to understand the percentages of a balanced diet.

**PROTEIN**
30% of daily intake

**CARBOHYDRATES**
40% from a variety of fruits, vegetables, and whole grains

**FATS**
30% from whole, healthy fats

## CARBOHYDRATES

**Plants:** Fruits, vegetables, grains, seeds, and legumes are packed with carbohydrates, fibre, vitamins, minerals, and prebiotics. Encourage her to eat a variety of colours to ensure she gets all the nutrients her body needs.

**Vegetables:** At least 3 cups of mixed vegetables daily.

**Fruit:** 2 pieces of fruit or the equivalent in berries.

### SUGGESTIONS: HOW TO EAT A 'RAINBOW' DIET

**Red:** Capsicum, beetroot, tomato, apples, raspberries
**Yellow:** Corn, banana, pineapple, capsicum
**Green:** Snow peas, asparagus, lettuce, broccoli, kiwi
**Orange:** Carrot, pumpkin, sweet potato, mangoes
**Purple:** Eggplant, purple sweet potato, blackberries
**Blue:** Blueberries
**Cream/Brown:** Mushrooms

## WHOLE FATS

Healthy fats are essential for maintaining hormonal balance and healthy skin. These include:

- Avocados
- Nuts and seeds
- Olives and olive oil
- Macadamia and avocado oil
- Coconut
- Fatty fish (salmon, sardines)
- Organic cheese (goat, sheep)
- Meat and chicken

## AVOID PROCESSED AND FAST FOODS

Processed and fast foods contain unhealthy trans fats that can disrupt hormones and harm skin and gut health. Consider these switches:

**Deep-fried foods**: Choose air-fried vegetables made at home. Use avocado or macadamia oil (more stable under high heat).
**Fast food burgers:** Make homemade burgers with fresh lettuce, tomato, and beetroot.
**Potato chips:** Try homemade sweet potato crisps in an air fryer.
**Packaged snacks**: Prepare a stockpile of homemade healthy snacks.
**Overcooked or burned fats**: When eating out, select your order wisely. Use safe cooking techniques at home with heat-stable oils like macadamia or avocado oil.

## PROTEIN

Protein is essential for building and maintaining strong muscles, which are crucial for an active lifestyle. Sources include foods that swim, walk, and fly. Choose fish, seafood, chicken, turkey, duck, beef, and lamb. Plant-based proteins like tofu, tempeh, nuts, seeds, and legumes should also be encouraged.

If your daughter follows a vegetarian or vegan diet (even occasionally), ensure she gets adequate protein at every meal. Tofu is a great option, and it's important to consult a nutritionist to ensure she's getting all the nutrients she needs, especially as she begins menstruating.

## ENCOURAGE BALANCED EATING

It can be frustrating when your teenager doesn't eat what you provide but be patient. You can hide vegetables in dishes like mince, or puree them into sauces (yes, like a toddler!). Ultimately, she will make her own choices, but you can remind her that food can be her best medicine, especially when her skin or hormones act up.

CASE STUDY | DR KAREN

# Hannah
## Puberty transition

I recall a conversation with my daughter, Hannah, around the time of her puberty about the importance of regular movement. To my surprise, she challenged me on my own lack of exercise, pointing out how the demands of my clinical practice had taken priority over physical activity. She suggested we find a regular activity to do together. Expecting she might choose a team sport like netball, indoor soccer, or canoeing, I gave her the task of deciding.

After nearly a week of consideration, Hannah, in her usual decisive manner, sat me down and said, 'Mumma, I've made a decision. I think we should do kickboxing together. There's a class this Thursday at the community centre, and I've already spoken to the trainer. We can start this week.'

At the time, I was in my mid-40s, and kickboxing wasn't the type of movement I'd imagined committing to for the next decade! But I had promised, so we began our kickboxing trial. This decision turned out to be life-changing for both of us. I entered menopause fitter than I had ever been, and Hannah gained a self-confidence that still serves her in her career and relationships. Our trainer, Vincent Perry, was an inspirational coach with a background as a registered nurse. He later became the co-author of my first book and remains a lifelong friend.

As a postscript, Hannah and I now hold brown belts in Escrima, also known as Arnis, a form of Filipino martial arts that focuses on stick fighting. The training emphasises speed, accuracy, and coordination through fluid, dynamic movements. It has become a moving meditation for us, as well as a respected form of self-defence. The skills Hannah developed during her puberty transition gave me peace of mind as she stepped out into the world as an independent young woman.

# MOVEMENT AND EXERCISE

Encouraging regular movement also helps your teen find a balance. It's important to avoid too little or too much activity, as both can affect her hormones. You will likely know what she enjoys—whether it's outdoor sports, walking the dog, or indoor activities like dancing or trampolining. There are plenty of ways to keep your teen active.

> **MODERATION IS KEY**
>
> Even simple activities, like walking to the bus, can help her achieve the recommended goal of 7500–10,000 steps a day.
>
> Even better, find an activity you can do with her. Try pickleball, tennis, or even deep water running. There's little chance to talk, although its time spent together that counts. Here we offer you some insights, we also provide a deeper dive in our Spotlight on Movement and Exercise on page 485.

### FOUR KEY AREAS OF MOVEMENT

**Strength**
Strength training supports muscles and joints. If she's lifting weights, make sure her form is correct to avoid injury. For guidance, an experienced trainer is ideal. Activities that build strength include:

- Lifting weights (including higher repetitions and less weight) for your teen is best done under the supervision of a trained professional
- Pilates, yoga, bodyweight exercises (push-ups, squats, lunges)
- Horse riding, surfing, cycling, swimming, team sports

### Flexibility

Flexibility keeps muscles balanced and supports good posture. Without it, joint and muscle pain can develop. Encourage:
- Stretching, yoga, Pilates
- Fun activities like hula hooping

### Cardiovascular exercise

Cardiovascular fitness is key for heart health and stamina. Encourage activities that get her heart rate up, but watch for over-exercising, which can disrupt hormones. Activities include:
- Dancing, skipping, brisk walking or running
- Swimming, sports that make her 'huff and puff'
- Weight training for an interval effect

### Stability and balance

Core strength and balance are essential for physical fitness and injury prevention. Proprioceptors in her joints help keep her steady and prevent injury. Activities that challenge stability include:
- Yoga, Pilates, core exercises
- Balancing on one leg or walking on narrow beams

> **A NOTE ON YOGA**
>
> Yoga and martial arts support strength, flexibility, fitness, and stability while also helping to manage stress. These practices will teach her to breathe through challenges, making it a valuable life skill. During her period, Yin or restorative yoga is preferred. (See Spotlight on Restorative Practices on page 372.)

## BALANCING ACTIVITY AND REST

While it's important for your teenager to stay active, rest is crucial for muscle repair, growth, and hormonal balance. Encourage her to listen to her body and rest when needed. Limit highly active pursuits to no more than two hours per day, especially during menstruation.

**EXAMPLE WEEKLY EXERCISE AND MOVEMENT SCHEDULE**

| DAY | EXERCISE | MINIMUM STEPS |
| --- | --- | --- |
| Day 1 | Cardio (moderate intensity, 20–45 minutes) | 7000 steps |
| Day 2 | Bodyweight strength training (30 minutes) or Pilates | 7000 steps |
| Day 3 | Rest or light stretching | 7000 steps |
| Day 4 | High-intensity interval training (15–20 minutes) | 7000 steps |
| Day 5 | Strength training (30–60 minutes) or Pilates | 7000 steps |
| Day 6 | Flexibility and balance exercises or active games | 7000 steps |
| Day 7 | Rest or light movement (easy walk or light play) | 7000 steps |

**TIP**

Gentle exercise can relieve period pain by relaxing uterine muscles. Encourage your teen to stay active, even with light movement such as a gentle walk or Yin yoga, or by sticking with their favourite sport or hobby.

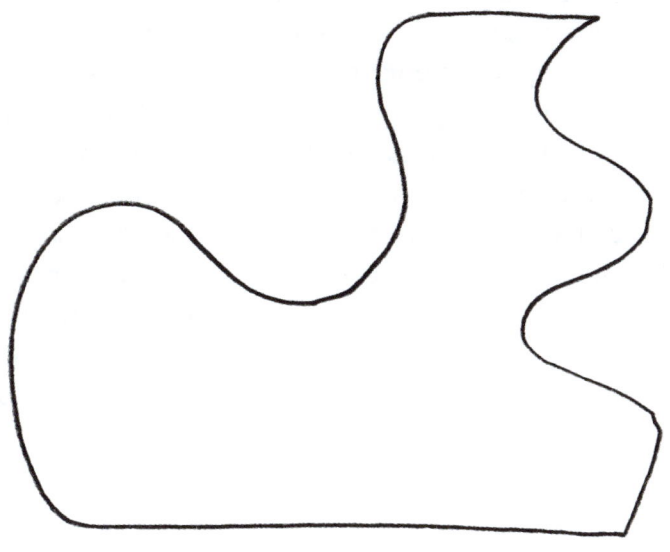

# A MESSAGE FOR PARENTS AND CARERS OF TEENAGERS

Supporting your daughter through puberty is a journey of patience, understanding, and love. Be patient and kind, establish fair boundaries, and communicate clearly. Importantly, make sure she feels that you have heard her and considered her viewpoint, that you see her challenges and remember that this time of life is not an easy time of life, she is not an adult yet. Feel with her, she needs you to understand her feelings. Remind her often that she is loved, she may scowl or demonstrate she doesn't care, yet research is clear, this is the most important aspect for her to feel safe. Show love in many ways, not just buying things for her. Listen to her stories, dreams, and fears, get involved and try to enjoy the things that light her up. Your most important role is to be consistent. Be the caring, loving mentor and family leader, she needs to feel safe and unconditionally loved.

This stage in her life is when she steps into the first phase of being a woman, an exciting time full of challenges and new experiences. She is waking up and growing up with a brain that is still under construction so choose your battles wisely. Your guiding light will make a difference, and if all else feels overwhelming, just love her. Remember that love is so much more than a romantic notion, it is also compassion, empathy, forgiveness, respect, trust and most importantly connection. As she moves into the next hormonal phase—the Fertile Years—a woman will emerge, a grown-up version of her childhood self, and who knows where her life will lead? This is a journey you are on together, and as she becomes an adult, relationships will mature, and you will continue to age and grow together. Who knows, one day she may be taking care of you!

# The Fertile Years

The Fertile Years can be fulfilling, challenging and powerful all at once as you balance the rhythm of your cycle with the demands of adult life. Let's explore what's normal and when to act or ask for help, with a look at the following topics:
- Fertility
- Your menses
- Your fertility checklist
- Taking care of yourself during pregnancy
- Your post-natal checklist

**Always fill your own cup first and allow the world to benefit from the overflow.**

LISA NICHOLS, MOTIVATIONAL SPEAKER

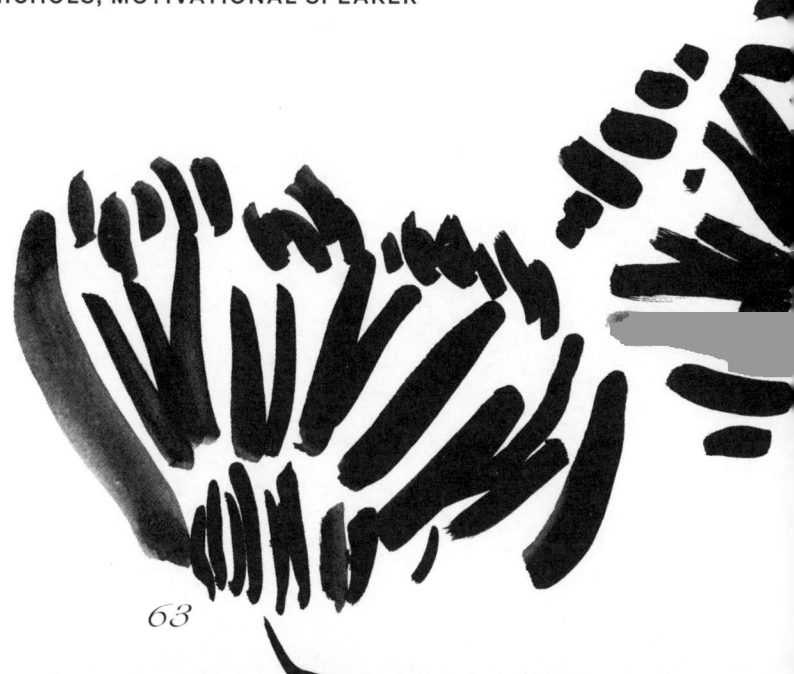

**DR KAREN:**

Have you ever wondered why a typically calm woman can transform into an irritable, restless being, akin to a 'she-wolf', just before her period? This question baffled me during the early years of my career in women's health.

Month after month, I encountered young women describing the same trio of symptoms—irritability, mood swings, and breast tenderness in the days leading up to their period. It was a story familiar not only through my patients but also through my own experience as a newly graduated doctor navigating the demands of a busy profession. I often reassured these women that their symptoms were within the realm of 'normal', advising their partners to tread carefully during 'that time of the month'. When nothing else seemed to help, I'd reluctantly reach for the prescription pad, offering the contraceptive pill as a solution.

It wasn't until the early 1990s, when I started to explore the intricate interplay of fertility hormones, that I began to understand the true origins of these premenstrual struggles. Armed with this new knowledge, I sought to empower women with solutions beyond pharmaceuticals.

There is now strong evidence that the notorious 'Jekyll and Hyde' transformation many women experience before their period is linked to an imbalance between oestrogen and progesterone. This brings us to a key principle: There is a difference between what seems 'normal' and what is 'natural'.

In short, it's not *natural* to experience these uncomfortable symptoms before your period, but over time, society has come to consider them 'normal'.

# NAVIGATING HORMONAL HARMONY DURING THE FERTILE YEARS

As we enter the Fertile Years, we embark on a journey of balancing life while maintaining hormonal harmony. In earlier times, 'maidenhood' referred to a virgin, marking the transition into the Fertile Years, typically from around 18 to 40 years of age. Formally known as pre-menopause, we prefer to call this phase 'the Fertile Years'—we think you'll agree, it's a much nicer term!

Times have certainly changed. In the past, women were expected to secure marriage prospects before turning 20, often in unions that were more about securing a home and financial stability than love. Back then, virginity was essential for these often-arranged alliances, and women's roles were restricted to reproduction and household duties. Records from Renaissance Italy even classified women as *bocche*—or 'mouths' to be fed—emphasising their perceived role as dependents and expenses of the family.

Women were once prized mainly for their fertility, with little consideration for their personal aspirations. Though the world has evolved, remnants of these old customs still exist in some cultures. In fact, as recently as the 1960s, Australian female government employees were forced to resign if they married or became pregnant.

As you move from puberty into the Fertile Years your body has matured hormonally. While it is biologically capable of pregnancy once menstruation begins, fertility truly peaks in the late teens and twenties, gradually declining as you approach 40 years of age. However, just because your body is primed for motherhood doesn't mean you're obligated to follow that path. Whether or not motherhood is on your radar, your body prepares for the possibility each month, setting the stage for conception through a finely tuned hormonal process.

Navigating contraception becomes important if motherhood isn't on the horizon. But before exploring the options for birth control, it's essential to understand the inner workings of your menstrual cycle. Knowledge is power and understanding your body's rhythms can help to prevent health challenges that often accompany imbalances.

> **TIP**
>
> Your menstrual cycle is a natural reflection of your overall health. Rather than viewing your period as a monthly inconvenience, see it as a vital sign of your wellbeing. A balanced cycle is your best protection from hormone-related conditions. Your cycle is a personal performance tracker, revealing how stress and lifestyle affect your body.

# THE DANCE OF OESTROGEN AND PROGESTERONE

Your body's hormonal system is a masterpiece of biological wisdom. The interplay between two key hormones, oestrogen and progesterone, choreographs the beautiful and complex rhythm of your fertility cycle. These hormones don't work in isolation; instead, they engage in a delicate dance, guiding you through the Fertile Years with precision.

Understanding this dynamic duo and how they fluctuate throughout your cycle is key to navigating hormonal harmony, whether you're considering pregnancy or simply aiming to balance your body for optimal health.

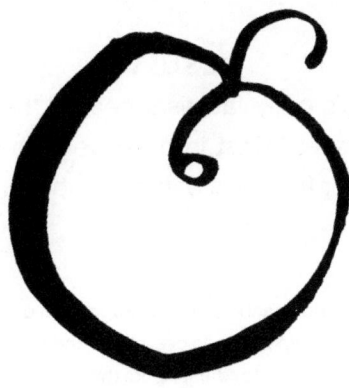

CASE STUDY | DR KAREN

# Amy

## Overtraining, period red flags, and visceral fat

At 34, Amy, a professional triathlete, was preparing for her final year of competition. Despite her rigorous training, she struggled with stubborn belly fat and a shortened period cycle. When she raised her concerns, her coach shockingly responded, 'If you're still having periods, you're not training hard enough.'

### ASSESSMENT

Though Amy had low body fat and excellent muscle mass, overtraining had pushed her into a chronic state of stress, elevating her cortisol levels. This was causing the belly fat and period changes. I explained how overtraining can break down muscle and collagen (cortisol is catabolic), weaken the immune system, and increase injury risks.

### SOLUTION

I recommended Amy reduce her training intensity by 20% and start taking withania (ashwagandha), a herb that helps regulate cortisol and supports the immune system.

### RESULTS

Within three months, Amy's belly fat disappeared, her periods normalised, and she avoided pre-race illnesses. Most impressively, she achieved one of her best personal performances after finding a balance between training and recovery.

> As you transition through each hormonal stage from puberty through to the Age of Wisdom, the partnership between oestrogen and progesterone remains vital—these hormones maintain a steadfast bond, their influence enduring even as your hormonal seasons change.

## THE ROLES OF THESE HORMONAL PROTAGONISTS

### OESTROGEN

- Acts as the guardian of bodily fluids, maintaining hydration and balance.
- Thickens the uterine lining in preparation for pregnancy.
- Enhances cognitive function, improving learning and memory.
- Fosters empathy, communication, and interpersonal bonds.
- Helps regulate appetite for a healthy relationship with food.
- Promotes restorative sleep for a rejuvenated mind and body.
- Supports bone density, safeguarding skeletal health.

### PROGESTERONE

- Balances oestrogen during the luteal phase, ensuring hormonal equilibrium.
- Supports the early stages of pregnancy, nurturing the embryo.
- Boosts thyroid function, optimising metabolism and wellbeing.
- Protects breast tissue and promotes overall health.
- Acts as a natural mood stabiliser and antidepressant, enhancing emotional resilience.
- Helps maintain fluid balance and hydration.
- Partners with oestrogen to protect bone health.

## EXPLORING THE MENSTRUAL CYCLE

Your menstrual cycle is a harmonious dance between oestrogen and progesterone, ideally lasting 28-30 days, driving physiological changes and hormonal fluctuations.

### KEEP A RECORD

We encourage you to keep a record of your menstrual cycle, whether written or digital. Apps include *MyNFM*, *Flo*, *Spot On* or *Clue*. For those exploring natural fertility or contraception we provide further recommendation later in this chapter (see Let's Get Pregnant (or Not) on page 94). However you choose to track your cycle, your record will serve as a compass, helping you identify patterns and understand the rhythms of your cycle.

In addition to its practical use, your record provides valuable insights for healthcare professionals. Be sure to document your mood, mental clarity, physical symptoms, and the length and regularity of your bleed. This information offers a roadmap for understanding hormonal dynamics, guiding hormonal testing, and shaping personalised recommendations.

## YOUR NATURAL MENSES

The menstrual cycle begins with menstruation, marked by low oestrogen and progesterone levels. Day 1 of your cycle is defined by the first appearance of bright red blood.

## THE EARLY FOLLICULAR PHASE (DAYS 1–5)

Day 1: Bright red blood signals the start of menstruation, typically lasting no more than five days.

Brownish spotting may occur up to 24 hours before or after the main flow—this is normal.

### PERIOD RED FLAGS

A 'natural' balanced menstrual flow should be easily managed with pads, tampons, or a menstrual cup, requiring a change every four to six hours. Red Flag includes a heavier flow with the following symptoms:

- Needing to change your tampon/pad more often than every three hours, especially on heavy days (Day 1 or 2).
- Heavy flow that lasts more than two days.
- Bright red blood lasting more than five days.
- Spotting lasting over a day after your period or starting more than a day before.
- Cycles shorter than 26 days.
- Blood clots in the toilet or on pads.

These signal hormonal imbalances, and the possibility of iron deficiency, or anaemia. Consult your healthcare provider and get your iron levels checked, ideally around Day 8, when iron levels are at their lowest. (See our Spotlight on Iron on page 449.)

## THE LATE FOLLICULAR PHASE (DAYS 6–14)

During this phase, oestrogen rises, thickening the uterine lining (the endometrium) in preparation for pregnancy. Around Days 12-13, a surge in luteinising hormone (LH) and follicle-stimulating hormone (FSH) triggers ovulation.

Oestrogen primes both the body and mind, enhancing cognitive function and physical performance. This phase also brings noticeable changes in vaginal mucus, which turns to a 'stretchy egg white' consistency, indicating fertility.

### NATURAL FERTILITY AND CONTRACEPTION

By tracking your cycle, you can identify fertile days (such as noticing changes in mucus or body temperature) to either plan conception or prevent pregnancy. For more on natural methods, see Let's Get Pregnant (or Not) on page 94.

### THE PILL

The Pill, introduced in the 1960s, remains a common contraceptive choice today. While it can help manage heavy bleeding or hormonal imbalances, it also disrupts the natural cycle by providing synthetic oestrogen and progesterone in a one-size-fits-all dose, (depending on the brand of Pill). The 'period' experienced on the Pill is a withdrawal bleed, not a natural menstruation. Finding the right Pill often requires trial and error, and symptoms you experience while on the Pill are due to the synthetic hormones, not your body's own imbalance. When you stop taking the Pill, it may take up to 12 months for your body to re-establish its natural cycle, important to know if you wish to conceive. (For other contraceptive options, see page 117.)

## OVULATION (DAYS 14–16)

Ovulation occurs as an egg is released and travels down the fallopian tube, ready for fertilisation. Oestrogen declines, and progesterone rises.

If fertilisation occurs, the embryo implants in the uterine lining, initiating pregnancy. Progesterone, supported by the *corpus luteum*, sustains early pregnancy until the placenta takes over at around three months. This process is a beautiful demonstration of nature's balance and resilience.

> **OVARIAN TEAMWORK**
>
> Each ovary typically alternates in producing eggs each month, but sometimes this process can cause discomfort. Some women experience pain at the site of egg release, known as the *corpus luteum*. If fluid builds up around the egg, it can lead to *mittelschmerz*—German for 'middle pain'—a bi-monthly surprise from the ovary.
>
> For those who find this discomfort particularly strong, relief may come from a herbal blend of Chaste Tree (*Vitex agnus-castus*) and Cramp Bark. This natural remedy has been effective for many women in easing ovarian pain. If you need relief, consider consulting your local naturopath for this soothing solution.

### THE LUTEAL PHASE DAY 18

In a healthy cycle, successful ovulation allows progesterone to take centre stage. Even if pregnancy isn't on the horizon, women with balanced hormones will experience a steady surge of progesterone throughout the second half of their menstrual cycle.

The graph below shows the typical levels of a woman in ideal hormonal balance.

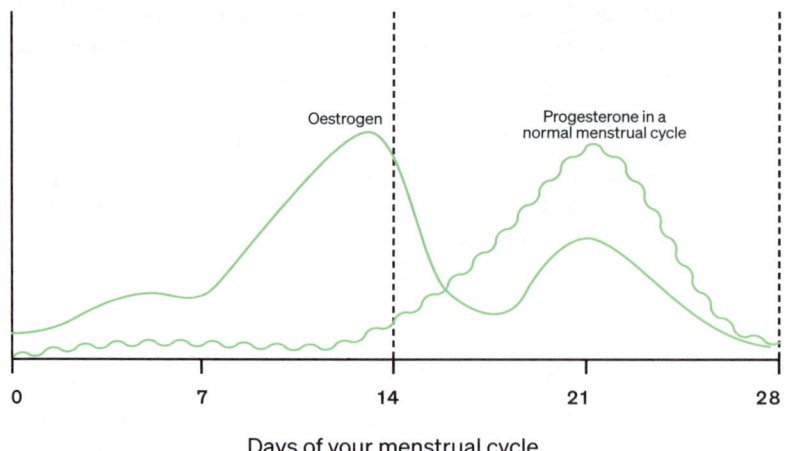

Days of your menstrual cycle

### DAY 21

Progesterone reaches its peak, making this an ideal time for hormonal blood tests to measure the balance between progesterone and oestrogen.

### DAY 28

If the egg remains unfertilised, hormonal signals trigger the start of a new cycle. The uterine lining is shed, marking the end of the cycle and the beginning of menstruation.

THE FERTILE YEARS

**DAY 28–29**

Oestrogen and progesterone levels decline, leading to menstruation and the start of a new cycle.

# Embrace the natural rhythm of your hormones as they ebb and flow; they are an essential part of your life's unique rhythm.

**SHARON KOLKKA**

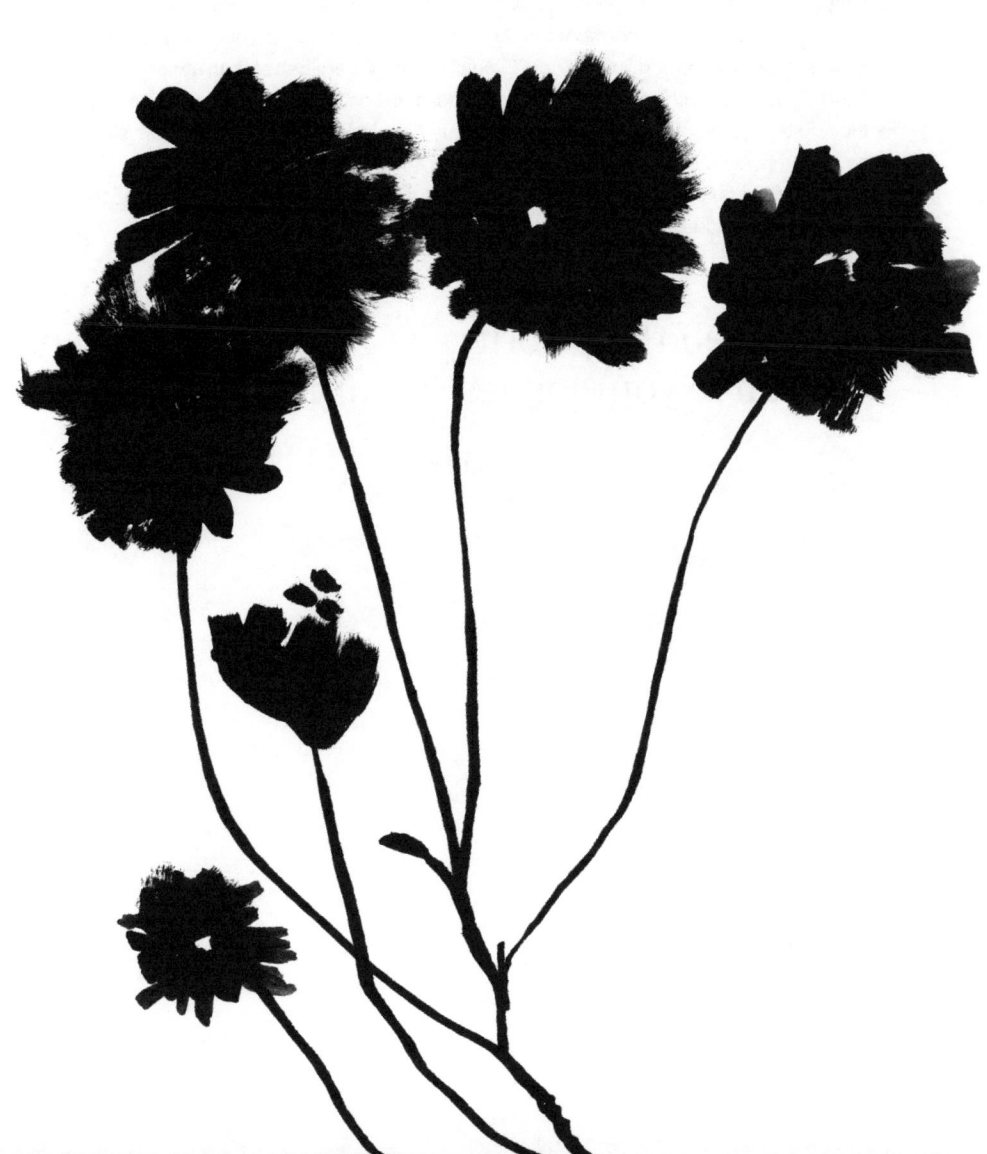

### GREEN FLAG PERIOD

A normal period, indicating balanced hormones.
- Should start with a clean flow of bright red blood lasting four to five days, with light spotting beforehand.
- Mild cramping on Days 1 and 2 is normal and can be eased with the herb Cramp Bark or mild pain relief.

### TIP

Achieving orgasm during menstruation can help relieve cramps by increasing blood flow and relaxing muscles.

### 'ME TIME'

Take time for yourself during menstruation. Life can be hectic, but your body needs rest and care to support a balanced hormonal cycle. Carve out moments for yourself throughout your cycle, especially during your period. Even short breaks are better than none.

Nurture yourself with warm, nourishing foods, a hot bath, or gentle restorative yoga. Reducing stress and intense exercise during this time is key to maintaining low stress hormone levels, which support the natural ebb and flow of your cycle.

For some guidance on relaxation visit Spotlight on Restorative Practices on page 372 for breathing techniques which may help.

> Make yourself the priority—at the end of the day, you're your longest commitment.
>
> **PASCALLE**

# OESTROGEN DOMINANCE

In a balanced menstrual cycle, oestrogen naturally dominates the first half, while progesterone rises in the second. However, if ovulation doesn't occur, the expected progesterone surge is absent, allowing oestrogen to continue at its usual level and dominate the second half of the cycle. When progesterone is lacking in the second half of the cycle, oestrogen remains unopposed. This imbalance triggers PMS (see Action Plan later in this section) and can lead to more complex issues, including:

- **Endometriosis:** see Spotlight on page 534.
- **Polycystic ovary syndrome (PCOS):** see Spotlight on page 546.
- **Premenstrual Dysphoric Disorder (PMDD):** A complex endocrine disorder that is beyond the scope of this book. We have provided, in the Resources section, a list of centres (in Australia, New Zealand and the UK) that specialise in this challenging hormonal condition. As a starting point follow the advice for PMS and reduce your exposure to xenoestrogen.

**Xenoestrogens and stress** amplify symptoms of PMS and PMDD. Eliminating these irritants is essential to restore hormonal balance. To read more on **Xenoestrogens** see the Spotlight on Managing Toxins on page 478 and don't forget to visit the Spotlight on Psychological Stress on page 290.

> **TIP**
>
> There is exciting new research extending the use of Chaste Tree as a herbal tool to treat PMDD symptoms. A study on the use of this herb showed nearly 60% of women with PMDD reduced their symptoms by half within two months. The daily dose of Chaste Tree (*Vitex agnus-castus*) is 1000 to 3000 mg each morning, taken continuously through the menstrual month.

> **A NOTE ON GPS**
>
> GPs are amazing, often seeing up to 40 patients a day. However, given their time constraints, it's unrealistic to expect them to solve complex hormonal issues in a 10-minute visit. Save GP appointments for when natural remedies have been exhausted. They can refer you to a specialist who focuses on women's hormonal health.

### THE PILL AND HORMONAL BALANCE

When hormonal imbalances become overwhelming, pharmaceutical options like the Pill can seem appealing. However, synthetic hormones may only provide short-term relief while blocking the body's natural hormonal resilience. Over time, this can lead to further imbalances, especially during perimenopause and menopause. Consider reserving pharmaceutical interventions as a last resort.

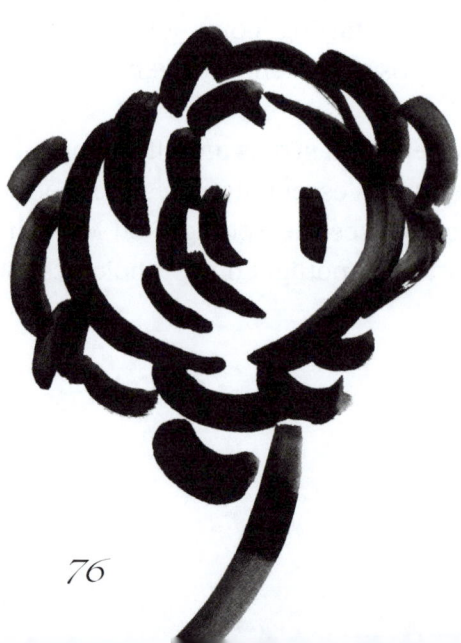

# PREMENSTRUAL SYNDROME (PMS)

PMS symptoms include:

- Sore breasts
- Cramps
- Heavy bleeding
- Clotting
- Frequent periods
- Mood swings
- Emotional irritability and intolerance

PMS is a 'Red Flag' signal for the need to restore hormonal equilibrium, and unchecked this imbalance can escalate into more complex conditions mentioned earlier, including cancer. Do not ignore the Red Flag symptoms: it's essential to act and reclaim your health. Part Two of this book provides deeper insights through Spotlight sections on Stress Management, Nourishment, Movement and Exercise, Sleep, and Rest—each a core element for achieving hormonal harmony, rooted in science, self-care and self-compassion. At the end of this chapter, a foundational Wellness Action Plan will guide you toward the Spotlight sections most relevant to your hormonal journey.

CASE STUDY | DR KAREN

# Jane

I could tell by the way she walked into my office that there were big problems. Jane sat down and burst into tears, apologising for taking up my time. Jane's husband was at his wit's end, and he had insisted she get a second opinion on her situation. He said he would do anything to have the old Jane back again. She had been to a couple of doctors who had done blood tests and said that her hormones were 'normal'.

Jane described the struggle with her hormones over several years, since the birth of her third child. I asked her if there was any time of the month when things were OK. She replied that the only time her family would get a glimpse of that old Jane was for a few days just after her bleeding stopped, 'After that the nightmare starts all over again.'

Jane told me how the rage would build up to the point where she felt frightened of herself and could only imagine the effect her behaviour was having on her children and husband. She had a good relationship with her husband, who she described as having the patience of a saint, 'but that patience is wearing very thin these days.'

I asked her if any other symptoms worried her in that second half of the cycle and she continued her story of hormonal havoc.

'My breasts get so sore and full that I can't even go to the gym. And I seem to be spotting for a few days before my period starts properly. It's much heavier than it was before I had the kids.'

When I asked for more detail about her bleeding she confirmed what I had suspected. Her periods were now six days long, instead of her normal five days and she had to change pads every 2 to 4 hours on her heavy days.

'Sometimes now I even have to get up during the night and change pads, otherwise ...'

I asked to see her previous blood pathology results and during which part of her menstrual cycle the blood was taken. Jane replied that she didn't recall, but thought it was shortly after her period as she had just recovered from a particularly heavy bleed and a bad episode of PMS had prompted the doctor's appointment.

After checking her over I sent her for more hormone testing, to be done precisely between Days 18 and 22 of her cycle, when her PMS symptoms were at their worst. From these tests, it was clear that her oestrogen levels were high, and progesterone had failed to rise, leading to oestrogen dominance.

## SOLUTION

Jane's first step toward hormonal health was understanding that her problem wasn't psychological—it was a hormonal imbalance disrupting communication between her brain and body. Read on to learn about hormonal imbalances and the solution to Jane's severe PMS. We also provide a Wellness Action Plan for PMS beginning on page 80.

### WARNING—STRESS ALERT!

Stress is a major saboteur of hormonal balance. The fight-or-flight response overrides the body's hormonal harmony, flooding the bloodstream with stress hormones that wreak havoc on everything from cardiovascular health to digestion. Stress is a top trigger for PMS symptoms, making stress management essential for hormonal health. Take proactive steps daily to reduce stress and protect your hormonal balance. (See Spotlight on Psychological Stress on page 290.)

### WHO TO CONSULT FOR FURTHER PMS SUPPORT

We believe in starting with natural remedies and lifestyle changes to address PMS. These approaches support the body's wisdom, helping to restore hormonal balance now and in the future, including perimenopause and menopause. Consulting a Traditional Chinese Medicine, Ayurvedic practitioner, or a naturopath can help create a personalised plan to gently restore hormonal harmony through diet, herbs, and adrenal support. For a more in-depth consultation, consider an integrative doctor who specialises in women's health. They can offer herbal remedies, supplementation, and bioidentical hormones if needed. Though these consultations may come at a higher cost, investing in your health is invaluable. (See the Resources section on page 691 for our recommendations.)

## WELLNESS ACTION PLAN
# PREMENSTRUAL SYNDROME (PMS)

> **TIP**
> You can also use this as the starting point to support PMDD.

## GUT HEALTH

Your gut and its microbiome have an intimate connection to the symptoms of PMS. Research out of Japan shows promise with a *Lactobacillus* probiotic supplement that has reduced the psychological symptoms of PMS. (See Core Food Principle Number 5 on page 396.)

## NUTRITION
Choose from these natural food sources:

**B1 (THIAMINE)**
- Wholegrains
- Fish
- Legumes
- Nuts and seeds
- Meats (especially pork)

**VITAMIN B1 AND B6**
Foods rich in Vitamin B1 (thiamine) and B6 (pyridoxine) can reduce both the psychological and physical symptoms of PMS, but supplemental B-vitamins can ramp up PMS.

**NATURAL FOOD SOURCES OF B6 (PYRIDOXINE)**
- Chicken breast
- Fish, especially salmon and halibut
- Vegetables: Potato, sweety potato, leafy greens like spinach
- Fruit: Bananas, avocado, prunes
- Legumes: Chickpeas, lentils, beans
- Nuts and seeds: Sunflower seeds, pistachios and sesame seeds
- Organ meats (liver)

> **TIP**
> If you have been prescribed a multi-B vitamin for other reasons, consider having a 'vitamin holiday' in the time leading up to your PMS symptoms.

Increase omega-3 oils in the second half of your cycle and incorporate as many PUFA-rich foods as you can—variety is the key here.

**INCREASE OLIVE OIL**
Replacing saturated fats with extra virgin olive oil (a monounsaturated fat) is a win-win for your hormones and overall wellbeing.

## WHAT TO AVOID

**Saturated fat:** Natural foods high in saturated fatty acids are OK in moderation (like delicious organic butter and cheeses), but if you tick the symptom box for PMS, these are best avoided at 'that time of the month'.

**Salty or high-fat foods:** Especially processed foods with added salt. These have been shown to increase both menstrual cramps and fluid retention.

**Alcohol**: Stop drinking leading up to the anticipated start of premenstrual symptoms. Alcohol can amplify the mood swings, and symptoms of irritability and anger. The catch is these may occur the day after imbibing as a delayed brain response to alcohol.

**Processed sugar:** Tricky for a lot of women, as the changing hormones of the premenstrual time also directly impact blood sugar/insulin pathways. Anticipate this time by making sure that healthy snack foods are on hand.

**Caffeine-related products:** Reduce coffee, chocolate, caffeine energy drinks, guarana-based energy drinks.

## SUPPLEMENTS

**Evening Primrose Oil:** For breast symptoms of congestion, fullness and tenderness. Take a total of 3000 mg divided over the day.

**Vitamin B6 (Pyridoxine):** This natural diuretic can be used to relieve fluid retention and reduce bloating. Cap dose at 100 mg daily.

> **TIP**
> Vitamin B6 is also a player in GABA hormone production, and this may be why a good dietary levels of Vitamin B6 can benefit severe PMDD.

**Phospholipid complex:** (sold internationally through Metagenics), it contains phosphatidylserine (active ingredient equivalent 100 mg per capsule). Take two capsules twice daily (400 mg total) in the luteal phase of the cycle.

**Zinc:** 30 mg of zinc gluconate daily. A 2020 study showed a decrease in both psychological and physical symptoms of PMS after 12 weeks.

## HERBAL OPTIONS

**St John's Wort (*Hypericum perforatum*):** The Flordis brand, Remotiv, is a high-quality option available over the counter in Australia, New Zealand, and the UK. Start with one tablet morning and evening, increasing to a maximum of three daily if needed. Avoid if taking antidepressants due to interactions.

**Chaste Tree (*Vitex agnus-castus*):** Supports progesterone. For PMS, take 1000 mg (dried herb equivalent) each morning.

**Chamomile:** Proven to help with PMS, it enhances sleep and offers anti-inflammatory, antioxidant, and antidepressant benefits. It is traditionally enjoyed as an evening tea.

## PSYCHOLOGICAL AND ALTERNATIVE THERAPIES

These support both PMS and PMDD.

Cognitive Behavioural Therapy (CBT)
Traditional Chinese Medicine (TCM)
Relaxation Techniques
Yoga
Acupuncture

## MEDICATION

**Luteal progesterone:** Taking a bioidentical form of progesterone during the second half of your cycle may benefit most women with simple PMS. The usual dose for PMS is 100mg daily for 10 to 14 days leading up to your period bleed.

**Oral contraceptive pill (the Pill):** This may be a good choice when contraception is an added consideration about the pros and cons of managing PMS symptoms.

## SURGICAL INTERVENTIONS

Endometrial ablation, a procedure that destroys the uterine lining, may relieve PMS symptoms, possibly by reducing monthly bleeding and allowing iron and nutrient levels to normalise. Speak to your doctor for advice and a referral to find out whether this is suitable for you.

# YOUR FERTILE YEARS OPPORTUNITY

The journey through your Fertile Years involves curiosity and openness—this time is an opportunity to learn more about your unique body. Paying attention to how stress, food, and lifestyle affect your cycle, moods, and libido offers you innate knowledge of what works for you and what interrupts hormonal flow. What works for one woman may not work for another, so listen to your body's cues.

Learning this vital information during these years assists you to transition into perimenopause and onto menopause and finally into the Age of Wisdom. So many women overlook the importance of establishing hormonal harmony in the Fertile Years as a strong foundation to deal with the hormonal changes ahead. Those that choose to ignore these vital signals from their body will realise in their 40s and 50s that their journey is more difficult. By nurturing your hormones with self-awareness, self-care, and wisdom, you'll emerge stronger and better prepared for the hormonal shifts ahead.

> Nurture your hormones with love, and they will nurture you with vitality.
>
> DR SARA GOTTFRIED

## WELLNESS ACTION PLAN
# THE FERTILE YEARS

Navigating the Fertile Years can be a juggling act, with life's demands often distracting you from self-care. Supporting your body with balanced nourishment, mindful movement, restorative sleep, and stress management is essential to maintaining hormonal harmony. Each choice helps build resilience and sustains wellbeing for the future.

### NOURISHMENT

This general nourishment plan (along with the information in our Spotlight on Nourishment page 393) is also suitable for Phase One and Phase Two of Perimenopause.

**SEASONAL, LOCAL, ORGANIC, WHOLE FOODS**

- Opt for nutrient-dense, seasonal foods to support a balanced hormonal ecosystem.

- Choose organic options wherever possible to reduce exposure to pesticides and other chemicals that can interfere with your hormonal balance and mood stability.

- Low-inflammatory and clean foods avoid unnecessary inflammation—minimise refined sugars and processed foods.

- Avoid or eliminate emulsifiers; these are hormone and gut microbiome disruptors. They are hidden in many processed foods like ice-cream, mayonnaise, and processed meats.

- Fermented foods: Gut-supportive foods like kimchi, sauerkraut, and yoghurt aid in hormone regulation by promoting a healthy gut microbiome.

- Fibre for oestrobolome support: Fibre-rich foods, such as vegetables, fruits, and whole grains, are essential for your oestrobolome—the gut bacteria responsible for metabolising oestrogen and ensuring it is safely eliminated. (Read more about the gut oestrobolome on page 424.)

- Phytoestrogen-rich foods: Include gentle, plant-based oestrogens like flaxseeds, soy, and legumes to support oestrogen balance and breast health, especially during natural fluctuations.

- Cruciferous vegetables (like broccoli, cauliflower and Brussels sprouts): These green and white powerhouses contain sulforaphane. (See pages 401 and 589 on this remarkable food molecule.) Aim for at least 1 serve (½ cup) every day for breast health and overall hormonal wellbeing.

- Progesterone-supporting foods: Avocados, nuts, and seeds contain healthy fats that support progesterone production, helping to balance oestrogen and promote calm.

- Magnesium for oestrogen metabolism pathways: Leafy greens, dark chocolate, and nuts provide magnesium, which supports the COMT enzyme (see Spotlight on Epigenetics page 269) aiding oestrogen clearance and supporting a balanced mood.

## EXERCISE PLAN
# HORMONAL BALANCE

The following exercise plan is specifically designed to match the ebb and flow rhythm of oestrogen and progesterone, as well as honour time for recovery during your menstrual cycle. We have also included the ideal foods for each week to support your training regime.

Most women exercise by repeating the same program week after week. This does not maximise the benefits of hormones that fluctuate, nor does it encourage your body to adapt to maximise your results.

In exercise science, periodisation to maximise results for athletes is an essential way to stimulate the body's natural adaptation response. This concept is often overlooked when training people who are not athletes. The mental and physical stimulation periodisation provides is key to maximising results.

Pilot studies using the idea of periodisation within a four-week menstrual cycle are discovering improved results physically, mentally and emotionally for women, while keeping hormones in balance. After reviewing the studies and considering the attributes of the ebb and flow of oestrogen, progesterone and testosterone, we outline a way to train to match your menstrual cycle. We believe the following exercise routine designed to meet your body's natural hormonal rhythm will maximise your efforts for your physical, mental and emotional wellbeing without under or overtraining.

This plan can be applied to all fitness levels, you just work to your body's current capacity and over time you will see improvements.

If you're a regular trainer, this may raise questions in relation to your usual approach. We encourage you to try this for three months faithfully and then review your performance, energy levels and hormonal symptoms, including any changes in your menstrual cycle.

Regardless of your purpose to train, muscle mass, strength, cardio and endurance are all required to support a fit, strong and healthy body. Burning fat is not about 'energy in vs energy out'. The balance of all your hormones affects your metabolic rate and you may find a different approach to your usual exercise regime (like having a week of rest during your menstrual cycle) works in your favour for a leaner stronger body and improved mental and emotional resilience.

### WEEK 1: MENSTRUAL PHASE (DAYS 1–7)
### TRAINING PHASE: REST AND RECOVERY

**Hormonal overview:** Oestrogen, progesterone and testosterone are at their lowest, gradually rising toward the end of the week. As a result, your energy may be lower at the start of your period, increasing as bleeding tapers off. See this week as your recovery week where your body resets itself and can build muscle and repair musculoskeletal damage. This also gives your adrenals a chance to recover, as it reduces the demand for stress hormones typically triggered by moderate to high-intensity exercise.

Your adrenals are your backup hormonal support and if they become overused can interfere with hormonal balance. We are also aiming to reduce cortisol surges in this phase, cortisol has been shown to elevate in training sessions longer than 30 minutes.

**STRENGTH**
- Gym: Days 1 to 5 take a rest from weight training.
- If you must train your muscles, focus on gentle, low-impact exercises using your bodyweight such as squats, lunges, push-ups with no weights, maximum repetitions (reps) of 30 (reps are the number of times you repeat an exercise).
- When bright red blood finishes, weight training and Pilates can be reintroduced, (intensity—lift weights to failure at 10 to 12 reps).

**PILATES**
- Ask your instructor to focus on low intensity—think rehab; no longer than 30 mins workout with 30 mins stretching to make up your 60 mins class.

**CARDIO**
- Keep cardio low impact during bright red blood loss (gentle walking/cycling) with a maximum of 30-min gentle training sessions.
- Increase intensity as your bleed stops if your energy levels rise. Shift the intensity to moderate intensity sessions which can include a 20 to 30-min run/jog/spin.
- Ideal activities: Qigong, restorative yoga, gentle walks in nature, meditation, intentional breathing, 'me time', movies with friends/family,

**FOOD FOR THIS PHASE**
- Reduce raw foods to minimal, instead choose warm nourishing soups, curries, casseroles, steamed and roast vegetables.
- Increase intake of foods containing iron:
  - Red meat (and liver, kidney if you enjoy)
  - Shellfish
  - Turkey
  - Spinach
  - Legumes
  - Pumpkin seeds
  - Quinoa
  - Broccoli
  - Tofu

## WEEK 2: FOLLICULAR PHASE (DAYS 8–14)
## TRAINING PHASE: STRENGTH

**Hormonal overview**: Oestrogen levels increase, which enhances energy, muscle recovery, and endurance. Testosterone peaks towards ovulation (around Days 13 to 14), optimising strength and power. This phase is about increasing your strength and power, with shorter bursts of very high intensity workouts.

**STRENGTH**
- Gym: This is a prime time for intense strength training to make you stronger and build bone.
- Incorporate heavy weights aiming for 3 to 5 reps while maintaining excellent form, use compound exercises that move more than one joint at a time for both lower and upper body (for example, squats, deadlifts, assisted chins).
- Try for your personal bests.
- Increasing strength prepares you for the next training phase; muscle and bone building.

**PILATES**
- Ask your instructor to focus on strength this week.
- Low reps at near maximum intensity.
- Focus on your personal weakest muscle groups, incorporate lower body, upper body and postural muscles.

**CARDIO**

This is the week for high-intensity cardio. Following your rest and recovery week last week, this is the time to push your cardio high-intensity limit.

- Phase Four anaerobic training.
- Keep workouts to high intensity, max out to your fitness level.
- This phase is shorter training duration—keep it to 20 to 30 mins.

Sample workouts: Interval training, walking hills, stairs, HIIT, cross fit, short fast sprints (walking or running), spin classes, swimming, and more challenging yoga such as Ashtanga.

**FOOD FOR THIS PHASE**
- Increase protein during this phase, ensure every meal includes adequate amounts.
- Keep to a low-inflammatory diet (lots of fruits and vegetables) to help manage any inflammation due to high-intensity training. (See Core Food Principles on page 396 for more detail.)

## WEEK 3: EARLY TO MID-LUTEAL PHASE (DAYS 15–21)
## TRAINING PHASE: BUILDING MUSCLE

**Hormonal overview:** Oestrogen reduces as progesterone rises significantly, boosting fat metabolism. There can be an increase in body temperature, making intense exercise feel slightly harder so back off the intensity and extend the duration of your training sessions. Testosterone starts to decline from ovulation, which is why we trained for strength last week.

**STRENGTH**
- Gym: Continue strength training.
- Reduce the weights to moderate and aim for higher repetitions to fail at 8–12 reps.

- This is the time to optimise stability and functional exercises.
- Focus on form and technique rather than maximum load.

**PILATES**
- Ask your instructor to focus on building muscle mass rather than brute strength.
- More repetitions and less weight (not muscular endurance).

**CARDIO**
Reduce your intensity this week.
- Phase Two Aerobic training.
- Moderate intensity and extend the length of your training session to 45–60 mins.
- Avoid excessive high-intensity sessions, the time for this was last week as higher progesterone this week can make recovery slower.

Sample workouts: Moderate-weight resistance training, steady-state cardio, Vinyasa flow yoga or Pilates for stability and recovery.

**FOOD FOR THIS PHASE**
- Focus on a balanced diet.

## WEEK 4: LATE LUTEAL/PRE-MENSTRUAL PHASE (DAYS 22–28)
## TRAINING PHASE: MUSCULAR AND CARDIO ENDURANCE

**Hormonal overview:** Progesterone and oestrogen begin to drop sharply; from Days 22 to 26/27. In this phase we focus on muscular and cardio endurance— as your period nears, we reduce the length of your training time. Think of petering off as you head to Day 1 again and resume the training regime for your bleed. A couple of days prior to your period you may notice some fatigue, bloating or mood changes. Include more gentle exercises that support mental wellbeing such as being in nature, meditation, Qigong and breathwork.

**STRENGTH**
- Lower weights with higher reps (20–25 to failure) deplete glycogen in muscles, supporting fat burning.
- Focus on mobility and stability work.
- This phase is suited to lighter resistance exercises or bodyweight movements that build muscular endurance.

**PILATES**
- Ask your instructor to focus on muscular endurance.

**CARDIO**
- Low-impact cardio Phase One is best.
- Low-impact endurance exercises such as hiking or flat cycling are beneficial.
- Lower intensity activities support stamina without draining energy.

**ENDURANCE**
- This is a good time for steady-state endurance activities that last up to or longer than an hour.
- Moderate-paced cycling, extended walks, runs or swimming that utilise fat as a fuel source.

Sample workouts: Mobility-focused strength circuits, brisk walking, low-impact cardio, low intensity extended jogs/walks. Yoga and Pilates focused on muscular endurance.

**FOOD FOR THIS PHASE**

You may feel hungrier during this phase due to your hormonal shifts.

- Focus on nutrient-dense foods rather than fast or processed foods.
- Choose home-made healthy comfort foods like mashed potato and veggies, mild curries etc.
- Healthy snacks such as nuts, hummus and crudités are preferred. Take the time to make your own biscuits, cakes, muffins to help support the need for more food or those times when you want something sweeter. Bio-hack your usual recipes. Try replacing the flour in cakes/muffins/biscuits with the same amount of almond meal (add in 1 tsp of baking powder) and replace sugar with maple syrup.
- Avoid sugary snacks as they will increase your hunger.

Our unique menstrual cycle-aware exercise approach helps you sync your training with your natural hormonal fluctuations, boosting both results and recovery, and essentially is designed to maintain hormonal balance. Remember to listen to your body and adjust based on personal energy levels, as individual responses can vary.

## THE IMPORTANCE OF QUALITY SLEEP

Sleep patterns vary across your cycle, with restful sleep being particularly crucial in the luteal phase. Consult our Spotlight on Sleep on page 351 for cycle-based tips to help you drift into deep, restorative sleep, such as reducing blue light exposure before bed and including calming nutrients like magnesium.

## STRESS MANAGEMENT TECHNIQUES

The Fertile Years often bring high-stakes responsibilities that can leave stress hormones running high. Elevated stress can lead to hormonal imbalances, especially affecting the adrenal glands and pathways tied to oestrogen and progesterone.

Integrating mindfulness practices like meditation, deep breathing, and gentle yoga can reset your stress response and promote a calm, balanced state.

**Epigenetic impact of stress:** Chronic stress can alter gene expression, increasing oxidative stress and potentially accelerating cellular ageing. Consider a daily antioxidant-rich diet (berries, leafy greens, and nuts) to counteract oxidative stress.

**Antioxidant 'housekeeping' enzymes:** Supporting antioxidant pathways through nutrient-rich foods and stress management can optimise their protective effects.

**COMT gene variants and stress:** COMT, the enzyme involved in processing stress hormones, is essential to a balanced mood and energy. If you find that stress impacts you more intensely, consider magnesium and other COMT-supportive nutrients to help maintain calm. (See more on COMT on page 224.)

## REDUCE TOXIN EXPOSURE

A personal care product audit is a great way to reduce daily toxin exposure. (Refer to our Spotlight on Managing Toxins on page 478.)

## OUR FINAL WORDS OF ADVICE

By tuning into these areas, you support your body's natural rhythm, giving it what it needs to thrive through the unique demands of the Fertile Years.

Work on establishing hormonal balance throughout your Fertile Years, as the foundations you lay during these years are well worth the investment in your 'self-care'. What you do now will either support you beautifully (or deliver a rough ride) as you move into the next three phases of your hormonal life.

Starting on page 119, discover everything you need to know about perimenopause and how to navigate the next part of your hormonal journey.

# LET'S GET PREGNANT (OR NOT)

*Fall in love with taking care of yourself.*
ROMA LEAF

To utterly understand the principles of conception and contraception, it is essential for you to pre-read the Fertile Years beginning on page 63. This section continues the story of the Fertile Years as we take a deep dive into pregnancy and contraception.

Nature gifts us with clear signs of fertility and learning to recognise these signals is key to understanding your body. This section is dedicated to exploring two paths:

- Maximising your chances of conception, or
- Avoiding pregnancy naturally without relying on medical contraception.

Whether you are planning for or preventing pregnancy, understanding these natural rhythms helps you make empowered choices about your body. We will uncover how to feel more connected with the brilliance of your body and its fertile potential, helping you embrace conception or your contraceptive journey with confidence.

> **IS EGG FREEZING WORTH IT?**
> Are you thinking about the possibility of pregnancy but not quite ready until after 30? It might be worth considering a proactive approach to your fertility. While it's possible to conceive into your 40s, it's important to know that egg quality peaks in your mid-to-late 20s. After your mid-30s, changes in egg quality can make it more challenging to conceive.
> If pregnancy isn't in your immediate plans but might be in the future, egg retrieval and freezing can be a fertility game-changer. Advances in IVF techniques are improving outcomes for pregnancies using frozen eggs. Taking steps now can give you more options down the road.

## GENETICALLY HARDWIRED FOR FERTILITY

Mother Nature designed the female body as a marvel of reproduction, genetically hardwiring it for the extraordinary journey of creating life. Whether you dream of nurturing new life or choose a different path, your body carries the ancient wisdom of fertility, driven by the primal instinct to perpetuate the human species. This potential remains extraordinary, regardless of how we identify. We understand this can be confusing if you struggle with fertility and hope the information in this chapter helps you.

It's said that subconscious behaviours can sometimes lead to unintended pregnancies—perhaps you, or someone you know, found themselves pregnant despite intentions otherwise. While some women may choose not to have children, others face the challenge of infertility, a poignant reminder that nature's plans don't always align with our own. But in most cases, the innate drive for reproduction remains strong, even against the backdrop of personal and global concerns.

Amidst the complexities of life, one truth stands; the call of fertility is embedded in our biology. By tuning into these natural rhythms, you can make empowered choices, whether you seek to conceive, or prevent pregnancy.

## EMBRACING THE FERTILITY DANCE

While fertility challenges are discussed more widely in the modern era, nature still provides us with tools to understand and enhance fertility. Factors such as lifestyle, diet, stress and your exposure to environmental toxins can influence your reproductive health.

A 1986 study comparing fertility rates in Japan found that women in Okinawa, a celebrated 'Blue Zone' region known for its long-living residents, had significantly higher fertility rates than the national average. Women aged 35 to 39 in Okinawa were twice as likely to conceive, and those aged 40 to 44 were three times more likely than their counterparts across Japan. While lifestyle factors in Okinawa play a role, the study underscores how health and environment impact fertility outcomes.

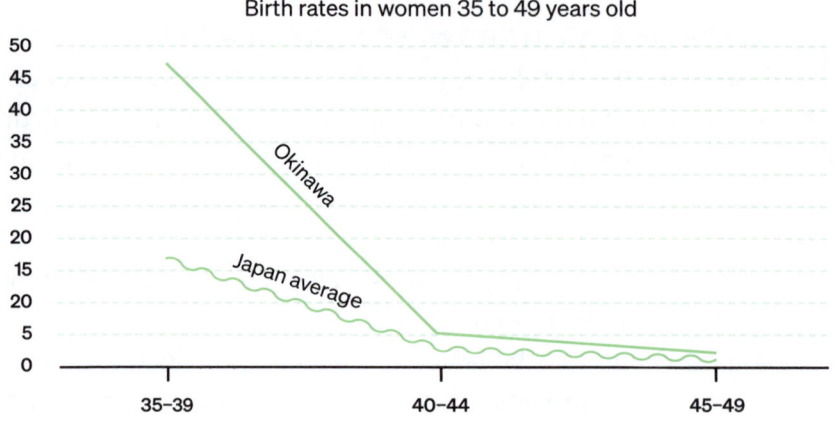

### LIFESTYLE AND FERTILITY

Natural fertility peaks in your 20s and starts to decline in your 30s. However, healthy lifestyle choices can help maintain fertility well into your 30s. Many women successfully conceive in their mid-to-late 30s and even early 40s without IVF. Focusing on supporting your natural cycle and cellular health in your early Fertile Years can boost your chances of conception later.

For more on how to support ovarian and egg cell health, see our Spotlight on Oxidative Stress on page 273.

# NATURAL FERTILITY: OBSERVING YOUR BODY'S SIGNALS

There are innate ways to observe your body's fertility.

- **Track your menstrual cycle**: Your most fertile window is usually around Day 14.
- **Take your temperature daily:** A rise in temperature can identify ovulation.
- **Check your vaginal mucus for changes**: Fertile mucus is typically clear and stretchy, like egg white.
- **Pay attention to the moon cycles:** You may spontaneously ovulate on the full moon, regardless of where you are in your cycle. The idea that spontaneous ovulation is linked to the full moon has roots in ancient beliefs.

### KEEPING A RECORD

The pioneer in natural fertility and contraception over 40 years is Sydney-based naturopath and herbalist Francesca Naish, who runs Australia's only clinic dedicated to helping people conceive naturally. We highly recommend her app, *MyNFM*, which offers comprehensive tools for tracking both menstrual cycle awareness and fertility, perfect for users focused on contraception or planning around ideal fertile windows. The app provides clear insights into your cycle, helping you understand your body's rhythms for both conception and natural fertility management. Read on to learn more about how to read the signs from your body.

### KNOW YOUR MENSTRUAL CYCLE

The most fertile window is during ovulation, typically around Days 12 to 15 of your cycle. Once an egg is released, it only survives for 12 to 24 hours. This makes your fertile window small, so it's important to take full advantage of it.

**TIP**

Sperm can survive for up to five days in a healthy vagina—this is important to know if pregnancy is not in your plans!

Leading up to Day 10, plan some self-care to make yourself feel beautiful. Get your hair or nails done, shave or wax, or treat yourself to whatever makes you feel sexy and confident. Plan some connection time with your partner, whether it's a date night, a cozy movie night at home, or simply enjoying quality time together. Keep things relaxed and avoid putting pressure on the moment—let intimacy happen naturally during this time. Neither of you need any pressure or stress that could interfere with conception.

### TAKE YOUR TEMPERATURE

Measure your basal body temperature using an ovulation thermometer before getting out of bed each morning. Your temperature will drop slightly just before ovulation, then rise by up to 0.5°C afterwards, signalling that ovulation has occurred. This thermal shift stays elevated until just before your period. If your temperature remains elevated for more than 20 days, it's a strong indication that you're pregnant.

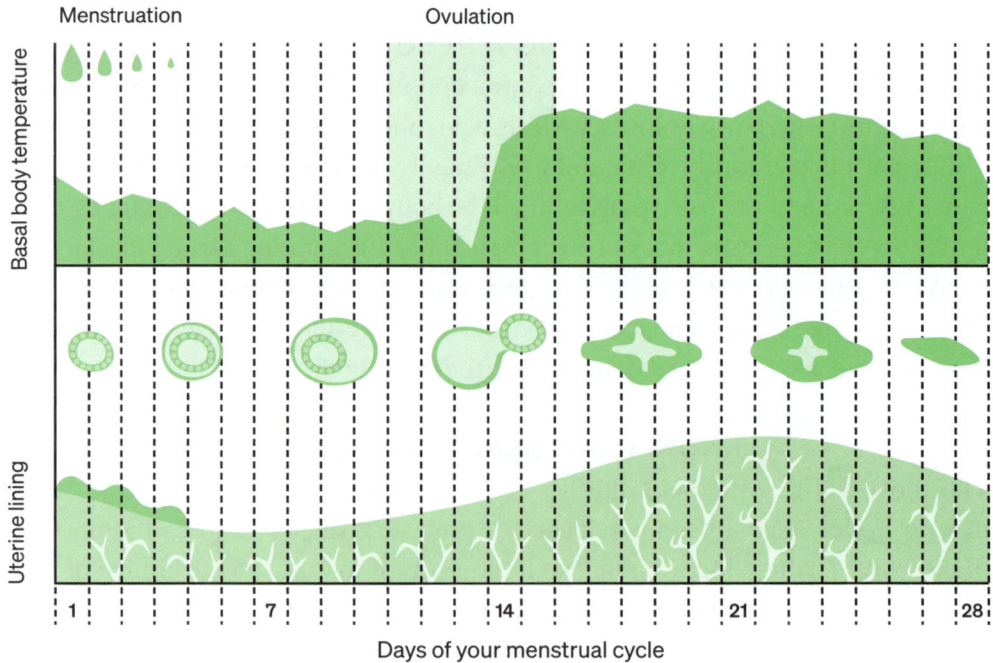

Around ovulation there is a surge in the luteinising hormone (LH) and follicle stimulating hormone (FSH) from the brain. LH activates receptors on the ovary to step up production of progesterone. As the name suggests, FSH gives the egg a nudge to be released in preparation for fertilisation.

### CHECK YOUR VAGINAL MUCUS

Nature provides a wonderful way of signalling your fertility through vaginal mucus.

- The best time to check it is in the morning before your first urination.
- Insert your index finger just inside your vagina and scoop out some mucus.
- Early in your cycle, just after your period, the mucus is usually thick, whitish, sticky, and slightly grainy—similar to the texture of hummus. If you try to stretch it between your fingers, it won't stretch.
- As you approach ovulation, the mucus changes, becoming thinner and more transparent.
- Around ovulation, it resembles clear, stretchy egg whites. This is a key sign that you're fertile. If you're trying to conceive, this is the time to have sex. If you're not planning to get pregnant, use a barrier method or avoid sex during this time.

### THE FULL MOON

Historically, a woman's menstrual cycle was called the 'moon cycle', as women would often cycle in sync with the moon before artificial lighting and synthetic hormones disrupted natural rhythms. Our ancestors lived in harmony with moonlight, stars, and firelight—natural sources of light that supported our circadian rhythm. This meant women often menstruated and ovulated together, leading to rituals and celebrations aligned with the moon's phases.

> **TIP**
> Today there is scientific evidence that the moon decreases melatonin in women—this occurs even when they are in a dark room with no moon light.

In many cultures, the full moon still symbolises new beginnings and significant events. It influences not only the tides but also fertility in humans and animals. Interestingly, it's believed that the full moon can trigger spontaneous ovulation, even if you're mid-cycle or on the Pill. This is why tracking the full moon can be helpful, even today. You can easily find moon phase calendars online and note the dates in your diary or digital calendar.

To maximise your fertility potential, watch for these signs:
- You're around Day 14 of your cycle.
- Your temperature has slightly risen.
- You notice egg-white stretchy mucus.
- There's a full moon or it's close to one.

When all the above signals align, your fertility is at its peak. Celebrate this natural connection and enjoy the process. Only women have the power to conceive, carry life within them, and give birth—a miraculous ability that should be honoured.

## KEEP YOUR EGGS CLEAN

Maintaining healthy eggs is crucial to optimising fertility. As women age, the processes that keep eggs 'rust-free', slow down, making it harder to conceive. Free radical damage due to reactive oxygen species (ROS) can affect your remaining egg supply, just like it affects other cells in your body.

Each month, your ovary prepares an egg (oocyte) that carries the potential for pregnancy. These eggs are susceptible to oxidative stress, so ensure your body has enough of these trace minerals:
- Manganese
- Selenium
- Iron

These are essential for maintaining healthy antioxidant pathways. (See Spotlight on Oxidative Stress page 273.)

# WHAT'S DISRUPTING YOUR FERTILITY?

Stress in all its forms is a major contributor to infertility, whether through:

**Psychological or psychosocial stress**: Chronic stress elevates stress hormones, shifting the body's focus toward survival rather than reproductive functions. (Read our Spotlight on Psychological Stress on page 290 and Restorative Practices on page 372.)

**Excessive exercise**: Over-exercising can lead to elevated cortisol levels, triggering the survival response and increasing oxidative stress, which can deplete resources essential for reproductive health. (Read our Spotlight on Movement and Exercise starting on page 485.)

**Oxidative stress:** Puts pressure on your entire system. (Read our Spotlight on Oxidative Stress beginning on page 273.)

**Environmental toxins**: Exposure to pollutants and endocrine disruptors can interfere with hormonal balance, undermining fertility. (Read our Spotlight on Managing Toxins page 478.)

These stressors increase inflammation, disrupting pathways vital to wellbeing and directly impacting fertility. For those hoping to conceive naturally, addressing these factors supports both maternal health and sperm quality.

# WHY PSYCHOLOGICAL STRESS IS YOUR SABOTEUR

From an evolutionary perspective, stress hormones like adrenaline are released as life-saving responses. Elevated adrenaline keeps the body in a heightened state of fight-or-flight, prioritising survival over reproductive functions. Over time, prolonged high adrenaline levels are joined by elevated cortisol, contributing to our chronic stress response. In ancient times, cortisol only became elevated due to war, drought, famine and life-threatening weather extremes. It is only natural, and it makes perfect sense, for our body to make the decision not to conceive because both pregnant mum and babies are vulnerable, and it is not a good evolutionary plan to reproduce while we are fighting and running for our life.

Today we drive the very same stress hormone pathways due to psychological stress—this kind of stress is a force to be reckoned with! Reducing stress hormones is the priority of every would-be mother. (Read our Spotlight on Psychological Stress on page 290.)

> **ADDRESS THE STRESS**
>
> Stress levels can not only affect your fertility, stress can also affect the development and epigenetic expression of your baby. High maternal stress has been linked to a reduction in nerve cells in the amygdala of newborns, a critical brain structure for processing emotions and social cues. Managing stress is especially important for women planning pregnancy.

CASE STUDY | DR KAREN

# Annie
### Fertility plan

A woman in her early 30s sat clicking away at her laptop while waiting for her consultation with me. Settling into my office chair, Annie began to share her story:

'Dr Karen, I hear you're really good with fertility issues. I'm needing to fall pregnant by October next year—can't be pregnant before July because I must be OK to travel overseas to a conference for work in March. My business is growing so fast that I won't be able to fit a pregnancy into my schedule the year after that. Problem is that my periods have been all over the place and I've missed the last two ...'

I looked across at this capable and organised young women and thought, 'This pregnancy is so not going to happen on her schedule.' I wasn't surprised to hear she squeezed a 45-minute spin class into every 12-hour workday, six days a week. She loved the post-exercise high, feeling like she could fly through her workload, and was pushing to do even more.

About a year ago, her periods became heavier (a telltale sign of declining progesterone, and oestrogen dominance), but now they'd stopped completely. I suspected her oestrogen had dropped, the body's final natural survival response to perceived danger and hardship.

The final piece of the puzzle? Her libido. Annie's lawyer husband, juggling stress of his own, wasn't troubled by her low sex drive—it suited them both for now.

With no period for two months, I ordered a fertility hormone profile. As I suspected, her results showed ultimate survival mode—low pituitary hormones (LH and FSH) suppressing oestrogen and progesterone to menopausal levels. Her testosterone—key for libido—was unrecordably low. Annie was, unfortunately, the perfect example of her ancestral pathways at work.

## SOLUTION

We worked on stress management and excessive exercise, limiting the spin classes to three times a week and adding yoga and breathwork. We also prioritised her sleep. I added herbal support (1000 mg of Chaste Tree each morning for a minimum of four months). A pregnancy didn't occur on her strict timeline. However, after making these lifestyle changes, Annie conceived naturally during a holiday in Fiji when her body finally got to rest. She went on to have two healthy children.

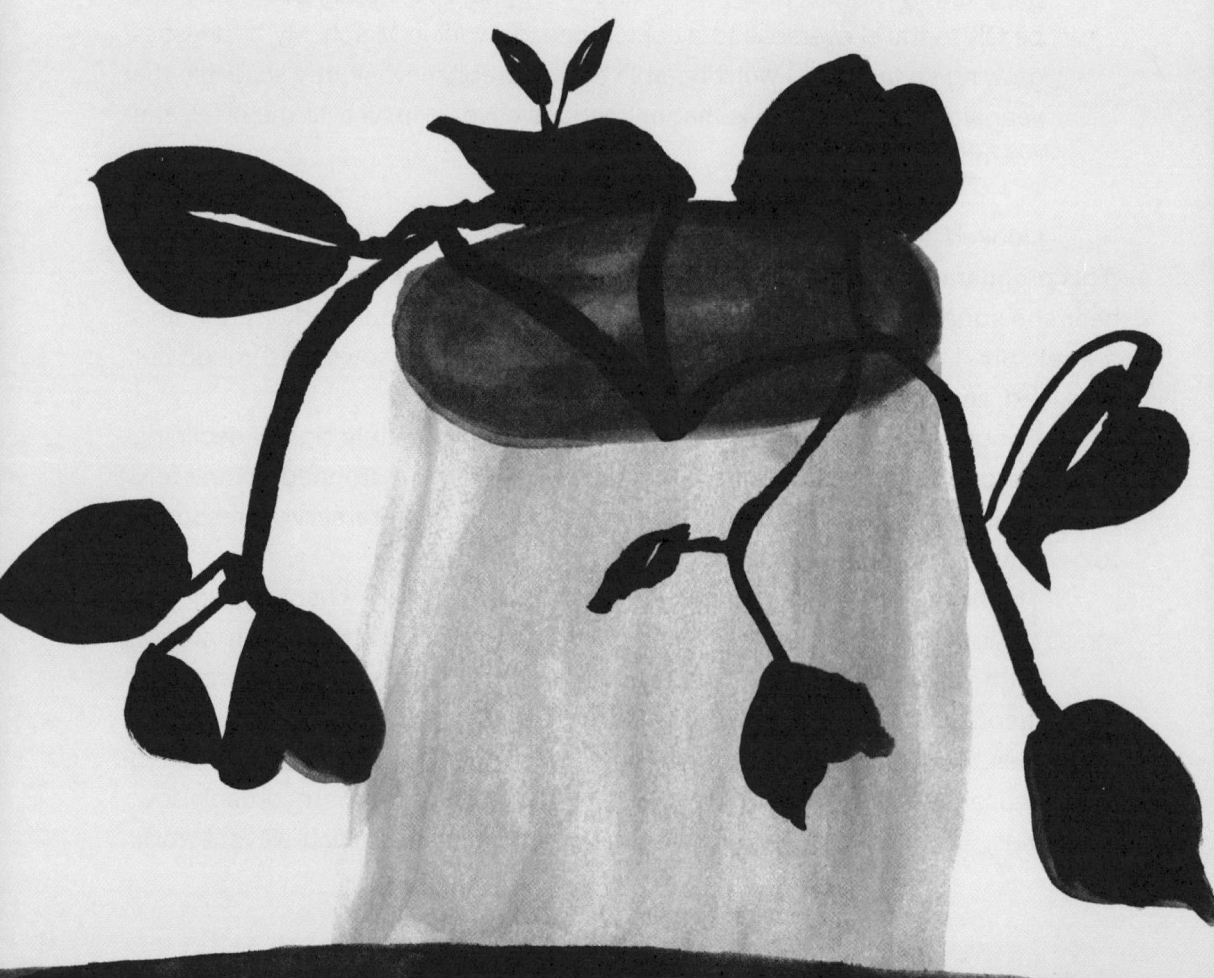

# IN VITRO FERTILISATION (IVF)

In vitro fertilisation (IVF) is a wonderful option for women who need additional support to conceive. It can also provide same-sex couples and single people with the joy and wonder of being a co- or solo parent. In these instances, these clinics can provide a safe, secure and legal way to ensure sperm and egg engage to produce another miracle, a beloved baby without any misunderstandings and the heartache of a donor changing their mind.

However, like many man-made methods, IVF is a double-edged sword and can be a very costly route on many levels. Financing the cost of multiple cycles and the roller coaster ride of these cycles emotionally can be very stressful, and stress is the enemy of fertility. A woman's body will resist and reject pregnancy when there is unrelenting stress present (read Marnie's story on page 106).

When conception does not happen or sadly miscarriage ends the hope of pregnancy, grief can forge a deep wedge in relationships, particularly the relationship to oneself and of course your partner. We recommend you seek a professional counsellor skilled to support you through this often-harrowing process.

Further, the extreme level of synthetic hormones required to push the female body beyond its natural ability can be overwhelming emotionally and physically with many women, although overjoyed to be a mother, find themselves dealing with a body and brain struggling to return to normality postpartum. (Read Leesa's story on page 106.)

Where possible, we recommend trying natural conception methods first, as discussed in this chapter, and consider IVF as a last resort—unless, of course, IVF is the only viable option based on your individual circumstances.

Regardless of the method—natural conception or IVF—pre-conception care supports your body physically and emotionally and increases the chances of a successful conception and pregnancy to full term. Read on for our Preconception Action Plan.

# Marnie's Story

'I initially thought IVF would be easy. As a same-sex couple, IVF was our path to parenthood. I had no known fertility issues, and my wife got pregnant with our daughter on her first embryo transfer. However, after four rounds of IVF (including two rounds where I had no embryos left by Day 5), three failed embryo transfers and one miscarriage, I began to lose hope that I would ever get pregnant with my own egg.

'After the fourth failed round, I switched specialists. Following a laparoscopy, I was diagnosed and treated for endometriosis. Despite this, my fifth round of IVF also resulted in no embryos. Feeling disheartened, my doctor and I agreed to give it one final, all-out attempt.

'Around that time, my mum gave me the book *How to Be Well* and introduced me to her friend Sharon Kolkka. I gladly accepted Sharon's invitation to meet and, during our conversation, she suggested several wellness changes to support my fertility journey. These included further reducing toxin exposure, seeing a naturopath, managing adrenal stress and letting go of the time pressure I was putting on myself. I am autistic and a lawyer, so I was really struggling with not being able to control when I would get pregnant.

'Meeting with Sharon felt like a turning point. I became one of my specialist's first patients to undergo ovarian rejuvenation where platelet-rich plasma (PRP) is injected into the ovaries. I also had further endometriosis removed. I consulted with an experienced naturopath who adjusted my supplements. While already living a low-tox lifestyle, I further scrutinised my diet and skincare. I adopted a largely anti-inflammatory diet, rich in whole foods, healthy fats, whole grains and pesticide-free produce, while avoiding red meat, alcohol and processed foods. I started meditating each morning and focused on reducing stress, despite juggling a toddler, a demanding career and neurodiversity.

'About three months later, I went through one last round of IVF. This time, I had four embryos make it to Day 5—double my previous best. A fresh embryo transfer led to pregnancy and my doctor placed me on an immune protocol to prevent miscarriage. Nine months later I gave birth to a beautiful healthy baby boy. And I still have three embryos in the freezer.'

# Leesa's Story

Leesa met her partner Will at the age of 42. After six months of trying to conceive naturally, they turned to IVF due to her history of endometriosis and fallopian tube insufficiency. Alongside IVF, Leesa incorporated acupuncture, naturopathy, and a strict anti-inflammatory diet for both her (and her husband) to follow.

After two rounds of Clomid and five rounds of IVF with multiple failed transfers, Leesa fell pregnant with twins at 44. Tragically, they lost one of the twins at eight weeks, which caused several hospital visits due to a haematoma near the placenta.

At 38 weeks, Leesa delivered a healthy boy via a scheduled C-section. However, by day four post-partum, she began experiencing severe symptoms: diarrhoea, anxiety, uncontrollable shaking, and a full nervous system meltdown. Despite having managed her IBS, endometriosis, and anxiety for over a decade through a gluten- and dairy-free, wholefood diet, her body seemed to crash.

The usual sleep deprivation, combined with the stress of delayed milk production, worsened her symptoms. She experienced extreme hunger, nausea, vomiting, insomnia, and an overall sense of being hungover. Her symptoms mirrored morning sickness but were accompanied by anxiety and sleeplessness. As the weeks passed, the bad days started to outnumber the good. With her partner back at work and little support, Leesa felt isolated and overwhelmed.

A GP prescribed antidepressants without any positive change. After several adjustments, Leesa realised they weren't the solution, as her distress wasn't about motherhood—it felt like her body had crashed. Eventually, she saw a medical doctor who specialised in post-natal depletion recovery. For the first time, she felt truly heard. The doctor explained post-natal depletion and the complex disruption of the hypothalamus-pituitary-adrenal (HPA) axis.

Tests confirmed Leesa had third-stage adrenal deficiency (low cortisol), leptin resistance, and borderline insulin resistance. With her doctor's guidance on nutrition, lifestyle changes, and supplements, she slowly started to recover. Her symptoms were further complicated by the onset of perimenopause, which intensified in the second half of her cycle. Recovery wasn't straightforward and there were many setbacks, but by the time her son turned two, Leesa began feeling more like herself again.

## POSTNATAL DEPLETION AND RECOVERY

Postnatal depletion is common in new mothers, particularly those with pre-existing health conditions like endometriosis or adrenal deficiency. Symptoms include extreme fatigue, anxiety and hormonal imbalances. Recovery involves addressing nutritional deficiencies, hormonal health, and managing stress.

IVF and pregnancy can be physically and emotionally demanding, but with the right support and holistic approaches, many women successfully conceive and recover from fertility treatments. Professional guidance and a balanced lifestyle can significantly improve the chances of a positive outcome.

## YOUR POSTNATAL CHECKLIST

- **Enhance nutrition:** Prioritise zinc-rich, iron-rich, and omega-3-rich foods, along with B-vitamins to support mood and hormone production.
- **Supplement:** Use an organic, plant-based vitamin supplement to optimise your health and breast milk quality.
- **Boost milk supply:** Add ½ teaspoon of nutritional yeast to your smoothies to support milk production.
- **Limit caffeine and alcohol:** Both can affect your sleep and your baby's sleep. If you indulge, do so right after breastfeeding to allow time for it to clear your system before the next feed.
- **Take time for yourself:** Spend 30-60 minutes daily on stress-reducing activities to enhance your wellbeing and increase breast milk production.
- **Rest:** Set aside time to do nothing, whether it's reading, meditating, or watching a movie.
- **Sleep:** Aim for short blocks of quality sleep (even three hours can help). Wake your baby for a final feed before bed to maximise sleep for both of you.
- **Housework can wait:** Delegate chores to focus on bonding with your baby. Consider hiring a housekeeper to take the pressure off maintaining 'Superwoman' status.

### UNLOCKING THE SECRETS OF IRON: A VITAL NUTRIENT

Iron deficiency—it's an unsuspecting foe lurking in the background of our busy lives. This humble mineral plays a critical role in over 90 biochemical processes within our bodies—talk about a multitasking marvel!

But here's the catch; when iron levels fall short, it's not just fatigue we're up against. It triggers a domino effect, leading to hormonal imbalances, autoimmune issues, and even the dark shadows of depression.

Women, often juggling multiple roles, are particularly susceptible to severe iron deficiency anaemia. Years of inadequate iron intake, compounded by heavy periods or regular blood donations, create the perfect storm for this silent assailant.

Listen to iron's subtle signals. In unlocking its secrets, you'll find one of the keys to restoring balance and reclaiming your vitality. (See Spotlight on Vitamins and Minerals on page 443.)

CASE STUDY | DR KAREN

# Sarah

## Pregnancy and post-partum recovery

Sarah has been my patient since she was 21, and we've maintained a good hormonal profile over the years. Throughout her adult life, Sarah was not on any hormonal contraception, and her cycles were regular, occurring every 28 days. She adhered to a mostly organic whole-food diet and minimised exposure to processed foods and chemicals in her household and skincare products.

In her early 30s, an AMH test revealed a low egg count for her age. I advised Sarah not to wait too long before considering pregnancy. At 33, she showed signs of HPA axis dysfunction (chronic stress) confirmed by low cortisol levels. She implemented lifestyle changes, cutting caffeine, prioritising rest, and adjusting to more restorative exercises. Additionally, she worked on dismantling internal beliefs contributing to adrenal burnout and successfully recovered within 12 months.

At 36, Sarah unexpectedly became pregnant on her wedding night. Despite some early bleeding and morning sickness, her pregnancy was smooth, and her son was delivered via emergency C-section at 41 weeks. With family support and a successful breastfeeding journey for three and a half years, Sarah felt back to herself around six weeks post-partum.

WELLNESS ACTION PLAN
# PRECONCEPTION

Preconception care is essential for both fertility and the epigenetic health of your future child. We recommend the following checklists as you embark on this journey:

## 1 MEDICAL AND DENTAL HEALTH CHECK-UPS

**Dental:** Address any issues before pregnancy and inform your dentist of your plans to conceive. Inflammation from gum disease may disrupt hormones and delay conception by up to two months.

**Medical conditions:** Ensure any pre-existing conditions (for example, diabetes, thyroid disorders) are well-managed.

**Medication review:** Consult your doctor about any medications you're taking to ensure they're safe for pregnancy.

**Cervical smear test:** Your vaginal health and cervix care are foundational to your fertility. (See more in our Spotlight on Your Cervix on page 511.)

**Herbs and supplements:** Check with your health practitioner to confirm that your current supplements are safe during pregnancy.

## 2 BLOOD TESTS

Ask for these tests via a referral from your healthcare provider:
- Full blood screen, iron stores, liver and kidney function
- Blood group and Rh factor
- STI screen, Hepatitis A/B, HIV, and syphilis
- Vitamin D, B12 (for vegans/vegetarians), thyroid function (TSH)
- Immunity to rubella and varicella (chicken pox)

> **ARE YOU A CAT PERSON?**
>
> Toxoplasmosis is a parasitic infection that can be transmitted by contact with cat faeces or undercooked meat. It can cause miscarriage, stillbirth, or birth defects if contracted during pregnancy. If you've had regular contact with cats, you may already have immunity. Ask your vet to check your cat for toxoplasmosis if you're planning to conceive.

## 3 LIFESTYLE MODIFICATIONS

When you know you're ready to conceive, give yourself around six months to allow your body to naturally find its balance. It's essential that your organs—liver, kidneys, heart, microbiome, and digestive system—function at their best. When your organs are healthy, you enhance your immune system and balance your hormones, which boosts your fertility.

Fertility and hormonal harmony rely heavily on balanced lifestyle choices. Excessive stress—both physical and psychological—can prevent pregnancy. Addressing these issues through lifestyle changes, stress management, and proper preconception care can significantly enhance your chances of conceiving and enjoying a healthy pregnancy.

By preparing your body before conception, you're creating a healthy environment for your baby to grow and develop with minimal complications and giving yourself the best chance to resist illness during pregnancy. This checklist is designed to help your body to achieve ideal cellular function, improve immune strength, and balance your hormones. We also suggest you remove irritants that could impede organ function,

### CLEAN FOOD

During preconception and pregnancy, it's essential to eat clean, nutrient-dense food. This means focusing on nutritional balance, as well as the quality of your food. Choosing clean, pesticide-free food is important.

> **WHAT IS 'CLEAN FOOD'?**
>
> Clean food is nutrient-dense, minimally processed, and free from harmful added chemicals. It supports overall health and fertility.

## CARBOHYDRATES (FRUITS AND VEGETABLES)
- Two-thirds of your plate should be filled with a rainbow of vegetables, while the remaining third should consist of animal protein (around 150 g).
- For your gut microbiome include starchy vegetables such as sweet potato and whole grains such as brown rice, oats and quinoa.
- If you're vegan or vegetarian, ensure you're getting sufficient vegetable protein and minerals, such as iron, for an upcoming pregnancy. It's worth consulting a naturopath or nutritionist to make sure you're getting enough nutrients from your daily intake, especially as you prepare for pregnancy.
- Aim for 3-5 cups of veggies each day and up to 2 pieces of fruit.
- While including a rainbow of veggies is important, anything green will help keep your liver clean.
- Ensure you include legumes, nuts and seeds.
- Also include fermented foods like kimchi, sauerkraut, miso, kefir, and kombucha for optimal gut health.

## PROTEIN
### WILD SEAFOOD IN AUSTRALIA: A GUIDELINE
- Sustainable, seasonal, wild-caught seafood is always the best option.
- When choosing fish, opt for small species like herring, pilchards, whitebait, and sardines. These are nutrient-packed, cost-effective, and unlikely to be farmed.
- Wild fish like snapper, barramundi, bream, and whiting are excellent sources of omega-3s and other essential nutrients.
- Sardines are not farmed and are a gold star choice for omega-3s. They are widely available fresh or in BPA-free tins.

### AVOID EATING BIG FISH
- Tuna, king mackerel, shark, swordfish, and tilefish are on the 'do not eat' list due to their high mercury levels, which can be harmful during pregnancy. This applies to other vulnerable groups too, such as young children, breastfeeding women, and older adults. Avoiding these species is an important step in your preconception care.

### CHICKEN
- Whenever possible, choose organic (ideally pasture raised) to avoid harmful chemicals.
- Wash chicken thoroughly before cooking to remove residual microplastics from packaging.

- Be cautious with 'free-range' labels, as they can be misleading. It's worth investigating the sourcing behind such claims to ensure you're getting the best quality.

**MEAT**
- Choose grass-fed, pasture finished.
- Reduce to one meat meal per week.
- Maximum 150 g per meal.
- Cut out processed meats such as salami and ham.
- Avoid nitrate-treated meat such as bacon (source nitrate-free instead).

**TO AVOID**
- **Processed food:** Processed and junk foods are full of additives that disrupt digestion, affect your gut microbiome, and overwork your liver and kidneys, leaving you with less energy.
- **Alcohol:** It's important to eliminate alcohol during preconception to allow your liver to cleanse and function optimally. Additionally, conceiving without alcohol in your system is critical, as research shows alcohol harms a developing foetus.
- **Caffeine:** This can reduce fertility by up to 50% in both men and women. It's best to significantly reduce or eliminate caffeine while trying to conceive, for both parents. (See more about caffeine in Sleep Saboteurs on page 357.)

**EXERCISE AND MOVEMENT**
Overtraining can push up stress hormones and sabotage your ability to conceive. Revise your routine; this isn't the time to increase your fitness level.
- If you enjoy running, keep your heart rate below 60% of maximum, limiting sessions to 30 minutes, three times a week.
- Reduce gym workouts to twice a week, reduce your weights and increase your repetitions for maintenance.
- Incorporate more restorative exercises like yin yoga, Vinyasa flow, Pilates, or gentle stretching routines.

**STRESS LESS**
This is the perfect time to activate your parasympathetic nervous system, what we call 'Blue Zoning'. (Read Spotlight on Restorative Practices on page 372).

- Consider learning meditation if you don't already practise it. The neurological rewiring meditation creates can help you stay calm and

responsive, which will be vital in early motherhood, particularly during sleep-deprived moments.
- Apps like *Headspace* or *Waking Up* are great resources to download and use at any time.
- Regularly practising long, deep breaths is another effective way to calm your nervous system, helping you remain centred and support your fertility efforts.

**PRIORITISE SLEEP**

Sleep is non-negotiable to your body. It is essential for stress management, and it is important to note that insomnia is inextricably linked to anxiety. Prioritise sleep (see Spotlight on Sleep page 351). Start by creating a relaxing pre-bedtime routine:

- Have a warm bath or hot shower, to raise your body temperature. Once you're in bed, your body will cool itself, which aids in falling asleep.
- Aim to keep your bedroom around 18°C for optimal sleep quality.
- Good sleep is essential for hormonal balance and conception.

**ADRENAL SUPPORT**
- Consider consulting a Traditional Chinese Medicine practitioner for acupuncture or acupressure to help balance your body's Qi and activate the relaxation response.
- Regular massages, facials or body treatments can also help reduce stress—just remember to inform your therapist that you're trying to conceive or may already be pregnant.

See our Spotlight on Adrenal Glands on page 334 for more information on keeping your adrenals healthy and strong.

**AVOID OVERHEATING**

In the first three months of pregnancy, avoid saunas, steam rooms, very hot baths, and overly hot thermal bathing to prevent raising your core temperature that may impact the early development of the growing foetus.

# NATURAL CONTRACEPTION

For those looking to avoid pregnancy naturally, follow the natural fertility information shared earlier in this chapter (page 97). You will need to know when you are fertile and avoid unprotected sex during these fertile windows and around the full moon (regardless of where you are in your cycle).

Remember, sperm can live in the vagina for up to five days, so be cautious if you're near ovulation when you have unprotected sex. While an egg only survives for 12-24 hours after ovulation, it's important to understand that your fertile window is brief but significant. This knowledge can empower you to avoid relying on hormonal contraception, putting control over your fertility back in your hands.

## PROTECTION BARRIERS

- If you're not using hormonal contraception, condoms are essential for preventing sexually transmitted diseases, especially during casual sex.
- In a committed relationship, some couples prefer going 'naked' or 'native.' It's important for your partner to understand your cycle and recognise when you're fertile. However, when you're fertile, your body produces pheromones that make you more attractive to your partner, so it's easy to forget the fertility plan! You'll both need to stay responsible, as your libido naturally peaks when you're most fertile.
- If you're both in sync and feel a natural desire to connect sexually, it's a good sign that you both have a healthy hormonal balance and libido.

## DIAPHRAGMS

Diaphragms have been used for centuries as a natural barrier method of contraception. They are shallow silicone domes with a firm rim that fits over the cervix. To use, apply spermicide or vitamin C cream to the dome, fold it in half, and insert it into the vagina, ensuring the rim covers the cervix. You won't feel it once inserted, and your partner won't notice it either due to its soft silicone material.

Leave the diaphragm in overnight so that the spermicide kills off all sperm before you remove it. Then simply wash and reuse. Diaphragms come in different sizes, so it's best to get fitted by a doctor or nurse at a family planning clinic.

For those seeking to avoid synthetic hormonal contraception, diaphragms are a great option. They offer natural protection without altering your body's hormones, allowing you to manage your fertility in a safe, effective way.

## OTHER CONTRACEPTIVE OPTIONS AND THEIR RELIABILITY

| METHOD | DESCRIPTION | EXAMPLES | RELIABILITY |
|---|---|---|---|
| Barrier Methods | Physical barriers to sperm reaching the egg | Condoms (Side effect: Physical reaction to the latex rubber. Source a silicone variety to reduce contact allergy) | 98% effective |
| | | Diaphragm (Side effect: Increased risk of urinary tract infections for women) | 94% effective when used exactly as instructed<br>83% effective in 'real life'<br>88% effective when used with spermicide |
| | | Cervical caps | Only 71% effective if used after giving birth |
| Hormonal Methods | Contains hormones to prevent ovulation and/or thicken cervical mucus to block sperm | Birth control pills, Vaginal ring (no longer available in NZ) | High—99% effective when used correctly |
| | | Hormonal patches (UK and USA only—marketed as Xulane) (Side effect: Risk of blood clots) | High—99% effective when used correctly |
| | | Depo-Provera 12 weekly injection (Uncommon side effects: Benign brain tumours (meningioma), increased risk of breast cancer, reduced bone density with long-term use) | More than 99% effective if given every 12 weeks |
| Intrauterine Devices (IUDs) | Small devices inserted into the uterus to prevent pregnancy | Copper IUDs | 99% effective |
| | | Hormonal IUD | More than 99% effective |

| METHOD | DESCRIPTION | EXAMPLES | RELIABILITY |
|---|---|---|---|
| Implants | Small rods placed under the skin that release hormones to prevent pregnancy | Implanon<br>Nexplanon | More than 99% effective |
| Sterilisation | Permanent procedures to block fallopian tubes (tubal ligation) or vas deferens (vasectomy)<br>(Side effects: Risk of infection, surgical risks higher for women) | Tubal ligation<br>Vasectomy | More than 99% effective |
| Emergency Contraception | Used after unprotected sex to prevent pregnancy — also called 'the Morning After Pill' | EllaOne<br>Contains Ulipristal Acetate | When used within 72 hours up to 98% effective—Remain effective up to 5 days (120 hours) after unprotected sex |
| | | Norlevo 1<br>1.5 mg tablet<br>Levonorgestrel | Must be used within 72 hours (3 days) of unprotected sex. |
| Natural Family Planning | Tracking menstrual cycle to determine fertile days and avoid intercourse during that time | Calendar method | 55%–95% effective, depending on commitment to follow the method. |
| | | Basal body temperature tracking | 76%–88% effective on its own.<br><br>Increased reliability when used with cervical mucus charting—apps like *Ovia*, *Flo* and *Clue* improve the reliability as a form of contraception, or as an aid to pregnancy if used 'in reverse'. |
| Spermicide Creams | Inserted into the vagina before genital contact with the penis.<br><br>Kills sperm on contact with the cream<br>(Side effect: Contact allergy—both male and female partners) | Often used with a diaphragm and condoms to increase reliability of barrier contraceptives | Used alone—with perfect use every time, 82% effective<br><br>Can enhance the reliability of barrier methods of contraception |
| Withdrawal Method | Withdrawing the penis before ejaculation to prevent sperm from entering the vagina | N/A | 78% effective—more effective if used with ovulation tracking and avoiding intercourse in the 5 days leading up to and during ovulation (96% effective) |

# Perimenopause

Now we begin our journey into perimenopause. We know it can be a bumpy ride, so buckle up and hold tight. Let's dive into the following topics:

- The science behind the beginning of this significant hormonal transition.
- The three phases of perimenopause.
- The distinct symptoms of each phase and how to navigate them.
- How to make informed choices about treatments and lifestyle adjustments.
- Evidence-based options for achieving hormonal balance.
- Herbal and lifestyle strategies to support wellness, with and without hormone replacement therapy (HRT).
- Practical tips and advice from our professional experience and personal journeys through perimenopause.
- Our Wellness Action Plan for a smoother transition through perimenopause.

**WELCOME TO PERIMENOPAUSE, THE AGE OF TRANSITION**

Perhaps you've just picked up this book, flipping straight to this page, desperate to understand what on earth is happening to your body—is it menopause or perimenopause? Or are you finally, completely losing your marbles? Can this book help? Yes. Yes, it can!

Trust us—we're here for you. While we can't offer a magic solution to skip this stage of your life, we do have solid advice and practical tips to help make it easier and less fraught. So, now that you've bought the book, head home, put your feet up, and let's explore this extraordinary time in your life together. You'll learn to see this transition through the lens of your incredible body. We have the information, solutions, and guidance to support you every step of the way. We've got you!

Or maybe you've had this book for a while, working through earlier chapters and wondering, 'What's next?' Suddenly, 'next' has arrived, and you're realising this is a completely different experience—hello, is this PMS 2.0, or something else? You're right—this is *not* your usual PMS. Welcome to perimenopause. And we're here, ready to guide you through this new chapter in your hormonal journey.

Take note. This is a significant time in your life.

Perimenopause can feel like a wild ride on a hormonal rollercoaster, where each twist and turn brings new challenges—physical, emotional, cognitive, and mood swings, all while managing the chaos of everyday life. Whether you're noticing subtle changes or you're already knee-deep in the whirlwind, this chapter is your guide through the ups and downs of this natural transition.

> Your hormones are not your enemies.
> They are the rhythm and melody of your
> body's symphony.
> DR CLAUDIA WELCH

## THE JOURNEY SO FAR:
## UNDERSTANDING YOUR HORMONAL HISTORY

Before delving into this chapter, it might be helpful to refer to the Fertile Years (from page 63), which acts as the origin story of your perimenopause journey (you might also enjoy revisiting puberty if you're a fan of backstories). These earlier chapters in your hormonal life set the stage, and your balance or imbalance during those years has influenced what you're experiencing now.

We strongly recommend continuing—or starting—a hormonal/period diary. This is crucial over the coming years to help track and navigate your hormonal highs and lows.

Perimenopause can begin as early as your 40s (and sometimes even in your late 30s, or even earlier in some rare cases), but the journey is as unique as you are. On any given day, up to 10 million women across Australia, New Zealand and the UK are walking this path with you.

## PERIMENOPAUSE: PUBERTY IN REVERSE

Remember puberty? The hormonal havoc, body changes, pimples, and the uncertainty of it all? Now, welcome to its reversal—you're entering perimenopause. And yes, it can be a rocky ride. How rocky it gets depends on how you approach, perceive, and work with your body through this natural transition as your Fertile Years wind down.

During puberty, your body was developing its hormonal pathways while your brain rapidly matured. Your hormones ramped up, transforming you into an adult, equipping you with everything you needed for sexual health and reproduction. You were a child, and then you became a woman, ready to navigate your reproductive years.

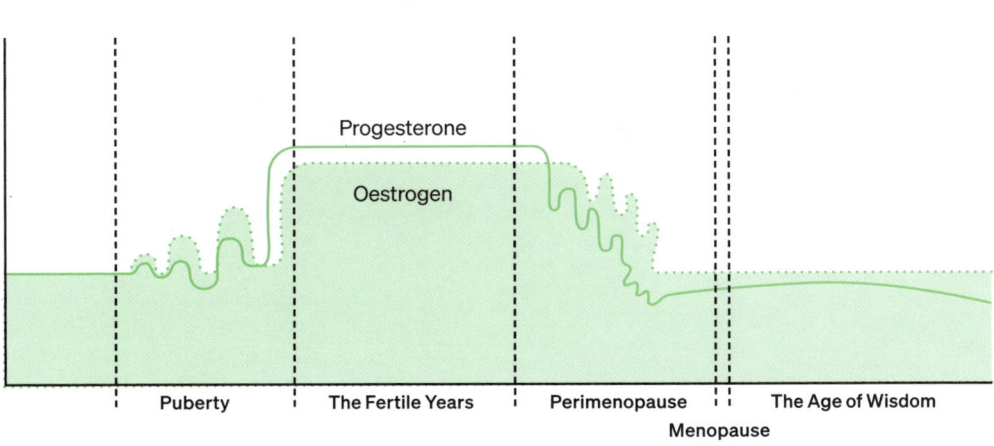

The five chapters of your hormonal journey

## PERIMENOPAUSE: THE DOWN RAMP

Perimenopause is the 'down ramp'. Your body is closing these factories and reducing the pathways, relying more on other factories (like your adrenal glands) that now need special support. Yes, your brain is also rewiring, and your nervous system is busy managing all these packing-up processes, and there are many moving parts to make this happen.

## TAKE A (VERY DEEP) BREATH: KNOWLEDGE IS POWER

Perimenopause stirs up a mix of emotions. For some, it brings feelings of loss—whether it's missed opportunities, longing for children, or the finality of family planning. For others, it can be a relief, a sense of freedom from reproductive responsibilities. *Whatever* you feel is valid. By understanding the changes in your body, you take control and step into your power.

Beyond perimenopause lies a life without periods, hormonal fluctuations, or menstrual management—an empowering time to connect more deeply with yourself. Yes, it takes work to get there, but we're here to help you through it.

## Do it for your future self.

### YOUR OVARIES: RETIREMENT IN PROGRESS

Think of your ovaries as diligent office managers. For years, they've handled your reproductive health, preparing eggs and maintaining balance. But now, they're heading for retirement. As your egg numbers decline, your ovaries signal their retirement to the brain's hypothalamus by failing to produce their usual surge of progesterone. For some women this retirement process can be quick and smooth, lasting only a few months. For others, it can be a lengthy, chaotic transition that stretches over a decade or more. During this time, you might notice the 'office' of your ovaries is, well, a bit of a mess.

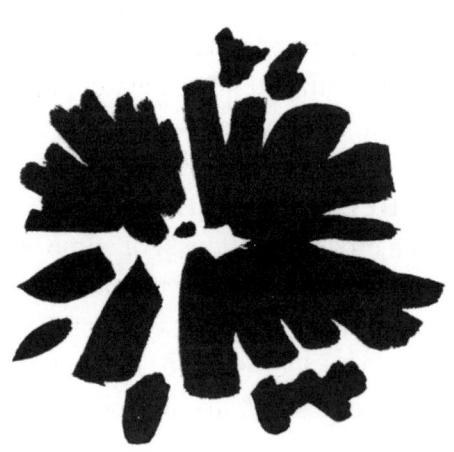

# WELCOME TO THE THREE PHASES OF PERIMENOPAUSE: TRANSITION TO MENOPAUSE

In this section, we aim to simplify the complex hormonal transition of perimenopause by breaking it down into three distinct phases. Our unique approach is designed to bring clarity, helping you identify where you are on your hormonal journey through this stage of life.

Why is this important? Because each phase of perimenopause comes with unique challenges and requires tailored treatment options. By understanding these stages, you'll be better equipped to navigate this change with confidence and control.

The three key phases of the perimenopause-menopause transition begin during your late 30s to early 40s.

**PHASE ONE:**
**EARLY PERIMENOPAUSE: PROGESTERONE DECLINE**

**PHASE TWO:**
**PERIMENOPAUSE: OESTROGEN DOMINANCE**

**PHASE THREE:**
**MENOPAUSE TRANSITION: LOWERED PROGESTERONE AND DECLINING OESTROGEN**

Each phase signals a shift in hormone levels and introduces new symptoms. This is tricky because it influences the way you feel and changes your treatment plan moving forward. That is, what works at the beginning of perimenopause will not work as you move towards menopause. When you have a clear understanding of these phases, you can have a more effective conversation with your health practitioner to manage your health and wellbeing as you transition into menopause.

## INTRODUCING THE PHASES

### PHASE ONE

This begins with a decline in progesterone. In this phase progesterone will often fluctuate from month to month. This is because you don't ovulate every month. Regardless of what's happening to progesterone, oestrogen is still hanging around at normal levels, and it takes charge, dominating the scene. You'll notice the signs—breast tenderness, mood swings—as if oestrogen has thrown a party after hours, while progesterone is nowhere to be found.

### PHASE TWO

As progesterone declines further, and the ovaries take regular holidays from progesterone production, oestrogen becomes the big bad boss, often throwing tantrums that feel like an out-of-control toddler. Welcome to Phase Two!

### PHASE THREE

And then, out of the blue, oestrogen throws in the towel and decides to take extended leave. You may notice this when you begin to experience the classic temperature changes or hot flushes, and perhaps sleepless nights. Just when you think you've adjusted, oestrogen might swoop back in for one last hurrah, filling your breasts with tenderness and giving you a rollercoaster of symptoms as the ovaries pump out a final surge. It's like they can't quite decide whether to shut down or give it one last spin!

If you were doing fine until hot flushes hit, followed by a missed period or two, you may have transitioned quickly through Phase One (low progesterone) and Phase Two (low progesterone plus the added challenge of oestrogen dominance) and are now experiencing the menopause transition, which is typically marked by declining oestrogen (Phase Three).

The following checklists will help you work out which phase of perimenopause you are currently experiencing. Adding to the chaos, you may find yourself ticking boxes in multiple phases, experiencing symptoms of oestrogen dominance one month, then oestrogen deficiency the next.

If you are resonating with the symptoms of Phase Three, the next chapter on the menopause transition may be more relevant to your current experience (covered from page 149). Either way, it's worth reading on to understand the intricate landscape of this hormonal journey. We outline the symptoms of each phase to help you recognise where your body is at any stage through perimenopause.

**PHASE ONE SYMPTOMS: PROGESTERONE DECLINE**
- ◯ Irritability and mood swings
- ◯ Headaches
- ◯ Fatigue
- ◯ Loss of libido
- ◯ Depression
- ◯ Anxiety
- ◯ Backache
- ◯ Bloating and fluid retention
- ◯ Weight gain (abdominal fat)
- ◯ Sore and/or lumpy breasts
- ◯ Sleep disturbance
- ◯ Erratic periods with less days between menstrual bleeds

**PHASE TWO SYMPTOMS AND SIGNS: OESTROGEN DOMINANCE**
Mark how many of these signs and symptoms you have experienced over the last three to six months:
- ◯ Heavy or prolonged menstrual periods
- ◯ Increasing breast tenderness or swelling may appear for the first time or get worse if you have a pattern of premenstrual breast pain or swelling
- ◯ Fluid retention—puffy hands, rings becoming uncomfortably tight, more ankle swelling
- ◯ Irritability and anger
- ◯ Weight gain, especially around the hips, thighs and abdomen
- ◯ Bloating

- Fibrocystic breasts (lumpy, tender breasts)
- Headaches or migraines, often linked to the menstrual cycle
- Mood swings or increased emotional sensitivity
- Decreased libido
- Increased risk of uterine fibroids
- Endometriosis flare-ups or worsening symptoms
- Hair thinning or loss
- Fatigue, particularly after eating
- Gallbladder issues and an increased risk of gallstones

**PHASE THREE SYMPTOMS: OESTROGEN DECLINE**
- Hot flushes and night sweats
- Vaginal dryness, itching, or discomfort during sex (vaginal atrophy)
- Bladder issues, including frequent urination, incontinence, or urinary tract infections
- Mood changes, including anxiety, depression, or irritability
- Difficulty concentrating or 'brain fog'
- Memory lapses
- Sleep disturbances (worsening insomnia and/or difficulty staying asleep)
- Pervasive fatigue
- Joint pain or stiffness
- Thinning skin and increased wrinkles
- Dry, brittle hair and hair loss
- Bone density loss, leading to increased risk of osteoporosis
- Palpitations or irregular heartbeats
- Dizziness or light headedness
- Weight gain, particularly around the abdomen
- Reduced breast fullness
- Decreased libido or sexual dysfunction

### WHAT'S HAPPENING TO YOU?

Your ovaries are packing up, but they're not in a hurry. You may oscillate between these phases; keep a hormone diary to help track your symptoms. Understanding the challenges of each phase can help you navigate perimenopause smoothly.

Perimenopause doesn't follow a strict timeline. Some women transition quickly, while others experience a mix of symptoms from all three phases over a longer period. As oestrogen declines, many women experience classic menopausal symptoms and increasingly absent menstrual bleeds, which means your body clock is ticking toward your menopause. Keeping a hormone diary and working with health practitioners will help you manage this hormonal journey with greater ease and insight.

# Phase One: Progesterone decline

**WHAT DOES PHASE ONE FEEL LIKE?**
As mentioned previously, one of the earliest signs that the ovaries are getting ready to retire is the decline in progesterone. This hormone plays a key role in stabilising your mood and balancing your cycle. As progesterone starts to dwindle, the hormonal balance is disrupted, setting the stage for physical and emotional changes that may leave you feeling a little out of sorts.

**MOOD SHIFTS AND EMOTIONAL UPS AND DOWNS**
One of the first boxes the ovaries pack is labelled 'mood stability.' As progesterone levels drop, mood swings and irritability can creep in. You might find yourself snapping at loved ones or feeling unusually emotional—like your nerves are suddenly a bit more exposed. That's the lack of progesterone at work. Without enough of this calming hormone, regulating emotions becomes tougher, leading to increased anxiety, tension, and even sadness or overwhelm. These feelings are often amplified in the second half of your cycle when progesterone would usually step in to keep things calm.

**RESTLESS NIGHTS AND FATIGUE**
As the ovaries pack up the 'sleep support' box, disrupted sleep becomes a common theme. Falling asleep might become more difficult or you may wake up in the middle of the night, unable to drift back to sleep. This ongoing battle with insomnia can leave you feeling foggy and exhausted during the day, no matter how many hours you spend in bed. Fatigue starts to set in, making even the simplest tasks feel more challenging than they used to be. We know progesterone is vital for a good night of sleep.

### IRREGULAR PERIODS

One of the hallmark signs that the ovaries are packing up is irregular periods. The ovaries may work overtime one month, giving you a shorter period one month, before seemingly going back to normal the next. These changes are normal but they can be unsettling if you've always had a predictable cycle. Look on this subtle change as a sign of the start of your perimenopause.

### PHYSICAL SYMPTOMS

As progesterone declines, you may experience breast tenderness, bloating, and water retention—symptoms that can make you feel physically uncomfortable on top of the emotional rollercoaster. These symptoms can remind you of the PMS you may have experienced during your Fertile Years—in a way, you're right. Both PMS and perimenopause are driven by declining progesterone. The key difference is while PMS in the Fertile Years is often linked to stress, the perimenopausal symptoms are part of the natural transition as your ovaries are preparing to retire.

For some lucky women, it may last only a month or two or go completely unnoticed in the busy-ness of life. For others it can drag on for years, before oestrogen deficiency symptoms start to scream.

### THE IMPACT ON YOUR WELLBEING

With the emotional highs and lows, restless nights, and physical discomfort, it's no surprise that perimenopause can start to chip away at your sense of wellbeing. You may feel like you're not quite yourself—you may feel less energetic, more irritable or just not as in control as you once were. The sense of being overwhelmed, paired with physical fatigue, can make even everyday tasks feel like a challenge.

CASE STUDY | DR KAREN

# Sandra

## Navigating early perimenopause in Phase One

Sandra was no stranger to juggling responsibilities as a 42-year-old mother of three. Between her three energetic children—the youngest just six years old—and her ageing parents needing more attention, Sandra's life resembled a never-ending relay race. She'd always prided herself on her ability to handle it all. 'I'm like a circus juggler', she joked in our first appointment, 'but lately I feel like I've dropped all the balls.'

Recently, something had shifted for Sandra. No matter how early she went to bed or how many cups of coffee she downed in the morning, she was exhausted. The kind of bone-deep fatigue that sleep couldn't seem to fix. She found herself wide awake at 3am, staring at the ceiling, mentally organising school lunches, parent-teacher meetings, and her mother's next doctor's appointment. 'I was awake worrying about why I wasn't sleeping', she confessed, half-laughing, half-serious.

When Sandra came to see me, her biggest concern was the fatigue. 'I don't feel like myself', she admitted, 'and I'm so tired, but I can't sleep!' Frustration was written all over her face. As we talked, something else stood out; her menstrual cycle had gone from a dependable 28-day routine to more of a wild card. 'Some months, it's like my period's in a hurry and shows up a week early. Other months, it's like it forgot and arrives fashionably late', she said with a wry smile.

Not only was her cycle unpredictable, but her periods were also heavier. Sandra described experiencing flooding—a sudden, intense flow that made it nearly impossible to keep up with her sanitary products. 'It's like a period party I didn't plan for, and it's showing up uninvited!' she quipped. This irregularity, combined with her insomnia and fatigue, pointed toward the beginning of her perimenopause— Phase One of her hormonal transition where progesterone levels start to drop in the second half of the menstrual cycle.

In Sandra's case, her body was sending signals loud and clear; it was time for a reset, a plan that would help her manage the hormonal rollercoaster of early perimenopause. We came up with a natural and holistic management plan, addressing her hormonal shifts, lifestyle, and stress management. As Sandra herself said, 'If I can handle three kids and two ageing parents, I can handle this!'

With that determined mindset, we moved forward to help Sandra reclaim her energy and wellbeing, one step at a time.

## DR KAREN'S PLAN FOR SANDRA'S PHASE ONE PERIMENOPAUSE

Sandra's journey began with understanding her body's changes. Blood tests confirmed low iron and low progesterone on Day 18, consistent with Phase One of perimenopause. Iron supplements and dietary changes became central to her treatment plan.

I formulated her plan based on our **Wellness Action Plan for Perimenopause Symptoms Phase One** (see page 132).

Sandra chose to support progesterone with a herbal tonic combining Chaste Tree (support for progesterone) and withania (a cortisol regulating herb).

Managing her stress—amplified by the demands of family life—was key, as stress often worsens hormonal imbalances. Our Spotlight on Psychological Stress beginning on page 290 offers further guidance on reducing stress for hormonal health.

To support her sleep, we introduced simple changes: a regular bedtime, less screen time before bed, and relaxation supplements (see our Spotlight on Sleep on page 351).

Embracing the transition as naturally as possible allowed Sandra to approach her symptoms with less anxiety and more empowerment. She learnt to anticipate heavier periods and prepare accordingly.

Sandra's experience with perimenopause had its challenges—this is a tricky time, yet by understanding the interplay between her cycles, stress, and symptoms, she regained control of her health. With practical solutions and a deepened awareness of her body's needs, Sandra could navigate this transition with resilience and grace, balancing family demands with self-care.

## THE JOURNEY FORWARD FOR PHASE ONE

We have some herbal advice for you over the next few pages. It is vitally important to note that herbs can be very potent and, in some cases, may interfere with medication or create sensitivity in some women. This is where you need to check in with your medical practitioner and have some savvy practitioners on your side! As with Sandra's story, the early warning signs are best treated holistically. Yes, it is possible to turn down the volume on your symptoms with a global approach of support from practitioners who have a special interest in women's health and the associated hormonal stages. While you may not need the following all at once, and may use them for different reasons, having a team of specialists who are all willing to work together is key.

The following list is worthwhile considering adding to your support team during this time:

- Naturopath
- Integratative doctor
- Traditional Chinese Medicine practitioner (one who focuses on all 5 Elements)
- Ayurvedic Doctor
- Counsellor or psychologist and, if necessary, psychiatrist.

## WELLNESS ACTION PLAN
# Perimenopause Symptoms Phase One

### PROGESTERONE DECLINE

#### HERBAL AND NUTRITIONAL SUPPORT

Herbal therapies can provide a gentle nudge to help balance your hormones. They support progesterone production and address stress, which often worsens hormonal imbalances. If you choose to approach this phase in a natural way, the following herbs have been proven to support progesterone levels during this early phase.

**Chaste Tree (*Vitex agnus-castus*):** This herb supports progesterone production and can help reduce symptoms of oestrogen dominance, such as mood swings and irritability. It is particularly effective in early perimenopause, as it promotes healthy levels of luteinising hormone (LH), and has been proven in studies to reduce prolactin levels (high prolactin is a natural part of the stress response and inhibits ovulation).

**Dosage:** A suggested dosage of 1000–2000 mg dried herb each morning throughout your cycle. This can help stabilise progesterone levels, reduce heavy bleeding, and even out any mood swings. It's nature's little helper, giving your hormones a boost when they need it most.

**Herbal mix for quality sleep:** If progesterone deficiency has you counting sheep way past your bedtime, a blend of hops, chamomile, ziziphus, and withania (ashwagandha) can work wonders. These herbs are known for promoting relaxation and restful sleep—because we all know a good night's sleep can make everything a little less, well, perimenopausal.

**Dosage:** An experienced naturopath can work with you to ensure the mix of herbs is right for your needs.

**Iron deficiency:** If you've noticed your periods getting heavier during perimenopause, you might also be feeling unusually tired or even run-down. This could be due to iron deficiency, which is common when menstrual bleeding becomes more frequent or intense. Iron deficiency isn't just exhausting—it also adds another layer of stress to an already hormonally stressed body.

> **TIP**
>
> Ask your doctor for a blood test to check your Full Blood Count and iron levels. To address this quickly, consider an iron infusion to get your iron stores back up quickly. The difference this can make to your brain power and energy levels can be remarkable. This is especially important if you are already showing signs of an iron deficiency anaemia. (See Spotlight on Vitamins and Minerals on page 443.)

Dietary changes are also crucial. We suggest considering including or improving these elements in your diet:

- **Focus on iron-rich foods such as red meat and poultry**: Packed with haem iron, these are easily absorbed by the body.
- **Leafy greens:** Think spinach, kale, and Swiss chard for non-haem iron and a vitamin boost.
- **Legumes and beans:** Lentils, chickpeas, and black beans are iron-rich plant options.
- **Nuts and seeds:** Pumpkin seeds and almonds can help keep your iron levels in check.

> **TIP**
>
> Remember to pair all greens with a little vitamin C (citrus fruits, anyone?) to help absorb all the iron goodness.

## STRESS MANAGEMENT

Stress affects the menstrual cycle through ancient survival mechanisms— see Spotlight on Psychological Stress on page 290.
- **Cognitive behavioural therapy (CBT):** Helps to develop effective coping strategies for managing stress and anxiety.

- **Mindfulness, meditation and breathwork:** These techniques are keys to promote relaxation and reduce the flow-on effects of stress on your body. (See Spotlight on Restorative Practices on page 372).

### LIFESTYLE SUPPORT
Supporting your wellbeing during perimenopause is about more than just supplements and hormone therapy. Lifestyle changes can have a huge impact on how you feel day to day.

**Stress management:** See above.

**Physical activity:** Follow our Hormonal Balance Exercise Plan on page 87 in the previous chapter, the Fertile Years. At a minimum some gentle, regular exercise—whether it's walking, yoga or swimming—can work wonders for your mood and stress levels. Plus, it's a great way to clear your head and feel more grounded.

**Sleep hygiene:** Establishing a calming bedtime routine can help with your sleep disturbances.
- Progesterone is a calming hormone, and when it's low, sleep can suffer. Ensure you're getting enough rest and try to go to bed and wake up at the same time each day. Speak to your medical practitioner for advice.
- Natural sleep aids like Valerian Root or magnesium glycinate may help.
- Slow down with a hot shower or bath, some herbal Tulsi tea, and keep screens out of the bedroom.
- Support your body's natural circadian rhythms. See Spotlight on Sleep on page 351.)

**Nutrition:** A balanced diet is key in this stage of life so the advice in the previous chapter the Fertile Years on page 85 remains relevant for Phase One and Phase Two of your perimenopausal hormonal journey.

### LISTEN TO YOUR BODY
As you implement these strategies, keep track of your symptoms and progress. Regular monitoring of your hormone levels and iron status will ensure that your plan is working effectively. And remember—perimenopause is a journey, not a sprint—so be patient with yourself as your body adjusts.

This holistic plan provides a balanced approach to managing progesterone deficiency in early perimenopause. Whether you opt for natural herbal support or bioidentical progesterone therapy (see Donna's story on page 138), the key is finding what works for you. With the right strategies in place, you can navigate this phase with confidence and stay in tune with your body's changing needs.

## Phase Two: Oestrogen dominance joins the party

Read through Lea's and Donna's stories, which give two different concerns and treatment plans for you to consider. We also provide the Wellness Action Plan for this phase on page 143.

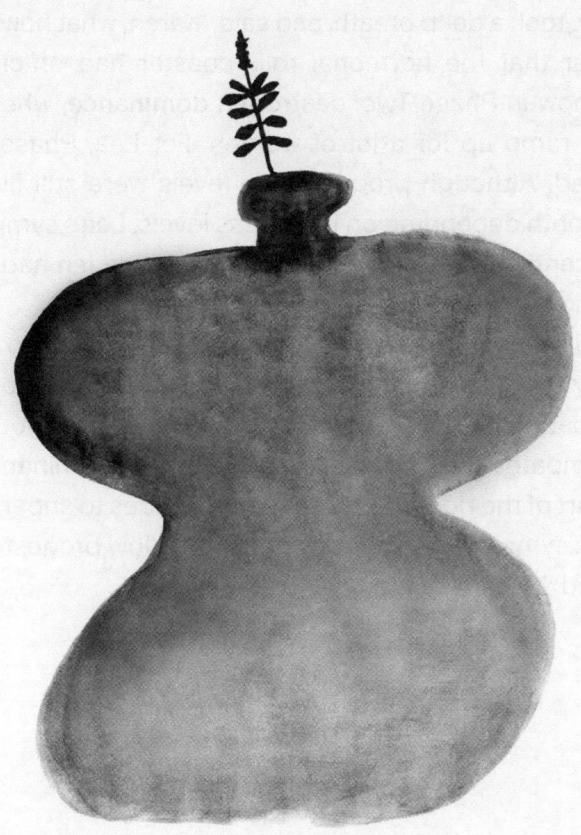

CASE STUDY | DR KAREN

# Lea
## Phase Two

Lea came to see me with that look in her eyes—the one I'd seen so many times before. You know the one: a mix of 'please tell me it's not going to get worse' and 'why is this happening to my body?' She had been sailing (well, sort of) through Phase One of perimenopause, the **progesterone deficiency phase**. We had tweaked her lifestyle, added some supplements, and after a bit of trial and error, she was feeling more balanced. But here she was, nearly twelve months on - this time, she plopped down on the chair, took a deep breath, and said, 'Karen, what *now*?'

It was clear that the hormonal rollercoaster had officially cranked up a gear. Lea was now in **Phase Two: oestrogen dominance**, where the hormonal symptoms really ramp up for a lot of women. For Lea, Phase One was a few bumps in the road. Although progesterone levels were still fluctuating a little from month to month depending on her stress levels, Lea's symptoms were very manageable. Recently things had changed now oestrogen had decided to turn up the volume. High!

Lea started rattling off her symptoms: 'My breasts are so sore I can't even look at a bra, my mood swings could scare off a lion, and don't even get me started on the bloating. By the end of the day, I look like I'm about to give birth.'

I smiled sympathetically. 'Welcome to oestrogen dominance', I said. 'You're officially at the part of the ride where your body decides to superimpose all those oestrogen-driven symptoms on top of your already low progesterone.'

She laughed. 'Great, I get to have *both* now?'

## DR KAREN'S PLAN FOR LEA'S PHASE TWO SYMPTOMS OF PERIMENOPAUSE

### A FOCUS ON OESTROGEN DOMINANCE

Lea knew the drill from Phase One and had been following her Wellness Action Plan for over six months, using Chaste Tree (*Vitex agnus-castus*) herb to support her progesterone. Now we had to tweak things to tackle both the low progesterone *and* the rising oestrogen. So, we sat down and revamped her management plan with a mix of science and common sense (and a dash of humour).

'I'm going to sound like a broken record here', I said, 'but we need to add more fibre in your diet to help your liver clear the extra oestrogen.'

- We added flaxseeds and more leafy greens and I asked her to leave the skin on all root vegetables like sweet potato.
- Supplements: We kept Chaste Tree in her regimen and introduced DIM (diindolylmethane)—a broccoli-derived supplement which helps metabolise excess oestrogen. It's like a natural detox for your hormones. We also added Evening Primrose Oil (1000 mg two to three times daily).

**Exercise:** Make it gentle. While Lea was already exercising, we upped her resistance training to help with the weight gain and added more gentle cardio like walking. There was no need to go hardcore, as her body was already working overtime. It was important to just keep things moving.

**Stress management:** Remember how stress ramps up cortisol, which competes with progesterone? We added a few extra minutes of mindfulness to her daily routine.

**Sleep and supplements:** Sleep was still an issue. I suggested continuing with bedtime magnesium glycinate to help her relax and added a supplement with Ziziphus herb.

Lea walked out of my office feeling lighter. The good news? By keeping her approach holistic and staying in tune with her body, she had the tools to ride through this phase, just as she had with Phase One. Her parting words were, 'At least now I know what's going on in my body, even though at times it feels like my hormones are throwing a rave party.'

## CASE STUDY | DR KAREN
# Donna
### A different journey through Phase Two Perimenopause

Donna, a 45-year-old teacher and the backbone of her small rural school, had always been known for her exceptional ability to juggle tasks. She balanced a classroom filled with children of various ages, managed administrative duties, and was admired by her colleagues for her efficiency and composure.

But recently, something had shifted. Tasks that once felt effortless now seemed overwhelming. Simple mistakes—misplacing documents, forgetting meetings, struggling to recall familiar students' names—were creeping into her routine. Beyond the memory lapses, Donna found herself increasingly short-tempered, snapping at her students in ways that felt entirely out of character. She had also begun experiencing intense breast tenderness, a new and unwelcome discomfort that added to her physical and emotional strain.

The final push to seek help came when a colleague gently asked if she was feeling well after she missed an important deadline. Alarmed, Donna arrived at my office, voicing a deep concern, 'I'm worried I might be getting early dementia.' She described how her once-sharp mind felt shrouded in fog, making it difficult to keep up with the demands of her job and leaving her feeling vulnerable and overwhelmed.

After listening to her concerns, it became evident that Donna wasn't dealing with early dementia but rather was in Phase Two of perimenopause. At this stage, progesterone levels are consistently lower than normal, but oestrogen remains relatively high, creating oestrogen dominance. This imbalance can exacerbate the symptoms like irritability, mood swings, brain fog, and the breast tenderness that Donna had been experiencing.

Donna had also noticed definite changes in her menstrual cycle, with her periods now arriving a few days earlier than her usual 28-day rhythm and a heavier period flow resulting in some night-time flooding.

## SUPPORTING COGNITIVE CHANGES

I asked Donna to have blood tests done around Days 16 to 18 of her next cycle. We did a Full Blood Count (anaemia screen) and checked oestrogen and progesterone, iron stores, vitamin D, liver and kidney function. At her review appointment, Donna's hormone results confirmed very low progesterone and high oestrogen levels in the luteal phase. Her iron stores were well below normal, and she showed a borderline iron deficiency anaemia. We organised an intravenous iron infusion to quickly optimise her iron levels. (See Iron in Spotlight on Vitamins and Minerals on page 449 for more on this essential nutrient.)

Helping Donna understand these hormonal shifts and their consequences gave her clarity that her symptoms were part of her perimenopause transition rather than cognitive decline. This reassurance restored a sense of control and resilience as she moved forward through this hormonal transition.

I started her on our Wellness Action Plan for Perimenopause Symptoms Phase Two to regulate her oestrogen levels (see page 143). Given the severity of her symptoms, I suggested we trial a monthly course of bioidentical progesterone replacement therapy, starting at Day 10 of her now 24-day cycle, continuing to the start of her next period bleed. The goal was to mimic her natural progesterone surge and to have a 10-day break from progesterone from the start of her period (Day 1 of her next menstrual month) and alleviate her symptoms.

### RESULTS

The results were nothing short of transformational. Within just a few weeks of starting the progesterone therapy, Donna noticed a profound difference. The fog that had clouded her mind started to lift, and she felt more like her old self. Her memory improved, her mood stabilised, and the irritability that had plagued her interactions with her students melted away. She even found herself enjoying teaching again, with the patience and composure she thought she had lost for good.

One day, a colleague jokingly asked if she had started taking Valium, noting the stark contrast in her demeanour. But Donna knew it wasn't a sedative that had brought her back to life—it was the simple yet powerful act of restoring her progesterone levels and rebalancing her hormones.

> **TIP**
>
> In the Fertile Years it is important to have blood tests done during the early luteal phase around Days 18 to 21. However, during perimenopause it's crucial to correlate blood tests with your monthly symptoms as this is when your bloods will show the true picture. Perimenopausal fluctuations can show normal levels one month at Days 18 to 21 and progesterone deficiency in next month's Days 18 to 21. This is the unpredictability of this perimenopause phase. Sometimes I just tell my patients to have the test done when they feel their symptoms are at their worst.

Donna's story is a powerful reminder of how hormonal changes during perimenopause can profoundly affect a woman's cognitive and emotional wellbeing. Her experience underscores the importance of recognising these symptoms as part of the perimenopausal transition and highlights the potential of bioidentical progesterone support to not only manage but transform the lives of women during this challenging time.

For Donna, what began as a frightening journey ended with the reclaiming of her health, career, and peace of mind—all through understanding and treating her progesterone deficiency.

A distinctive element of Donna's story was the cognitive symptoms that severely impacted her ability to function, which is common in many women. Since her oestrogen levels were just outside the high end of the normal range, no oestrogen replacement treatment was needed in Phase Two. However, it was essential for Donna to understand that regular reviews and adjustments would be crucial as she progressed toward Phase Three and menopause.

> **TIP**
>
> Many medical practitioners miss **Phase Two of perimenopause** and jump into **Phase Three** treatment options often prescribing both oestrogen and progesterone. In some cases, following hysterectomy, only oestrogen is prescribed. In Donna's case, prescribing oestrogen would not have solved her issues as her oestrogen was dominant. Interestingly her local GP had previously suggested that she try antidepressants. As Donna had such a profound response to bioidentical progesterone is it clear that antidepressants were not a part of her solution.

Donna's experience highlights the profound impact of bioidentical progesterone on brain function and overall wellbeing during perimenopause Phase Two. To support her transition, she adopted our holistic Perimenopause Wellness Action Plan on page 143 which addressed her hormonal needs, supported brain health, and empowered her with the knowledge to manage her symptoms effectively.

With bioidentical progesterone replacement, natural GABA support, and a comprehensive lifestyle approach, Donna not only felt a profound improvement but also gained a deeper understanding of her body's changes.

Thanks to this tailored approach, Donna continued to thrive in her career and personal life, feeling empowered and equipped to navigate perimenopause with resilience and confidence.

> **CAN I GET PREGNANT DURING PERIMENOPAUSE?**
>
> Yes, pregnancy is still possible during perimenopause, though it becomes less likely as you reach your mid-to-late 40s. However, it's not impossible.

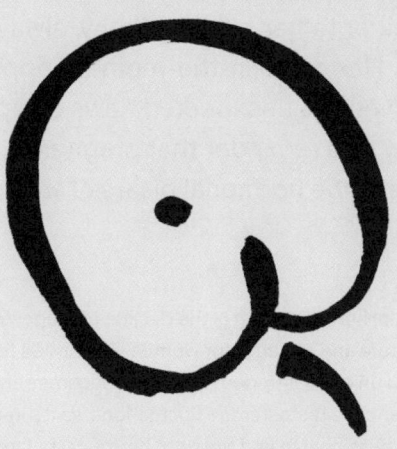

## CASE STUDY | DR KAREN
# Cathy

Cathy, a resilient country woman, had raised five healthy children and maintained a low-stress lifestyle, even during challenging times, such as droughts on the farm. She lived mindfully, making good lifestyle choices. After naturally conceiving her last baby at 42, she declined contraception postnatally, planning to breastfeed for two to three years, as she had done with all her previous children.

At 46, Cathy came to see me, having missed two periods. Assuming she was approaching menopause, I was surprised when she mentioned her breasts were incredibly sore, and she asked if she could be pregnant. A quick urinary test confirmed it; Cathy was pregnant, with an ultrasound revealing a due date just after her 47th birthday.

Her pregnancy was smooth and given that her previous labour had lasted less than an hour, Cathy opted to spend the last month of her pregnancy in town for convenience. A week before her due date, we admitted her to the antenatal ward.

I vividly remember the morning Cathy gave birth. After finishing my rounds, I watched her make herself a cup of tea and join me at the nurses' station for a chat. In the middle of our conversation, Cathy felt her first contraction. We helped her to bed, where she placed her tea on the bedside table and calmly lay down. After just five contractions—one of which broke her waters—Cathy delivered a beautiful, healthy baby girl.

As she reclined back onto her pillows, Cathy, always composed, finished her now-warm cup of tea. Her calm, in-the-moment approach to life and birth will always stay with me. Even the unexpected news of a pregnancy at 46 didn't shake her. I share this story as a reminder that pregnancy is still possible in your 40s for women who embrace the hormonal pillars of wellness.

### TIP

In perimenopause, the initial hormonal shift is the decline of progesterone. Supplemental progesterone is often safe and effective for women in their 40s to restore balance. Oestrogen is rarely needed unless oestrogen deficiency becomes an issue (Phase Three). Some women also experience testosterone fluctuations, so it's important to consult a healthcare professional to find the right hormonal balance for you.

## WELLNESS ACTION PLAN
# Perimenopause Symptoms Phase Two

### BIOIDENTICAL LUTEAL PROGESTERONE REPLACEMENT

For women experiencing significant symptoms, bioidentical progesterone during the luteal phase can effectively address the hormonal imbalances of Phase Two. Key benefits include:

- **Enhanced brain function**: By replenishing progesterone, GABA activity in the brain is supported, which aids in mood stability, cognitive clarity, and anxiety reduction. (Read our Spotlight on GABA for Relaxation on page 667.)
- **Improved sleep**: Progesterone's calming effects promote deeper, restorative sleep, essential for cognitive and emotional health.
- **Cycle regulation**: Stabilising menstrual cycle length to a regular 27 to 28-day range can help preserve iron stores.

### HERBAL SUPPORT FOR HORMONAL AND EMOTIONAL BALANCE

For mild progesterone deficiency symptoms, herbal support (as outlined in Phase One on page 132) may provide sufficient relief until Phase Three.

- **Withania (ashwagandha)**: This adaptogen herb helps manage stress, supports adrenal health, and enhances hormonal balance.
- **Passionflower**: Known for its calming properties, passionflower can ease anxiety and support better sleep.
- **St John's Wort**: This powerful herb supports mood hormones that regulate nervous system pathways and can aid in symptoms of anxiety and low mood. (See page 169 for more on this herbal option.)

## GABA SUPPORT STRATEGIES

Low progesterone in Phase Two can reduce GABA signals, increasing cognitive symptoms and anxiety. The following strategies can help boost GABA naturally:

- **Magnesium supplementation**: Magnesium is essential for GABA production and has natural calming effects. (See our Spotlight on Magnesium, page 462).
- **L-Theanine**: This supplement is particularly helpful during high-stress periods, supporting calm and reducing anxiety and can be found in black and oolong tea.
- **Mindfulness practices:** Stress management through mindfulness and meditation can help regulate the nervous system and promote GABA production.

## NOURISHMENT

- Emphasise whole foods, leafy greens, healthy fats (fish, avocados, nuts), and lean proteins to support hormone health and brain function.
- Follow the nourishment advice in the previous chapter, The Fertile Years, on page 85 as well as Core Food Principles on page 396.

## MOVEMENT AND EXERCISE

- Prioritise moderate activities like walking, yoga or swimming.
- Avoid high-intensity exercise, which raises cortisol and can worsen hormonal imbalance.
- We encourage you to follow the unique hormonal exercise plan outlined in the previous chapter. It is important however that you monitor your hormonal signs and symptoms. When your periods become irregular, we suggest you then start following this amended weekly program to suit your hormonal transition. You will notice we have deleted any endurance exercise during this time in your hormonal life. You can keep the intensity in your workouts—the key is to reduce your duration.

### TIP

Strength training can include Pilates. Because the intensity is medium, a Pilates class can extend to one hour. This is because Pilates incorporates a variety of approaches designed for physical balance. In essence this is the ideal activity to maintain your strength and hormonal balance during perimenopause.

| DAY | EXERCISE | MINIMUM STEPS |
|---|---|---|
| Day 1 | Cardio (run, brisk walks or cycling, 30 minutes) | 7000 steps |
| Day 2 | Strength training (30 minutes) | 7000 steps |
| Day 3 | Yoga or active stretching | 7000 steps |
| Day 4 | Cardio interval training (short bursts high intensity, 10-15 minutes) | 7000 steps |
| Day 5 | Strength training (30 minutes) | 7000 steps |
| Day 6 | Flexibility exercises (yoga or Pilates) | 7000 steps |
| Day 7 | Rest or light activity (leisure walk or stretching) | 7000 steps |

## MINIMISE YOUR EXPOSURE TO XENOESTROGENS

It's time to have to have *that* talk. Have you heard about the chemicals known as **PFAS** and **xenoestrogens**? They're the unwelcome guests at your hormonal party, wreaking havoc on your body's receptor sites. Every cell in your body has these 'docking stations' where hormones connect and give their instructions. But thanks to the Pandora's box of environmental chemicals unleashed since the 1940s, we now have what's affectionately called 'forever chemicals'—so named because these chemicals don't break down and decompose, making them hard to avoid completely. However, reducing your exposure wherever possible can make a real difference to your passage through perimenopause and menopause passage.

**Xenoestrogens** are chemicals that mimic oestrogen, sneakily docking onto your oestrogen receptor sites—whether it's your breast, uterus, or brain cells—and bombarding your body with extra oestrogen signals. It's like adding fuel to the fire when your progesterone is already struggling to keep things balanced. (For tips on reducing PFAS and xenoestrogens, see Spotlight on Managing Toxins on page 478.)

## YOUR DETOX PATHWAYS

As you transition through perimenopause, menopause, and beyond, your body's natural detox systems begin to slow down, thanks to the ageing process. If you've inherited less efficient detox pathways (thanks, genetics), all toxins and man-made chemicals can have an even greater impact. This is why it becomes more important than ever to tighten your lifestyle boundaries (such as caffeine, alcohol and your exposure to toxins) as you move through perimenopause. (For tips on supporting your body's natural 'housekeeping' detox pathways, see our Wellness Action Plan— Reducing Oxidative Stress on page 282.) The goal is to lighten the load and give your body the support it requires for hormone balancing.

## EDUCATION AND SELF-MONITORING

Understanding hormonal fluctuations and the impact of progesterone and oestrogen on mood and cognition is essential for managing Phase Two. Self-monitoring of symptoms, cycle patterns, and mood helps you stay attuned to your body's responses and needs.

## ONGOING MONITORING AND SUPPORT

**Phase Two Perimenopause** involves hormone fluctuations that require regular check-ins with your healthcare practitioner. Periodic adjustments to your plan ensure you stay well-supported as you move toward menopause and the oestrogen deficiency of Phase Three.

Perimenopause is a highly individual experience, with each woman facing a unique blend of hormonal changes, physical symptoms, and mood shifts. There is no one-size-fits-all roadmap, as the onset and progression of symptoms can vary widely.

As seen in Sandra's story on page 129, the first sign of perimenopause may be a drop in energy levels and changes in your menstrual cycle, as progesterone levels fluctuate from low to normal month to month. While cycle changes are a common early sign, they're easy to overlook in a busy life. This is why tracking both your cycle and symptoms is so helpful—it lets you recognise gradual shifts over time. Lea's perimenopause journey (page 136) highlighted the disruption of Phase Two oestrogen dominance, reminiscent of the PMS of the Fertile Years.

In Donna's case (page 138), mood and cognitive changes were the most noticeable symptoms, while subtle shifts in her menstrual cycle might have gone unnoticed if not for the emotional and memory challenges. These stories illustrate how differently perimenopause can present for each woman.

Ultimately, your perimenopausal journey is uniquely yours.

When you approach a doctor with symptoms of Phase One or Phase Two perimenopause, many practitioners will simply check your oestrogen levels to reassure you that you're not in early menopause. But, if you're seeking answers about perimenopause, that's not really addressing the right question. During perimenopause, the focus should be on identifying hormonal imbalances, particularly with progesterone, as oestrogen levels often remain normal at this stage. Timing of the test is vital—if the bloods are not taken in the luteal phase (between Days 18 to 22) where we expect to see progesterone surging, the blood tests are a waste of time.

Obviously, the interpretation and timing are critical. A doctor who specialises in women's health will know the difference. (See our Resources section on page 691 for more information.)

Your attitude toward perimenopause can shape your entire experience. Instead of seeing this stage as an ending, view it as a transformative phase—an opportunity for personal growth and self-discovery. This time offers the perfect chance to reassess your health goals, evaluate your lifestyle, and make choices that promote wellbeing. Whether it's through regular exercise, balanced nutrition, or simply giving yourself permission to rest and reflect, prioritising self-care can make a huge difference.

## Perimenopause is a natural progression, a testament to the resilience of your body.

As we get ready to move onto the final phase of perimenopause, let's recap the distinct phases of this hormonal journey. The first two phases are defined by dropping progesterone levels and surging oestrogen, creating a cocktail of symptoms like irregular periods, mood swings, and stress overload. During this time, the goal is to balance progesterone while keeping oestrogen in check.

However, as you move deeper into this journey, the hormonal tides shift again. Oestrogen dominance gives way to oestrogen deficiency—Phase Three—signalling the arrival of menopause just around the corner. This transition can feel like you are entering uncharted waters, and it requires a clear understanding of your body's changing needs. Supporting progesterone remains crucial, and as oestrogen levels drop and your periods become more erratic, how you approach hormonal support will need to evolve.

Recognising the importance of this shift, we've dedicated the next chapter to **Phase Three—The Menopause Transition**. In this chapter, we'll guide you through the changes that come with moving on from perimenopause and through the door of menopause, helping you navigate this new terrain with clarity and confidence. We'll explore how to adjust your approach to progesterone and oestrogen support and take a deep dive into the pivotal decisions around oestrogen treatment. By fully understanding these changes, you'll be better equipped to manage this phase of your hormonal journey with information that helps you find the path that's right for you.

We promise you. It's all going to be okay, this is not permanent.

# Menopause

This chapter contains a lot of information for you! You may want to read this entire chapter from the beginning to the end, which we think is the best approach. Alternatively, you may want to jump into specific sections that provide you with an explanation and solutions to menopausal symptoms. This chapter will guide you through your final phase; your passage through menopause. We encourage you to read the previous chapter **Perimenopause** to understand **Phase One** and **Phase Two** as this will give you the back story to understand **Phase Three: Menopause**—which is your transition into this hormonal part of your life. Let's explore these topics:

- A history of menopause
- What is menopause?
- The symptoms of menopause
- Phase Three of the perimenopause-menopause transition
- Signs you're in menopause transition
- Troubleshooting menopause symptoms
- Remedies for menopause symptoms
- Your Wellness Action Plan

# WHAT IS MENOPAUSE? AN OVERVIEW

This final leg of perimenopause is the biological journey that eventually leads you to the medical label of 'menopause'. This becomes your label when you have marked 12 months since your last period (if you can keep track!).

This transition typically occurs between ages 45 and 55, though your personal timeline may vary due to a combination of genetics, lifestyle and health history. While saying goodbye to your periods means no more cramps, bloating or worrying about birth control, it also marks the start of a new chapter—one that invites more 'me time' and the chance to finally put yourself at the top of the priority list.

One of the more emotional aspects of menopause can be the grief associated with the finality of the end of reproductive capability; menopause is the final moment when this is no longer an option. This realisation can evoke a range of emotions, from sadness and loss to a sense of relief and acceptance. The end of fertility can bring a sense of closure, but it may also trigger reflections on ageing, personal identity, and life's transitions. If this is you, know that you are not alone.

Menopause affects women mentally, emotionally as well as physically which is why it is called 'the Change'. Some evolution of self is required, and each woman walks this path in her own unique way.

We hope our advice and solutions offer you the support you need. We also encourage you to seek like-minded friends and develop communities with positive perspectives that support you and your tribe through this change.

This part of your hormonal journey is **Phase Three: Menopause Transition**. You've made it through the rollercoaster that was Phase One and Two of your perimenopausal journey and now you've arrived at the pathway leading to your rite of passage that is menopause itself.

# Phase Three: Declining oestrogen

No, this isn't just a new chapter about the end of your periods; it's an entirely different story for you to write, and it comes with its own unique set of challenges and, dare we say it, rewards.

You've either come to the end of perimenopause, or fast approaching it, when low oestrogen takes centre stage, and progesterone waves a slow, dramatic goodbye. The gaps between your periods are likely becoming longer, and keeping a journal of your symptoms might just save you from wondering, 'Am I there yet?'

Think of it as a roadmap to the finish line, preparing you for the entry into the Age of Wisdom. The profound changes that follow the end of perimenopause and the beginning of menopause shape the next phase of your life. It signifies the conclusion of one chapter in your hormonal life and the beginning of another.

The very word 'menopause' can strike fear in even the most organised and capable woman. Horror stories abound, urban myths lead the way into what may happen, and you may feel that you are not ready to face this. We understand, we've been there, and we both have the T-shirt!

In this chapter, we'll explore how to navigate the quirky mix of symptoms that come with low oestrogen—from night sweats that have you tossing off the covers, to that charming 'brain fog' that leaves you wondering why you walked into the room. But don't worry, there's a method to this hormonal madness, and you'll learn how to support your body through it all. We'll also look at how this stage fits into the bigger picture of your transition from perimenopause into menopause, and beyond, into what we like to call the Age of Wisdom—or, as some prefer, The Age of 'Why Did I Put That in the Fridge?'

If you are struggling with the symptoms of this pivotal and final hormonal transformation, the information in this chapter is your game-changer to navigating these shifts. We'll explore how your brain health is affected during this transition and, more importantly, how you can support it. You'll also discover why body fat doesn't seem to settle where it used to (and what you can do about it). In the pages ahead, we'll explore the 'when' and 'how' of hormone replacement therapy (HRT). Some Australian practitioners now refer to it as Menopausal Hormone Therapy (MHT), but most women are more familiar with the term HRT, which is the term we use throughout this book.

We'll explore your options for managing low oestrogen levels, and the domino effect that creates the mood and brain changes of menopause but don't forget—those pesky progesterone deficiency symptoms are still lurking in the background!

Think of this as your guide to stepping into this phase with knowledge and confidence. You'll understand how these changes unfold, but more importantly, you'll know how to manage them with grace and resilience.

## Let's dive in—you've got this!

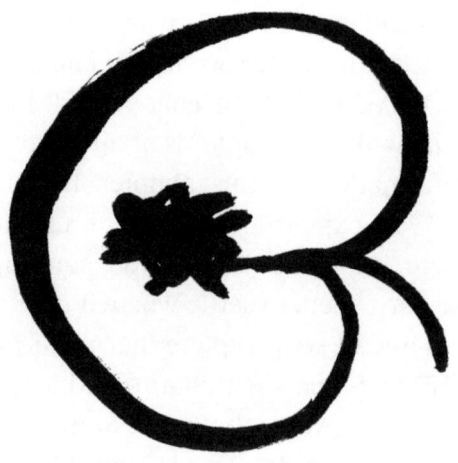

# A HISTORY OF MENOPAUSE: THE ORIGINS OF HYSTERIA AND HYSTERECTOMY

Patriarchal societies have long overlooked or trivialised the experiences of women during key hormonal changes. The ancient Greeks coined the term 'hysteria', believing that the uterus (*hystera*) was the root cause of psychological symptoms in women. This led to the medical practice of 'hysterectomy'—the removal of the uterus—as a so-called cure for hysteria.

Fast forward to today, hysterectomy is no longer performed for such archaic reasons, but the word persists in medical jargon. Now, they are mostly performed for conditions like premenstrual dysphoric disorder (PMDD) and endometriosis. However, the historical roots reveal a longstanding societal discomfort with women expressing strong emotions or challenging behaviours—especially during hormonal transitions such as menopause.

In earlier times, a woman moving through menopause and stepping out of a submissive role may have been deemed 'hysterical' for daring to assert herself. Rather than understanding these changes as part of a natural hormonal shift, society sought ways to 'control' this perceived loss of composure.

### WHAT IF MEN HAD HORMONAL TRANSITIONS LIKE WOMEN?

Imagine how quickly medical advancements might have progressed if men experienced dramatic hormonal fluctuations like women do during menopause. What if the solution to outbursts of rage or anger triggered by testosterone surges was castration? Absurd as it sounds, this scenario mirrors the hysterectomy response to women's emotional and hormonal changes.

The differences between men and women extend far beyond the X and Y chromosomes. Women are hormonally and biochemically unique, with intricacies that reach into nearly every system of the body. Yet historically, women's hormonal transitions—particularly menopause—have been misunderstood, often minimised, or even mocked.

Today, women are standing up, demanding better recognition of their complex hormonal make-up and more tailored solutions to manage these transitions. But despite some progress, women still face an uphill battle.

## MENOPAUSE AWARENESS TODAY

In Australia, female politicians have made significant strides toward better support for women in perimenopause and menopause. In November 2023, they successfully campaigned for a Senate inquiry into menopause and perimenopause, highlighting the medical profession's lack of understanding and the scarcity of treatment options for women navigating these transitions.

This inquiry underscored the financial cost to the Australian economy due to menopause-related symptoms affecting women's ability to remain active in the workforce. These politicians advocated for more research, better resources, and increased awareness among healthcare providers. Similar shifts can be seen in the UK where the government in October 2024 appointed their first Menopause Employment Ambassador.

As more women demand recognition of the unique challenges they face, the medical community is slowly catching up. With more clinical trials including women, and growing awareness of the importance of tailored treatments, the future looks promising. We're on the cusp of a shift where women's health is no longer an inconvenient exception but a vital area of focus in medical research and healthcare.

Menopause may still be a daunting transition for many women, but with ongoing advocacy and a more informed medical community, women can look forward to more understanding, more options, and better care for this significant phase of life.

## THE GENDER GAP IN MEDICAL RESEARCH

For much of history, women have been largely excluded from medical research. This wasn't necessarily due to sexism but rather due to the cost and complexity of accounting for fluctuating female hormones in clinical trials. Since women's hormone levels can vary daily, including them in studies was often seen as a complication that skewed data.

As a result, most of the drugs and treatments prescribed to women have been tested primarily on men. This is particularly concerning given the substantial differences between the sexes in how hormones affect not just reproduction but a broad array of bodily systems, including the cardiovascular, immune, metabolic and endocrine systems.

Thankfully, this is beginning to change. In recent years, there has been an increasing focus on women-only research, as it's become clear that women often experience different symptoms and respond differently to treatments than men. For example, women often show different symptoms during heart attacks, which historically were diagnosed based on male symptoms.

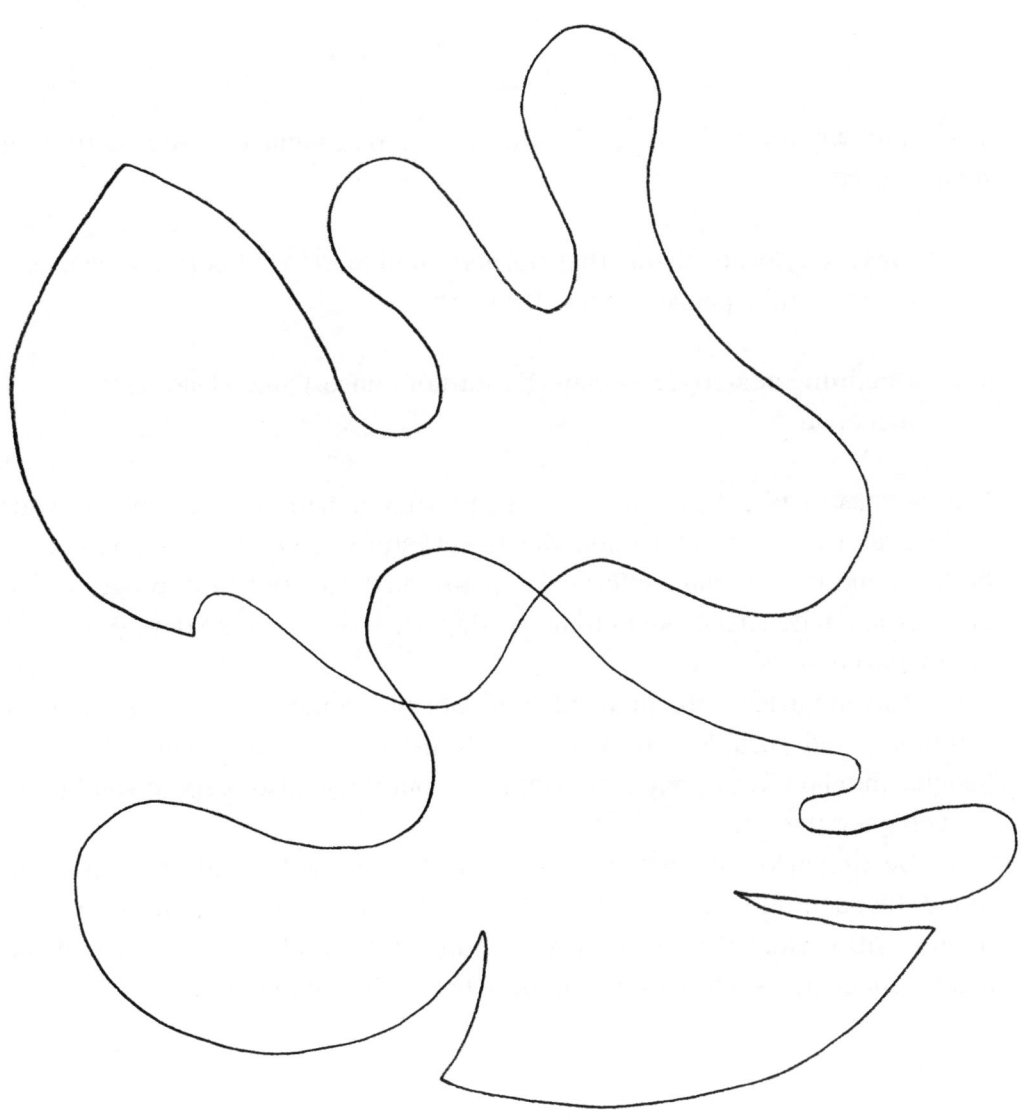

# THE SYMPTOMS OF MENOPAUSE

There are two key shifts in your hormonal balance, signalling your entry into menopause.

> **Lowered progesterone** that starts from Phase One of perimenopause. (See Perimenopause on page 119.)

> **Declining oestrogen** signals the start of Phase Three—leading to menopause.

During Phase Three, you may notice a pattern of absent periods, only for your cycle to return as oestrogen production tries to stumble along. It's as though your body is making a last-ditch effort to keep up, and during this time, progesterone and oestrogen deficiency symptoms overlap, leading to a range of physical and emotional changes.

As you navigate the final stage of your hormonal journey, tracking your symptoms and periods can be incredibly helpful. Not only will it give you insights into how your body is transitioning, but it will also prepare you for the next chapter: the Age of Wisdom.

Oestrogen loss impacts more than just your periods. It affects your brain, mood, bladder, and vaginal health. You might notice mood swings, anxiety, depression, vaginal dryness or even bladder issues, all of which signal the significant changes many women experience in this chapter of life.

## PHASE ONE SYMPTOMS THAT PERSIST THROUGH TO PHASE THREE—LOW PROGESTERONE

- Irritability and mood swings
- Headaches
- Fatigue
- Depression
- Anxiety
- Backache
- Bloating and fluid retention
- Weight gain (especially around the abdomen)
- Sleep disturbances
- Loss of libido

## PHASE THREE SYMPTOMS OF OESTROGEN DECLINE

- Hot flushes and night sweats
- Vaginal dryness, itching, or discomfort during sex
- Bladder issues, such as frequent urination or urinary tract infections (UTIs)
- Mood changes, including anxiety, depression, or irritability
- Difficulty concentrating, also known as 'brain fog'
- Memory lapses
- Sleep disturbances (trouble staying asleep or worsening insomnia)
- Fatigue
- Joint pain or stiffness
- Thinning skin and increased wrinkles
- Dry, brittle hair and hair loss
- Bone density loss, increasing the risk of osteoporosis
- Palpitations or irregular heartbeats
- Dizziness or light-headedness
- Weight gain, especially around the abdomen
- Reduced breast fullness
- Decreased libido or sexual dysfunction

Over the next few pages, we'll go through each one, offering practical strategies to help you manage them and step into the next stage of life with confidence.

## CASE STUDY
# Dr Karen
### My early encounters with oestrogen deficiency

I can clearly remember when things began to shift around the age of 47. In hindsight, it was likely the stress from my busy professional life that triggered a few missed periods earlier than expected. My cycles would disappear during overwhelming times at work and return when things calmed down. I was proactive in supporting my progesterone levels by using a blend of herbs like Dong quai and Chaste Tree, with a touch of St John's Wort when stress or sleep issues popped up. Thanks to these early interventions in my 40s, I didn't find the low progesterone phase too troubling.

In my mid-40s, I had taken up mixed martial arts—a form of moving meditation—that helped keep me fit and manage abdominal fat. Though looking back, I realise that a more restful meditation might have been more supportive during that phase.

Then came the low oestrogen phase, and that's when things started to really change. One of the first signs was how my favourite glass of red wine began to betray me. I'd toss off the blankets all night, even in winter. It became clear that my body didn't handle alcohol like it used to. While I didn't struggle with the cognitive fog many of my patients describe, my memory was affected. I'd lose track of my car keys and sunglasses, double-book appointments, and forget to note things in my diary, leading to more than a few mix-ups.

To manage the night sweats, I started avoiding alcohol on nights when I needed to be sharp the next day. If there was a weekend event, I'd take St Mary's Thistle to support my liver ahead of time. But as I edged closer to menopause, I realised the impact on my sleep wasn't worth it. Often, I became the designated driver—a small price to pay for a good night's rest.

Even now, I still 'run hot', and my trusty personal fan is never far from my handbag—a constant companion that helps me keep my cool.

# A NEW BEGINNING

As oestrogen takes its final bow, you may encounter new challenges such as Karen did with giving up red wine (most of the time!). Here are some of the symptoms and hurdles you might face on your journey through menopause. The more you understand these changes—and accept them as a normal part of the process—the easier it will be to embrace this new chapter of life.

Over time, you'll discover strength within yourself that you may not have known existed. Think of this as a chance to be bold, to face uncertainty head-on, and to embrace a new hormonal, emotional, and physical life.

### ARE WE THERE YET?

Your periods may start playing hide and seek, showing up sporadically and never quite on time. While symptoms of progesterone deficiency—like mood swings and restless nights—haven't disappeared, you're now also facing the challenges of oestrogen deficiency. This brings a fresh set of surprises; from hot flushes that feel like an internal furnace, to night sweats that may have you reconsidering your love of blankets.

For some, this phase is a gentle winding down, manageable with a few lifestyle adjustments. For others, it's more of a 'What fresh hell is this?' kind of experience. Don't lose heart! You're not alone, and you're still in transition. The key is learning how to adapt to these new oestrogen levels while figuring out what your body needs as you inch closer to the big M (menopause).

Let's work our way through the symptoms and give you solutions and fixes along the way, starting with those classic hot flushes, which almost every woman will experience at some stage in her menopausal rite of passage.

Hot flushes are like your body's thermostat throwing a tantrum—one minute you're perfectly comfortable, and the next, you're a human furnace. It's as if your internal heater suddenly cranks up to full blast, and you're left wondering whether it's time to invest in industrial-strength fans!

## The good news is, you're not powerless.

**CASE STUDY | DR KAREN**

# Sally

## A gentle way to navigate Phase Three oestrogen deficiency

Sally, at 50, has always prioritised her health. She's the kind of woman who seems to glow with energy and purpose, whether she's demonstrating the perfect plank for a client or making dinner for her family. With two teenagers, a husband she adores, and a part-time job as a personal trainer, she's kept her lifestyle active and has never been one for excess—minimal alcohol, a balanced diet, and a natural ability to manage stress. Life felt in balance, and yet ... along came unmistakable symptoms that didn't quite fit.

It started subtly—a hint of vaginal dryness here and there, something she hadn't really felt before. Then came the hot flushes. Nothing major, but frequent enough to make her day feel ... off. Especially during her training sessions, the heat would seem to amplify, leaving her in a sudden sweat. 'It's like my body just decides to hit the sauna button on its own', she joked. But as much as she could laugh it off, the flushes were irritating enough to bring her to my office.

### SOLUTION

I reviewed Sally after she had completed some bloods test and a routine bone density scan. Sally's blood results showed a suboptimal vitamin D at 76 nmol/L, under the threshold shown to fully support bone density. Her bone density scan results were reassuringly normal. With Sally's healthy habits and relatively mild symptoms, we decided to explore natural options before considering oestrogen replacement therapy. Here's the approach we crafted together:

- **Vitamin D support:** I suggested she start a vitamin D3 supplement of 1000 IU daily to achieve a target range between 100 to 180 nmol/L. (Read more on vitamin D in our Spotlight on page 445.)

- **Herbal support:** I gave her a herbal tonic based on adaptogens and cooling herbs to help smooth out those flushes. Sage, a trusted herbal ally, offers gentle but effective support for hot flushes. Along with red clover, and black cohosh these herbs have a solid history of use for managing menopausal symptoms, providing mild oestrogenic support without being overly stimulating.

- **Phytoestrogen-rich foods:** Given Sally's enthusiasm for lifestyle-based health choices, incorporating phytoestrogens was a natural next step. Foods like flaxseeds, chickpeas, and soy products can subtly support oestrogen levels by providing plant-based compounds that mimic its effects. With her active life, these could be seamlessly added into her diet, giving her body a little extra support.

- **Temperature control techniques:** Since Sally's hot flushes seem to flare up during her training sessions, we discussed a few cooling techniques. Practising paced breathing during her sessions can help calm her internal thermostat, and wearing moisture-wicking fabrics can keep her feeling cooler. Adding a floor-based fan in her workspace offers a constant flow of cool air, making it easier to handle those heat waves. Keeping a cooling cloth or spray nearby was another practical tip to help her manage those surprise sauna moments.

Sally's stress levels were well-managed, a testament to her balanced approach to life. With this tailored plan in place, she left our session feeling encouraged. There was no need for big hormonal changes just yet—just some gentle support to help her body glide through this phase with grace and a little more comfort.

For women like Sally, supporting her with lifestyle tweaks may be all that she needs. However, research shows there are proven benefits for the use of bioidentical oestrogen and progesterone support for a period of time in the menopause transition. In Sally's case, given her normal bone density results the risk- benefit consideration was not strong for hormone replacement just yet, but I reminded her that my door was open for her at any time to review her choices.

# LET'S TALK ABOUT HORMONE REPLACEMENT THERAPY (HRT)

As oestrogen continues its graceful exit, you might start wondering if HRT is the right option for you. HRT can help relieve common menopause symptoms such as hot flushes, night sweats, vaginal dryness, and mood swings. However, this isn't a one-size-fits-all solution. It's essential to have an open conversation with your healthcare provider to determine if HRT suits your symptoms, risks, and overall health.

If your symptoms are interfering with your daily life, HRT might be worth considering. After all, you deserve to feel like yourself again. However, if your symptoms are manageable with lifestyle adjustments, you might decide to skip HRT. Sometimes, pharmaceutical options are presented as a catch-all solution, but it's essential to listen to your body to determine what works best for you.

Important considerations:

- Hormone replacement generally benefits those women with low hormone levels with menopausal symptoms.

- HRT can be life-changing for some women, offering significant relief from challenging symptoms.

### SAFETY

Reassuring new data from long-term research shows that bioidentical HRT is safe for most women. It's essential for you to read the Our Love-Hate Relationship with Oestrogen (page 172) because timing of oestrogen replacement is crucial, and this chapter offers easy-to-understand facts to help you make an informed decision.

## CASE STUDY | DR KAREN
# Miranda

Like many women, Miranda experienced intolerable hot flushes that began to impact every aspect of her life, from sleepless nights to the struggle of staying comfortable during the day.

Miranda, at 47, was navigating the challenging Phase Three. With the surprise arrival of her daughter two years ago—as an unexpected but very welcome gift in her mid-40s—she felt she never fully recovered after her pregnancy. In retrospect, Miranda's low mood postnatally would have qualified for a diagnosis of postnatal depression. The two years leading up to her first appointment with me were classic low-progesterone years. Miranda put these symptoms of low mood, reactivity and poor sleep down to baby brain and her busy life. She was prompted to seek help when she noted that her periods were skipping every second or third month. The menopause penny dropped when the hot flushes hit, coming in waves and bothering her intensely for weeks, only to vanish suddenly. Then night sweats had become a frequent visitor, especially when she indulged in a glass of wine during the evening. These symptoms have wreaked havoc on her sleep, leaving her feeling tired, exhausted and irritable. To make matters worse, her once-active sex life has dwindled to nothing.

Life at home wasn't offering much respite. With two teenage boys going through their own hormonal storms and a demanding toddler, the household was often fraught with tension. Miranda was still working full-time, but barely coping. She managed several staff members, but her professional facade crumbled at times—particularly when the hot flushes struck during the day, causing her to sweat profusely and needing to change her blouse, leading to embarrassing situations at work.

During her consultation, Miranda initially focused on her hot flushes and night sweats, but as the conversation progressed, she burst into tears, revealing the emotional toll this was taking on her. She scored highly on a depression checklist, highlighting the need for a comprehensive approach to her care.

## SOLUTION: DR KAREN'S PHASE THREE PLAN FOR MIRANDA

**Hormone Replacement Therapy (HRT):** Oestrogen Replacement Therapy (also called HRT) can be highly effective in women like Miranda with symptoms that tell me she is significantly deficient in oestrogen while also struggling with her mood and mental health. For Miranda, HRT could significantly improve her quality of life by stabilising her hormone levels and reducing the intensity of symptoms like hot flushes, night sweats, and support brain and heart health through this final rite of passage to the Age of Wisdom.

Risks/benefits: HRT is well-known for its effectiveness in alleviating hot flushes and night sweats. It can also improve mood, energy levels, and sleep quality, which are significant concerns for Miranda. There is also evidence from long-term studies that women with severe oestrogen deficiency symptoms may have a reduced long-term risk of dementia by starting oestrogen around menopause, a welcomed positive benefit. It's important to discuss both benefits and potential risks; the science shows it is also important to marry oestrogen with a body/bioidentical progesterone, even in women who have had a hysterectomy, as most women will benefit from both hormones in different ways (read more about HRT on page 172).

In Miranda's case, her severe oestrogen deficiency symptoms were impacting her quality of life and work performance daily. She elected to start a combination of oestrogen and progesterone. A low-dose, transdermal (skin patch) oestrogen combined with body/bioidentical oral progesterone offers a safer profile, particularly concerning cardiovascular risk in women prescribed oral oestrogen medication.

**Herbal supplements: (St John's Wort):** Considering Miranda's high depression score, I suggested that Miranda start St John's Wort, proven to alleviate mild to moderate depression and improve mood. St John's Wort doubles as both a serotonin and a dopamine support herbal, a valuable combination at menopause. We did discuss a trial of antidepressants from the SSRI family (for serotonin support), but I also discussed the expectation the HRT would start to improve her low mood—and Miranda elected to try the herbal first.

Miranda's journey through perimenopause was filled with both physical and emotional challenges that tested her limits. But by creating a personalised plan—complete with hormone therapy, herbal supplements, nutrition tweaks and practical tricks for managing those infamous hot flushes—she found her way back to feeling like herself again.

With ongoing support and tweaks to her plan, she navigated this transition more comfortably, finding resilience to cope amidst her work life and family challenges.

## We talk about supportive foods and lifestyle changes in detail later in this chapter.

### SURPRISE, SURPRISE

As progesterone fades and oestrogen packs up and starts its exit out the office door, your symptoms start to shift. Say goodbye to sore, lumpy breasts and the rollercoaster of erratic periods—well, almost. You might still get the occasional surprise period that resets your 12-month countdown to earning your 'menopausal badge of honour'. And just when you think you're in the clear, your breasts start aching after months of no bleeding. It's Mother Nature's way of saying, 'Surprise!'

The one-foot in, one-foot out stage does come with questions and uncertainty. In the beginning when you miss a period you may wonder if you're pregnant (do a test if you're worried). When you have another period, it may not come in the usual monthly cycle (we encourage you to keep your menstrual diary going until you earn your menopausal badge).

The change is individual.

To navigate this unpredictable phase, it's wise to keep some sanitary items handy for a couple of years, which can be quite annoying. Many women have experienced the exasperation of being caught off guard at a function, thinking, 'WTF? I thought I was past this!'

Behind the scenes, your oestrogen levels are falling and surging as the ovaries intermittently clock in and out of work. Eventually, the ovaries pack up every box, and the production of oestrogen declines to a non-reproductive level, marking the end of your periods.

BEWARE ... the villain of menopause is stress!

# Dr Karen's Story
## Menopause transition

At 48, I found myself in menopause almost without noticing, having bypassed the early perimenopausal phases entirely. Focused on running my integrative medical clinic and managing a team of 15, I missed the early signs. It was only when my favourite glass of shiraz began triggering hot flushes that I realised my hormones were shifting. I credit my skilled in-house acupuncturist and naturopath for smoothing over the symptoms I had overlooked.

As the demands of my practice intensified approaching the December holidays, my resilience faltered. Feeling overwhelmed, I reached out to Sharon, my co-author and best friend. At the time, she was the General Manager at Gwinganna Lifestyle Retreat. She arranged for me to stay at Gwinganna for a full week of respite, free from responsibility and mobile phones. In that nurturing environment, I felt myself unwind and reconnect.

On my last day, my first period of the year arrived unexpectedly, reminding me that I'd need to restart my 12-month count toward menopause. Fast-forward 12 months, and once again, the holiday stress had me calling for help. Sharon welcomed me back to Gwinganna for another restorative retreat, and, as fate would have it, my period returned on the last day—this time, it would be my final one.

Back at work, I consulted my acupuncturist and naturopath for some herbal adjustments to support my hormonal balance and manage stress. Looking back, I'm still amazed at how completely my cycle rebooted with the removal of external stress.

Now, apart from the occasional hot flush, I've transitioned into my hormonal rest phase. Embracing the Age of Wisdom, I find myself appreciating the calmer, more introspective side of life that comes with being on the other side of menopause.

While spending time at a health retreat can work wonders, we understand that stepping away for a full week may not be realistic, or affordable for some women juggling busy lives, families, and careers. But the good news is, you don't need a whole week to give yourself the time and space your body needs to reset. Even micro breaks can make a big difference in reducing stress, supporting hormones, and helping you reconnect with yourself. You will find some practical, achievable options to create your own 'mini retreats' on page 306.

> ## We need to do a better job of putting ourselves higher on our own 'to do' list.
> **MICHELLE OBAMA**

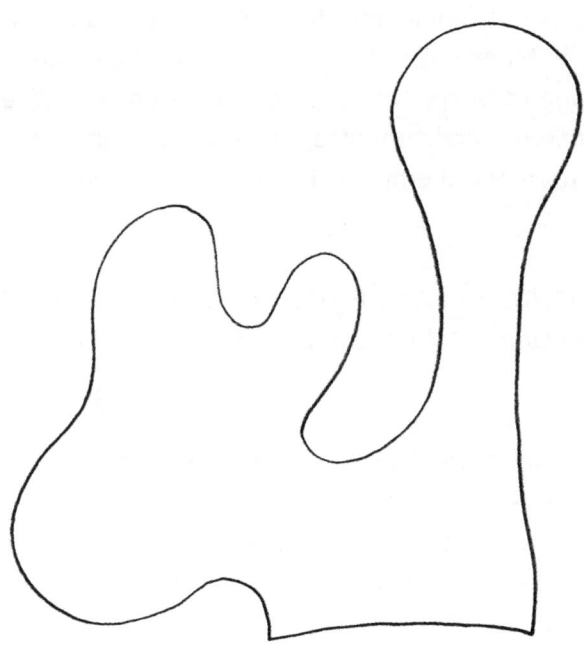

CASE STUDY | DR KAREN
# Helen

Helen, now 50, came to see me as she said her hormonal balance seemed 'off'. She is a very successful, informed woman and had a great deal of knowledge about hormones and lifestyle balance. She was confused and just did not understand, even with all that she knew, how to get the right answers to her questions, it seemed each medical doctor she consulted had conflicting advice. And it did not seem to fit with her understanding of what to do for hormonal balance.

Her doctor had put her on hormone replacement therapy (HRT) two years prior, initially starting with a combination of oestradiol patches and cyclical Prometrium (a bioidentical progesterone). This effectively addressed her hot flushes and night sweats but did not resolve her insomnia. After a diagnosis of endometrial hyperplasia (unhealthy thickening of the lining of the uterus) her specialist added a Mirena IUD for endometrial protection. Helen continued to use the oestrogen therapy and Prometrium each day. When we spoke her primary concerns were persistent sleep disturbances and cognitive fog, as well as balancing her hormone therapy with cancer risk. Together we agreed on the following action plan.

**HORMONAL BALANCE AND DUTCH TEST ANALYSIS**
DUTCH test (Dried Urine Test for Comprehensive Hormones) to get a complete picture of her:

- **Oestrogen metabolism:** The DUTCH test identifies how Helen's oestrogen is being metabolised via either:
  a. The protective 2-hydroxyestrone pathway, or
  b. The more harmful 16-hydroxyestrone pathway.

- **Cortisol rhythm:** Her sleep disturbances may be related to high cortisol levels, especially if they spike in the evening. The DUTCH test gives us a detailed view of her daily cortisol pattern, which could explain the insomnia and stress.

### DNA ASSESSMENT OF COMT AND CYP1B1 SNPs

In addition to the DUTCH test, Helen had a DNA analysis to evaluate:

- **Her COMT pathways:** Helen had a COMT variant that reduced her ability to clear hormones like oestrogen, dopamine and adrenaline, contributing to her cognitive symptoms and potentially her insomnia.

- **CYP1B1:** Variants in this detox gene pathway compounded the effect of her COMT gene variant, further impairing her body's ability to metabolise oestrogen safely. This could impact breast health as she moves through menopause.

## SWITCH PROMETRIUM DOSING TO NIGHT FOR SLEEP SUPPORT

Helen was taking Prometrium daily. Given the sedative properties of progesterone, which naturally promotes slow-wave sleep, switching to night-time dosing maximises its benefits for sleep.

### ST JOHN'S WORT (REMOTIV BY FLORDIS) FOR SLEEP AND COGNITIVE SUPPORT

To further support Helen's sleep and cognitive function, she started to take Remotiv, a standardised extract of St John's Wort. This herb works through both serotonin and dopamine pathways to:

- Boost serotonin levels, helping regulate mood and promoting melatonin production, which is essential for sleep.

- Support dopamine balance, helping with the cognitive fog Helen is experiencing, while also improving her emotional wellbeing.

## MELATONIN SUPPLEMENTATION FOR SLEEP AND METABOLIC SUPPORT

In addition to Remotiv, we added a low-dose melatonin supplement (2 mg) to further enhance sleep:

- Melatonin can improve both sleep onset and quality, particularly in menopausal women whose natural melatonin levels decline with age.

- Studies show that melatonin can also aid in weight management and insulin sensitivity, which is important as menopause often disrupts metabolism.

## HERBAL SUPPORT FOR CORTISOL AND STRESS MANAGEMENT

The test revealed elevated cortisol levels. We added withania (ashwagandha) and Schisandra to her plan:

- Withania helps lower cortisol and improves sleep quality, especially in women dealing with stress-induced insomnia.

- Schisandra supports the adrenal glands and helps regulate stress hormones, while also promoting daytime energy and night-time relaxation.

## LIFESTYLE AND NUTRITIONAL SUPPORT

To support overall wellbeing, I recommended the following lifestyle adjustments:

- **Regular exercise:** Continue her aerobic activity like walking or swimming to boost cognitive function and improve sleep.

- **Sleep hygiene:** Establishing a regular bedtime, avoiding electronics an hour before bed, and creating a calming bedtime routine.

- **Diet:** Adding foods rich in melatonin—such as pistachios, cherries, and walnuts—to her evening meals for added sleep support.

Support breast and endometrial health with phytoestrogen foods:

- **Soy products:** Tofu, tempeh, edamame, miso, soy milk
- **Nuts and seeds:** Flaxseed, sesame and sunflower seeds, almonds, walnuts
- **Legumes:** Chickpeas, lentils, beans,
- **Whole grains:** Oats, barley, wheatgerm
- **Fruits:** Apples, plums, berries, peaches, pomegranates
- **Vegetables:** Carrots, alfalfa sprouts yams, garlic, parsley

## MONITORING AND FOLLOW-UP

We planned follow-up assessments every 6 months to monitor her hormone levels, cortisol, and breast/endometrial health. Regular breast exams and breast screening will be necessary, as well as ultrasound scans to ensure the Mirena IUD continues to protect her from endometrial hyperplasia as per her gynaecologist's recommendation

This management plan balances hormone therapy with natural supports like St John's Wort and melatonin to improve Helen's sleep and cognitive function.

By continuing to monitor her progress with the DUTCH test and symptoms, we can adapt her treatment as necessary to ensure optimal wellbeing throughout menopause.

### TIP—DR KAREN

In my work with women's health, the DUTCH test has been a practical and insightful tool for tracking hormonal shifts through life's transitions. It conveniently measures hormone metabolites and cortisol rhythms, offering a window into both reproductive balance and stress resilience. While large-scale validation studies are still emerging, the DUTCH test is widely used in medical research and can be a powerful guide when interpreted alongside clinical insight.

# HORMONE REPLACEMENT THERAPY (HRT)

Before we dive into your Wellness Action Plan for menopause, let's explore how oestrogen replacement, a key component of Hormone Replacement Therapy (HRT), may support your transition through this phase.

### OUR LOVE-HATE RELATIONSHIP WITH OESTROGEN

Our natural oestrogen, a hormone with a complex and evolving roles, has been supporting us from puberty through to the Fertile Years. As menopause approaches, declining oestrogen levels bring hormonal shifts that affect the brain, heart and bones.

The history of HRT has been tumultuous. In 2002, studies linking it to increased breast cancer risk created widespread panic, and prescriptions plummeted. Today, bioidentical oestrogen and progesterone offer safer alternatives. Studies suggest that bioidentical hormones may even lower breast cancer risk compared to synthetic options.

### TIMING IS CRUCIAL

Starting bioidentical HRT within the first year of menopause can reduce dementia risk and support cardiovascular health. However, after age 60, or beyond 10 years post-menopause, oestrogen may drive inflammatory pathways, increasing risks of dementia and breast cancer. This 10-year 'hormonal window' is a critical period for safely reaping oestrogen's protective benefits.

> **TIP ONE**
>
> If you experienced early menopause, the 10-year guideline may not apply to you. We recommend reviewing your ongoing use of HRT with your health practitioner as you approach 60 years of age.

### TIP TWO

This advice also extends to women thriving on HRT well into the Age of Wisdom. At this stage, it's important to reassess cognitive health risks, such as a family history of dementia, and weigh them against the continued support HRT provides for your heart and bones. Emerging research suggests this 'safe window' of opportunity may be more flexible for some women, making regular reviews even more essential to assess the risks and benefits of continuing HRT.

### TIP THREE

Choose transdermal or sublingual delivery to avoid the increased risk of thrombosis associated with the oral tablet form of HRT.

Your health journey is shaped by lifestyle choices far more than genetics. Discuss HRT with a doctor interested in women's hormonal health to explore whether it fits your unique needs during this pivotal transition into wisdom and wellness.

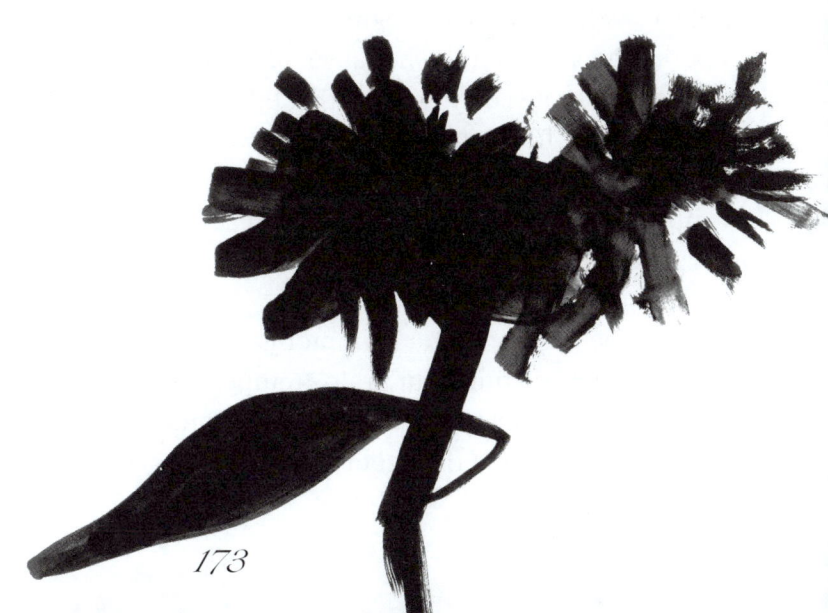

WELLNESS ACTION PLAN
# MENOPAUSE

Menopause is a journey marked by unique and diverse symptoms that don't follow a one-size-fits-all pattern. Each woman experiences this transition differently, with a unique blend of hot flushes, mood shifts, sleep disturbances, and energy changes that create her own 'menopause signature.' That's why a rigid, one-size-fits-all approach isn't the answer. Instead, the following solutions and wellness advice empowers you to tailor your own Wellness Action Plan with solutions that align with your specific symptoms and challenges. By selecting from a range of effective bio-hacks, you can build a personalised toolkit that supports you through this transition—embracing menopause as a passage uniquely yours, guided by your own needs and wellbeing.

## UNDERSTANDING HOT FLUSHES AND NIGHT SWEATS

Hot flushes. Night sweats. Those sudden, fiery waves that leave you flushed, drenched, and wondering if you're losing your mind—sound familiar? You're not alone. These intense heat surges are a common experience for many navigating perimenopause and menopause, often arriving at the worst times—like during a meeting or just as you're drifting off to sleep.

Thankfully, there are many ways to manage these symptoms, from lifestyle tweaks to targeted therapies. It's not just about cooling off; it's about supporting your body from within. Options range from HRT and herbal remedies like black cohosh to complementary therapies like acupuncture, all offering ways to regain control.

These 'vasomotor symptoms' are triggered by fluctuating oestrogen levels, which disrupt your brain's temperature regulation. Think of your internal thermostat receiving mixed signals, prompting blood vessels to expand, triggering heat, and then cool down as your body attempts to reset.

Deep in the hypothalamus, the kisspeptin, neurokinin B, and dynorphin (KNDy) neurons act as your body's thermostat. Oestrogen normally keeps these neurons in check, maintaining smooth temperature control. But as oestrogen declines during menopause, these neurons become overactive—like a thermostat set too high—causing hot flushes and night sweats.

Progesterone also plays a role, sending cooling signals. As it declines this cooling signal diminishes When both oestrogen and progesterone wane, this balance shifts, and the brain's thermostat loses its main sensors, leading to those intense waves of heat. Understanding this mechanism can help you navigate this phase with greater clarity—and, importantly, remind you that you're far from alone.

### BEDTIME AND BEDROOM HACKS

Create a cool sleep environment and consistent routine with the following:

- **Temperature control:** Keep your bedroom cool, ideally between 16-20°C. Consider using a small personal fan next to your bed or air conditioner.
- **Cooling bedding:** Opt for breathable, moisture-wicking sheets and pyjamas made from natural fibres like cotton, linen or bamboo.
- **Chill pillow:** Invest in a cooling pillow (latex, feather and down) or use a gel pad on your pillow to help keep your head cool. Synthetic memory foam mattresses and pillows tend to keep you too hot.
- **Bedtime routine:** Maintain a consistent sleep schedule, going to bed and waking up at the same time every day to support your circadian rhythm, your body's internal clock.

See Spotlight on Sleep on page 351 for comprehensive sleep tips.

### FOODS THAT HELP SETTLE HOT FLUSHES (A LOT!)

- **Phytoestrogens:** Incorporate soy-based foods like tofu, tempeh, and edamame, which contain isoflavones that can mimic oestrogen in the body and may help reduce hot flushes. Rich in lignans, flaxseeds may have a mild oestrogenic effect, potentially helping to alleviate symptoms.
- **Water-rich foods:** Cucumber, watermelon, and celery can help keep you hydrated, crucial for temperature regulation.

## AVOID OR MINIMISE

- **Avoid alcohol:** The bottom line in menopause is if you drink, you'll flush! Yes, we know we are pushing it! It's your choice to make, but we suggest you experience the difference going teetotal makes to your hot flushes and their intensity.

During menopause your liver is under the pump, clearing and cleansing hormonal residue in your body and is helping with the recycling of oestrogen. A clean liver is a must for a smooth passage through menopause. But that's not all. Alcohol also disrupts REM sleep, so you might find yourself waking up in the early hours, feeling anxious or stressed as your cortisol levels spike. By mid-afternoon, the fatigue from both the alcohol and poor-quality sleep hits, leaving you craving another drink just to push through.

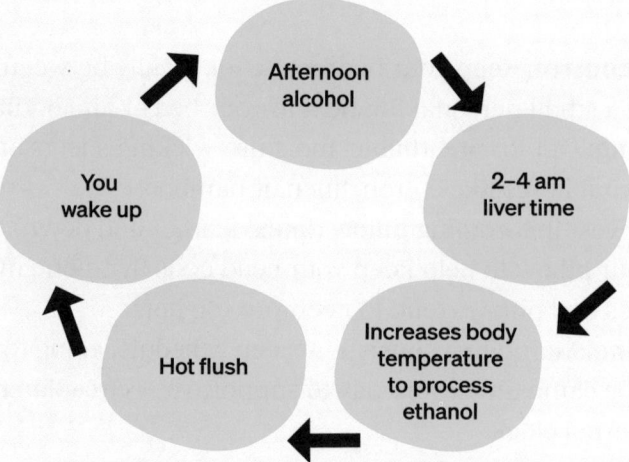

It's a vicious loop—alcohol messes with your natural sleep patterns, ramps up stress hormones, and tempts you to reach for it again for short-term relief. (See Spotlight on Alcohol on page 287 and Liver Care on page 592.)

- **Spicy foods:** Spices like chili and pepper can increase body temperature and trigger hot flushes. Opt for milder flavours.
- **Processed sugars:** High sugar intake can lead to blood sugar spikes, potentially worsening symptoms. (See our guidelines for supporting a healthy blood sugar/insulin dance on page 566.)

**HERBAL SOLUTIONS**

The following herbs have a strong traditional use for hot flushes, along with some recent evidence supporting their traditional uses:

- **Magnolia bark** may help modulate the hyperactivity of KNDy (thermostat) neurons caused by reduced oestrogen levels. By calming the nervous system, it can reduce the overactive signalling that leads to hot flushes and night sweats.
- **Liquorice root** has mild oestrogenic effects which may help balance the hyperactive KNDy neurons, reducing the intensity of vasomotor symptoms like hot flushes.
- **Passionflower's** calming effect on the nervous system might help soothe the overstimulated KNDy neurons, thereby improving sleep and reducing the anxiety that can exacerbate menopausal symptoms.
- **Ginger's** anti-inflammatory and neurotransmitter-modulating properties could indirectly influence the KNDy system, potentially helping to stabilise mood and sleep, which are often disrupted by the same neural mechanisms involved in vasomotor symptoms.
- **Black cohosh** is a popular herbal remedy that may reduce the frequency and intensity of hot flushes, though its precise action on the body remains unclear. A study in the *Journal of Obstetrics & Gynaecology* found that combining black cohosh with St John's Wort was more effective than black cohosh alone, significantly easing menopausal symptoms like hot flushes. Side effects were minimal, affecting only 0.16% of participants (those with liver issues should avoid black cohosh).

  - A 2022 study also found no adverse effects for women with breast cancer using black cohosh. In fact, it slightly reduced the cancer marker Ki67 in women who used it for three weeks before surgery, suggesting potential benefits for those with a history of breast cancer.

- **Red clover (*Trifolium pratense*)** is available in pharmacies as Promensil. A popular herbal remedy in North America, red clover has long been used to support women's hormones, and science backs up its effectiveness.

- Numerous studies show it can significantly reduce hot flushes. In one notable 2005 study, women took 80 mg of red clover isoflavones daily (Promensil brand). After four months, those on Promensil saw a 44% greater drop in hot flushes compared to the placebo group—a significant difference! Red clover also supports bone density during menopause, making it a valuable ally for women in this transition.

- **Soy isoflavones** can significantly reduce the frequency and severity of hot flushes in menopausal women, particularly in those with higher baseline levels of hot flushes, as demonstrated in a 2009 clinical trial.
- **Maca (*Lepidium meyenii*)** root has evidence-based benefits in reducing the frequency of hot flushes and other menopausal symptoms, suggesting its potential as a natural alternative for hormone replacement therapy.
- **Dong quai (*Angelica sinensis*)** can be used in combination with other herbs. A randomised controlled trial assessed the efficacy of Dong quai in combination with other herbs for menopausal symptoms. While Dong quai alone has mixed results, when used in combination, it showed promise in reducing hot flushes.
- **Evening primrose oil** is rich in gamma-linolenic acid (GLA). It may help with hormonal balance and reduce hot flushes, though evidence is mixed.

For direction and dosage of the above herbs, always consult a healthcare professional to ensure the herbs you choose are safe and effective for you.

**TIP**

An experienced naturopath can create herbal tonics tailored to your unique needs, taking your medical history into account.

## HORMONAL PHARMACEUTICALS FOR HOT FLUSHES

### HORMONE REPLACEMENT THERAPY (HRT)

Uncontrollable hot flushes are one of the main reasons women turn to HRT. (See page 162 for more details on HRT.)

- **Bioidentical hormones:** Custom-compounded bioidentical hormones that may include bioidentical progesterone, oestrogen and testosterone are an option for those seeking a more individualised and cost-effective approach, available through integrative doctors (see Resources on page 691).

### NON-HORMONAL PHARMACEUTICALS

- **Selective Serotonin Reuptake Inhibitors (SSRIs):** Low doses of the SSRI family of antidepressants can be effective in reducing hot flushes. Ideally this would not be prescribed as the first response.
- **Gabapentin:** Originally used for nerve pain, gabapentin has been found to help reduce hot flushes, especially at night.
- **Veoza (Fezolinetant):** Targets the KNDy neurons to alleviate vasomotor symptoms without oestrogenic effects on the body. Fezolinetant is a new drug designed to ease hot flushes, night sweats, and insomnia by targeting KNDy neurons in the brain. Unlike oestrogen, it works only on this specific neural pathway and doesn't act as a hormone. This means it won't affect breast tissue or other cells in your body, making it a safer option for menopausal symptoms compared to hormone therapies. Fezolinetant works by blocking NK-3 receptors, helping to reduce these symptoms.

### WELLNESS AND LIFESTYLE BIO-HACKS FOR HOT FLUSHES AND NIGHT SWEATS

- **Regular physical activity** can help regulate body temperature and reduce the severity of hot flushes. Aim for at least 30 minutes of moderate exercise most days of the week.
- **Yoga, meditation and mindfulness** have been shown to reduce stress and improve the management of menopausal symptoms. See Spotlight on Restorative Practices on page 372.)

# VAGINAL DRYNESS, ITCHING, OR DISCOMFORT DURING SEX

Even some women taking HRT may find that 'down below' still needs a little extra help!

### SUPPORT YOUR VAGINAL MICROBIOME

Think of your vaginal microbiome as a delicate garden, and like any good gardener, you want to avoid harsh chemicals. Steer clear of strong soaps, fragrances, and even chemical-heavy laundry detergents that could throw your vaginal ecosystem out of balance. Choose gentle, natural alternatives to give those struggling vulval and vaginal cells some well-deserved TLC.

### COCONUT OIL: YOUR NEW BATHROOM ESSENTIAL

Here's a fun and practical bio-hack; move that bottle of organic coconut oil from the kitchen to your bathroom! After showering, while your skin is still damp, apply a small amount around the vulval area, then pat dry to avoid excess oiliness. Coconut oil is naturally antibacterial, anti-fungal, and acidic, making it a great match for your vaginal microbiome. Reapply as needed, but stick to simple, organic oils—coconut or olive oil are perfect—and avoid products with extra chemicals or fancy price tags unless prescribed by your doctor.

### COCONUT OIL FOR SEX

Coconut oil is also a fantastic, long-lasting natural lubricant. A little goes a long way, which is big win compared to those gel-based lubes that give up after 30 seconds. This is especially useful for women who can't use oestrogen products due to medical conditions. It's edible and you get comfort and hydration without the chemicals—win-win!

### VAGINAL OESTROGEN CREAM (OESTRIOL)

If you need extra help, ask your doctor about vaginal oestrogen cream. E3 (oestriol) is a good option, it's a milder form of oestrogen that effectively relieves vaginal dryness. In Australia, New Zealand, and the UK, it's available by prescription as Ovestin. It can also be compounded into a different base, like rosehip oil, by a compounding pharmacy. This low-dose, targeted cream delivers the oestrogen your vaginal tissues need to stay healthy and comfortable. For more details and application tips, check out our Spotlight on Pelvic Wellness on page 501).

Keep smiling—onwards!

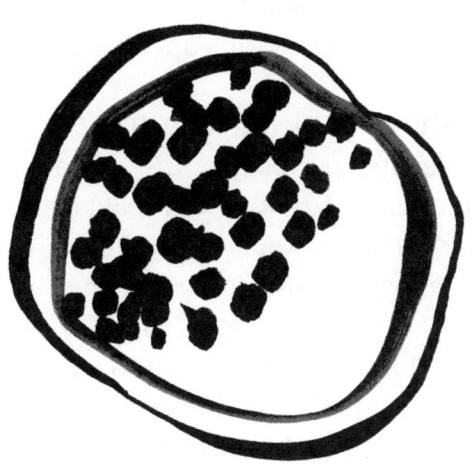

# THE BLADDER DIARIES

Surviving the urge, the dribble, and the dreaded urinary tract infections (UTIs), this hormonal ride can get a little rocky. Bladder problems can sometimes feel like your body's playing a cruel joke—hang in there, we have ways to outsmart it.

Thinning of the urethra and loss of muscle tone can cause urinary incontinence and frequent UTIs. Any activity that forces you to use your core muscles helps to keep your pelvic floor strong—the electrical circuit activating the core muscles also activate your pelvic floor muscles, so if you train one, you train both! Remember to orgasm—this can be the nicest way to train! Here are some more practical bio-hacks to keep your bladder in check.

### HYDRATION—DRINK SMART, NOT LESS

Contrary to what you might think, cutting back on water isn't the answer. In fact, dehydration can irritate your bladder and make you feel like you need to go even more. The key is balance. Aim for 6-8 glasses of water a day and keep sipping throughout. Your bladder prefers a steady flow, not the flood that comes when you down a litre after forgetting to drink anything all day.

### CULL THE CAFFEINE (AND OTHER IRRITANTS)

We know, coffee is life, but your bladder may not agree. Caffeine, alcohol and fizzy drinks are notorious for irritating your bladder and making incontinence worse. Try swapping coffee for water or herbal tea—your bladder will breathe a sigh of relief, and you might just reduce those mad bathroom dashes.

### URINARY ALKALINISERS—SOOTHE THE BLADDER

If you're feeling the burn, it might be time to give your bladder a little TLC with urinary alkalinisers. Foods like bananas, melons and potatoes are naturally alkaline and can help calm down an irritated bladder. Or, for a quick fix, over-the-counter products like Ural dissolve in water and can soothe things from the inside out.

### TOPICAL VAGINAL OESTROGENS—HORMONAL HELP

The drop in oestrogen levels can weaken the tissues around your bladder and urethra. Topical vaginal oestrogens (like creams, rings, or tablets) can help rejuvenate those tissues, improving bladder control. Consult your doctor to see if this is a good option for you—it could be just the hormonal boost your bladder needs.

> **TIP**
> If you do use the Oestradiol vaginal tablet, be wary of using it at bedtime, as the change in oestrogen (even when oestrogen is increasing) can trigger a hot flush. This doesn't happen with the Oestriol cream, as this form of oestrogen does not talk to your thermostat.

### PROBIOTICS—FRIENDLY BACTERIA TO THE RESCUE

A healthy vaginal microbiome doesn't just keep things balanced down there—it also helps protect against recurrent UTIs. Incorporating probiotic-rich foods like yoghurt, kefir, or supplements can help maintain a strong defence line. If you can deal with the mess, inserting a little yoghurt into your vagina can really help - Look for yoghurts with strains like *Lactobacillus rhamnosus* or *Lactobacillus reuteri* for extra support.

> **TIP**
> Source a large (20 ml) syringe to make insertion easier—visit a horse veterinary supply or stockfeed centre and ask for their largest syringe. Perhaps don't share why you need it!

### CRANBERRY (THE RIGHT KIND)

Cranberry products have long been praised for UTI prevention, but here's the trick; it needs to be the unsweetened, concentrated kind—no sugary cranberry cocktails! Cranberry supplements or pure cranberry juice help prevent pesky bacteria from sticking to your bladder walls. Ellura, a high-quality, standardised cranberry extract by Flordis, has solid evidence supporting its ability to reduce UTIs caused by the most common culprit, *E. coli*. It is available over the counter at most pharmacies.

## SURGICAL OPTIONS

If all else fails, there are surgical options to consider. Urethral bulking agents or sling procedures can provide support to your bladder and prevent leaks. These are typically last-resort options, but it's good to know there's a backup plan if you need it. Consult your doctor to explore these possibilities.

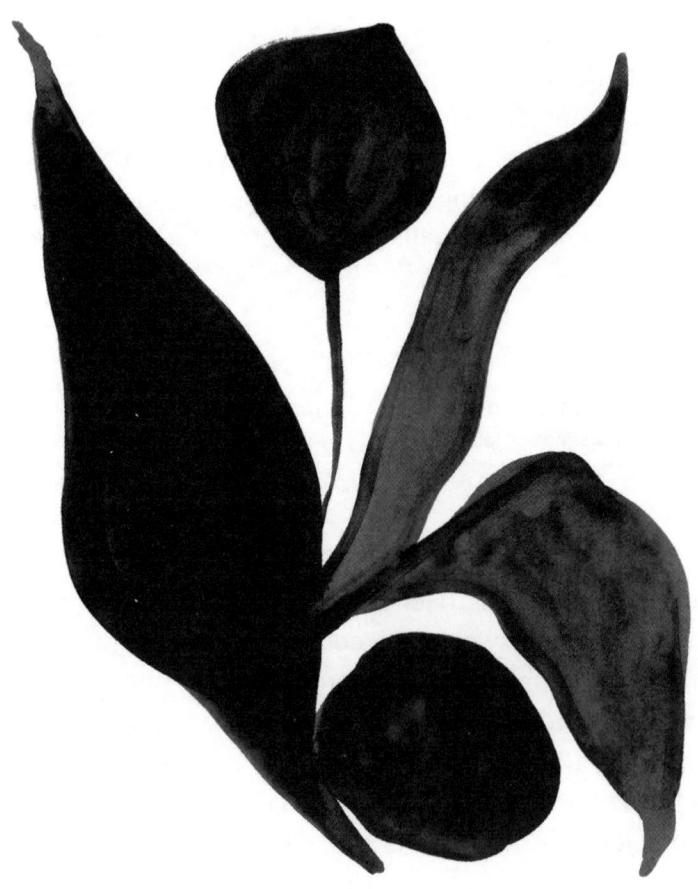

# MOOD CHANGES, INCLUDING ANXIETY, DEPRESSION AND IRRITABILITY

As oestrogen deficiency deepens, mood changes—such as anxiety, depression and irritability—can become one of menopause's most frustrating challenges. These shifts stem from complex interactions between fertility hormones (oestrogen and progesterone) and key mood neurotransmitters like serotonin, dopamine, and GABA (covered in Part 4).

Depending on your genetics, lifestyle, nutrition, and stress, your support plan may vary. Here's an overview of effective strategies to support your mood through this phase.

### STRATEGIES TO SUPPORT YOUR MOOD DURING MENOPAUSE

#### NUTRITIONAL SUPPORT

Nutrition plays a major role in mood hormone balance. Omega-3 fatty acids, B-vitamins (especially B6 and B12), magnesium, and zinc are key nutrients that help support neurotransmitter function. Omega-3s, for example, are known to boost serotonin levels, while magnesium supports GABA, the calming neurotransmitter.

#### MOOD SUPPORT FOODS

As you navigate menopause, diet plays a key role in supporting mood. Specific nutrients help regulate neurotransmitters like serotonin, dopamine, and GABA, stabilising emotions and reducing anxiety, irritability, and even depression:

- **Omega-3s:** Found in sardines and other oily fish, walnuts, and chia seeds, these essential fats support serotonin and reduce brain inflammation linked to mood disorders.
- **B-vitamins:** B6, B9 (folate), and B12 aid mood regulation. Sources include leafy greens, eggs, lentils, and fortified cereals for plant-based diets.
- **Magnesium:** Known as the 'calming mineral', magnesium in pumpkin seeds, almonds, and dark chocolate helps relax anxiety by regulating GABA.
- **Tryptophan:** This amino acid boosts serotonin and is found in turkey, eggs, cheese, and oats. Pairing with complex carbs like sweet potatoes enhances its effect.
- **Fermented foods:** Probiotics in yoghurt, kimchi, and miso support gut-brain health, enhancing mood.
- **Dark leafy greens:** Spinach and kale are rich in folate, supporting dopamine, which lifts mood.
- **Antioxidants:** Berries, green tea, and brightly coloured vegetables combat oxidative stress and inflammation in the brain.
- **Proteins:** Lean sources like fish, beans, and Greek yoghurt help stabilise blood sugar, preventing mood swings.
- **Hydrating foods:** Cucumbers, watermelon, and oranges support hydration for mental clarity. Including these foods daily can help stabilise mood and enhance wellbeing. Each woman's menopause journey is unique, and these options provide flexible, targeted support. For more details, explore our complete section on mood hormones and menopause.

### EXERCISE FOR DOPAMINE AND SEROTONIN BOOSTS

Physical activity is one of the most effective ways to naturally boost mood. Exercise increases serotonin and dopamine levels, helping to combat feelings of depression and anxiety. Simple activities like walking, yoga, or swimming can have a powerful impact on mental wellbeing.

### NATURE

A balm for your nervous system. Research shows that spending time outside daily supports mood, circadian rhythm, and mental health. In the morning, step outside and tip your face to the sky, letting sunlight filter into your eyes for at least five minutes (even on cloudy days). Before sunset, do the same to take in the waning light. Adding simple breathing techniques as you invite sunlight into your eyes encourages your brain to release the neurochemicals needed for happiness and contentment. Consistency is key.

### STRESS MANAGEMENT: MIND-BODY TECHNIQUE

Since stress can magnify mood swings, it's essential to manage it. Mindfulness practices like meditation, yoga, and intentional breathing exercises can help reduce stress hormones like adrenalin and lower overactive cortisol. Less stress hormones means a more balanced mood. (See Spotlight on Restorative Practices on page 372.)

### SLEEP SUPPORT

Poor sleep can worsen mood disturbances, so prioritising good sleep hygiene and habits is vital. Creating a calming bedtime routine, considering techniques like cognitive behavioural therapy for insomnia (CBT-I), and keeping your sleep environment restful can help ensure you get the sleep your brain needs to regulate mood. (See the Sleep section on page 351 for more information.)

### HORMONE REPLACEMENT THERAPY
### (ALSO CALLED MENOPAUSE HORMONE THERAPY, OR MRT)

HRT can stabilise mood by replenishing declining oestrogen and progesterone, supporting serotonin and thyroid health. While it's not suitable for everyone, consult your healthcare provider to explore if it's right for you.

### SUPPORT THYROID HEALTH

Maintaining mood stability during menopause relies on thyroid health. The progesterone-thyroid connection means that foods rich in iodine, selenium, and zinc can support thyroid function, and addressing thyroid imbalances can make a difference. (See Spotlight on Core Food Principles on page 396.)

### SUPPLEMENTS FOR MOOD AND THYROID SUPPORT

Certain supplements can provide extra support during menopause. Adaptogens like withania (ashwagandha) help manage cortisol and stress, while 5-HTP and St John's Wort may support serotonin levels.

# BRAIN FOG, MEMORY LAPSES AND FOCUS DURING MENOPAUSE

Now let's turn our attention to the very real issue of changes in focus, concentration, and brain fog—because, let's be honest, losing your train of thought mid-sentence or struggling to stay focused has become the new normal during menopause. It's not just a momentary lapse; it's a whole new challenge to navigate.

> Menopause brain: It's like your train of thought derails, and sometimes you forget there was ever a train to begin with.
>
> **UNKNOWN**

### BRAIN FUEL AND ENERGY NEEDS IN MENOPAUSE

The research is clear; your brain no longer relies on glucose as its primary fuel. For lasting brain power and healthy cognition, fats—specifically ketones—become the driving force behind cognitive function from menopause through the Age of Wisdom.

Healthy fats, like those found in avocado, fatty fish and olive oil, help your brain transition from relying on glucose to using ketones for sustained energy and mental clarity. So, skip the sugar, and embrace good fats that truly fuel your brain and body for the long haul. Learn more about the brain changes in your menopause transition on page 637.

## DOPAMINE HACKS:
## BOOST YOUR BRAIN'S MOTIVATION AND FOCUS

Dopamine, the neurotransmitter for motivation, focus, and reward, can leave you feeling sluggish and unfocused when low. Luckily, there are easy ways to boost it naturally.

- **Protein-rich foods:** Dopamine is made from tyrosine, found in protein-rich foods like chicken, turkey, eggs, tofu, and fish. Eating these supports dopamine levels and enhances focus.
- **Exercise:** Physical activity, from brisk walks to weight training, increases dopamine production, boosting both mental and physical health.
- **Celebrate small wins:** Achieving small goals releases dopamine, so set manageable tasks and check them off for a natural dopamine boost

## OMEGA-3 FATTY ACIDS: BRAIN FOODS FOR CLARITY

> **TIP**
>
> Healthy oils are non-negotiable if you want to thrive through the menopause transition and into the Age of Wisdom. For more omega-3 options, see our list in Spotlight on Nourishment on page 393.

## MAGNESIUM: CALM YOUR MIND, BOOST YOUR MEMORY

Magnesium plays an essential role in regulating neurotransmitters and supporting brain function. It helps reduce stress and anxiety, both of which can cloud your memory and focus. Magnesium-rich foods include spinach, pumpkin seeds, almonds, and dark chocolate (chocolate can help but ditch the sugar!).

## MINDFUL MEDITATION

Mindfulness and meditation have been shown to improve attention, memory, and cognitive flexibility. At this time in life, it is essential to take just 10 minutes a day to practise meditation. Studies show you will grow your brain's grey matter and enhance your ability to focus and reduce stress. Apps like *Headspace*, *Calm* or *Endel* can guide you through simple meditation exercises. See our Spotlight on Restorative Practices on page 372.)

## BRAIN-BOOSTING FOODS

**Fuel your focus:** Certain foods are known to support cognitive function and memory and adding them to your diet can help counteract the brain fog of menopausal symptoms.

- **Blueberries**: Packed with antioxidants, blueberries have been shown to improve memory and brain function.
- **Dark leafy greens**: Spinach, kale, and broccoli are rich in brain-boosting nutrients like folate and vitamin K, which help support cognitive health.
- **Walnuts**: High in DHA, a type of omega-3 fatty acid, walnuts are excellent for brain health and can help improve memory.

## ADAPTOGEN HERBS: STRESS MANAGEMENT FOR THE BRAIN

Adaptogens like withania, rhodiola, and ginseng help regulate hormones like cortisol, which can interfere with memory and focus. These herbs work by supporting the body's stress response, helping to keep you calm, clear-headed, and focused.

## KEEP YOUR BRAIN IN GEAR

Dehydration can impair cognitive function and exacerbate brain fog, so stay hydrated throughout the day. Drink plenty of water (aim for at least eight glasses of filtered water throughout your day) and incorporate hydrating foods like cucumbers, watermelon, and oranges to help your brain stay sharp.

> I made it a rule that whenever my focus started to wander (and trust me, that happened a lot while writing this book) I would get up, stretch, drink a glass of filtered water to rehydrate, and have a quick game of tug-of-war outside with my gorgeous puppy, Kozi. That combo of movement, hydration and play was like a shot of dopamine to my brain, and before I knew it, my focus would snap back on like a light bulb!
>
> DR KAREN

### MENTAL WORKOUTS: KEEP YOUR BRAIN ACTIVE

Just like your body, your brain needs regular exercise to stay fit. Challenge your brain with puzzles, memory games, or even learning a new skill. Apps like *Lumosity* (Dr Karen's favourite) offer fun ways to keep your brain engaged.

### INTERMITTENT FASTING: A KETONE BOOST FOR YOUR BRAIN

Intermittent fasting encourages your body to produce ketones, which can provide a more efficient fuel source for your brain than glucose. This can help improve mental clarity and focus, especially during menopause, when brain energy shifts from relying on glucose to using ketones. Consider incorporating intermittent fasting into your routine to boost brain function and reduce fog. (See our Wellness Action Plan for Supporting Brain Health on page 639.)

By incorporating these brain bio-hacks into your daily routine, you can help support your memory, boost focus, and clear away brain fog as you navigate the cognitive changes of menopause. With the right combination of nutrition, lifestyle changes, and mental exercises, you'll stay sharp and focused well into the Age of Wisdom.

### SLEEP DISTURBANCE

This is often a symptom of Phase Three oestrogen decline. We suggest you begin with reading our Spotlight on Sleep page 351 and Spotlight on Melatonin on page 367. Should you need extra support with this key hormonal pillar see your health practitioner for more advice on pharmaceutical options that may help you through this transition.

# MENOPAUSE MAKEOVER: WHEN HAIR THINS, SKIN DRIES AND JOINTS CREAK

There is a strong connection between the changes in hair, skin, and joints during menopause, and it all boils down to the drop in oestrogen. As oestrogen levels decline, it affects the collagen and elastin in your skin, the hydration and health of your hair, and the cartilage that cushions your joints. Basically, oestrogen is like your body's beauty and flexibility serum, and when it starts to fade, things can get a little creaky and dry!

- **Hair**: With less oestrogen, hair can become thinner, drier, and even start falling out, while testosterone steps up to give you a few more facial hairs than you'd prefer.

- **Skin**: Oestrogen helps maintain skin elasticity and hydration, so as it drops, you might notice more wrinkles, sagging, and overall dryness.

- **Joints**: The decline in oestrogen also reduces the protective cartilage in your joints, leading to more stiffness and aches, especially in areas like the knees and hips.

### BIO-HACK: COLLAGEN AND OMEGA-3s

A helpful bio-hack for these changes is boosting collagen production and reducing inflammation with collagen supplements and omega-3s. Collagen supports skin elasticity and joint cushioning, while omega-3s (from fish oil or flaxseeds) reduce inflammation and keep skin hydrated. Add strength training to support bones and muscles.

Hormone Replacement Therapy (HRT) supports key structures during menopause, but to get the best results, your body needs the right raw ingredients for oestrogen to work effectively. Even with healthy oestrogen levels, maintaining hair, skin, and joint health depends on proper nutritional support.

So, while oestrogen may be packing up the office, a combo of collagen, omega-3s, and smart lifestyle tweaks can keep you strong, glowing, and flexible!

#### USE SUN PROTECTION (EVERY DAY!)

Protecting your skin from UV rays is essential. Use a broad-spectrum sunscreen with at least SPF 30 daily, even on cloudy days. Natural zinc or rosehip oil-based options offer sun protection without harsh chemicals.

Rosehip oil has compounds that absorb some UV radiation, plus antioxidants to neutralise free radicals and boost hydration for skin repair.

Topical vitamin C also shields skin from sun damage, supports collagen, and reduces hyperpigmentation. It works best with other antioxidants like vitamin E and should be fresh—cream-coloured, turning brown as it loses potency. Discard vitamin C products once they change colour. Oil-based vitamin C serums offer longer-lasting protection and should appear golden when fresh.

Wear protective clothing, hats, and sunglasses when spending extended time outdoors.

> **TIP**
>
> Make sure to avoid any creams with the paraben family as an ingredient, as this has been shown to increase the risk of sun cancers with sun exposure. Check the product label.

#### CHOOSE GENTLE SKINCARE PRODUCTS

Use skincare products that are gentle and formulated for sensitive or ageing skin. As you age the natural oil production in the skin reduces—your skin will need more oil-based moisturisers to compensate for this. Avoid harsh chemicals and fragrances that can irritate the skin and add the extra burden of chemical rubbish for the housekeeper enzymes of skin cells to deal with.

#### CONSIDER TOPICAL HORMONES TO SUPPORT SKIN HEALTH

An integrative doctor can talk to you about facial creams containing the oestrogen oestriol (E3) a very skin-supportive type of oestrogen which is okay to use for the rest of your life. (See Dr Karen's favourite face cream recipe on page 370).

Topical melatonin in cream form has an extra benefit for skin health outside of its sleep supportive role—see our Spotlight on Melatonin (page 367) for more information on this hormone and its incredible support for women's health.

#### BIOTIN AND SILICA

These nutrients are stars for healthy hair, skin, and nails. Biotin strengthens your hair and nails, while silica supports collagen production, promoting firmer skin and more resilient hair. Look for supplements or foods like leafy greens, oats, and seeds to boost these.

#### VITAMIN D AND CALCIUM

Essential for bone health but also play a role in supporting healthy nails and joints. Vitamin D helps your body absorb calcium more efficiently, reducing joint stiffness.

#### ANTIOXIDANT-RICH FOODS

Load up on foods rich in antioxidants like berries, green tea, and dark leafy greens. They fight oxidative stress that contributes to skin ageing and joint inflammation. Bonus: They keep your hair and nails stronger too!

#### STRENGTH TRAINING

Don't underestimate the power of strength training! Regular resistance exercises boost collagen production, support joint and bone health, and even help keep your hair looking thicker by promoting better circulation.

Together, these bio-hacks can work wonders alongside HRT or natural oestrogen support, giving you the building blocks your body needs to maintain that glow from the inside out.

#### A SPECIAL MENTION OF HYALURONIC ACID

This hydration powerhouse helps maintain skin moisture and supports joint lubrication. You can take it in supplement form or find it in skincare products to plump up your skin. That said, if you don't address your body's hydration needs, hyaluronic acid won't work for you.

## Without water, hyaluronic acid is just another moisture myth.

Applying this product to dehydrated skin might make your skin texture and appearance worse instead of better. It's not that the product isn't working—expensive or not, you don't need a miracle serum to see results. What you *do* need is to put in the effort to stay hydrated because without proper hydration, even the best product can't perform.

## JOINT HEALTH, OSTEOARTHRITIS AND HYALURONIC ACID

There is growing evidence to support the use of oral hyaluronic acid (HA) supplements for joint health, particularly in managing conditions like osteoarthritis. While more large-scale studies are needed to establish long-term benefits, several clinical trials and research studies have shown positive effects:

- **Joint lubrication and pain relief:** Oral HA supplements are believed to help by increasing synovial fluid in the joints, which acts as a lubricant, helping to reduce friction between bones. This can ease joint pain and improve mobility, especially in conditions like osteoarthritis.

- **Anti-inflammatory effects:** Oral HA has been shown to have anti-inflammatory properties that may help reduce swelling and pain in the joints.

- **Cartilage protection:** HA can also help protect cartilage from further damage, which is crucial in managing joint conditions like osteoarthritis, where cartilage breakdown contributes to pain and stiffness.

Oral HA is absorbed into the bloodstream and makes its way to the joints, where it rehydrates cartilage and reduces friction—think of it as a little moisture boost for your joints. This process can relieve pain and stiffness, especially in weight-bearing joints like the knees.

While it's not a cure-all, studies suggest that oral HA supplementation can enhance joint lubrication, reduce pain, and support joint health. It's a beneficial addition to your joint-care routine, especially for those managing osteoarthritis or the natural discomfort that comes with ageing.

## BONE DENSITY SUPPORT

For an in-depth look at how to protect and strengthen your bones during menopause, see our Spotlight on Bone Care, page 612.

# PALPITATIONS OR IRREGULAR HEARTBEATS— WHAT'S GOING ON?

During menopause, many women experience heart palpitations or an irregular heartbeat. These can feel like your heart is fluttering, racing, or skipping beats. While it can be unsettling, it is a common symptom of menopause and often related to the hormonal changes taking place, particularly the drop in oestrogen.

## WHY DOES THIS HAPPEN?

- **Oestrogen and your heart**: Oestrogen helps regulate blood vessels and maintains the balance of stress hormones like adrenaline. As oestrogen levels decline, it can lead to changes in how your heart responds to stress, making it more sensitive to the effects of adrenaline, which can trigger palpitations.

- **Progesterone's role**: Progesterone is often referred to as the 'calming' hormone due to its ability to help soothe the nervous system, reducing anxiety and promoting relaxation. This makes progesterone particularly important in helping manage stress and anxiety, which can reduce the frequency of heart palpitations during menopause. It also enhances the action of GABA (gamma-aminobutyric acid), a neurotransmitter that has calming effects on the brain. (See Spotlight on GABA on page 667.)

- **Adrenaline and stress**: During menopause, fluctuations in adrenaline levels can cause your heart to race or beat irregularly. Since oestrogen usually plays a calming role on your nervous system, lower levels of this hormone can increase sensitivity to stress, anxiety, or excitement. Think of it as your body's fight-or-flight response kicking in when it doesn't need to, contributing to an increased possibility of anxiety and panic attacks.

- **Hot flushes and palpitations**: Hot flushes can also trigger a sudden spike in heart rate. When your body feels overheated, it may compensate by making your heartbeat faster to cool down.

- **Electrolyte imbalance**: The hormonal shifts of menopause can lead to changes in how your body manages hydration and electrolytes (like potassium and magnesium), which play a role in maintaining a steady heartbeat.

> **IMPORTANT!**
> If palpitations persist—or if they're accompanied by any discomfort such as pain, tightness, squeezing or burning in the upper body, neck, jaw or arms, or symptoms like dizziness or shortness of breath—it's important to check in with your doctor.

## BIO-HACKS TO HELP

By making a few lifestyle adjustments and managing your stress, you can help calm your heart and navigate menopause more comfortably.

- **Manage stress:** Since adrenaline plays a role, managing stress is key. Practising relaxation techniques such as deep breathing, meditation, or yoga can help regulate your stress response and keep palpitations at bay.

- **Magnesium and potassium**: These minerals help regulate heart rhythm. Adding magnesium-rich foods like spinach, almonds, avocados, and potassium-packed foods like bananas and sweet potatoes, can support a healthy heartbeat. Supplements may also be helpful but check with your health practitioner first.

- **Hydration**: Drink enough water throughout the day. Dehydration can exacerbate heart palpitations and cause electrolyte imbalances.

- **Cut back on stimulants**: Caffeine, alcohol, and sugary foods can trigger palpitations, especially when you're already more sensitive to adrenaline. Try reducing these, especially in the afternoon and evening, to see if it helps calm your heart.

- **Exercise smart**: Gentle, regular exercise, such as walking or swimming, can improve overall cardiovascular health and reduce the likelihood of palpitations. Just make sure to avoid sudden bursts of high-intensity activity when starting a new exercise regime, which might temporarily worsen symptoms.

- **Cooling strategies**: Since hot flushes can trigger palpitations, managing them with lightweight clothing, cooling fans, or even herbal remedies (like black cohosh) can help reduce both the flushes and accompanying heart symptoms.

- **Sleep and rest**: Lack of sleep can increase stress levels and sensitivity to adrenaline. Aim for a regular sleep routine 7-9 hours of sleep each night to help your body recover and reduce the frequency of palpitations.

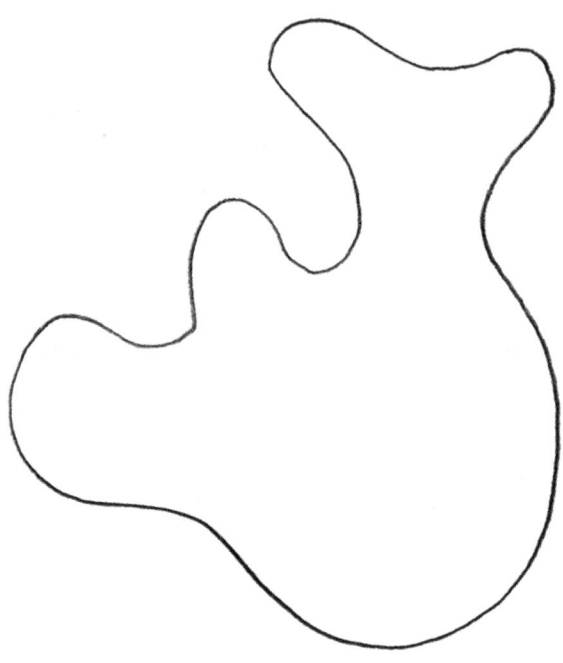

## CASE STUDY | DR KAREN
# Molly
### Menopausal palpitations

Molly was in her late 40s when she came to see me, distressed by debilitating heart palpitations. Her heart seemed to race for no reason, leaving her anxious and unable to sleep. Concerned, I organised for Molly to have an extensive cardiovascular check up with a local cardiologist—fortunately the results came back clean—no significant heart issues were found. Yet, the palpitations persisted, creating a heavy sense of unease.

After discussing her symptoms and lifestyle, we decided to try a small, continuous dose of bioidentical progesterone. Progesterone is a natural calming agent for the nervous system and can help balance out the hormonal fluctuations that trigger palpitations and anxiety.

Apart from palpitations, Molly didn't experience typical menopausal symptoms like hot flushes. However, as she entered Phase Three, she noticed rising anxiety. Since hot flushes weren't an issue, Molly chose to skip oestrogen therapy, preferring to avoid extra hormones unless necessary.

Within weeks, her palpitations vanished. Her journey wasn't over, though. Twice, she ran out of progesterone, and each time, the palpitations returned. After the second instance, she knew her body needed this balancing hormone. Now, she always keeps a fresh supply, and her symptoms remain under control.

Molly's story shows how progesterone can effectively ease menopausal symptoms like anxiety and palpitations, helping her enjoy this phase without the disruption of racing heartbeats.

# DIZZINESS AND LIGHT-HEADEDNESS IN MENOPAUSE

Feeling dizzy or light-headed during menopause can be disorienting and concerning but it's a common symptom linked to the hormonal changes that occur during this transition. Let's break down what's going on and how you can manage it.

## HORMONAL CAUSES OF DIZZINESS IN MENOPAUSE

- **Oestrogen fluctuations**: Oestrogen plays a key role in regulating the nervous system and blood flow. During menopause, fluctuating and declining oestrogen levels can affect your cardiovascular system, causing dips in blood pressure and reducing blood flow to the brain. This can lead to feelings of dizziness or light-headedness.

- **Progesterone decline**: Progesterone has a calming effect on the nervous system and when levels drop, can lead to increased anxiety or feelings of unease, which may also cause dizziness. Additionally, lower progesterone can affect your sleep, which can make dizziness worse due to fatigue.

- **Adrenaline and stress**: The hormonal shifts of menopause can increase cortisol and adrenaline, which can make you feel light-headed, especially if you're experiencing stress or anxiety. The fight-or-flight response activated by these hormones can leave you feeling off-balance and jittery.

- **Blood sugar swings**: Oestrogen also influences insulin sensitivity and how your body processes glucose. During menopause, blood sugar levels can fluctuate more easily, leading to episodes of dizziness, especially if you haven't eaten in a while or have consumed sugary foods.

- **Dehydration**: Hormonal changes can alter your body's ability to retain water, leading to dehydration, which is a common trigger for dizziness and light-headedness.

## BIO-HACKS TO MANAGE DIZZINESS

- **Stay hydrated**: One of the simplest but most effective ways to reduce dizziness is to make sure you're drinking enough water throughout the day. Herbal teas and hydrating foods like cucumbers and watermelon can also help.

- **Balanced meals**: To avoid blood sugar swings, eat balanced meals with protein, fibre, and healthy fats. This helps maintain stable glucose levels throughout the day and can prevent episodes of light-headedness caused by dips in blood sugar.

- **Breathwork, mindfulness and meditation**: Stress and adrenaline can exacerbate dizziness—add relaxation, meditation, breathing techniques or yoga to your day to help calm your nervous system.

- **Support your adrenal health:** Adaptogen herbs like withania (ashwagandha) and rhodiola can help balance cortisol levels and support adrenal health, which in turn reduces stress-related dizziness and low blood pressure.

- **Get moving (gently!)**: While intense exercise might not be the best option when you're feeling dizzy, gentle physical activity, like walking or stretching, can improve circulation and blood flow, which helps reduce light-headedness. Avoid sudden movements or standing up too quickly, which can trigger dizziness.

- **Magnesium supplements**: Magnesium helps regulate the nervous system and supports healthy blood pressure, both of which can reduce dizziness. Foods like leafy greens, nuts, and seeds are excellent sources, or you can try a magnesium supplement to ensure you're getting enough—see more on magnesium on page 464 in our Spotlight on Vitamins and Minerals.

- **Regular sleep**: Since fatigue can worsen dizziness, aim for good quality sleep by establishing a calming bedtime routine. Herbal teas like Tulsi, chamomile or valerian root can help you unwind, and reducing screen time before bed can improve sleep quality—you know the drill. All things sleep can be found on page 351.

- **Check your iron levels**: Low iron levels, or anaemia, can also contribute to dizziness, especially in menopausal women. If you're experiencing frequent episodes of light-headedness, it may be worth checking your iron levels with your doctor.

### WHEN TO SEEK HELP

While dizziness is often related to the hormonal changes of menopause, persistent or severe symptoms should always be discussed with your health practitioner to rule out other underlying conditions like cardiovascular or thyroid issues. By managing stress, staying hydrated, and supporting your hormonal balance with these bio-hacks, you can reduce dizziness and stay more grounded through the ups and downs of menopause!

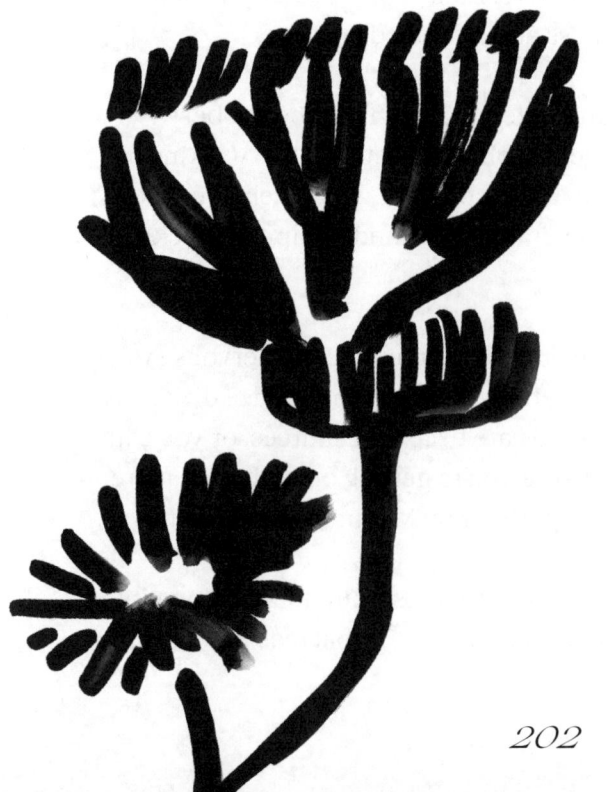

# LET'S TALK ABOUT BODY FAT

Or, more specifically, let's talk about the changes of fat distribution particularly around the abdomen that so many women talk about when discussing the M-word.

First things first. Let's celebrate those hips and thighs! A little extra fat in these areas is not just normal, it's protective. Studies show that women with a BMI of around 26—which often includes a bit more fat around the hips and thighs—have a lower mortality rate than those with very low body fat. Fat stored in the lower body isn't associated with the same health risks as abdominal fat; in fact, it can help protect against certain diseases, including cardiovascular conditions.

### WHY PEAR-SHAPED BODY FAT IS NOT THE ENEMY

Fat stored in the hips, thighs and buttocks has a different metabolic effect than fat stored around your middle. Body fat around the hips and thighs tends to act as a buffer, keeping excess fat from accumulating in more harmful areas, like around your organs. Women with more fat in the hips and thighs generally have better insulin sensitivity and lower risk of metabolic disorders compared to those with central obesity (apple-shaped belly fat). So, having a bit of extra cushion in the lower half is not a bad thing—it's a natural and healthy part of your body's design.

### THE PROBLEM WITH BELLY FAT

When it comes to central obesity—fat around the middle—things get a bit trickier. Excess belly fat is closely tied to insulin resistance, a condition where your body struggles to properly manage blood sugar, which can lead to weight gain, fatigue, and eventually Type 2 diabetes. Belly fat also increases the risk of heart disease and other metabolic disorders. This is where balance becomes key; embracing your body's natural fat distribution while avoiding the health risks associated with abdominal fat.

## INSULIN RESISTANCE: THE BIGGER PICTURE

Since insulin resistance plays such a key role in central obesity and overall health, we've dedicated a whole chapter to breaking down the science and offering practical solutions. (See Spotlight on Insulin Resistance on page 564.) By managing insulin sensitivity, you can help prevent belly fat accumulation and maintain a healthy balance between lower body fat and overall health.

Move throughout the day. Even light movement—like taking a quick walk or standing up every hour—can help keep insulin levels stable. Sedentary habits are strongly linked to insulin resistance and central obesity, so try to stay active in small ways throughout your day.

## ADJUST YOUR STORY

Feeling more conscious of ageing can create a domino effect to your self-worth developing feelings of inadequacy or loss of attractiveness. The story you tell yourself about this transition and the changes you see and feel in your body is super important. Your inner story is a powerful tool during the ageing process. It's essential to cultivate a narrative of success and transition, rather than focusing solely on external measures like mirrors or scales. By shifting your attention toward embracing ageing positively, you can support your overall wellbeing. This means viewing each phase of life as an opportunity for growth, rather than dwelling on physical changes.

Promoting a healthy lifestyle through balanced nutrition, regular exercise, and mental health practices creates a strong foundation. But beyond the physical, cultivating a mindset that appreciates inner strength, resilience, and the wisdom that comes with age is equally vital. This shift in perspective helps to reinforce the belief that ageing is not something to fear but to embrace, and your energy is better spent on what you can do to live vibrantly.

Ageing with intention means understanding that while your body may change, it doesn't define your sense of self or success. Rewriting your inner story to one of vitality and possibility can transform your approach to ageing, focusing more on the richness of experience and personal fulfillment rather than just appearance or numbers.

It is true your body is less forgiving at this time of life, so enjoy life knowing that for good health and vitality, healthy lifestyle choices with consistency is key.

Confront and reshape any negative body image thoughts and actively work to develop your self-esteem during the changes you notice. Society often places high value on youth—remember, your role is to challenge this outdated paradigm and take pride in your achievements as a mother, grandmother and professional. Rejoice in your successes no matter how big or small, and the support you may have offered to your workplaces, friends and families. This period offers you an opportunity to embrace a more mature physical body, to care for yourself with loving kindness and work positively to accept the changes you observe in the mirror regarding any changes to your overall appearance.

## BIO-HACKS TO MAINTAIN HEALTHY FAT DISTRIBUTION

- **Exercise smart:** See our Exercise Plan for menopause later in this chapter on page 209.

- **Balance blood sugar:** Since insulin resistance is the key player in belly fat gain, stabilising your blood sugar is crucial. Eat balanced meals with plenty of fibre, lean protein, and healthy fats to avoid blood sugar spikes. Avoid processed carbs and sugars that can promote fat storage around the abdomen.

- **Healthy fats for hormone and brain health:** Incorporate foods rich in omega-3 fatty acids, like fatty fish, flaxseeds, and walnuts, to help manage inflammation and support hormone balance. These healthy fats are also key for maintaining healthy cell function and fat distribution. (See our Spotlight on Nourishment on page 393.)

- **Stress:** Chronic stress and poor sleep are notorious for raising cortisol levels, which in turn can lead to fat gain around the belly. Use the stress-management techniques in Spotlight on Psychological Stress on page 290.

- **Sleep:** Prioritise quality sleep to regulate your body's natural circadian rhythm. contributing to the sleep disturbances. (See our Spotlight on Sleep on page 351.)

- **Exciting news on melatonin:** The levels of your sleep hormone melatonin, decline significantly during menopause, Emerging research suggests melatonin may play a bigger role than just sleep—it might also influence bone health by supporting bone remodelling and potentially offering protection against osteoporosis. Supplementing melatonin can improve sleep quality and also to help reduce the risk of fractures and support bone health.

And there's more! Since 2021, emerging research has uncovered a fascinating link between melatonin and body composition during menopause—especially when it comes to managing weight gain. In particular, studies suggest that melatonin may help counteract the increase in abdominal fat that's so common after menopause. In animal models simulating menopause by removing the ovaries, melatonin supplementation not only improved sleep but also significantly reduced visceral fat, especially around the belly. Researchers believe melatonin may influence metabolic rate, fat distribution, and insulin sensitivity, making it a powerful ally for midlife weight maintenance. And because melatonin is considered a safe supplement with a well-established sleep profile, human studies are now ramping up to see if these same benefits apply to women in menopause—so stay tuned.

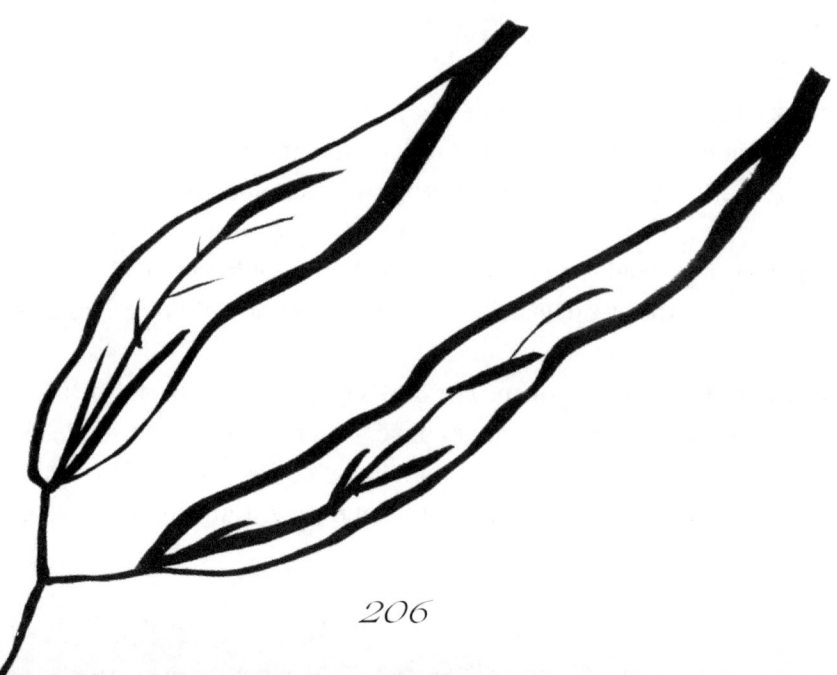

# WHAT'S HAPPENING TO MY BREASTS???

As if hot flushes and mood swings weren't enough, now your breasts seem to be staging a disappearing act. One day, you're filling out your favourite bra, and the next, you're wondering who let the air out. This reduction in breast fullness is a completely normal part of menopause, and there are good reasons why it happens. Less commonly the opposite can happen, and you may find yourself more endowed after menopause if your body decides to use your breasts as an extra fat store, leading to a little oestrogen production boost for your breasts—it's a lottery! Make sure you read our Spotlight on Breast Care on page 569 to keep your breasts healthy though these hormonal changes and for the rest of your life.

## WHY ARE MY BREASTS SHRINKING?

The answer is simple: hormones. Oestrogen, the hormone that helps keep your breasts plump and perky, naturally declines during menopause. With less oestrogen, your fat and glandular tissue decreases, which leads to a reduction in breast size and fullness. On top of that, the loss of collagen reduces skin elasticity, which means things may start heading south a bit faster than you'd like.

## COPING WITH THE CHANGES

### BRA REBOOT

It's time to ditch those old bras and invest in some new, supportive ones. Look for sports bras or non-wired supportive bras that provide comfort and lift without compressing your breast tissue. You might find yourself going down a cup size but up a band size, as your ribcage can expand slightly with age.

### EXERCISE FOR PERK

While you can't stop gravity, you can firm up the muscles underneath your breasts. Strength training—think push-ups and dumbbell presses—will tone your pectoral muscles and give your chest a natural lift.

### POSTURE MAKES PERFECT

This is where the magic happens. Don't think about putting your shoulders back—think about putting your breasts forward (that is, lead with your heart). Proper posture can make a world of difference, both in how you carry yourself and how your breasts look. A good physio can guide you on how to align your body to enhance both appearance and health.

### MOISTURISE AND MASSAGE

Keep the skin on your breasts hydrated and healthy with moisturisers rich in vitamin E or shea butter. A little self-massage can also boost circulation and help you stay connected to your changing body. Use this as an opportunity for self-breast examination (more in our Spotlight on Breast Care on page 569).

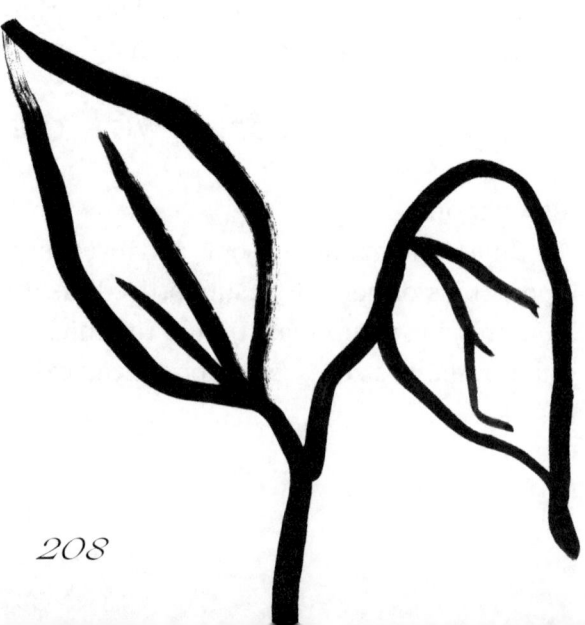

EXERCISE PLAN

# FOR MENOPAUSE AND THE AGE OF WISDOM

To begin this conversation, we encourage you to read our deeper dive in our Spotlight on Movement and Exercise on page 485. It is important for you to understand that exercise and movement are different yet intrinsically connected.

The following addresses the fact that menopause brings physical changes that can impact muscle mass, bone density, heart health and even balance. Tailored exercise can counteract these effects, boosting cardiovascular health, building bone strength, improving balance, and enhancing overall wellbeing. Research shows two major focus points for you to work on:

1. **VO₂ MAX**
2. **STRENGTH TRAINING**

1. $VO_2$ max is the maximum amount of oxygen your body can use during intense exercise. It's a key measure of cardiovascular fitness and reflects how well your heart, lungs and muscles work together. For menopausal women, maintaining or improving $VO_2$ max is essential because it helps boost energy, supports heart health, and counteracts age-related declines in stamina. Improving $VO_2$ max can be as simple as adding interval training (short bursts of intense activity) to your routine, which strengthens the heart, enhances oxygen delivery, and contributes to overall vitality and longevity.

2. Strength training involves exercises that build muscle and bone strength by using resistance like weights, bands or even body weight. Typically, this involves training in a gym, Pilates or any form of exercise that improves strength. Strength training enhances your ability to lift heavier weights, execute movements in yoga or aerials (silk training) and forces your muscles

to become stronger for you to advance your practice. For menopausal women, it's essential because it helps maintain muscle mass, supports bone density to prevent and help reverse osteoporosis, and improves joint stability helping you to keep your stability and balance as you age to reduce falls. Regular strength training boosts metabolism, enhances balance, and increases energy, which can counteract many age-related physical changes.

We have provided a two-program approach designed for both beginners and those with an existing routine. In addition to the information below, if you have already been flagged at risk of low bone density or have a history of bone fractures the specific information in our Spotlight on Bone Care (page 612 ) is an important inclusion in your unique menopause Wellness Action Plan.

## PROGRAM 1: BEGINNERS

If you are new to training, we suggest you work in a Pilates group or hire an exercise physiologist well-versed in the benchmarks for physical longevity. Should you wish to step on the path on your own, Google the exercises so you know how to perform them correctly and listen to your body. This program introduces foundational exercises to build strength, increase balance, and enhance cardiovascular fitness. The goal is to establish a consistent routine to address menopausal symptoms and create a sustainable and safe exercise habit.

## PROGRAM 2: MAINTENANCE

For those who already have a routine, this program will provide more advanced techniques to maximise strength, cardiovascular endurance ($VO_2$ max), and stability. This plan helps you to maintain bone density, preserve muscle, and improve heart health over the long term. The goal in menopause and through the rest of your life is to preserve and protect your health and wellbeing. Training too hard and too often can produce results in the short term, however long-term issues may not be worth the risk. Endurance sports should be avoided due to wear and tear on joints and an increase in inflammation that can lead to issues that include arterial plaque and adrenal overload, to name a few. While it may seem okay to train like a man or the same as when you were 30 to 40, now is the time to take a small step back to pace your body to last for the rest of your life.

## PROGRAM 1: BEGINNERS

**Frequency**: 3 days a week with rest days in between.

### BEGINNER WEEK 1-4: FOUNDATION BUILDING

- **Warm-up**: Gentle cardio (walking, cycling or marching in place) (5-10 mins)
  **Strength exercises**: (2 x per week)
    - **Bodyweight squats**—2 sets of 10-12 reps (improves leg strength and stability)
    - **Wall push-ups**—2 sets of 8-10 reps (upper body strength)
    - **Standing calf raises**—2 sets of 10-12 reps (strengthens calves and improves balance).

- **Balance exercise**: (2 x per week)
    - **Single-leg stand**—Hold one leg up without it touching the other leg or the floor for 10-20 secs per leg, repeat 2 times each side. Hold onto a wall if needed at the beginning.

- **Cardio**: (1 x per week)
    - **Brisk walking**—20 mins, gradually increasing intensity to improve heart rate and cardiovascular health. To increase intensity, add hills or stairs into your walk.

### BEGINNER WEEK 5-8: BUILDING MOMENTUM

- **Warm-up**: Same as above but increase to moderate intensity (5-10 mins).
- **Strength exercises**: (2-3 x per week):
    - **Bodyweight standing lunges**—2 sets of 10-12 each leg.
    - **Dumbbell deadlifts**—2 sets of 8-10 reps (incorporate light weights such as 5 kg to build muscle).
    - **Modified push-ups**—2 sets of 8-10 reps (on knees if needed).
    - **Seated row with resistance band**—2 sets of 10 reps (for back and shoulder strength). Anchor the resistance band on a table leg.

- **Balance exercise**: (2 x per week)
  - **Heel-to-toe walk**—2 sets of 10 steps per leg adds core stability. Heel-to-toe walking is a balance exercise where you walk in a straight line, placing the heel of one foot directly in front of the toes of the other with each step.

- **Cardio**: (1 x per week)
  - **Incline walking or light jogging**—25 mins, gradually increase incline or pace.

## PROGRAM 2: REGULAR EXERCISERS MAINTENANCE

**Frequency:** 4–5 days a week with 2 rest days.

### WEEKLY ROUTINE

- **Warm-up**: Dynamic stretching and light cardio (for example, brisk walk or light jog) (5-10 mins)
- **Strength training**: (3 x per week)
  - **Deadlifts (using moderate weights)**—3 sets of 8 reps (focuses on bone health and back muscle strength)
  - **Lunges**—3 sets of 10 reps per leg (balance and leg strength)
  - **Overhead dumbbell press**—3 sets of 8 reps (improves shoulder strength and stability)
  - **Plank**—Hold for 20-30 secs, repeat (strengthens core stability)

- **Balance and Stability**: (2 x per week)
  - **Single-leg balance with eyes closed**—10 secs per leg, repeat 2 times (challenges stability)
  - **Side leg raises**—2 sets of 15 reps per leg (hip stability)

- **Cardio and VO$_2$ max training** (1-2 x per week).
- **Interval training**: Alternate 1-2 min of high-intensity activity (for example, fast walk, jog, stairs etc. with 2 mins of lower intensity. Repeat for 20–25 mins. This boosts cardiovascular health and improves VO$_2$ max.
  - **Low-impact cardio option:** Cycling or elliptical, 30 mins at moderate intensity, maintaining heart rate in a target zone (60–70% max heart rate).

> **TIP**
>
> To calculate your aerobic zone, use this formula:
> VO₂ MAX = 60-70% x (220 minus your age).

- **Stretching and flexibility (all programs):** Flexibility work keeps joints and muscles pliable, which is essential as your body ages and changes hormonally.
    - End each workout with stretching for at least 5-10 mins.
    - Focus on major muscle groups.

Each program emphasises consistency and gradual progression. As with all exercise routines, please consult with a healthcare provider or trainer to ensure these exercises are suitable, especially if new to exercise or if you have existing physical conditions that limit your movement and function.

## SEXUAL HEALTH

Maintaining vibrant sexual health through this transition is outlined in the Melbourne Women's Midlife Health Project, which offers valuable insights. Following Australian women aged 45-55 over eight years, the study showed that sexual dysfunction rose from 42% to 88% as women moved through menopause, with declines in oestrogen (not androgens, like testosterone) closely linked to these changes.

After menopause, women may experience reduced arousal, interest, and activity frequency. Vaginal dryness and painful intercourse (dyspareunia) became more common, with some noting that their partner's sexual performance also affected their experiences! Lower sexual functioning scores from a women's perspective were tied to greater distress, highlighting the emotional impact of these shifts.

# WHERE HAS MY LIBIDO GONE?

When you're in menopause, sex drive may take a backseat or feel like it's vanished—and that's completely normal. For some it may be important and for others it is not a priority. Every woman's experience is unique, with no 'right' way to feel about it.

Some women rediscover their libido like a lost treasure on a beach in Fiji, right next to their favourite book, and their person.

Sex drive is a complex issue impacted by stress, relationships and your declining hormones. Libido is supported by your testosterone levels being in optimal range—however there is more to the testosterone story. (See our Spotlight on Testosterone on page 673.)

We interviewed several women about their experiences with libido as they moved into the menopause transition. Read their stories to discover different perspectives—do any of these resonate with you?

### LINDA'S STORY

'Once I reached menopause, the desire to engage in any kind of sexual activity holds literally zero interest for me now. At the moment I am single, so I don't really care. Sex never enters my mind and to be honest, I am relieved that my hormones are not ruling my desire to have sex to "scratch the itch".

'As a heterosexual woman I would love to find a partner. It would be great to have someone to share my life, although I am noticing that I am seeking different things in men these days. I finally feel free from being sexually attracted to men as the main criteria, I can literally see though men's charms and they seem to hold no power over my emotions now, which is a relief.

'It's like I have been given a superpower to see the sexual attraction of younger people, girls and women being manipulated and manipulating, while the boys and men are so strongly driven by their testosterone, they have no self-awareness they are literally being manipulated by their own hormonal urge, no wonder they make bad choices too often—scary!

'Now I am seeking companionship; someone who sees me for who I really am and accepts my need for space to explore finding my joy in life, so compatibility has overridden sexual attraction. I do worry though, what happens when I find a nice man to share life with when I do not feel like sex, does this ever change?'

### KATIE'S STORY

'I used to have a huge libido and loved sex, couldn't get enough of it! Over the course of my relationship with my partner, one of the most positive aspects of our relationship was we matched each other in our sex drive. We were so sexually active, playful, explorative, and loved to push the boundaries safely in our intimacy. Since menopause my libido has dropped significantly and while I am still attracted to my partner, it is obvious we no longer seek the same level of sexual activity. I feel just awful, like somehow, I am failing the relationship, yet I just can't help it. To be honest I am terrified my partner will seek relief elsewhere (even though we love each other dearly) because I do understand what a high sex drive feels like. We are arguing because of my insecurity, I would be devastated if my partner was to seek sex elsewhere because I am not interested. What can I do?'

### ASH'S STORY

'I can remember a time in my life where walking down the street would attract attention from potential partners. I admit to getting a bit of a thrill and feeling attractive to the opposite sex even though often I would play it cool. At parties and events, I did alright and had no problem attracting a date. As a single menopausal woman today though, this just does not seem to happen. As much as men are happy to talk to me, they just don't seem to be that interested in women my age. I have noticed this is in sync with my waning menstrual cycle and wonder if there is any evidence to support my theory? I take care of myself and look younger than my age, but this does not seem to be enough. I want to feel like sex, and I want to feel that my partner is attracted to me. What can I do?'

### MARY'S STORY

'I am in a same-sex relationship and my wife is younger than me. She does not seem to find me sexually attractive anymore. She tells me she is still deeply in love with me yet does not feel a desire to initiate sex. She tells me that it is because she understands menopause, we have read the literature together about a loss in libido and she says she doesn't want to put pressure on me. I know her, yes, she still loves me, yet I think she is no longer attracted to me sexually and is happy to "do it herself". Is there anything I can do?'

### SARAH'S STORY

'I am 38 years old; I have just gone through chemo and now find myself in chemical menopause. It has been the most horrendous few years; my gorgeous boyfriend has been a saint through the horror diagnosis and treatment. I am now in recovery, I want our old life back, I want to move on. My sex drive is gone, like nil, nada. I love my boyfriend so much and at 39 he has a very strong libido. We have tried, I just can't seem to get into the swing of regular sex. Why do I just want to cuddle and not have sex with him? Help, what can we do to save our amazing relationship?'

### BIO-HACKS TO BOOST YOUR LIBIDO

The following bio-hacks are solutions to the above stories and will help you to discover what you can do if you are interested in rediscovering your libido. It is safe to say though, you may never reach the same level of libido you once enjoyed in your Fertile Years. Yet, you can still enjoy a good sex life—it's about finding the balance that suits you, and if you have one, your partner.

Hormonal Replacement Therapy (HRT) can significantly boost libido for some women. If low testosterone is detected on hormone testing, then bioidentical hormones compounded for your unique needs can support more than just the low oestrogen levels. For more information on this option, see Spotlight on Testosterone on page 673.

### VAGINAL COMFORT SUPPORT

Try organic coconut oil and read more on page 180.

### LOW OESTROGEN

A big part of the issue! So vaginal oestrogen creams or pessaries, like Ovestin, can help restore vaginal comfort and make intimacy feel good again. These local treatments can be a game changer. Even if you're using oestrogen creams, adding lubricants like coconut oil for intimacy can make all the difference.

### HERBS THAT HELP

Try over-the-counter or naturopathically prescribed herbal remedy of horny goat weed extract 500 to 1000 mg per day—start low and increase.

### BODY IMAGE BOOSTERS

Libido is also associated with how you feel about yourself. Feeling good about your body can do wonders for your confidence in the bedroom. Small lifestyle changes like regular exercise, eating a balanced diet, and finding clothes that make you feel fabulous can help boost your self-esteem. Also, don't underestimate the power of good lighting and a flattering mirror!

### MINDFULNESS AND COMMUNICATION

Libido isn't just about physical readiness—it's mental too. Practising mindfulness or relaxation techniques can help reduce stress and anxiety about your libido, which can take the wind out of your sails. Open communication with your partner about how you're feeling can also remove some of the pressure and lead to a more enjoyable, intimate connection.

## MAINTAINING OR INCREASING SEXUAL ATTRACTIVENESS: THE PHEROMONE STORY

As we age, it's easy to assume that our declining sexual attractiveness is purely based on changes in physical appearance. But there's more to this story.

During our Fertile Years women emit chemical signals known as pheromones (men do too). These natural attractants can affect not just us, but the people around us. For instance, you might have noticed that if you lived with another menstruating woman, your cycles may gradually sync up—this is a result of the power of pheromones.

However, as we reach menopause, our pheromone production declines. No longer sending out signals of fertility, we lose some of the unconscious cues that previously made us more sexually attractive to potential partners.

It's not just about how we look—it's also about how we smell, or in the case of menopause, how we don't smell. This subtle shift in scent can contribute to partners or potential partners being less attracted (outlined in some of the stories earlier), and it's completely unrelated to physical appearance.

### THE GOOD NEWS

Did you know you can buy pheromones online and use them, either in raw form or mixed with your perfume, to bring back those chemical cues. Pheromones can subtly signal to partners that you're still sexually active and ready for intimacy.

> **PHEROMONES AND DR WINNIFRED CUTLER**
>
> This isn't just a gimmick. Dr Winnifred Cutler, a biomedical researcher, discovered human pheromones in 1986, igniting a wave of media attention. She explains:
>
> 'Throughout the animal kingdom, females emit sex attractants that cause males of the same species to approach. By the late 1970s, pheromones were even used in pest control to lure animals and insects into traps. In 1986, my colleagues and I proved that human pheromones exist and can be applied topically to mimic natural effects. This discovery was groundbreaking in understanding this component of sexual attraction in humans.'
>
> Dr Cutler's research led to the creation of pheromone-based products that are bottled as unscented fragrance additives. These products are available online at Athena Institute (athenainstitute.com).

> **FROM SHARON K**
>
> Over wine with my besties, we wondered why no one flirted with us anymore. I shared that after menopause, we stop producing pheromones—cue gasps, giggles, and a pact: I'd test synthetic ones from the United States. No online dating (that won't work), just added drops to my natural perfume. Three months later—four dates! No lasting romance but definite extra attention. My brother-in-law even suggested I 'dumb down' to attract men. Nope! I'll take pheromones over that any day. Might just reorder … for science!

# ORGASMS:
# TO BE OR NOT TO BE

The story of the Big O continues into menopause. Research suggests that up to 15% of women have never experienced an orgasm in their life even through clitoris or G-spot stimulation. This is due to many reasons including physical disability, surgical removal of the clitoris, religious beliefs around self-stimulation, as well as inexperienced sexual partners or the just plain selfish ones!

If you've never experienced an orgasm and are physically able, it's worth exploring ways to discover what works for your body. Speak with a healthcare provider or specialist if physical conditions or health concerns are a barrier. For those able and whose beliefs permit, consider self-exploration through clitoral or G-spot stimulation, which are two primary pathways to orgasm.

Tools and devices designed for this purpose, such as vibrators or G-spot stimulators, can provide support. These can be purchased discreetly online. Remember, exploring your body is a personal journey, and there is no 'right' way—it's about understanding what feels good for you.

Orgasms, apart from being an extraordinary feeling in our body that makes us gasp in ecstasy, offer a wide range of biochemical and physiological benefits for all women, especially menopausal woman. Experiencing an orgasm contributes to better physical health, and improved overall quality of life highlighting the importance of maintaining a healthy sexual life during and after menopause.

## THE PROVEN BENEFITS OF ORGASMS

From a biological perspective there are significant benefits for you to reach orgasm regularly.

### HORMONAL BALANCE

- **Endorphin release:** Orgasms stimulate the release of endorphins in your body, which are natural pain relievers and mood elevators. This can help you to counteract any mood swings and depressive symptoms that can be associated with menopause.

- **Oxytocin increase:** The hormone oxytocin, known as the 'love hormone,' is released when you orgasm. It promotes feelings of bonding; most importantly it reduces your stress levels (your body can't be in ecstasy and be stressed at the same time). Oxytocin can help your body counteract the decline in oestrogen levels that occurs during menopause. (See Spotlight on Oxytocin on page 683.)

- **Testosterone levels:** Regular sexual activity, including orgasms, can help you to maintain testosterone levels, which are important for both your libido and energy levels, and helps you to build and maintain muscle mass in your body. (More on this in the Spotlight on Testosterone on page 673.)

### CARDIOVASCULAR HEALTH

- **Improved circulation:** Orgasms increase blood flow to your pelvic region and throughout your body, which can contribute to your cardiovascular health. Enhanced circulation helps to deliver nutrients and oxygen to your tissues more efficiently.

- **Heart rate and blood pressure:** The increase in heart rate during sexual activity with or without a partner can act as a form of passive or active exercise, which may help to maintain healthy blood pressure and reduce your risk of cardiovascular decline.

### PELVIC FLOOR HEALTH

Orgasms trigger pelvic floor muscle contractions, helping to strengthen these essential muscles. A strong pelvic floor supports urinary and bowel control, which often weaken during and after menopause.

Sexual arousal and orgasms also boost blood flow to the vaginal area, enhancing lubrication and easing vaginal dryness, a common problem in menopausal women.

### MENTAL AND EMOTIONAL HEALTH

- **Stress reduction:** Orgasms trigger the release of several neurotransmitters, including dopamine and serotonin, which promote your feelings of happiness and relaxation.

- **Improved sleep:** The release of oxytocin and endorphins during orgasm can also promote better sleep, anything that supports sleep during menopause is more than important to include in your life.

### COGNITIVE BENEFITS

Regular sexual activity, including orgasms, has been linked to better cognitive function and memory.

### PAIN RELIEF

Orgasms release endorphins, which act as natural painkillers and may help alleviate chronic pain conditions like migraines or arthritis, which are common during menopause. If you still have one foot in the perimenopausal phase, orgasms can help reduce menstrual cramps and discomfort by increasing blood flow and releasing endorphins.

### OVERALL QUALITY OF LIFE

**Enhancement of sexual wellbeing**: Maintaining sexual activity and experiencing orgasms can improve your sexual satisfaction and wellbeing. This can lead to you having a positive body image and greater confidence.

### RELATIONSHIP BENEFITS

Regular orgasms can strengthen intimate relationships by fostering closeness and emotional bonding, which can be particularly valuable during the transitional period of menopause.

# WHAT IF NOTHING SEEMS TO WORK?!

> If there is a tsunami in my town,
> I will blame it on menopause!

**CHARMAINE YABSLEY**

If you're tearing your hair out, screaming that nothing is working, and wondering what on earth can you do and where to turn for help, we're here for you. We have created the following emergency management plan to help you find *you* again.

### WHAT'S YOUR THERAPEUTIC BANDWIDTH?

Each woman will have a different response to treatments of all kinds from herbal to pharmaceutical.

For some women, such as Dr Karen, the bandwidth is very narrow. In other words, deviating in any way from a prescribed treatment (higher or lower, natural, or pharmaceutical) will create a wave that goes either above or below their ideal bandwidth.

For others, such as Sharon K, their therapeutic bandwidth is wider and any deviation from prescribed treatment (higher or lower) hardly registers a wave because they have more wriggle room within their bandwidth for fluctuations.

This means:
- Women with a narrower bandwidth will be more sensitive to fluctuations of any hormones, resulting in symptoms.

- Women with a wider bandwidth can get away with deviations without noticing any shift in wellness or symptoms.

Your individual bandwidth is affected not just by prescribed treatments, it is also affected by your unique genetic landscape and how purely you apply your Hormonal Health Pillars. In other words, some women are much more sensitive to the impact of menopause and the fluctuations of hormones during this time. Even the smallest increase of oestrogen (either naturally produced or through hormonal replacement) can throw a wave outside your bandwidth, pushing symptoms of irritability and anger. Even with a constant daily dose of oestrogen replacement, there will be fluctuations in the level of oestrogen from day to day depending on stress levels, gut health, sleep quality and nutrition.

## SUPPORTING HORMONES

These hormonal fluctuations don't just affect oestrogen and progesterone; they impact a range of your supporting hormones as well. The interplay between hormones like dopamine, GABA, and serotonin adds complexity to the puzzle of menopause. The hormonal shifts that come with menopause can set off a chain reaction, negatively influencing these support hormones, too.

### NARROW THERAPEUTIC BANDWIDTH

If you suspect you have a narrow (or narrower) therapeutic bandwidth, you may be more sensitive to changes in your biochemistry—and, unfortunately, to lifestyle choices, too. Any deviation to your nutrient intake, your gut microbiome, or sleep quality, is likely to affect you more than it would someone with a broader bandwidth. A high-stress day, a sleepless night, or even that extra glass of wine, can leave you wondering if this is a new kind of hormonal havoc—and if it will ever go away.

We know it is hard; however, the first place to start is to take an honest look at your Hormonal Health Pillars (see our Spotlights in Part 2) and ask yourself: Am I doing enough in each area, or can I make improvements to support my genetics and my narrow bandwidth?

These pillars lay the foundation for lifelong hormonal balance, and without them, no herbal or pharmaceutical intervention can fully compensate. With a narrower bandwidth, you have less wriggle room. It also means that keeping your supporting hormones in balance is an important part of the puzzle.

A third consideration in some women who having disappointing responses to menopause treatment is 'oestrogen sensitivity'. This can go undetected within the mainstream arena but is well documented in research.

## OESTROGEN SENSITIVITY

Sensitivity can lead to severe symptoms from small doses due to genetic, epigenetic, or metabolic differences. Some women's cells are highly responsive to oestrogen due to increased receptor sensitivity, leading to strong physical and emotional symptoms from small hormone doses. If this is you, even small doses of oestrogen can create a wave that pushes out of your narrow bandwidth. And, if your oestrogen dips for any reason, the wave drops below your bandwidth leaving you with symptoms like hot flushes and mood swings. The narrow bandwidth is out of your control; however, it does mean you need to focus on the elements that are in your control, such as your Hormonal Health Pillars.

## FACTORS CONTRIBUTING TO OESTROGEN SENSITIVITY

- **Genetic variants:** Certain genes, like COMT and CYP1B1, influence oestrogen breakdown. Variants in these genes can cause more potent oestrogen metabolites, intensifying symptoms like breast tenderness, mood swings and bloating, even with low doses. Gene expression can vary over time, even day to day, affecting oestrogen pathways and causing fluctuating sensitivity, especially in menopause.

- **Receptor sensitivity:** Some women's cells are highly responsive to oestrogen due to increased receptor sensitivity, leading to strong physical and emotional symptoms from small hormone doses.

- **Different forms of HRT:** Not all oestrogen types and delivery methods work the same. Oestradiol patches or gels are bioidentical but can still cause overstimulation, while transdermal creams may release more gradually and are sometimes better tolerated.

- **Environmental oestrogens:** Xenoestrogens in plastics, cosmetics, and foods mimic natural oestrogen and accumulate in the body, potentially compounding symptoms for sensitive individuals.

ACTION PLAN
# WHEN NOTHING SEEMS TO WORK

**FIRST STEPS**

1. Tighten the Pillars of Hormonal Health (Part 2):
   - Remove alcohol and caffeine altogether for at least six weeks and monitor the difference.
   - Reduce your exposure to xenoestrogens to reduce oestrogen sensitivity. (Read more on page 478.)

2. Optimise the function of your support hormones. See Part 4 to explore these supporting hormones in detail. A deep dive into these sections may offer 'ah ha' moments where you can make some adjustments and find some relief.

3. Investigate the possibility of oestrogen sensitivity.

Here are some strategies for managing oestrogen sensitivity. For many women a standardised delivery of hormones via patches can work effectively, however for others the delivery needs to be more of a drip feed approach.

- Start with micro-doses and adjust gradually.

- A good option is to consider is low-dose bioidentical hormones and opt for transdermal creams, which deliver a gentler dose over the day:
   - Source a doctor experienced in bioidentical hormone replacement who works with a compounding pharmacy for further guidance.
   - Under their guidance—Starting hormones with very low doses and increasing slowly can help reduce reactions because it will minimise fluctuations in your dose over 24 hours.

- It also gives you the option to deliver your daily dose as a twice daily application (half dose morning and night).

- Branded HRT (Hormone Replacement Therapy) delivered by the transdermal patch is a one-size-fits-all and may be more suited to women with a wider bandwidth. Note: The delivery of hormones via the patches will fluctuate over the week from day one and then become less as the days progress before you change to a new one.

- Note that oral oestrogen tablets give you a high level within an hour or two of dosing and will decrease over the day—this can impact your ability to keep levels within your therapeutic bandwidth. Note: When the oestrogen waves goes above or below your bandwidth you will have symptoms.

### GUT HEALTH

Support gut health with:
- Fibre
- Probiotic foods such as yoghurt and kimchi
- Eating an anti-inflammatory diet helps regulate oestrogen by improving gut microbe metabolism (your 'oestrobolome').
- Phytoestrogen foods to help your body regulate oestrogen messages in your cells. Consume foods like soy, flaxseeds and edamame. (See page 404 on these important hormone balancing foods.)

### SUPPORTIVE NUTRIENTS

These nutrients can aid oestrogen metabolism, potentially reducing symptoms:
- Magnesium
- B-vitamins
- Antioxidants foods like berries, apples and citrus fruits
- Sulforaphane-rich foods: Cruciferous vegetables like broccoli and Brussels sprouts. Note: You can get sulforaphane in supplement form from your health care provider.

### BALANCE OESTROGEN WITH PROGESTERONE

Progesterone helps balance oestrogen's effects, and it should be individually tailored.

> **TIP**
>
> If you have had a hysterectomy, you may not have been offered progesterone as a part of your hormone replacement—this needs to be reviewed.

Menopause can be a walk in the park for some and for others a nightmare that needs to be managed on a day-by-day basis. It's worth acknowledging that some days simply won't be easy. On those tougher days, give yourself permission to throw your hands up and admit, *this is hormonal hell, and I need a break.* These are the days to find 5 to 10 minutes to meditate and practise 2 to 5 minutes of cyclic breathing (page 383) throughout the day. We give you permission to be remind yourself that it's okay; this is one hard day, and it will pass. Be kind to yourself in these moments and maybe go out and buy yourself a new pair of shoes!

### EARLY, SURGICAL OR MEDICALLY-INDUCED MENOPAUSE

For some women, menopause doesn't follow the usual timeline. Instead of arriving gradually, it can come on suddenly due to surgery, medical treatments, or even unexpectedly during what seemed like a normal journey through the Fertile Years. Whether menopause is induced by surgery (like the removal of ovaries, called an oophorectomy) or medical treatments like chemotherapy, the hormonal shift can be fast and intense, making it more challenging than the gradual progression of perimenopause.

Natural menopause before age 45 presents its own unique challenges. Early menopause can occur in three ways:

- Premature menopause (before age 40)
- Early menopause (between ages 40 and 45)
- Induced menopause (typically from surgery, chemotherapy, or radiation treatment).

Each type comes with different hormonal changes that can affect health both before and after periods stop. Even a hysterectomy that leaves the ovaries intact can reduce ovarian function over time. Grouping all these experiences under the label 'menopause' doesn't fully capture the nuances of what each woman may face. The transition is abrupt, leaving many women dealing with physical, emotional, and cognitive hurdles much earlier than expected.

## CASE STUDY | DR KAREN
# Kirsten
## Oophorectomy for severe endometriosis

Kirsten was 38 when I met her. She had already been through a lot; severe endometriosis had shaped much of her adult life. After years of pain, surgeries, and trying every treatment available, she decided to undergo an oophorectomy (removal of her ovaries). She cherished motherhood with her 12-year-old daughter but was struggling with daily pain.

The surgery relieved her endometriosis, but it thrust her into surgical menopause—a rapid hormonal shift. Kirsten had expected symptoms like hot flushes, mood swings, and night sweats. What worried her more were the long-term effects of losing her ovarian hormones at such a young age, especially how this would impact her ability to be present for her daughter and what it meant for her bone, brain, and heart health.

Unlike other cases, Kirsten didn't have to worry about cancer, which gave us more flexibility in addressing her hormone loss. Hormone replacement therapy (HRT) was an option, and given her age, the benefits of replacing oestrogen far outweighed the risks.

### HORMONE REPLACEMENT OPTIONS

**Oestrogen Replacement Therapy** (ORT): With her ovaries removed, Kirsten no longer produced oestrogen. ORT was essential for managing her symptoms and protecting her long-term health. Research shows that younger women who undergo surgical menopause benefit from oestrogen replacement to maintain heart and bone health. We chose transdermal oestrogen patches, a safe and effective method that reduces the risk of blood clots compared to oral oestrogen.

**Progesterone supplementation:** Since Kirsten still had her uterus, it was important to balance oestrogen with progesterone to protect against endometrial hyperplasia (thickening of the uterine lining). We used bioidentical progesterone, which not only safeguarded her uterus but also helped stabilise her mood.

### BONE HEALTH AND HEART PROTECTION

With no oestrogen, Kirsten's bone density was a primary concern, as she was at higher risk for osteoporosis. We developed a bone health plan with weight-training exercises, calcium and vitamin D supplementation, and regular bone density scans. Heart health was also a focus, as women who experience early menopause are at higher risk of heart disease. A combination of oestrogen replacement and a healthy lifestyle helped manage these risks.

Kirsten regained control of her body and life. The focus shifted from daily pain management to enjoying her daughter's teenage years and looking forward to her own future. Menopause wasn't the end for her—it was a new beginning.

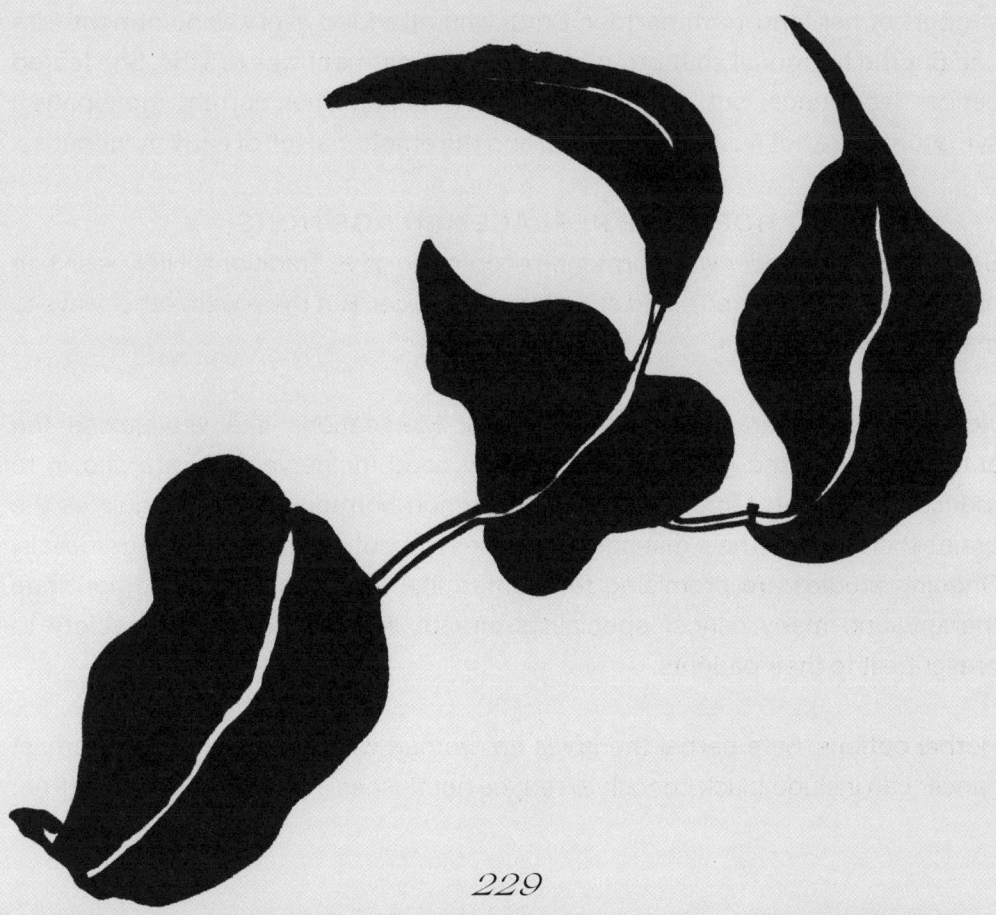

**CASE STUDY | DR KAREN**

# Beth

### Hormonal support after surgery for hormone-receptor positive breast cancer

Beth, 29, came to see me just four months after a hormone-receptor positive breast cancer diagnosis. She was understandably overwhelmed, concerned about her fertility, and grappling with the sudden hormonal shift from cancer treatment.

Before surgery, Beth's oncologist had recommended freezing her eggs, which gave her hope for starting a family one day. She had the unwavering support of her long-term partner, Brad, who attended every appointment with her. But the hormonal shift brought on by her treatment was drastic. She feared cancer recurrence, but we also needed to manage her current menopausal symptoms, like hot flushes, bone loss, and the emotional toll of early menopause.

### HORMONE REPLACEMENT OPTIONS

Because Beth's cancer was hormone-receptor positive, traditional HRT wasn't an option, as any oestrogen could stimulate the cancer. But there were other ways to manage her symptoms.

**Non-hormonal therapies for hot flushes:** Medications like venlafaxine (an antidepressant) and gabapentin (originally used for nerve pain) are shown to reduce hot flushes. More recently, Veoza, a non-hormonal option, regulates the brain's thermostat to help manage hot flushes without increasing oestrogen levels. Ongoing studies are promising for women like Beth, who can't use hormone therapy, and many cancer specialists already feel confident in its safety to prescribe it to their patients.

**Herbal options:** Safe herbal therapies for women with hormone-positive breast cancer can include black cohosh to reduce hot flushes and phytoestrogens (from soy or flaxseeds) to soothe oestrogen deficiency symptoms. Beth enthusiastically embraced flaxseeds as a new kitchen staple after learning about their potential benefits for both low oestrogen symptoms and breast cancer outcomes.

**Bone health:** Without oestrogen, Beth was at risk of bone loss, so we included calcium, vitamin D, and weight-training exercise in her plan. We also considered red clover, available in products like Promensil, which supports bone density and is safe for women recovering from breast cancer.

**Fertility preservation:** With her eggs frozen, Beth had time to consider future family planning. While hormone replacement was off-limits for now, advancements in fertility treatments offered hope for the future.

Beth's journey was one of resilience. Though HRT wasn't an option, we found ways to manage her symptoms and protect her long-term health. Her determination to live fully, despite these challenges, was inspiring.

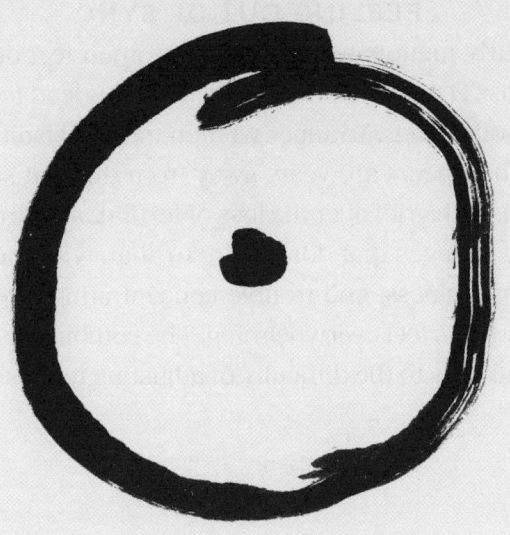

## THE FUTURE *CAN* BE BRIGHT

Kirsten's and Beth's stories highlight that, whether natural, surgical or medically-induced, menopause brings its own set of challenges. But with the right support, there are solutions that can help you face these transitions with resilience and, most importantly, hope. Every woman's journey is unique, and investing the time to find the best approach for your situation is key to thriving through menopause.

## THE SUDDEN LOSS OF HORMONES: IMMEDIATE CHALLENGES

When ovaries are surgically removed or shut down by medical treatments, oestrogen and progesterone levels plummet almost instantly. While natural menopause tends to unfold gradually, the abrupt hormonal drop in surgically or medically-induced menopause can hit like a hormonal freight train, leaving you overwhelmed by intense symptoms.

- Hot flushes and night sweats tend to be more severe and frequent, as your body hasn't had time to adjust to the loss of oestrogen.

- Vaginal dryness and sexual discomfort can appear quickly, reducing libido and making intimacy more challenging.

- Sleep disturbances become common, with night sweats and general hormonal fluctuations often wreaking havoc on sleep.

## FEELING OUT OF SYNC

Being thrust into early menopause can make women feel out of sync with their bodies and emotions. The sudden hormonal shift can lead to heightened anxiety, depression, and mood swings. Younger women may feel isolated as they navigate menopause while their peers are years away from this transition. The emotional toll can be profound, with grief over the loss of fertility, an abrupt end to menstrual cycles, and physical changes that don't seem to align with their age.

Brain fog, forgetfulness, and trouble concentrating often come on fast and can make even daily tasks feel overwhelming. The combination of emotional stress and cognitive decline adds to the difficulty of adjusting to these sudden changes.

## HORMONAL DEFICIENCY

Early menopause creates hormonal deficiencies at a time when the body would typically still be producing oestrogen and progesterone in full force. These deficiencies bring long-term health risks:

- **Heart health:** Oestrogen helps protect the cardiovascular system. Without it, younger women face an increased risk of heart disease, making heart-healthy habits essential.

- **Skin and hair:** Oestrogen also plays a role in skin elasticity and hair health. The sudden hormone drop can lead to dry skin, wrinkles, and thinning hair; changes that seem premature for younger women.

- **Bone density:** Oestrogen is crucial for maintaining bone strength, and its sudden loss can lead to rapid bone density decline, making younger women more vulnerable to osteoporosis and fractures.

## FINDING SUPPORT AND BALANCE

Surgical or medically-induced menopause in younger women requires a holistic approach to manage symptoms, support emotional health, and protect long-term wellbeing. Here's how to approach this transition:

## HORMONE REPLACEMENT THERAPY (HRT)

For many younger women, HRT is recommended to replace the lost oestrogen and progesterone unless contraindicated for medical reasons. HRT not only helps with symptoms like hot flushes and night sweats but also plays a key role in protecting bone density and heart health. The earlier menopause occurs, the more important it is to consider hormone replacement to maintain overall health.

## BONE HEALTH SUPPORT

Calcium, vitamin D, and weight-training exercises are essential for protecting bone density. Your doctor may also recommend regular bone density scans to monitor changes and prevent osteoporosis.

### EMOTIONAL AND MENTAL HEALTH SUPPORT

Therapy, support groups or connecting with other women who've experienced early menopause can help manage the emotional impact. Finding a supportive community or professional guidance can make a huge difference in coping with the challenges of early menopause.

### LIFESTYLE ADJUSTMENTS

Regular exercise, a nutrient-rich diet and stress management practices can significantly improve physical and emotional wellbeing. Staying active and connected with your body helps you regain a sense of control during a time that may feel overwhelming.

### RECLAIMING YOUR POWER

While early menopause can be challenging, it's not the end of your vitality. In fact, it can be a time to reclaim your health and focus on what your body needs now. By understanding the physical, emotional, and cognitive impacts of early menopause, you can embrace this phase with strength and resilience.

## This journey may not be one you expected but by understanding the physical, emotional and cognitive impacts of early menopause, you can take control, prioritise yourself and thrive.

# OUR FINAL WORDS ON MENOPAUSE

If you're wrapping up this chapter now, here are some final words. Menopause can often coincide with other significant life changes, such as children leaving home (empty nest) or career transitions. It can also arrive at a time when your parents may need more medical care and support from you. Often big decisions are harder to make when menopause delivers the pangs of emotional sensitivity. Marriage breakdowns can deliver emotional wounds and financial challenges.

We hope that learning more about menopause has empowered you with knowledge to feel more in control. Remember, your hormonal landscape is shifting, impacting brain functions that influence your thoughts and perceptions. If this time feels overwhelming, don't hesitate to seek support from healthcare providers, support groups, or counselling to help navigate the emotional journey. This phase will pass; for many, those unsettling thoughts and feelings calm down as they move into the Age of Wisdom. Everyone's experience is different—some may find this transition smoother, while others face more challenges.

Be proactive in supporting yourself; engage in regular exercise, enjoy a nutritious, balanced diet, and find stress-relieving activities like yoga or meditation to enhance emotional wellbeing. Sharing your feelings and experiences with your partner, friends, or family members can also provide comfort and support as they gain a better understanding of what you're going through.

Here's the reality; life unfolds, and so does menopause, and you can face both. If it all feels like too much at times, remember your resilience as a woman. Take small moments, even five minutes, to pause, breathe, and create space for yourself to recharge and process everything life throws at you.

It's also common to feel a shift in how you view yourself, perhaps wondering if you're still 'enough' or grappling with questions about identity and purpose. Menopause can stir feelings of lost femininity or vitality, which may impact your confidence. Know that as your hormones stabilise, these emotions will ease, and you'll find your rhythm in this new phase. Menopause marks the beginning of the Age of Wisdom. It's a time of freedom and self-discovery, so hang in there—see you on the other side!

# The Age of Wisdom

### Actually, life is beautiful, and I have time.
**GINGER PARRISH**

Welcome—finally—to your last hormonal chapter, medically referred to as post-menopause. We invite you into our tribe and hope you will join us in what we prefer to call the Age of Wisdom. Language is everything and how we refer to ourselves and each other in this final chapter either empowers us or puts us in a box.

Let's explore these topics:
- Celebrating the end of menstrual cycles
- Adjusting your view on ageing
- Your Wellness Action Plan to thrive
- Medical and naturopathic actions to manage your wellbeing
- Spiritual connection and growth.

## I believe that it's a privilege to get older. Not everyone gets older.
**CAMERON DIAZ**

If you haven't already, we recommend revisiting the previous chapter on menopause, as some of the advice remains relevant. Whether your menopausal journey was smooth or challenging, you've arrived at a new beginning. We hope you've earned your 'menopausal badge of honour' after one year without a period, with a blood test confirming elevated FSH levels, signalling that transition. Now, let's embark on a sacred mission of self-care to ensure smooth sailing through the seas of age.

This time of life is often misunderstood and undervalued. We hope to inspire you to evolve in ways you never thought possible. The winding path through this new garden of life holds many surprises—if you're curious and open to new adventures, what lies ahead will be incredibly rewarding. Our aim is to shift the narrative, celebrating the Age of Wisdom as a vibrant new beginning. Yes, there are challenges, but there are also countless joys and benefits that this stage of life brings.

The Age of Wisdom marks a significant evolution in a woman's life, a time when the brain undergoes fascinating transformations. As oestrogen and progesterone decline to a harmonious balance, the brain recalibrates. There may be a poetic pause between thought and speech—where the word is right there, but it's taking the scenic route to your lips. Yet beneath the surface, clarity sharpens. Many women find that, with a healthy lifestyle, this phase brings emotional resilience and focus. The brain sheds clutter, revealing a more decisive mindset— one that feels deeply empowering and invites engagement with life in richer, more meaningful ways.

Emotionally, this phase can be liberating. Freed from the hormonal fluctuations that characterised the fertile and perimenopausal years, many women experience a greater sense of stability and self-assurance. This is an ideal time for reflection, setting new goals, and embracing passions that may have been put aside. The wisdom gained from years of experience, combined with emotional balance, can lead to richer relationships and a deeper connection with yourself.

It is also time to face some of the realities of life and build resilience. Ageing is kinder to some and more challenging for others. This is the time of life when your friends, partner or siblings, may experience health challenges that can deeply affect your emotional state. It is important to seek support through friends, a trusted counsellor or support groups to help you find the smoothest path forward when unplanned events shake your tree of life. All emotions are relevant, they are biochemical explosions in your body that you literally feel. These feelings are your body giving you feedback about your life and some of these feelings are harder to navigate than others.

## CELEBRATING THE END OF MENSTRUAL CYCLES

One of the most celebrated benefits of menopause is the end of menstrual periods. No more monthly cycles mean saying goodbye to menstrual everything, tampons/cups/pads, cramps, premenstrual syndrome (PMS), and the complete inconvenience of managing menstruation. One day you'll suddenly realise you had forgotten you ever bled! This freedom allows you to reclaim the time and energy you spent in pain or dealing with a monthly bleed and allows you to focus on activities and pursuits that bring you joy and fulfillment. The cessation of periods is not just a physical relief but also a symbolic release from the reproductive demands of earlier years, opening space for new experiences and adventures.

In this chapter, we will delve into the science behind these changes and provide practical advice on how to navigate the Age of Wisdom with grace and confidence. We will celebrate the physical, emotional, mental, and spiritual transformations that come with this stage of life and offer insights into how to harness your feminine power to live your best life. Much of this journey is embracing growth, opportunity, and profound joy. You can write your story your way, celebrating a vital and enriching new phase in your life.

> Life can begin anew, if you let it.
> BROOKE BALDWIN

> In remembering that nothing is separate, she came home to herself. Her truest power was not control or perfection, but the quiet, unshakable love she chose to give herself—again and again.

### CHANGE YOUR VIEW ON AGEING

Ageing gracefully means extending your health span, not just your lifespan. In the Blue Zones—regions like Japan, Costa Rica, Italy, Greece and parts of California—people live to be 100 and beyond. The secret isn't their geography, it's their lifestyle. Residents of Blue Zones have low rates of cardiovascular disease, cancer, dementia and diabetes.

Often when we ask, 'Who wants to live to be 100?' many people frown. The common perception is that old age brings frailty, dementia and dependence. Unfortunately, in the West, we often associate ageing with a longer disease span rather than a longer health span.

However, in the Blue Zones, people perceive ageing differently. They see 90-year-olds and centenarians still physically active and mentally sharp. For them, the idea of living to 100 is not only possible, but also desirable.

It's easy to attribute Blue Zone longevity to factors like clean air and water, yet Loma Linda, California—a Blue Zone on the outskirts of Los Angeles in San Bernardino County—shares the same air and water as its surrounding areas. Unlike the rest of San Bernardino County, where degenerative disease rates match the American average, Loma Linda stands out with a high percentage of centenarians and significantly lower rates of degenerative disease.

The difference lies in lifestyle. Loma Linda is home to a close-knit Seventh-day Adventist community who follow a fresh, plant-based diet, abstain from smoking and alcohol, exercise regularly, and maintain strong community bonds. They experience lower stress, which contributes to their remarkable longevity, often living to a healthy 100 and beyond. Perhaps most strikingly, they view this as normal; their perception of ageing is rooted in health, vitality, and community support.

To embark on your own journey of graceful ageing, start by changing any negative biases you may hold about growing older. Ageing can be full of vitality, yet it requires self-care, regular check-ups, and a commitment to balance, especially as your hormone levels decline.

Let's begin with the practical aspects—your body is ageing, and it needs support through a healthy lifestyle.

### ADRENAL HEALTH

Now that your ovaries have fully retired, other parts of your body take up the mantle to provide you with hormones every day. Your adrenal glands have been supporting you hormonally all through your life as back up to your ovaries, now they take centre stage. We can't state strongly enough how imperative it is for your health and wellbeing that your adrenals are robust and fully functioning with little to no fatigue. Please read Spotlight on Adrenal Glands page 334 and, if required, visit a naturopath or TCM practitioner to maintain or restore your adrenal health.

You also may notice a thickening around your middle; this is normal, providing it is within a healthy range. The fat cells of your torso are also supporting you hormonally by making oestrogen, working in partnership with the adrenal glands that supply the raw ingredients.

## If you are still grappling with seemingly residual menopausal symptoms, refer to our Action Plan, 'When nothing seems to work' on page 225.

## THOSE PESKY HORMONES

Hormones are chemical messengers, so even in this stage of life we still need oestrogen and progesterone and the sidekicks, testosterone, melatonin, oxytocin, and many others. The difference is you will produce them (or need to take them) in reduced levels. With ovaries in retirement, you no longer have hormonal surges taking the lead role. Think of a calm sea—this is how your hormones should be now—level, and constant, active in a supportive health role rather than the stars of the reproductive show.

The first thing you may notice (without the hormonal fluctuations that drove your moods previously with PMS, perimenopause, and menopause) is that you may be experiencing a calmer sense of self, and you may feel less reactive to tiny irritations. Where once the sight of something could set your pulse racing and your tongue wagging, now you probably feel less reactive and may even think, 'Whatever'. For the first time in your adult life, you are fully in control of your emotions and are unable, or do not want to, blame your hormones anymore. Now is the time to outgrow the reactivity of youth and cultivate wisdom to respond more calmly and positively to life.

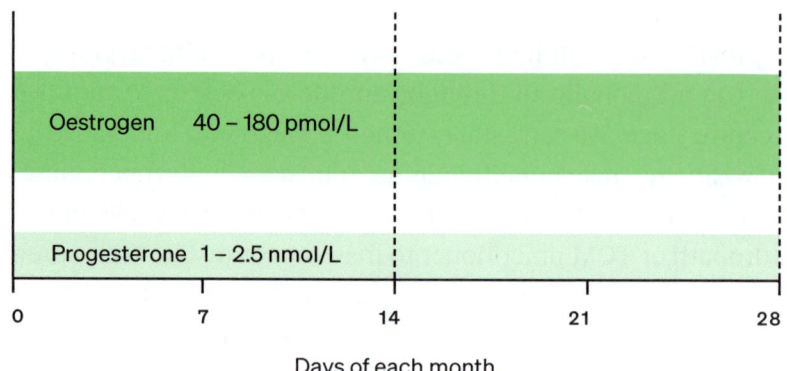

THE IDEAL HORMONE LEVELS FOR THE AGE OF WISDOM

Oestrogen 40 – 180 pmol/L

Progesterone 1 – 2.5 nmol/L

Days of each month

**TIP**

After menopause, oestrogen does not fall to zero. When the transition into the Age of Wisdom is smooth, oestrogen can settle at levels similar to those seen early in a menstrual cycle, where it can drop to around 110 for the week of bleeding, before rising to a peak of 1650 pmol/L.

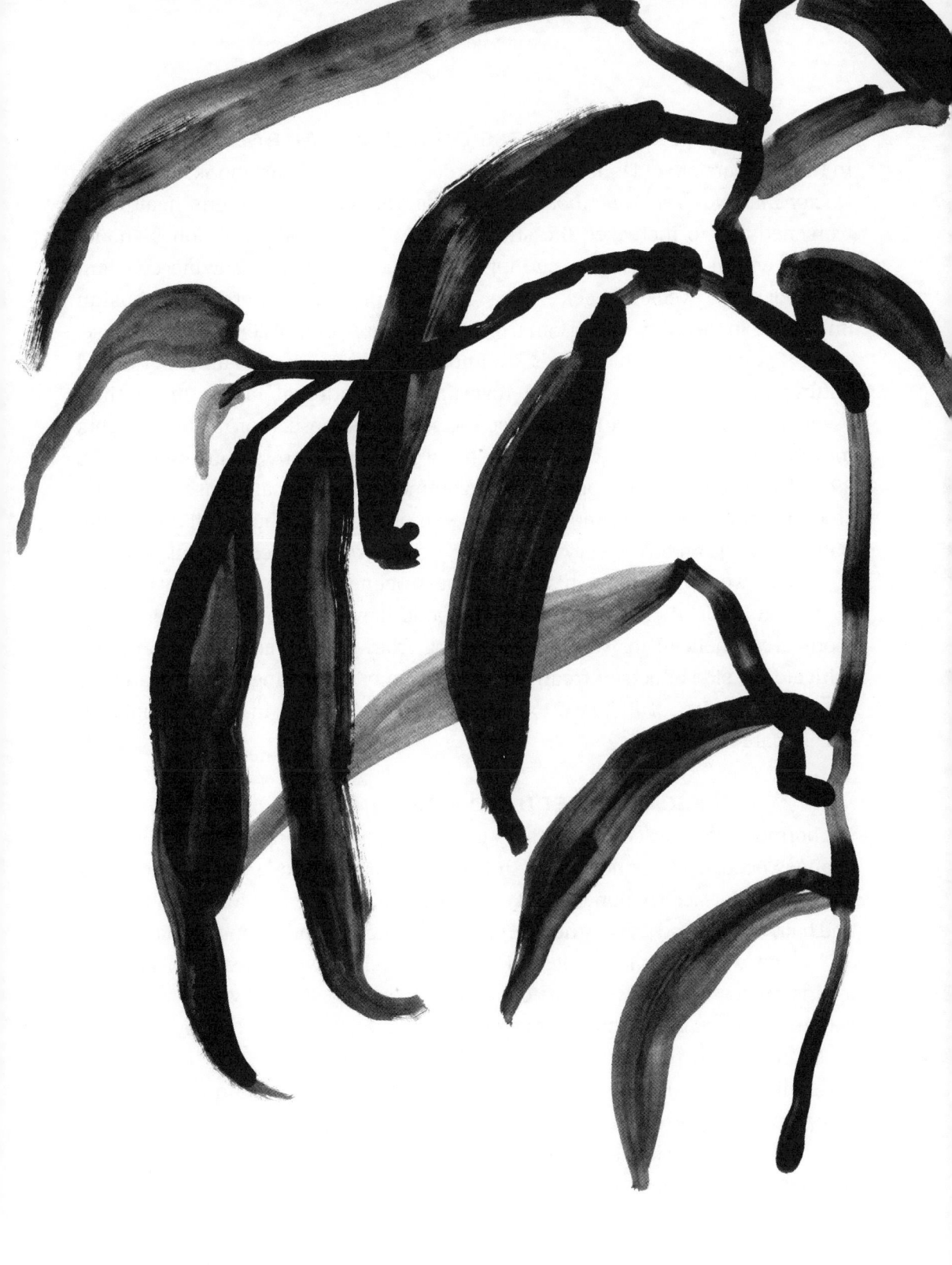

## THE IMPACT OF STRESS ON HORMONAL BALANCE

In the 30 years since Dr John R. Lee wrote his revolutionary book, *What Your Doctor May Not Tell You About Menopause*, the state of women's health has worsened due to increased life stress. Ideally, your fertility hormones should remain within the normal range for this stage of your life, staying constant day-to-day and week-to-week. Any significant decline or increase signals an imbalance in the body, which can trigger symptoms reminiscent of menopause.

If you notice such changes, it's important to consult with an experienced naturopath, as stress might be diverting your adrenal glands from their essential hormonal work to prioritise the stress response. (For further insights into managing stress, see Spotlight on Psychological Stress starting on page 290.) This is also why we previously recommended seeing a counsellor to help smooth emotional highs and lows. Some emotions take a huge toll on adrenal pathways and can be the very reason why your hormones become imbalanced.

For women with a history of oestrogen-sensitive cancers, keeping oestrogen levels in check is crucial. The good news is that phytoestrogen-rich foods are beneficial for women recovering from breast cancer and can help mitigate the side effects of treatments like hormone-blocking drugs, improving day-to-day quality of life. (We explore this in more depth in our Spotlight on Breast Care page 569.)

## EFFECTS OF REDUCED HORMONAL BALANCE

As hormone levels decline in the Age of Wisdom, a range of physiological changes occurs. These hormonal shifts affect various body systems, including cardiovascular health, bone density, metabolism, muscle and joint health, skin and hair, vaginal and urinary health, cognitive function, mood, and sexual health.

However, this is not a 'death knell'. Research shows that we can slow the ageing process and actively participate in our own health and vitality. Step one is understanding these changes and acknowledging that these changes are very real. Fortunately, proactive steps, such as maintaining a healthy lifestyle and combining medical interventions with supportive therapies, can help manage symptoms and preserve overall wellbeing.

It is never too late to change habits and adopt new perspectives. Let's take up the gauntlet and let's live life well!

## WELLNESS ACTION PLAN
# AGE OF WISDOM

As you enter the Age of Wisdom, it's essential to recognise the physiological changes that naturally come with reduced hormone levels. The good news is with mindful choices, you can address the following common challenges and enhance your overall wellbeing.

As in menopause, every woman's journey is shaped by her distinct blend of wisdom, resilience, physical changes and evolving perspectives. That's why a one-size-fits-all approach doesn't fit here either. The following wellness insights offer you the tools to create your own Wellness Action Plan for this stage of your life so you can embrace this time with balance, vitality and confidence.

By selecting from a variety of strategies and bio-hacks, you can build a toolkit that truly reflects your needs, supporting your wellbeing as you navigate this period—embracing the Age of Wisdom as a passage uniquely yours, guided by your body, mind and spirit.

We suggest you read the rest of this book, but specific information may be helpful for you during this stage on the following pages and sections:

- Blood pressure and cardiovascular health page 244
- Your cholesterol levels page 244
- Bone health page 245
- Changes in fat distribution page 245
- Insulin resistance page 245
- Muscle and joint health page 246
- Joint pain and stiffness page 246
- Cognitive function and mood page 247
- Mood swings and depression page 248
- Vaginal changes page 249.

## BLOOD PRESSURE AND CARDIOVASCULAR HEALTH

### INCREASE IN BLOOD PRESSURE

Oestrogen has a protective effect on the cardiovascular system, including promoting vasodilation (widening of blood vessels) and maintaining healthy blood vessel function. The reduction in oestrogen levels can lead to the narrowing of blood vessels and an increase in blood pressure.

The risk of developing hypertension (high blood pressure) increases, and this can contribute to a higher likelihood of cardiovascular diseases such as heart attacks and strokes.

**SOLUTION**

- **Regulate your stress response:** Stress is one of the most common and reversible causes of high blood pressure. Getting a handle on stress regulation to manage blood pressure will show benefits for both heart and brain health.
- **Optimise magnesium:** This mineral relaxes the smooth muscle around arteries allowing them to regulate blood pressure. See more on magnesium in our Spotlight on Vitamins and Minerals on page 464.)

### CHOLESTEROL LEVELS

Lower oestrogen levels can negatively affect your cholesterol profile, which is something your doctor will monitor during routine health checks as you age. These changes often include an increase in low-density lipoprotein (LDL) cholesterol—known as 'bad' cholesterol—and a decrease in high-density lipoprotein (HDL) cholesterol—'good' cholesterol. Elevated LDL levels can lead to plaque build-up in the arteries, increasing the risk of heart disease and stroke.

> **TIP**
> There's more to cholesterol than just 'good' and 'bad'.

It's important to note that LDL cholesterol also has a good and bad side. Cardiologists are increasingly measuring lipoprotein(a), as high levels of this are recognised as an independent risk factor for heart disease.

**SOLUTION**

Reducing stress is crucial for lowering cholesterol levels. Stress hormones can cause inflammation in the arteries, prompting cholesterol to patch the damage, which contributes to arterial stiffness and narrowing. Focus on stress management, along with dietary shifts—reduce fried and fatty foods and increase whole fats like olive oil, nuts, seeds and avocados. Omega-3 oils are a hero for your heart, shown to reduce unhealthy levels of triglycerides in your blood. (See Our Core Food Principles on page 396 and Psychological Stress on page 290.)

### BONE HEALTH

Oestrogen plays a critical role in maintaining bone density by inhibiting bone resorption (breakdown). As oestrogen levels decline, the risk of osteoporosis—characterised by weak and brittle bones—increases, making women more susceptible to fractures.

**SOLUTION**

Simple and proven strategies can help maintain and improve bone density. See our Spotlight on Bone Care on page 612, for more information about the new evidenced-based approach.

### WEIGHT GAIN AND CHANGES IN FAT DISTRIBUTION

Hormonal changes can lead to a slower metabolism and changes in body shape. Reduced oestrogen levels contribute to a shift in fat distribution, with more fat being stored in the abdominal area (as mentioned previously, a little is normal). However, too much abdominal fat is associated with a higher risk of insulin resistance, fatty liver changes, diabetes and heart disease.

**SOLUTION**

Remember how powerful food is in helping here. A balanced diet with a healthy gut is far better at preventing chronic disease than any pharmaceutical drug. (See Our Core Food Principles on page 396.)

### INSULIN RESISTANCE

Lower oestrogen levels can impair the body's ability to respond to insulin, leading to insulin resistance and higher blood sugar levels. This increases the risk of developing Type 2 diabetes after menopause.

**SOLUTION**

Careful management of diet and lifestyle is key. (See Spotlight on Insulin Resistance on page 564 and Nourishment on page 393.)

### MUSCLE AND JOINT HEALTH

Oestrogen helps maintain muscle mass and function. Reduced oestrogen levels can lead to a gradual loss of muscle mass (sarcopenia), affecting strength, mobility, and overall quality of life.

**SOLUTION**

Now is the time to embrace resistance training and cardio. Start slow and build strength. Join a group, hire a trainer, and use tracking devices for motivation. Vitamin D is essential for bone health, reducing fractures and the risk of falls. Also, ensure optimal magnesium levels for better muscle performance. (See page 247 for an exercise plan, review the Spotlight on Movement and Exercise on page 485 and review our magnesium deficiency checklist on page 465.)

### JOINT PAIN AND STIFFNESS

Oestrogen's anti-inflammatory properties help protect joints. Its decline can lead to increased joint pain and stiffness, affecting daily activities.

**SOLUTION**

Keep muscles strong and flexible through regular stretching and specific care of your fascia, the connective tissue over muscles. Some say fascia holds past emotional pain, so stretching it is important for physical, emotional and spiritual wellbeing. Increase omega-3 fats and decrease omega-6 fats to reduce inflammation. Eat an anti-inflammatory diet (refer to our Spotlight on Nourishment starting on page 393) and incorporate joint mobilisation exercises and insure adequate magnesium. Also try contrast bathing (see page 375) to reduce inflammation.

## EXERCISE PLAN
# AGE OF WISDOM

At this stage in life, strength and cardiovascular fitness should be your focus for the rest of your life. We encourage you to work with a trained professional to get your started or review your current exercise program. See our TIP for the best options as they will be able to introduce you safely to new exercise regimes that counteract the effects of diminished oestrogen on your bones, joint and muscles.

- Your hormones have now flatlined so increasing intensity in your cardio workouts is encouraged.
- Try to fit in 2 to 3 cardio workouts a week; ideally swimming, walking or other activities that do not put too much pressure on your joints.
- Aim to maintain range of motion in your joints, and work on strength and mobility exercises to maintain bone and muscle health.
- Yoga is the perfect exercise for life—try to engage in both restorative or yin yoga as well as more challenging classes that encourage you to improve your balance and maintain rotation of the spine.
- Take up Pilates to help with pelvic floor and core muscle strength.
- Join a gym and start lifting weights. Begin light and increase under the guidance of an experienced trainer.

### TIP

If you have arthritis, it is essential to move your joints and keep your muscles strong to support damaged joints. There is a sweet spot in stimulating bone density without overtaxing your joints. Exercise physiologists, physiotherapists and Level Two Trainers are specifically trained as musculoskeletal holistic specialists and they are your best support crew if you require guidance. We strongly advise you seek support to ensure you:

- Start correctly
- Perform exercise with correct form and technique
- Offer enough diversity to stimulate your body
- Maintain bio-mechanical balance, avoiding injury, joint and muscle pain.

### COGNITIVE FUNCTION AND MOOD

Oestrogen has neuroprotective effects and supports cognitive function. Lower levels can affect memory and concentration.

**SOLUTION**

See the Wellness Action Plan Supporting Brain Health on page 639 for tips on supporting brain health through diet and lifestyle changes. Eager to know more? We recommend reading *The XX Brain* by Dr Lisa Mosconi (see Recommended reading on page 690), whose research on female dementia offers valuable insights.

### MOOD SWINGS AND DEPRESSION

Oestrogen regulates neurotransmitters like serotonin and dopamine, which are crucial for mood stability. Lower levels can cause mood swings, irritability, and a higher risk of depression.

**SOLUTION**

Diet plays a vital role in mood regulation. Incorporating certain foods can help balance hormones, support brain health, and reduce inflammation.

- **Phytoestrogen-rich foods**: Phytoestrogens mimic oestrogen and can help ease mood swings and depression. Include soy products (tofu, tempeh, edamame), flaxseeds, and legumes (chickpeas, lentils) in your diet.
- **Omega-3 fatty acids:** Crucial for brain health, omega-3s can reduce depression and support neurotransmitter function. Include chia seeds, sardines and walnuts in your meals.
- **B-vitamins:** Essential for brain health and neurotransmitter synthesis, B-vitamins can improve mood and combat depression. Whole grains, leafy greens, and lean proteins like free-range chicken and eggs are great sources.
- **Magnesium:** Magnesium helps nerve function and energy production. Nuts, seeds and dark chocolate (in moderation) can boost mood by supporting serotonin production.
- **Antioxidants:** Antioxidants protect brain cells and reduce inflammation. Berries (blueberries, blackberries) and fermented foods (yoghurt, miso, sauerkraut) support mental health through the gut-brain connection.
- **Herbs and spices:** Turmeric and saffron have natural mood-boosting properties. Use turmeric in cooking or supplements (with black pepper for better absorption), and add saffron to dishes for flavour and mental health benefits.

For a deeper understanding of hormones and mood, turn to page 185.

## OTHER CHALLENGES IN THE AGE OF WISDOM

The following challenges are residual problems that begin in the menopause transition and may continue. For details and solutions refer to the following pages within the Menopause chapter:

**SKIN AND HAIR HEALTH PAGE 192**
**VAGINAL HEALTH PAGE 180**
**URINARY HEALTH PAGE 182**
**SEXUAL HEALTH PAGE 214**

## VAGINAL CHANGES

### DRYNESS AND IRRITATION

The low vaginal oestrogen levels from menopause onward results in a loss of hydration, blood flow and nourishment for the vaginal and vulval cells. When oestrogen levels decline from menopause and beyond, the vaginal wall becomes thinner (atrophic). This thinning reduces the number of cell layers, leading to a less robust barrier of protection against the outside environment.

After menopause, there is reduced collagen and elastin production, making the vaginal tissues less flexible and more prone to dryness and irritation.

Oestrogen influences the function of Bartholin's glands (located near the vaginal opening) and mucus-secreting glands on the cervix that helps lubricate the vagina. Lower oestrogen levels reduce the activity of these glands, leading to decreased mucus production and contributing to vaginal dryness.

### IMPACT ON THE VAGINAL MICROBIOME

The vaginal microbiome, dominated by lactobacilli, is essential for maintaining vaginal health. Oestrogen supports the growth of lactobacilli by providing glycogen as a prebiotic sugar—the food of choice for the *Lactobacillus* family. A decrease in oestrogen disrupts this balance, leading to a less favourable environment for lactobacilli and a potential increase in the overgrowth of unhealthy bacteria, which can make symptoms of dryness and discomfort worse.

A combination of these changes results in a less lubricated, more fragile, and less elastic vaginal environment, contributing to the symptoms of vaginal dryness and discomfort. (See Phillipa's story on page 250 for some tips on how to pre-empt this common problem after menopause.)

## CASE STUDY | DR KAREN
# Phillipa
### Cervical smear success with coconut oil

Phillipa, in her late 50s, came to me for her first cervical smear since entering menopause. Her last attempt five years ago had been traumatic, with a cold metal speculum and discomfort that caused her to stop the procedure. She was not interested in taking Valium to calm her before the test, or starting oestrogen replacement therapy as suggested by her previous doctor.

As a female GP with years of experience, I used a small, well-lubricated plastic speculum, a pillow to raise her hips, and guided her through deep breathing. In less than 20 seconds, the procedure was complete, and Phillipa left my office relaxed.

However, her smear results showed 'severe atrophy of cervical cells' due to lack of oestrogen, making it impossible for the lab to analyse the sample—a six-week course of vaginal oestrogen was recommended. Phillipa had previously tried vaginal oestrogen with negative side effects, so I suggested using organic coconut oil daily after showering to hydrate her vaginal tissues.

Six weeks later, her follow-up smear was smooth and pain-free, and her results came back completely normal: 'Well-oestrogenised hydrated cervical cells, with no evidence of cervical dysplasia.' The natural approach had worked where pharmaceuticals had been uncomfortable for her.

Note: Thanks to modern cervical screening methods, which focus more on detecting high-risk HPV strains, post-menopausal atrophy is less likely to interfere with test results.

## MEDICAL CHECKLIST
# AGE OF WISDOM

It's important to maintain regular check-ups and blood tests to monitor your overall health and wellbeing. The following tests can provide insights into vital health markers and help track trends over time:

- **Insulin/blood sugar levels:** To monitor for insulin resistance or Type 2 diabetes.
- **Kidney and cardiovascular health:** Blood tests to check kidney function, cholesterol levels, and other markers of cardiovascular health.
- **Inflammation markers:** To assess overall inflammatory response in the body. Your naturopath or healthcare practitioner can help interpret these results and suggest gentle, supportive options to maintain your wellbeing. Keeping track of these trends over time can help ensure stability and good health as you age.
- **Regular cervical smears:** If you've had normal results throughout your life, you can celebrate your final smear around age 70, guided by your doctor or health nurse.

| TEST NAME | WHAT DOES IT TEST FOR | MEDICALLY ACCEPTABLE | IDEAL RANGE | UNITS |
|---|---|---|---|---|
| Bicarbonate | Alkalinity | 20 - 32 | Higher than 29 | mmol/L |
| Uric Acid | Metabolic Syndrome | 0.150 - 0.400 | Less than 0.3 | mmol/L |
| Creatinine | Kidney Function | 45 - 85 | Less than 80 | umol/L |
| eGFR | | >59 | Higher than 90 | mls/min |
| Glucose Fasting | Fasting Blood Sugar and Insulin | 3.6 – 6.0 | 3.5 – 5.0 | mmol/L |
| Serum Insulin | | Less than 25 | Less than 10 | microIU/L |
| CRP | Inflammation | Less than 5 | Less than 1 | mg/L |

## THE IMPORTANCE OF C-REACTIVE PROTEIN TESTING

The commonly ordered C-Reactive Protein (CRP) test provides a score as low as 5 but it won't quantify lower scores. To determine whether your CRP is below 5—ideally less than 1, which indicates a low cardiovascular risk—your doctor must specify a **Highly Sensitive CRP (HsCRP)** test. This is particularly important for those with high cholesterol but no history of heart disease, as it helps assess your true cardiovascular risk.

## NATUROPATHY CHECKLIST FOR LONG-TERM WELLNESS

Your health practitioner can help create a personalised management plan and advise on optimal review intervals for your nutritional and hormonal health. If you're addressing hormonal imbalances or nutritional deficiencies, check in with your practitioner every four to six months. Regular reviews will help you stay on track with your wellness goals and ensure key health markers remain in the ideal range. Use the following table as a reference guide and reminder after formulating your ongoing checklist with your health practitioner.

| KEY HEALTH MARKERS AND SUPPORT | REVIEW INTERVAL | COMMENTS |
| --- | --- | --- |
| Digestion | | |
| Immune System | | |
| Dietary Support | | |
| Gut Health | | |
| Adrenal Support | | |
| General Heart Health—Blood Pressure | | |
| Inflammation Markers (for example, C-Reactive protein) | | |
| Supplement Review and Supply | | |
| Lifestyle Recommendations | | |

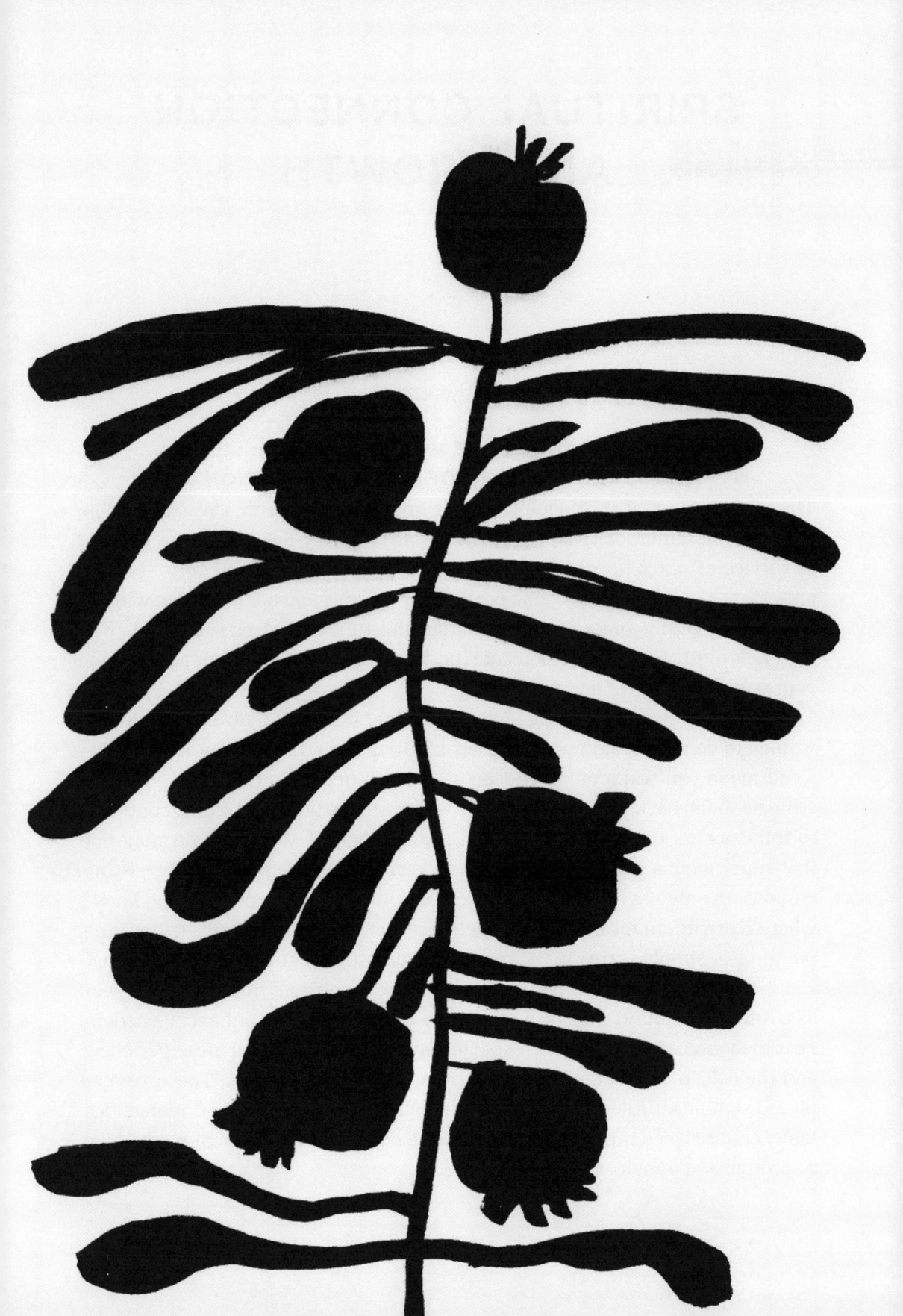

# SPIRITUAL CONNECTION AND GROWTH

### EMBRACING THE AGE OF WISDOM: A SACRED JOURNEY OF TRANSFORMATION

The physical care of your ageing body is important. However, this stage of life is also about embracing aspects of yourself that may have been put on hold in service of other needs. As you age, your skin stretches and your youthful appearance changes. When you accept the inevitable and acknowledge without fear you are getting older, you can embrace this time of life and seek wisdom as your new kind of beauty. We dedicate the final pages of this chapter to exploring your passage to power and wisdom.

In times past, before the age of farming, it was the job of menopausal women to care for children while their mothers slept. Even today, it's said that a full moon can wake us from deep sleep, and under its influence, we often struggle to fall back asleep. The moon, which affects tides and crops, continues to influence us throughout life. Well into the Age of Wisdom, you may find that super moons still have the power to keep you awake. Instead of resisting, embrace the moon's influence and celebrate this passage to power. Who knows what creativity might emerge during these moonlit wake cycles—try writing, painting, or simply sitting in the moonlight, breathing, reflecting, and creating.

The transition from menopause, in ancient spiritual traditions, was seen as a time of profound transformation, spiritual growth, and enhanced wisdom. Post-menopausal women were respected and honoured for their life experiences and their deep connection to the spiritual and natural worlds. These women played significant roles as keepers of knowledge, healers, and spiritual guides. Many cultures recognised this natural phase not just as a biological event but as a spiritual and transformative milestone.

## ANCIENT TRADITIONS OF THE WISE WOMAN

In many ancient cultures, such as Celtic and Greek, women's lives were viewed through the lens of the Triple Goddess: Maiden, Mother, and Crone. The Age of Wisdom marked the transition to the Crone phase, symbolising wisdom, inner strength, and spiritual maturity. The Crone, a wise elder, held the collective knowledge of the community, often respected as a healer with wisdom of herbs and childbirth. These post-menopausal women were revered for their life experiences and their ability to offer guidance and counsel.

> ### HERBAL LORE
>
> In early European societies and their colonies, wise women passed herbal knowledge down the matriarchal line. Many of these wise women understood the importance of a clean home, often using a broom and keeping cats to deter vermin. Sound familiar? The archetypal witch was once simply a woman who birthed babies and practised herbal lore—respected and trusted within her community.
>
> As patriarchal power grew, these women became a target of suspicion. They held healing knowledge and community trust—threats to rising male dominance. Women's lore excluded men, just as women were long excluded from men's lore.
>
> Religious movements misused the voice of Pope John VIII, who affirmed the existence of witchcraft but didn't condone the hysteria that followed. His decree was misinterpreted by those wanting to control communities and erode trust in women healers. Fear spread like wildfire. Wise women were branded as witches—accused of being in league with the devil—and burned alive in acts of religious frenzy.
>
> Even cats, once companions in cleanliness, were condemned and killed, disrupting the natural balance. Without them, rats and fleas overran cities—some say helping spread deadly plagues.
>
> The archetype of the witch—peasant clothes, broomstick, and a cat—endures. Much of Europe's herbal wisdom was lost as surgeons and Western medicine rose to dominance. Yet, the lore never truly died. Slowly, it re-emerged through naturopathy and modern herbal medicine, blending traditions from around the world.
>
> Ayurvedic medicine, standing strong and proud, still thrives in Indian hospitals, alongside Western medicine. Traditional Chinese Medicine, too, remained intact and today offers a holistic voice in preventative health—especially in hormonal wellbeing.
>
> It's through these ancient and modern natural therapies that we access nature's best medicine—grown by the living, breathing intelligence of Earth, who feeds and supports us to live and thrive.

## RITES OF PASSAGE AND SPIRITUALITY

Apart from humans, there are very few animals on the planet that live long after their fertility has passed. Whales and elephants are two that spring to mind. The older females are key to the success of the males and younger members of the family unit. They are prized for their extraordinary knowledge and memory;

they remain to mentor and pass on their wisdom to the next generations. So do human women!

Many ancient cultures honoured menopause as a powerful rite of passage, marking a woman's transition into a new, respected phase of life. Ceremonies celebrated her contributions and recognised her emerging role as an elder. These rituals often symbolised spiritual renewal—shedding the old and embracing a deeper, more intuitive identity. In some traditions, menopausal women were believed to gain heightened mystical powers and a stronger connection to the spiritual realm. Their wisdom bridged the physical and the divine. In Ancient Greece and Rome, postmenopausal women often held spiritual roles—such as oracles or priestesses—respected for their insight, maturity, and freedom from fertility's earthly ties.

> **MODERN-DAY WOMEN'S LORE**
>
> Why do we humans pretend we know it all, when we've only lived a moment in the vast life of our planet? 'She'—Mother Earth, as the ancients knew—is where true wisdom lies. Not on the internet nor in books or the societal narrative. Helpful, yes—but not the whole story. Wisdom lives in our connection to ourselves and the natural world. It's in what we see, feel, smell, hear and touch in the ever-present Now. When we trust this deep knowing, we awaken to our conscious connection with all that exists—and remember we are already whole. Everything else is illusion. Our time-travelling minds keep us trapped in outdated beliefs, conditioned responses, painful memories and imagined futures. Escape. Wake up! Come home to your true self—and live authentically.

> Healing began the moment she stopped abandoning herself. By facing what she had long avoided and embracing all that she is—
> light, shadow, longing and truth—
> she finally found her way home.

Many ancient cultures, such as Native American and Aboriginal Australian traditions, linked women's menstrual cycles to the moon, recognising a sacred synchronicity. Menopause was seen as a shift into the Age of Wisdom —a time of deeper alignment with nature. Seasonal metaphors likened it to autumn, a time of harvest, reflection, and inner growth.

In Hinduism and other spiritual traditions, menopause marked liberation from earthly duties, offering space for spiritual focus. Buddhist and Taoist paths saw post-menopausal women as having greater clarity for meditation and higher consciousness.

Often revered as healers and wisdom keepers, elder women held vital roles in many Indigenous cultures—passing down herbal, spiritual, and cultural knowledge to ensure the continuity of ancestral wisdom through generations.

### FORGIVENESS

Forgiveness is a process of setting yourself free—releasing hatred, revenge and resentment, which are toxic to your body. These harsh feelings flood your body with harmful biochemicals—it's said to be like drinking poison and expecting the person who wronged you to die. Consult a compassionate therapist if you need help processing your emotions and finding freedom.

> The only work that will ultimately bring any good to any of us is the work of contributing to the healing of the world. The first step in forgiveness is the willingness to forgive.
>
> MARIANNE WILLIAMSON

### YOUR JOURNEY TO AWAKENING

It's time to explore your wise feminine power. At this stage of your life, you have the unique opportunity to embrace your accumulated wisdom and experience, supporting and mentoring younger generations. Consider storytelling, genealogy, and creativity as ways to pass on your knowledge and heritage.

### MODERN-DAY STORYTELLING AND LEGACY

Engage in storytelling sessions with younger generations to share family history, cultural traditions, and life lessons. Explore your family's genealogy, document stories, and research ancestry to provide a deeper connection to your roots. Encourage younger women to journal and write, fostering communication and understanding across generations.

## CREATIVE AND HEALTH PRACTICES

Learn or teach traditional crafts, write a book or blog, share your natural remedies and holistic practices, and consider exploring yoga, meditation, or breathwork. These practices promote mental and physical wellbeing and help you connect with your inner wisdom and the natural world.

### WRITING AND JOURNALING

Write a book or start a blog or Substack about what you love: cooking, gardening, career moves—anything that makes your heart sing. Share your knowledge on being the best mother or grandmother, or even how to hide vegetables in meals! Creativity is key, and whether it's for your family, friends or a wider audience, all is welcome. (See our Sacred Journey section on page 259.)

Encourage younger women to journal or write about their experiences. Share your own writings, memoirs or poetry. Writing is a powerful way to reflect on life and sharing fosters communication and understanding.

### PROMOTE HEALTH AND WELLNESS PRACTICES

Pass down knowledge about natural remedies, herbal medicine, and holistic health practices. Share what worked for you, your grandmother's advice, and the traditions that make you laugh. Promoting natural health practices can offer alternatives and empower others to consider preventative health strategies. Explore natural cleaning solutions too—like oil of clove for mould, and vinegar, salt and dishwashing liquid for weed control. Share your research and findings!

### YOGA AND MEDITATION

Consider becoming a yoga or meditation teacher—it's never too late! If you think your body has limitations, starting a practice will do wonders, and you can share what you learn with others. These practices are beneficial for mind-body wellness, stress reduction and mindfulness. Daily meditation and breathwork are essential at this stage of life. (Refer to pages 381-392 for more details.)

An observational study even suggests that a week of intense meditation focused on cellular health can block viruses from entering cells. *Source* is a documentary that offers insight into this. Please note, it is meant for individual reflection and not as medical advice (sourcethefilm.org).

# SACRED JOURNEY

In honour of our past matriarchal lines and the wise women who came before us, we invite you to join a three-month sacred journey. Our intention is to deepen your connection to yourself and everything that cannot be bought or owned. You will know when the time is right for you to begin, whether on your own, with friends or in a women's circle. Start when you can commit to completing the sequence once a week for 12 weeks. This transformative experience will connect you with yourself, nature and your inner wisdom.

Your journey includes weekly practices, ceremony, and ritual, all immersed in nature to reflect the ancient women's bond with Mother Earth. These practices engage all your senses and offer a weekly mindful experience. They're progressive, cultivating sacredness, healing and growth.

Listen to your body, mind, and spirit. If it feels right, keep a journal—write, draw or sketch your observations before and after the journey.

We don't subscribe to the mystical image of witches. We believe all women have an innate intuition, an instinct, a natural state of wisdom. In a busy world, many have forgotten this inner knowing. Our hope is to awaken this spirit, showing you that you are part of something whole—the intelligence of love that permeates all things.

> Love is what we are born with.
> Fear is what we learn. The spiritual journey
> is the unlearning of fear and prejudices and
> the acceptance of love back in our hearts.
> Love is the essential reality and our
> purpose on Earth.
>
> **MARIANNE WILLIAMSON**

## MONTH 1:
## AWAKENING YOUR SENSES AND CONNECTING WITH NATURE

### WEEK 1: GROUNDING AND EARTH CONNECTION
**Practice:** Earth Embrace Ceremony
**Location:** A quiet outdoor space, like a garden or park

**RITUAL**
- **Preparation:** Gather natural elements like stones, leaves, or flowers.
- **Ceremony:** Write down any fears or limiting beliefs on paper. One by one, throw them into the fire, visualising each one transforming into positive energy. Watch the flames dance, feel the warmth, and imagine the fire igniting change within you.
- **Reflection:** Write about the transformations you hope to achieve and how releasing the old has empowered you.
- **Sensory focus:** Touch (earth), smell (nature), hearing (sounds).

### WEEK 2: WATER CLEANSING AND EMOTIONAL FLOW
**Practice:** Water Ritual
**Location:** Near a natural body of water

**RITUAL**
- **Preparation:** Collect a small bowl of water, essential oils (like lavender or eucalyptus), and a candle.
- **Ceremony:** Light the candle beside the water, and add a few drops of oil. Dip your hands into the water, feeling its coolness as it flows through your fingers. Visualise the water cleansing away emotional blockages or negativity. Splash the water on your face and hands, and relax.
- **Reflection:** Write about the emotional burdens you've let go of and how you feel now.
- **Sensory focus:** Touch (water), smell (essential oils), sight (water reflections).

### WEEK 3: AIR AND BREATH OF LIFE
**Practice:** Wind Meditation and Breathwork
**Location:** A breezy outdoor space (beach, hilltop, park)

RITUAL:

- **Preparation:** Bring a scarf or shawl and a notebook.
- **Ceremony:** Sit comfortably, focus on your breathing, letting it sync with the rhythm of the wind. Visualise the wind carrying away stress or anxiety.
- **Reflection:** Write about how the experience of breathing with the wind has impacted your sense of peace and clarity.
- **Sensory focus:** Touch (wind), hearing (wind sounds), feeling (breath, wind).

### WEEK 4: FIRE AND INNER TRANSFORMATION
**Practice:** Fire Rebirth Ceremony
**Location:** A safe outdoor space for a small fire

RITUAL:

- **Preparation:** Gather twigs, leaves, and pieces of paper to burn.
- **Ceremony:** Write down fears on paper and burn them, visualising transformation.
- **Reflection:** Write about the changes you hope to achieve and how releasing the old has empowered you.
- **Sensory focus:** Sight (fire), touch (warmth), smell (smoke).

## MONTH 2:
## DEEPENING CONNECTION AND PERSONAL TRANSFORMATION

### WEEK 5: CONNECTING WITH ANIMALS AND INNER WISDOM
**Practice:** Animal Spirit Journey
**Location:** A peaceful, natural area with wildlife

RITUAL

- **Preparation:** Bring a journal.
- **Ceremony:** Observe animals quietly and choose one you feel drawn to. Reflect on how its qualities may relate to your life.
- **Reflection:** Write about the wisdom this animal may have offered you.
- **Sensory focus:** Sight (animals), hearing (animal sounds), feeling (connection).

### WEEK 6: PLANTING SEEDS OF INTENTION
**Practice:** Seed Planting Ritual
**Location:** A garden or place where you can plant

**RITUAL**

- **Preparation:** Gather seeds (herbs, flowers, or vegetables), soil and a small shovel.
- **Ceremony:** Hold the seeds in your hand and set an intention—peace, love, strength or whatever you wish to grow in your life. Plant the seeds, imagining your intention taking root in the Earth. Water them, and commit to nurturing both the seeds and your intention as they grow.
- **Reflection:** Write about your intentions and how you'll nurture them in your life, just as you would care for the seeds.
- **Sensory focus:** Touch (soil), sight (planting), smell (earth).

### WEEK 7: MOON PHASES AND FEMININE ENERGY
**Practice:** Moonlight Ritual
**Location:** A space with a clear view of the moon

**RITUAL**

- **Preparation:** Bring a blanket, candle, and notebook.
- **Ceremony:** Meditate on the moon's phases and how they reflect your own monthly cycles. Visualise the moonlight filling you with calm.
- **Reflection:** Write about how the moon's phases resonate with your life changes.
- **Sensory focus:** Sight (moonlight), feeling (calm), reflection (inner cycles).

### WEEK 8: HEALING WITH HERBS AND AROMATICS
**Practice:** Herbal Infusion and Scent Ceremony
**Location:** A quiet space

**RITUAL**

- **Preparation:** Gather herbs into a teapot to prepare an herbal infusion.
- **Ceremony:** Pour boiling water over the herbs and let them steep. Inhale their scent and focus on their calming, healing energy as you sip slowly.
- **Reflection:** Write, draw, or create something symbolic of how the herbs made you feel, noting any insights or sense of wellbeing.
- **Sensory focus:** Smell (herbs), taste (infusion), touch (warm cup).

## MONTH 3:
## INTEGRATION, CELEBRATION, AND WISDOM SHARING

### WEEK 9: WALKING MEDITATION AND EARTH GRATITUDE
**Practice:** Sacred Nature Walk
**Location:** A natural trail, forest or park

**RITUAL**
- **Preparation:** Choose a safe trail and bring a small bag to collect items.
- **Ceremony:** Walk mindfully, collecting meaningful natural items (leaves, feathers). Pause to breathe deeply, listen to nature's sounds, and express gratitude for the Earth's gifts.
- **Reflection:** Create a small nature altar and write about your walk and what you're grateful for.
- **Sensory focus:** Sight (nature), hearing (sounds), touch (collected items).

### WEEK 10: SACRED DANCE AND MOVEMENT
**Practice:** Move or Dance of the Elements
**Location:** A free-moving space indoors or outdoors

**RITUAL**
- **Preparation:** Play music representing the elements (earth, water, air, fire).
- **Ceremony:** Begin in stillness, feet grounded, sensing the Earth.
  - For Earth, move slowly, feel your weight, imagine roots anchoring you.
  - For Water, flow with soft, wave-like movements.
  - For Air, dance lightly, led by breath, as if carried by the breeze.
  - For Fire, move with intensity—fast, dynamic, igniting your inner flame. Let music guide you as you embody each element through movement and presence.
- **Reflection:** Sit quietly after your movement. Close your eyes and sense the energy of each element within you. Then write, draw, or create something from your experience. Note which element you felt most connected to, and how it moved or stirred something in you.
- **Sensory focus:** Hearing (music), touch (movement), sight (visualising the elements).

### WEEK 11: VISION QUEST AND INNER JOURNEY
**Practice:** Inner Vision Quest
**Location:** A quiet, secluded natural area

**RITUAL:**

- **Preparation:** Prepare a small backpack with water, a journal, and a blanket. Choose a place that feels sacred and safe to you, such as a forest clearing or a secluded hilltop.
- **Ceremony**: Find a comfortable place to sit or lie down. Set your intention—perhaps clarity, guidance, or inner wisdom.
  - Close your eyes, breathe deeply and allow your body to soften.
  - Begin your inner journey: Visualise walking through a landscape that feels sacred—forest, desert, ocean, wherever calls you.
  - Notice any animals, symbols or figures that appear—they may carry meaning.
  - Stay in this meditative state for 30-60 minutes. Let your vision unfold gently. Trust what arises.
- **Reflection:** Write, draw or make something about your vision quest experience. Describe the journey, symbols or messages you received, and any insights or feelings that arose.
- **Sensory focus:** Sight (inner vision), feeling (relaxation), hearing (nature).

### WEEK 12: CREATING A PERSONAL SACRED SPACE
**Practice:** Building your Sacred Focus Point
**Location:** A serene indoor or outdoor area

**RITUAL**

- **Preparation:** Gather meaningful objects that represent your journey over the past three months, such as stones, feathers, shells, candles or photos.
- **Ceremony:** Choose a quiet space and cleanse it with sage or incense. Create a focus point with meaningful objects—include representations of earth, water, air, fire and personal symbols of growth. Spend time here daily—light a candle, meditate or sit in silence. Use this space to reflect, set intentions and connect with your inner wisdom.
- **Reflection:** Write, draw or make what this sacred space represents and how it helps you feel connected to your journey inward.
- **Sensory focus:** Sight (objects), smell (incense or candles), touch (sacred items).

**FINAL REFLECTIONS AND CELEBRATION**
**Practice:** Completion Ceremony
**Location:** A joyful, sacred space

**RITUAL**
- **Preparation:** Plan a celebration to mark the completion of your sacred journey. Invite close friends or family members to join you if you wish.
- **Ceremony:** Hold a closing ceremony to reflect on your three-month journey. Share insights, light candles, and speak words of gratitude for your growth. Celebrate with a joyful act—plant a tree, dance, or release something symbolic. Honour your transformation and the deeper connection you've cultivated with yourself and those who've shared the path.
- **Reflection:** Write, draw or make a final journal entry about the journey, your feelings about completing it, and your intentions for carrying this wisdom forward into your life.
- **Sensory focus:** All senses (celebration activities), sight (candles, nature), feeling (joy and connection).

By following this three-month sacred journey, you will cultivate a deeper connection with yourself and nature. Embrace your inner wisdom, and step confidently into your role as a mentor, guide, teacher, or leader.

> *Our deepest fear is not that we are inadequate. Our deepest fear is that we are powerful beyond measure. It is our light, not our darkness that most frightens us.*
>
> **MARIANNE WILLIAMSON**

By embracing this sacred journey, you can step into your role as a mentor, guide, teacher, or leader with confidence and grace—empowered by the accumulated wisdom of your life and the deep connection to the Earth and your inner self.

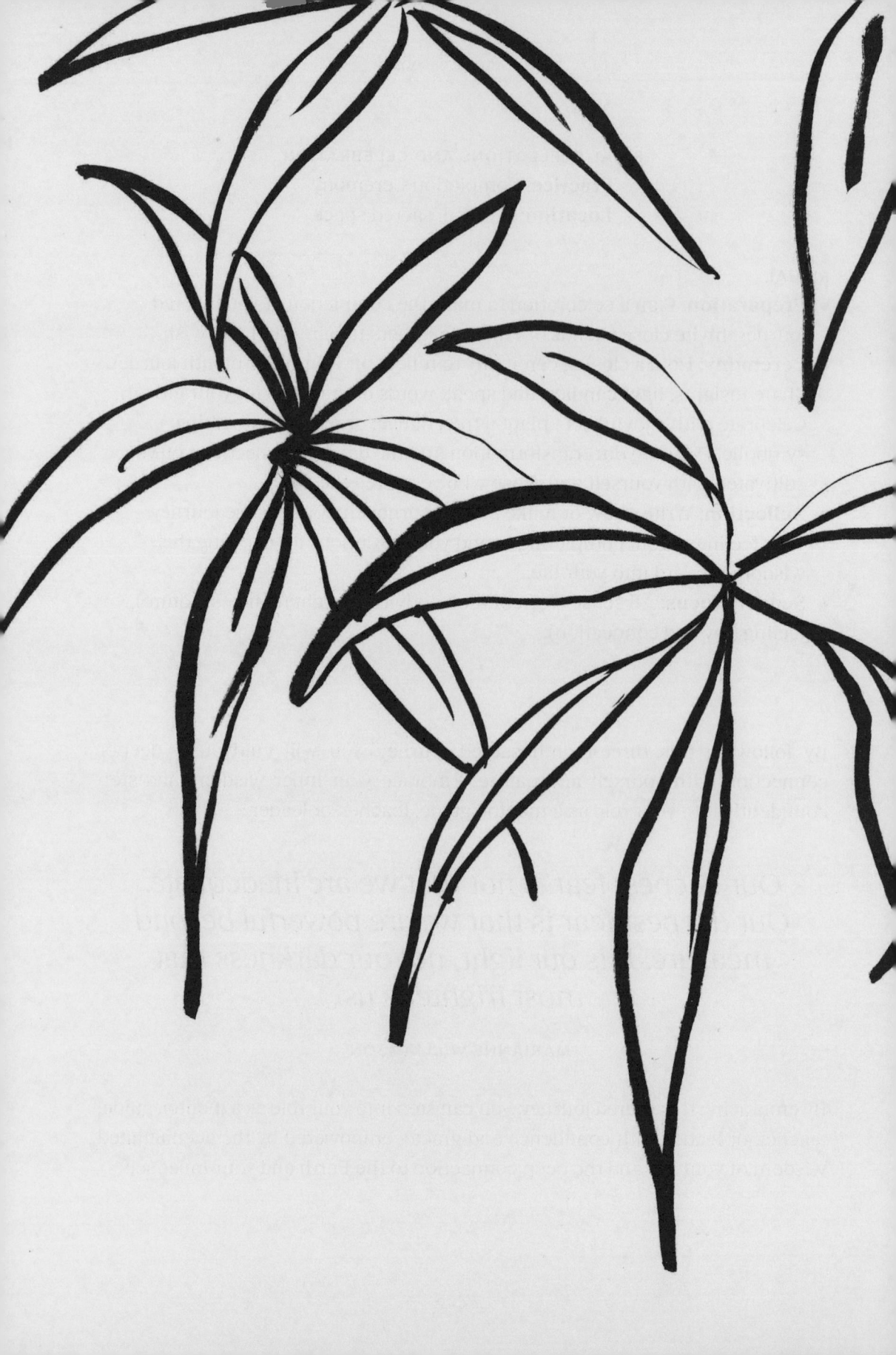

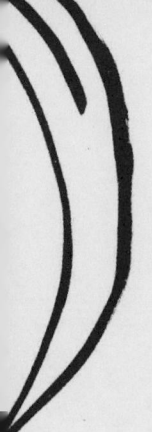

# 2. YOUR HORMONAL HEALTH PILLARS

Welcome to Part Two, where we focus the Spotlight on the Hormonal Health Pillars that form the foundation for balanced hormones. This section is all about turning knowledge into action, providing you with practical, evidence-based strategies to integrate these principles into your life. Consider this your guide to building resilience, restoring balance, and taking proactive steps toward hormonal and overall wellbeing at every stage of your hormonal journey.

**SPOTLIGHT ON:**

EPIGENETICS PAGE 269
OXIDATIVE STRESS PAGE 273
ALCOHOL PAGE 287
PSYCHOLOGICAL STRESS PAGE 290
ADRENAL GLANDS PAGE 334
CORTISOL PAGE 342
TULSI HERBAL TEA PAGE 349
SLEEP PAGE 351
MELATONIN PAGE 367
RESTORATIVE PRACTICES PAGE 372
NOURISHMENT PAGE 393
VITAMINS AND MINERALS PAGE 443
MANAGING TOXINS PAGE 478
MOVEMENT AND EXERCISE PAGE 485

## SPOTLIGHT ON
# Epigenetics

### No-one is you—that is your superpower.

**KARI GRASL**

#### EPIGENETICS AND HORMONAL HEALTH:
#### FROM CONCEPTION TO THE AGE OF WISDOM

The genes we inherit from our parents are fixed for life—one set from mum, another from dad. However, post-birth experiences, lifestyle choices, and stress levels influence how these genes are read and how they support or hinder our daily lives.

For instance, certain genes in some families can dictate a child's susceptibility to stress, Type 2 diabetes, or obesity. It can also determine the likelihood that you may face the same hormonal hurdles as your mother, aunt or sister. The final decider, however, is how well you support these genetic pathways to be the best and most efficient version of themselves through the lifestyle decisions that you make and the food you eat every single day.

Epigenetics is the study of how our cells read and use the genetic messages passed down through generations. It focuses on how the genes we inherit from our parents are either expressed (turned on) or silenced (turned off) through a layer just above the genes, called the epigenome. Much of modern genetic research now explores this layer of gene control, as well as the lifestyle and environmental factors that influence it.

## EPIGENETICS AND WOMEN'S HORMONAL HEALTH

The link between epigenetics and women's hormonal health highlights how lifestyle choices—both our own and those of our ancestors—can shape our wellbeing by impacting the epigenome. Western diets and modern, fast-paced lifestyles have deviated a long way from the natural rhythms of our ancestors. Today's constant stress and reduced physical activity has led to subtle shifts in the epigenetic layer, driving inflammation and contributing to chronic diseases and hormonal imbalances that more and more women experience.

Where and how we live, our lifestyle choices as young adults, and even the choices made by our grandparents can affect our hormonal journey from puberty through to menopause and beyond.

Epigenetic changes can also be passed down through multiple generations. For example, if your grandmother smoked during pregnancy, it may increase your risk of developing asthma. This underscores the long-term impact of lifestyle choices on gene expression and hormonal health across generations. Let's look at how epigenetic factors affect the different stages of your hormonal journey.

## PUBERTY

Puberty marks a critical phase of development where your body undergoes rapid hormonal shifts, shaping not only your physical growth but also influencing your long-term health. During this time, your genetic blueprint interacts with environmental factors, triggering processes that shape your future health—this is where epigenetics comes in. While you can't change your DNA, you can influence how genes are activated, especially during sensitive hormonal stages like puberty.

Key lifestyle factors, including diet, stress management, sleep, and toxin exposure, significantly impact your epigenetic landscape. Poor nutrition or chronic stress during puberty can alter gene expression, increasing the risk of hormonal imbalances or chronic inflammation later. Conversely, adopting healthy habits early can build resilience, reducing the risk of conditions like polycystic ovary syndrome (PCOS), mood disorders or other hormonal challenges.

## THE FERTILE YEARS

The rise in autoimmune diseases during our fertile years is deeply linked to epigenetics. This phase of life creates a 'perfect storm' of hormonal stress, nutritional deficiencies (such as low levels of zinc and iron), and imbalances in oestrogen and progesterone. These factors interact in complex ways, heightening the risk of autoimmune conditions, especially during the postnatal period. Understanding how these elements interact is key to maintaining hormonal balance and preventing health issues later in life.

## PERIMENOPAUSE

During perimenopause, epigenetics plays a key role in how your body navigates hormonal shifts. Lifestyle choices like diet, physical activity, stress management, and toxin exposure directly influence gene expression, affecting symptoms and overall health during this transition.

A diet rich in antioxidants and anti-inflammatory foods—such as fruits, vegetables, whole grains, and healthy fats—can support genes that regulate inflammation and oxidative stress, helping to ease symptoms like hot flushes, mood swings, and weight gain. (See our Spotlight on Nourishment page 393 for advice.) In contrast, a diet high in processed foods, sugar, and unhealthy fats may trigger unfavourable gene expression, worsening symptoms and increasing risks of chronic conditions like cardiovascular disease and osteoporosis.

Stress management is equally important, as high stress levels can lead to chronic inflammation, hormonal imbalances, and negative epigenetic changes. By adopting healthy habits and coping strategies, you can optimise your epigenetic profile, alleviate symptoms, and support a smoother transition into menopause. (See Spotlight on Oxidative Stress on page 273 and Psychological Stress on page 290 for advice on how to become more stress resilient.)

## MENOPAUSE

Epigenetics plays a pivotal role in how the body responds to hormonal changes and how external factors can influence overall health during the menopause. Lifestyle choices, including nutrition, physical activity, sleep and stress management can have a profound effect on gene expression, potentially mitigating some of the common symptoms associated with menopause.

A diet rich in antioxidants and omega-3 fatty acids can promote healthier gene activity and help combat inflammation, which may alleviate symptoms such as mood swings and hot flushes. (See Part One—Menopause on pages 175, 186 and 188 for advice on your food choices during menopause.) Engaging in regular physical activity not only supports hormonal balance but also enhances mood and cognitive function through positive epigenetic modifications. Conversely, negative influences like chronic stress, poor dietary habits and environmental toxins can lead to unfavourable epigenetic changes, increasing the risk of conditions such as heart disease and osteoporosis.

## THE AGE OF WISDOM

Post-menopause marks a significant transition in a woman's life, as hormone levels stabilise after the fluctuations of perimenopause and menopause. Epigenetic mechanisms, such as DNA methylation and histone modification, can influence how genes are expressed, affecting various biological processes, including metabolism, immune response, and cellular ageing.

In the Age of Wisdom, the decline in oestrogen levels can lead to an increased risk of chronic conditions like cardiovascular disease, osteoporosis, and cognitive decline. However, epigenetics offers a pathway for intervention. Lifestyle factors, such as a nutrient-rich diet, regular physical activity, and stress reduction techniques, can positively influence gene expression. For example, consuming a diet high in fruits, vegetables, whole grains, and healthy fats has been associated with beneficial epigenetic changes that support heart health and reduce inflammation. (Turn to Our Ten Core Food Principles on page 396 for more in-depth advice.)

It's also important to maintain a healthy weight during these years. Engaging in resistance training can help improve bone density and metabolic health, counteracting some of the risks associated with post-menopause. On the other hand, adverse factors such as smoking, excessive alcohol consumption, and chronic stress can trigger negative epigenetic changes, potentially exacerbating health issues. (Our chapter on the importance on exercise during the Age of Wisdom begins in Part One on page 247.)

### AGEING AND GENETIC EXPRESSION

As we age, our cells continually regenerate and duplicate our genetic 'instruction manual.' However, each time this occurs, there is a chance for errors, leading to less efficient cell function. Processes like cellular repair and detoxification slows, which becomes more noticeable with age. For example, the alcohol tolerance we once had in our youth fades, and a night of celebration in our 60s may leave us feeling the effects much more acutely. This is because our detox pathways aren't as efficient as they once were.

See our Spotlight on Alcohol (page 287) to help you understand the impact of alcohol on your brain body and hormonal system.

# SPOTLIGHT ON
# Oxidative Stress

There are many different types of stress that can tip a woman's hormonal balance off course, but one of the most disruptive—and least understood—is oxidative stress. In this section, we'll explore exactly what oxidative stress is, what causes it, and how it quietly unpacks the delicate harmony between your hormones. Most importantly, we'll share practical solutions to help you reduce oxidative stress and restore a stronger foundation for lifelong hormonal health and general wellbeing.

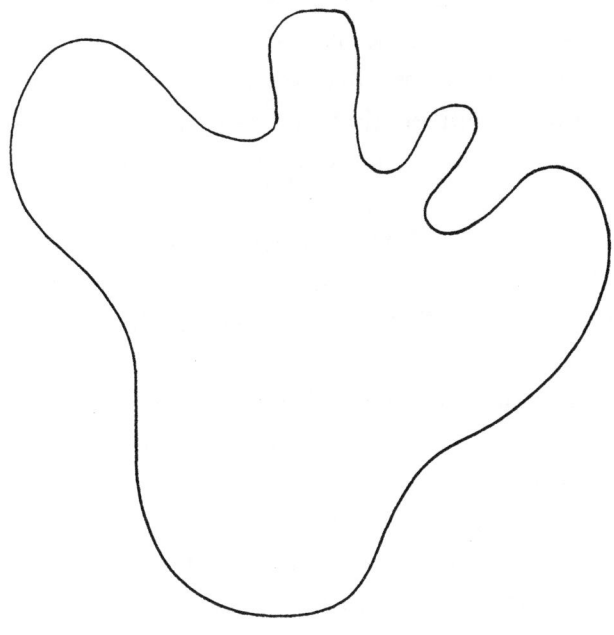

# THE DIFFERENT TYPES OF STRESS

When we think of stress, we often picture that heart-racing feeling before a big meeting or the constant juggle of life's demands. But stress is far more than just a mental or emotional response—it affects your body in multiple ways that are interrelated.

### YOUR EPIGENETIC STRESS LOAD

On a fundamental level, your ability to respond to stress is written into your genetic code. Let's talk about gene variations—small differences in our DNA that can affect how well we handle stress. Some women are born with variations that make it harder to process stress hormones, which can leave them more vulnerable to the negative effects of stress.

These stress response genes can be further influenced by the experiences your mother and grandmother had with stress during their childhood and fertile years, thanks to epigenetic changes passed down through generations (as discussed in our previous Spotlight on Epigenetics).

### OXIDATIVE STRESS

In addition to that, we also must deal with stress on a cellular level. This type of stress is called 'oxidative stress', which is like rust forming in the inside of cells within body organs. Free radicals, unstable molecules, build up from things like energy production and environmental toxins. Normally, our antioxidant housekeepers (more on them soon) clean up these free radicals, but for some women, certain gene variants slow down this clean-up crew, allowing oxidative stress to pile up and make things worse.

It doesn't stop there. Nutritional deficiencies, chemical exposures, and poor lifestyle choices add even more pressure. Our bodies need the right amount of vitamins, minerals and antioxidants to function properly, and when we're running on empty, it's like trying to run a marathon without fuel—eventually, something breaks down.

**PSYCHOLOGICAL STRESS**

Then there's psychological stress—the anxiety that gnaws at us and triggers hormonal shifts. Note that genetics continues to play a part in your stress response. Variants in the COMT gene, which helps break down stress hormones like adrenaline and noradrenaline, can slow this process, leaving some women stuck in a stress cycle that's harder to escape.

Here's the tricky part—when your body experiences psychological stress, it ramps up cortisol levels to catabolic emergency levels. Now acting as a secondary stress hormone, every molecule of cortisol is broken down inside your cells, and leaves behind two free radicals, which contribute to oxidative stress. This extra load on your system doesn't just stop there—it can fuel hormonally driven imbalances, creating a cycle where cellular stress amplifies the risk of disease. By understanding how this cycle works, you can take steps to protect your health and break the pattern. (More on this in our Spotlight on Psychological Stress on page 290.)

By focusing on reducing psychological stress, you can break the cycle and stop feeding the fire that drives oxidative stress. Read on as we drill down into the causes and challenges providing you with deeper solutions and nutritional interventions to help douse any oxidative stress and build cellular resilience from the inside out.

# THE IMPACT OF ALL KINDS OF STRESS ON OUR EPIGENOME

Elevated cortisol acts as both an epigenetic switch and a volume control. Once activated by the body's stress response, unfavourable genes can be expressed loudly, for example, with a diagnosis of an autoimmune disorder like severe rheumatoid arthritis.

On a positive note, managing our body's stress response effectively is part of the solution to turning down the volume on unfavourable genes, improving our chances to experience remission from disease. Learning and building good stress management strategies can be an invaluable investment in our hormonal and overall wellbeing. A high burden of stress hormones puts another demand on cell cleanup pathways, as free radicals are generated in the process of our cells having to deal with adrenaline surges and a build-up of elevated cortisol.

# OXIDATIVE STRESS EXPLAINED

As science delves deeper into the origins of chronic diseases, one thing is clear; many diseases begin with a tiny spark of inflammation, often driven by oxidative stress. Think of it as a slow-burning fire within our cells, quietly causing damage long before symptoms appear. For women, this is particularly important because oxidative stress plays a major role in health challenges like breast and ovarian cancers, endometriosis, thyroid dysfunction and cognitive decline.

Imagine a healthy cell being attacked from the inside by **free radicals**, also known as **reactive oxygen species (ROS)**. These free radicals are produced as part of daily cellular waste (rubbish) and are normally neutralised by your body's housekeeping antioxidant enzymes (more on that soon). But when too many free radicals build up, they overwhelm the cell's ability to neutralise the damage—and your cell begins to rust from the inside out.

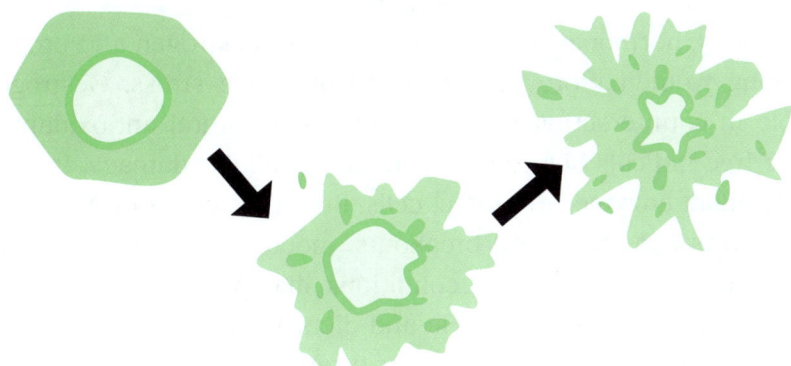

This damage may affect the nucleus (where your genetic blueprint is stored), and the cell membrane (which helps the cell function normally). As the harm escalates, the cell sends out an SOS to the immune system. What begins as a small spark becomes a fire. For women with certain genetic vulnerabilities, this fire can spread, leading to unhealthy tissue and an increased risk of cancer. In other women, the immune system gets confused, tagging healthy cells as damaged, which may trigger an autoimmune attack. This is how oxidative stress can spiral, deeply affecting your health.

### YOUR HORMONES AND OXIDATIVE STRESS

Oestrogen is a powerful ally in protecting women from oxidative stress, acting as a natural antioxidant by neutralising free radicals (ROS) and boosting key antioxidant enzymes like superoxide dismutase (SOD) and glutathione peroxidase (GPx). This protection is especially important during the Fertile Years when oestrogen levels are higher, helping maintain cell health and reducing the risk of oxidative stress-related diseases such as heart disease and cognitive decline. Other hormones also play a role. Progesterone has anti-inflammatory properties that calm oxidative damage. Melatonin is a potent antioxidant that declines with age. DHEA supports immune function and reduces oxidative damage, and insulin helps manage oxidative stress by regulating blood sugar. Together, these hormones work to keep oxidative stress in check throughout a woman's life.

### OXIDATIVE STRESS THROUGH YOUR HORMONAL JOURNEY

As women move through the different stages of life each phase brings its own unique hormonal shifts, and with those changes come challenges to cellular health.

### PUBERTY

During puberty, hormonal surges, particularly of oestrogen and progesterone, make young women more vulnerable to oxidative stress. Oestrogen plays a key role in counteracting this by acting as a natural antioxidant, helping neutralise free radicals before they can cause cellular damage. It also boosts your antioxidant enzymes to protect cells. But in the chaos of hormonal shifts, oxidative stress can still cause breakouts, mood swings, and in some cases, contribute to the incubation of conditions like polycystic ovary syndrome (PCOS) and endometriosis. Lifestyle and dietary choices at this stage set the foundation for managing oxidative stress throughout life.

### THE FERTILE YEARS

During your Fertile Years, oestrogen protects you from oxidative damage by preserving egg quality and supporting fertility. Its antioxidant effects slow egg ageing, improving conception chances and reducing early pregnancy complications. However, unmanaged oxidative stress can disrupt hormone balance, affecting fertility, menstrual cycles, and contribute to conditions like adenomyosis and fibroids. Just as some women show signs of ageing externally, oxidative stress can prematurely age your eggs. Managing oxidative stress is vital for fertility, slowing skin ageing, and reducing chronic disease risks.

Progesterone also plays a key role. With anti-inflammatory effects, it acts like a fire extinguisher, calming inflammation caused by oxidative damage and supporting cellular health.

### PERIMENOPAUSE

As perimenopause nears, hormonal shifts, especially oestrogen dominance in **Phases One and Two** (higher oestrogen with low progesterone), fuel oxidative stress. This 'perfect storm' can increase risks to breast cells, which divide faster under high oestrogen, amplifying free radical damage and the risk of breast cancer.

Oxidative stress also worsens symptoms like weight gain, mood swings, and irregular cycles. The thyroid is especially vulnerable, with oxidative damage triggering conditions like Hashimoto's thyroiditis. Hormonal fluctuations during this stage make managing oxidative stress critical for overall health.

### MENOPAUSE

With menopause comes a significant drop in oestrogen, and with it, a rise in oxidative stress. Oestrogen's protective antioxidant effects fade, leaving cells more vulnerable. Without the hormonal shield of oestrogen, cells dehydrate, becoming more like sultanas than the plump grapes they once were. This cellular dryness contributes to the visible signs of ageing, such as wrinkles and reduced skin elasticity, as well as vaginal discomfort.

The stakes are higher for your heart and brain, as oxidative stress increases the risk of heart disease and cognitive decline without oestrogen's antioxidant shield. Declining melatonin, a key antioxidant, further weakens your defences against oxidative damage. Managing oxidative stress during menopause is essential for both appearance and long-term health.

### THE AGE OF WISDOM

In this stage, defences against oxidative stress decline further as oestrogen, progesterone, and DHEA levels drop. This raises the risk of chronic diseases like heart disease, arthritis, diabetes, and immune dysfunction. Without oestrogen's protection, ovaries become more vulnerable to oxidative stress, heightening the risk of ovarian cancer, especially in the first decade post-menopause. (See Ovarian Health on page 524.)

Focusing on oxidative stress management and maintaining balanced insulin levels is vital. High insulin leads to oxidative damage through advanced glycation end products (AGEs). Proper insulin and blood sugar regulation reduce oxidative burden, supporting health in this phase of life.

### THE GOOD NEWS

To keep oxidative stress in check within our cells nature has given us two tools:

1. A genetic blueprint that tells you how to make and maintain three housekeeping teams of enzymes whose only job is to mop up the free radical that cause oxidative stress inside our cells, neutralising the threat.

2. Food containing antioxidants: These molecules are literally the antidote to intracellular damage caused by oxidative stress, and powerful enough to protect you from diseases like cancer, dementia and diabetes.

### CELL HOUSEKEEPING

Imagine your cell is a household—a relatively clean house still produces waste that needs to be removed every day. The dust and grime that builds up is manageable if cleared regularly but can become a much bigger task if left for weeks and can even encourage disease as old food waste decays. This is exactly what happens within the home of your body cells. There is a background of activity for every cell as they go about the daily business of maintaining your body. Some cells create hormones for you. Others, like liver cells have a special role in clearing toxins, especially alcohol, while also needing to protect themselves from damage.

Your body's natural cleanup crew is composed of antioxidant enzymes.

There are three key 'housekeeping' families:
- **Manganese superoxide dismutase (MnSOD):** Powered by manganese, this enzyme protects against oxidative damage.
- **Glutathione pathway**: Selenium is essential for this enzyme to work efficiently in detoxifying your cells.
- **Catalase:** This iron-driven enzyme neutralises harmful molecules to maintain cellular health.

Some women have inherited variations in their genetic blueprint that give them instructions to produce more efficient housekeeping enzymes to keep cells clean. If you are one of these lucky ones, then your playground for 'breaking the rules' of good health choices is a little bigger. If you inherit less efficient versions of these antioxidant enzymes, you may pay a heavier price for stepping outside the boundaries of healthy habits. However, none of us can rest on our laurels—as we age, these antioxidant processes inevitably slow down. Nutritional gaps and unbridled stress will make all women more vulnerable, some earlier in life than others.

### THE CORTISOL-OXIDATIVE STRESS CONNECTION

Cells that process cortisol are highly vulnerable to oxidative stress from the free radicals this process generates. While not all cells carry this burden, cortisol regulation occurs in the adrenal glands and liver, as expected. Surprisingly, kidney, fat, brain and breast cells also process cortisol, producing two potent free radicals (superoxides) for every cortisol molecule. This cortisol-breast connection explains why breast cells are so vulnerable to unhealthy changes. This can happen under long-term stress, which produces elevated cortisol and drives oxidative stress.

## WELLNESS ACTION PLAN
# REDUCE OXIDATIVE STRESS

By implementing the following plan, you can keep your cells clean, reduce oxidative stress, and improve your overall health. The steps ahead aren't complicated, yet breaking old habits can be challenging.

These actions will pave the way for a healthier future, helping protect your cells and support your wellbeing as you navigate life, all the way to your Age of Wisdom.

There are three steps to improve the efficiency of these cellular cleanup teams:

1. **Reduce the production of free radicals:** Less rubbish produced, less cleaning work to do.
2. **Provide the nutritional support that drives them to work efficiently:** Your trace minerals.
3. **Increase your antioxidant-rich foods:** This reduces the load for your housekeeping enzymes.

Now let's drill down into the details:

### REDUCE DAILY PRODUCTION OF FREE RADICALS

Producing free radicals can overwhelm the system, leaving more 'rubbish' behind. The key is to lower the amount of rubbish generated in the first place.

**ACTION STEPS**

- **Reduce alcohol consumption:** Alcohol metabolism generates free radicals. Cutting back lightens the load for your body's cleaning crews, allowing them to focus on more important tasks. (Read more on alcohol in our Spotlight on Alcohol on page 287.)

- **Manage psychological stress:** Chronic stress ramps up cortisol, which in turn increases free radical production. Managing stress helps reduce the oxidative mess, giving your antioxidant team some relief. (Our Spotlight on Psychological Stress starts on page 290.)

- **Minimise chemical exposure:** Everyday chemicals in products can generate free radicals. Choosing natural alternatives means less debris for your body to clear. (Read more on how to reduce your toxic load on page 483).

- **Avoid processed and fried foods:** These foods introduce unhealthy fats (such as trans fats) and additives, creating extra waste.

- **Avoid cigarette smoke:** Smoking floods the body with free radicals, overloading your system. Take extra care with second- and third-hand smoke exposure as these can often be worse.

- **Sensible sun exposure:** UV rays from too much sun create a cascade of free radicals. Find practical tips on skincare on page 193.

- **Balanced exercise and movement routine for your hormonal stage:** Over-exercising produces cortisol, adding to free radical load. (Read more on page 485.)

**NUTRITIONAL SUPPORT THAT DRIVES YOUR ANTIOXIDANT HOUSEKEEPING TEAM**
Increase the minerals manganese, selenium and iron—they are non-negotiable support nutrients for your antioxidant enzyme team.

**ACTION STEPS:**
- **Manganese:** Increase intake of mussels, brown rice, pineapple, nuts like hazelnuts and pecans, and spinach.

- **Selenium:** This mineral is crucial for your antioxidant housekeepers and multitasks as a thyroid and pregnancy support nutrient. Increase these foods: Brazil nuts (the richest natural source of this essential mineral), seafood like sardines, prawns, shrimp and white bait (a favourite for our New Zealand tribe).

- **Iron:** Crucial throughout all phases of your hormonal journey and, as with any nutrient, the 'more isn't better' rule applies—finding your sweet spot is key, so avoid supplementing without a good reason. Have your iron levels checked, and review the information in Spotlight on Iron on page 449 to optimise iron levels.

### INCREASE YOUR ANTIOXIDANT-RICH FOODS

**ACTION STEPS:**

Here are the top 10 antioxidant-rich foods that can help reduce oxidative stress, particularly supporting breast, ovarian, and overall hormonal health:

- **Berries (blueberries, strawberries, raspberries)**—Packed with vitamin C and flavonoids, they help combat oxidative stress and support hormonal balance.
- **Dark leafy greens (spinach, kale)**—Rich in vitamins A, C, and E, these greens promote detoxification and protect hormone-producing cells.
- **Nuts (especially almonds and walnuts)**—High in vitamin E, which is essential for protecting cell membranes from free radicals—especially helpful for brain, breast and ovarian health.
- **Turmeric**—Contains curcumin, a powerful anti-inflammatory antioxidant that supports hormonal health and reduces oxidative damage.
- **Cruciferous vegetables (broccoli, cauliflower, Brussels sprouts)**—Rich in sulforaphane, which helps detoxify oestrogen and supports breast health.
- **Pomegranate**—Rich in polyphenols and ellagic acid, pomegranates have strong antioxidant properties that support breast and ovarian health by reducing oxidative stress and helping to regulate oestrogen levels
- **Avocados**—High in healthy fats and glutathione, an important antioxidant that helps protect cells from oxidative damage.
- **Citrus fruits (oranges, lemons, grapefruits)**—Loaded with vitamin C, which helps neutralise free radicals and supports collagen production, essential for skin and tissue health.
- **Tomatoes**—Rich in lycopene, an antioxidant linked to reduced risk of breast and ovarian cancers.
- **Flaxseeds**—Contain lignans and omega-3 fatty acids that support hormonal balance and reduce oxidative stress, particularly in breast tissue.

Incorporating these foods into your diet can help protect your cells from oxidative stress and support overall hormonal health.

> **TIP**
>
> Feed your body with powerful nutrients, and watch it transform oxidative stress into strength.

### SPECIFIC HERBAL SUPPORT

**Sulforaphane (EnduroCell):** There is solid evidence supporting the use of natural therapies that support antioxidant and liver detox pathways. Sulforaphane, an extract from broccoli sprouts activated by its enzyme myrosinase, has been shown to reduce oxidative damage in ovarian cells—an exciting discovery. Traditionally used to help balance oestrogen dominance, sulforaphane also acts as a SOD inducer, enhancing your body's natural antioxidant defences and improving the efficiency of cellular cleanup, ultimately reducing the burden of oxidative stress.

**GliSODin:** A powerful plant-based antioxidant enzyme made from French melon extract, combined with a wheat protein called gliadin to improve absorption in the body. This makes it more effective at neutralising harmful free radicals, especially in hormone-sensitive areas like the breasts, ovaries and skin.

These products are available online or through naturopathic and integrative doctors.

## YOUR OXIDATIVE STRESS CHECKLIST

The Wellness Action Plan on page 282 is your *starting point* to reduce oxidative stress—use it as a foundation and layer additional strategies based on the following checklist. Remember, not every tip will apply to every woman. This checklist will help you personalise your plan and direct you to relevant chapters for further action. If you have multiple vulnerabilities, you'll need to put in more effort to control oxidative stress and protect your health and wellbeing throughout your hormonal journey.

- **Are you experiencing disruption in your oestrogen levels?** Oestrogen is your top antioxidant hormone. Symptoms of oestrogen dominance or deficiency can be found on page 75, along with solutions and support.

- **How healthy is your liver?** The liver works together with your antioxidant housekeeping families. Its detox pathways are essential for metabolising and recycling fertility hormones, and safely clearing out chemicals and toxins. (For more on liver support, see Liver Care on page 592.)

- **Medical history?** If you have the following medical conditions, be sure to focus on the information in the relevant chapter
    - PCOS (page 546)
    - Endometriosis (page 534)
    - Insulin Resistance (page 564)
    - Cancer (see Breast Cancer on page 578 and Ovarian Health on page 526.)

As you progress from your Fertile Years to the Age of Wisdom, revisit this list. Your vulnerabilities will shift with fluctuations in your oestrogen levels, gut health and nutritional choices—adjusting your approach will help you minimise the risk of hormonal challenges along the way.

Throughout each hormonal phase, from puberty to menopause, oxidative stress influences health outcomes. Hormones like oestrogen, progesterone, melatonin, DHEA, and insulin provide protective layers, but as they decline, managing oxidative stress is crucial for cell protection and hormonal balance.

## Start today!

Adopting small, daily habits early, such as healthy eating, stress management, and self-care, sets a strong foundation for long-term health. It's never too late.

SPOTLIGHT ON
# Alcohol

**LET'S TALK ABOUT ALCOHOL**

While social gatherings bring friends and family together to connect and relax, they often centre around sharing a favourite wine or cocktail. While we all enjoy these times of fun and celebration it is essential to be very aware that alcohol is not as harmless as it may seem. When it comes to alcohol, its impact on women's hormones and overall health should not be taken lightly. Certain cells are particularly vulnerable to the oxidative stress caused by alcohol, creating a domino effect on hormonal balance.

**Liver:** Responsible for metabolising alcohol, the liver endures oxidative stress, which disrupts hormone metabolism. It's crucial for breaking down excess hormones like oestrogen, but alcohol puts your liver under pressure, which throws a massive curve ball on your hormonal balance. Women battling symptoms of oestrogen dominance will amplify their symptoms as alcohol adds fuel to the fire.

**Breast cells:** These are highly sensitive to alcohol. As the liver processes alcohol, acetaldehyde—a harmful byproduct—reaches breast tissue, causing oxidative stress and increasing oestrogen levels, which can raise the risk of breast cancer. In Australia the Cancer Council warns that even small amounts of alcohol increase cancer risk, and the risk escalates with higher consumption. The Council does not provide a guideline for safe consumption. Alcohol also reduces your ability to absorb folate, which is vital for DNA repair and breast health.

**Heart, immune and kidney cells:** Alcohol stresses heart muscle cells, raising cardiovascular disease risks. Immune cells and kidneys also struggle, especially as hormonal changes occur with age. The kidneys, crucial for blood pressure and fluid balance, face added strain.

## HOW MUCH ALCOHOL IS OKAY?

Sadly, the information on the damage alcohol does to our bodies means our 'normal' alcohol habits have to change. If you are healthy and want to stay that way, limit alcohol to one standard drink per day (this is about half a bottle of wine each week). Your liver will thank you for one or two days off each week.

Binge drinking more than four drinks in any one day is even worse for your hormonal and general health—there is an increased risk of breast cancer of nearly 30% and increased risk of heart attack close to 70%.

### 'STANDARD DRINK' DEFINITIONS:

In Australia and New Zealand, a standard drink contains 10 g of pure alcohol. The UK adopts even tighter guidelines, defining a standard drink as just 8 g, (nearly half the 14 g used in the USA).

One standard drink of 10 g equates to:
- 250 ml of beer (5% alcohol content)
- 100 ml of wine (13% alcohol content)
- 30 ml of distilled spirits (40% alcohol content).

### INDIVIDUAL CONSIDERATIONS:

Personal health, family history and advice from healthcare professionals play a vital role in shaping decisions about alcohol consumption. Recent guidelines from the World Health Organization (WHO) and other health authorities stress that no level of alcohol is completely safe. There is growing evidence linking even moderate intake to serious health risks like cancer, liver disease, cardiovascular problems, and mental health disorders. In short, alcohol disrupts hormonal harmony and your wellbeing, making balance harder to maintain.

While an occasional drink may be fine, be mindful of its impact on your hormones and overall wellbeing no matter your hormonal stage of life. If you are struggling with hormonal health, chronic disease or already feel that alcohol is impacting your life and relationships then you may need to tighten the boundaries on alcohol or stop altogether. This is especially relevant in Phase Three of perimenopause, through the menopause transition.

# If you're struggling to manage symptoms, try planning a 'dry month' and see how your body feels after giving it a well-deserved holiday from alcohol.

Should you find your relationship with alcohol to be problematic, be honest with yourself. Be brave and seek support from a recognised support group listed in our Resources section on page 691.

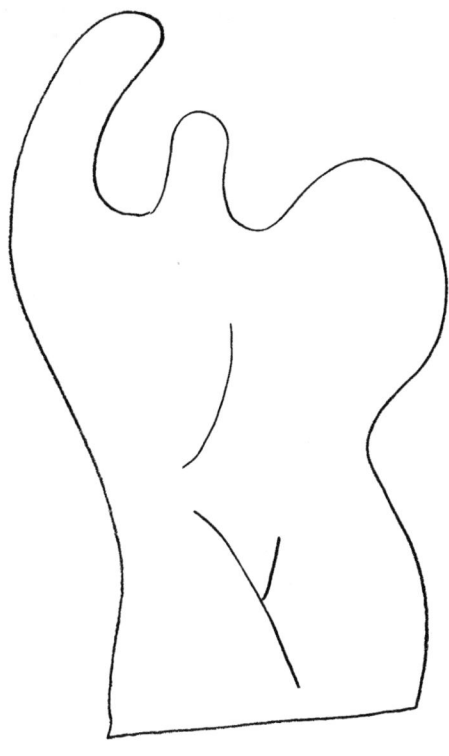

## SPOTLIGHT ON
# Psychological Stress

Psychological stress is a universal experience that transcends all stages of life. While the pressures we face may vary—a teenager preparing for final exams, a woman dealing with fertility issues—the core truth remains the same. Regardless of the pressures, learning to moderate our body's stress response is essential as we age. These pressures include emotional challenges, self-doubt, financial, work and family pressures along with every curve ball life throws our way.

Learning self-management tools that support us to become resilient in the face of these challenges will help us to moderate and manage our body's stress response more effectively—this is a superpower worth learning and practising.

# LET'S TALK ABOUT STRESS!

Our goal is to guide you in transforming stress from something that controls you into a force you can manage, ultimately leading to better hormonal health and optimal wellbeing.

### STRESS: THE HORMONAL DISRUPTOR

Stress is one of the primary disruptors of hormonal balance, particularly during key hormonal stages such as puberty, your Fertile Years, perimenopause, and menopause. Excessive stress hormones, like adrenaline and cortisol, can wreak havoc on progesterone and oestrogen levels, contributing to conditions such as PMS, endometriosis, PCOS and even cancers. In menopause, stress amplifies symptoms like hot flushes, brain fog, and increases the risk of serious conditions like dementia and osteoporosis. Therefore, managing stress is vital to maintaining hormonal balance and reducing oxidative stress.

## UNDERSTANDING EUSTRESS AND DISTRESS

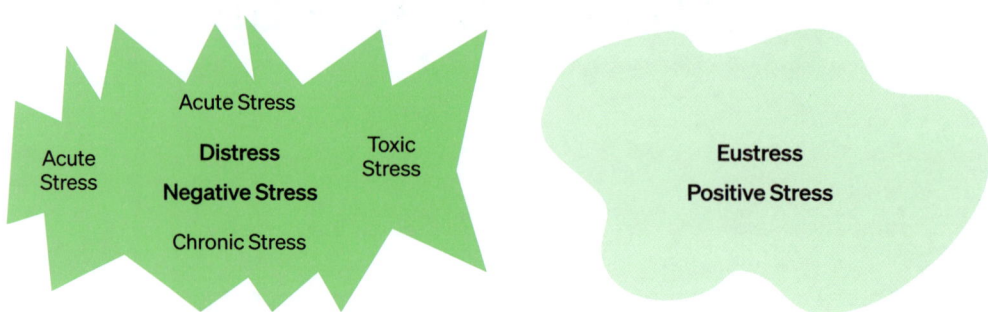

### EUSTRESS
Not all stress is harmful. Eustress, or positive stress, is a healthy level of stress that motivates and excites you. This is the stress that drives you to meet deadlines or achieve goals. We refer to this as the 'Purple Zone' (more on this later) where stress hormones are more regulated, keeping you productive and engaged.

### DISTRESS
Distress, on the other hand, is referred to as the 'Red Zone' (more later). This feels overwhelming, as it causes the body to continuously flood with stress hormones, leaving you feeling anxious, reactive and unable to cope. Chronic distress can disrupt the body's natural processes, leading to long-term health issues like hormonal imbalances, metabolic disruptions, oxidative stress, and a weakened immune system. Distress is women's greatest adversary.

### ACUTE AND CHRONIC STRESS
Acute stress occurs when you face a sudden event—like someone tapping you on the shoulder unexpectedly, a mouse darting between your legs as you clean, or receiving shocking news. In these moments, your body floods your bloodstream with adrenaline, triggering an automatic reaction. If such moments are rare, your body recovers quickly.

Chronic stress, however, is ongoing. It's the stress that accumulates over time due to incessant worrying, work pressures, financial worries, or difficult relationships. Chronic stress keeps your body on high alert, disrupting your hormones and overall health. This chapter will help you recognise when stress turns toxic and how to intervene.

### REAL VS IMAGINED STRESS

Your brain doesn't know the difference between what's real and what's imagined. This is why you can feel anxious just by imagining a stressful situation. Similarly, if you close your eyes and focus on imagining eating a very sour lemon, you will probably salivate even though the lemon is not real. Your thoughts and perceptions are a key moderator (or activator) of your ability to avoid toxic stress.

### THE NERVOUS SYSTEM: YOUR PATH TO BALANCE

#### YOUR JOURNEY TO SELF-REGULATION

Psychological stress is not life-threatening stress. Even if we think any situation is critical or serious, if it is not a life-or-death situation, it is categorised as psychological stress. This can be caused by many events in life; relationship challenges, work pressures, family illnesses, grief, and loss etc. However, the research is clear, how you think about what is happening, can either turn the volume up (activating toxic stress) or down (maintaining eustress). So, even if the situation is dire, your thoughts, perceptions and emotional regulation have the power to escalate or regulate your stress response.

> A common exception is domestic violence, a multifaceted complex stress. Should any woman find themselves a victim of this insidious horror we strongly encourage seeking professional support. (See our Resources section on page 691 for more information.)

In this chapter, we've set the stage for your self-revolution. By learning to self-regulate, you can break the cycle of toxic stress, improve your hormonal health, and enhance your wellbeing. The following chapters will guide you through practical tools and exercises to help you stay balanced, even in the face of life's pressures.

### HOW TO BALANCE YOUR NERVOUS SYSTEM

To begin (or continue) your journey of self-revolution you need to be able to self-regulate in difficult situations and this begins with understanding your body.

There are two branches to your nervous system:

1. SYMPATHETIC
2. PARASYMPATHETIC

They each play a different role to activate your body's systems. One branch (sympathetic) is designed to keep you safe, and the other branch (parasympathetic) is designed to keep you healthy. In today's fast-paced, pressurised world we are often pushed into the sympathetic branch in a perceived need for safety. Unfortunately, we often fail to balance the system by not activating the parasympathetic branch often enough, thereby sacrificing our health. This chapter will help you to understand more about the two branches and how to find the balance in order for you to keep your entire body's system, including your hormones, balanced.

To keep this simple, we have provided a colour-coded way for you to become aware of what part of the nervous system you are in. This way you can learn how to self-manage and regulate your hardwired stress response into a zone of productivity and the zone of healing.

### SYMPATHETIC NERVOUS SYSTEM

Let's start with the sympathetic branch (think S for Stress). This is the only branch that can activate your adrenal glands to enable you to produce the stress hormone adrenaline and elevate cortisol. We would like you to think of the sympathetic nervous system in two colours.

1. RED ZONE
2. PURPLE ZONE

#### THE RED ZONE

This is where your blood stream is 'dumped' with a significant amount of stress hormones and as a result you experience 'acute' or 'toxic distress'. This is your body's very clever survival tactic (in the event of life-threatening danger) to allow you to fight-or-flight to survive. Stress hormones are very powerful chemical messages that create priority urgency in your body. They make you very reactive and are designed to save your life. Problem is, you can activate this ancient hardwired system when you are not in mortal danger and probably do it unconsciously when someone takes your car park at the shopping centre.

Think of the Red Zone as Code Red in your body, everything else gets put on hold and your behaviours and communication get hijacked. You become very egocentric and lose your sensitivity to the feelings of others. You also become very narrow in thinking (fight-or-flight), which is what the Red Zone is designed for—to get you out of danger.

### THE PURPLE ZONE

Purple is Eustress. Your brain will activate the ideal 'drip feed' of stress hormones to enable you to stay grounded and maintain your centre. In the Purple Zone you are more in tune with others, you think more globally, which allows you to respond positively to your challenges. This is ideal to keep you motivated, collaborative and creative.

### THE PARASYMPATHETIC NERVOUS SYSTEM

The other arm of the nervous system is the parasympathetic—we refer to this as the Blue Zone.

### THE BLUE ZONE

Think P for Peace, as the parasympathetic has no capacity to activate your adrenal glands. Therefore, you are unable to make stress hormones when this part of your nervous system dominates. Often called the 'rest and digest' system, this is where your body recovers and repairs itself. This is your very own extraordinary healing system, inbuilt and part of your body's innate wisdom. All you need to do is activate this part of your nervous system and your body knows what to do—it's hardwired into your genes.

## Your body is only ever in one Zone at any one time, yet it can move from one Zone to another very quickly.

Remember the Zones in this way:

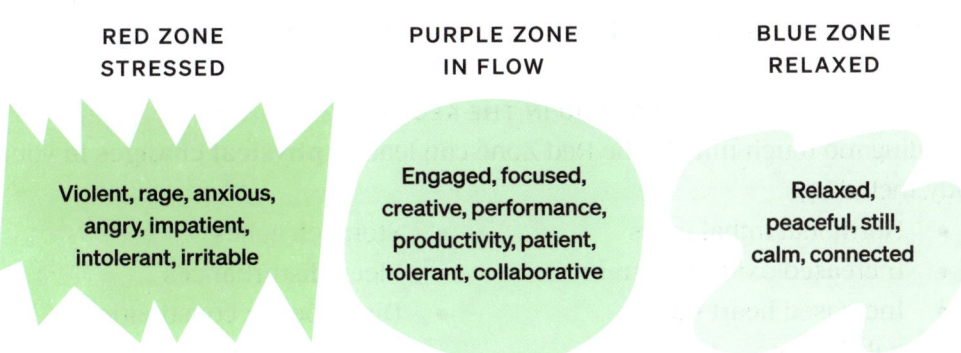

| RED ZONE<br>STRESSED | PURPLE ZONE<br>IN FLOW | BLUE ZONE<br>RELAXED |
|---|---|---|
| Violent, rage, anxious, angry, impatient, intolerant, irritable | Engaged, focused, creative, performance, productivity, patient, tolerant, collaborative | Relaxed, peaceful, still, calm, connected |

**Red:** A 'dump' of too many stress hormones resulting in you losing your centre and becoming too reactive.

**Purple:** A 'drip feed' of stress hormones—not too much, not too little—to keep you motivated, grounded, and centred.

**Blue:** No stress hormones. Ideal for you, rest and relax, and give your body time and space to recover and heal. This is the only part of the nervous system where all the healing activation happens. Without Blue Zoning, true healing, recovery and hormone balance cannot happen.

## WHAT CAN THE ZONES FEEL LIKE

### RED ZONE

Imagine waking in the morning, your eyes still closed, already preoccupied with the day ahead. The persistent buzz of worry might sound like, 'So much to do, so little time'. This kind of thinking is perceived by the brain as a threat, propelling you into the Red Zone within milliseconds.

Really? Yes! Simply thinking can elevate you to the Red Zone.

The brain continuously interprets messages and images from the mind, distinguishing between safe and unsafe thoughts. Often, it activates the Red Zone as if confronting a genuine threat.

The brain cannot differentiate between what is real and what is imagined. Have you ever woken from a nightmare? Notice how your heart races, your breathing quickens, and you feel disoriented and scared? You're in bed, physically safe—unless someone unexpected is in the room. Your physical location is secure, but the mental stimulus from your subconscious has triggered the Red Zone. This phenomenon occurs in conscious states as well; you might be physically safe, yet your mind is overwhelmed with unhelpful or ruminating thoughts.

### ARE YOU IN THE RED ZONE?

Spending too much time in the Red Zone can lead to **physical changes** in your body, including:

- Hormonal imbalances
- Increased oxidative stress
- Increased heart rate or palpitations
- Higher blood pressure
- Muscle tension
- Frequent illnesses
- Stomach aches
- Sleep disturbances
- Diarrhoea or constipation
- Fatigue or exhaustion
- Headaches
- General aches and pains
- Changes in appetite or weight

**Mental and emotional signs** of extended time in the Red Zone may include:
- Irritability
- Impatience
- Intolerance
- Frustration
- Anxiety, fear, or worry
- Feeling overwhelmed
- Anger or rage

Other signs might be:
- Sadness
- Crying
- Loss of pleasure in previously enjoyed activities
- Feelings of depression
- Hopelessness
- Difficulty retaining information
- Unwanted repetitive negative thoughts
- Poor concentration
- Scattered thoughts

Reacting from a brain hijacked by perceived danger can adversely affect your behaviour, hindering your communication and negotiation skills. You might find yourself feeling panicky, uncertain, or overly reactive to both minor and significant issues.

Do you overreact when your kids leave the fridge door ajar? Have you felt frustrated or shouted at them? Are you easily irritated by coworkers' minor mistakes? These examples illustrate how small irritations can amplify when you're in the Red Zone.

### WHY YOU NEED TO DE-STRESS

Your body is not designed to spend excessive time in the Red Zone. Think of it as an emergency lane with flashing lights and warning signals. Prolonged time in the Red Zone can deteriorate your physical, mental, emotional, and hormonal balance.

### HOW TO EXIT THE RED ZONE AND FIND YOUR CENTRE

1. Name the emotion you're experiencing (for example, anger, frustration).
2. Practice cyclic breathing for 10 cycles (see Breathwork on page 383).
3. Observe your thoughts and perspectives (see Self-Revolution on page 309).
4. Suspend judgement—you might be missing relevant information or context in your reactive state.
5. Repeat from Point 1 until you feel centred again.

## Today, I will not stress over things I can't control.

**SHARON KOLKKA**

**PURPLE ZONE**

In the Purple Zone, you may feel:
- Motivated
- Creative
- Focused
- Calm
- Patient
- Tolerant
- Cooperative
- Collaborative
- Respectful

The Purple Zone is where productivity and performance thrive. In this state, you find your 'centre', approaching work and family challenges with calm enthusiasm, patience and tolerance. Here, you're motivated, open to others' ideas, and engaged in creative collaboration.

    To maintain this mindset, self-regulation is essential. Staying in the Purple Zone while getting things done is key to achieving good health, productivity, and performance in your daily life.

## Time is urgent, let's slow down.

**AFRICAN SAYING**

This quote may seem contradictory, but when we mindfully approach our to-do lists while maintaining the Purple Zone, we create space for new insights. Instead of reacting impulsively, as we might in the Red Zone, the Purple Zone offers clarity, creativity, and ingenuity—tools that help us navigate life's challenges from a fresh perspective.

## We cannot solve our problems with the same thinking we used when we created them.

**ALBERT EINSTEIN**

## MAINTAINING THE PURPLE ZONE AT WORK

Neuroscience shows that our attention spans wane after about 90 minutes. Even if you feel productive, mistakes and lapses in creativity can occur without these necessary breaks.

To stay focused and in the Purple Zone, set a timer for 90 minutes. After this period, take a short break to stretch, hydrate with water or herbal tea, and engage in intentional breathing to dip into the Blue Zone. This practice prevents you from slipping into the unproductive Red Zone.

## THE BLUE ZONE

Your body maintains a baseline level of cortisol, which is aligned with your natural circadian rhythm. Importantly, it's physically impossible to produce adrenaline or increase cortisol levels in this part of your nervous system—and that's a good thing!

In the Blue Zone, you're likely to feel:
- Peaceful
- Relaxed
- Calm
- Reassured
- Patient
- Loving
- Creative
- Content
- Able to gain perspective

Spending time in the Blue Zone allows your body to:
- Balance hormones
- Neutralise oxidative stress
- Build and enhance your immune system
- Protect gut microbiome
- Improve sleep quality
- Enhance nutrient absorption
- Heal and repair cellular functions
- Foster a sense of contentment and relaxation
- Increase telomerase production (more on this in the next chapter)

Being calm and relaxed is your natural state, so aim to spend ample time in the Blue Zone.

> **HOW TO RECHARGE YOUR BLUE ZONE**
>
> Consider your time in the Blue Zone like charging your digital devices. Just as your phone requires regular recharging to function optimally, your body also needs time to recharge and repair.
>
> If your phone runs low on battery, you'll likely scramble to find a charger to get it working again. Similarly, when your energy levels dip, you might reach for caffeine, sugar, or other stimulants to get through fatigue. However, if you don't recharge your body properly, you'll lack the energy needed for healing and replenishment.
>
> When your phone's battery is nearly depleted and you can only charge it for five minutes, you can expect limited functionality. The same applies to your body. You need sufficient time in the Blue Zone to fully recharge.
>
> The busier you are, the more you need to prioritise time in the Blue Zone to balance your nervous system.

### DO YOU SPEND ENOUGH TIME IN THE BLUE ZONE?

While quality sleep contributes to your time in the Blue Zone, it's not enough on its own. You need additional time for rest and recovery from your busy life. This can include small breaks throughout your day as well as larger blocks of time dedicated to recharge. (See our Wellness Action Plan activating your Blue Zone on page 373.)

### YOU'VE GOT A FRIEND IN ME

The Blue and Purple Zones work with support from the prefrontal lobe—your brain's 'CEO'. This area helps manage impulsive reactions, keeping you out of the Red Zone and in the Purple Zone when you are getting things done.

When activated, the prefrontal lobe enhances optimism, collaboration, creativity, curiosity, and openness. It enables you to handle complex tasks, engage in deeper learning, and approach challenges philosophically.

Your CEO and 'social' brain help you return to the Blue Zone, fostering safety and emotional intelligence. This awareness enables meaningful connections and a deeper sense of purpose, leading to a greater appreciation of life.

Research shows that regular meditation increases prefrontal lobe activation, promoting calm. (See page 386 for more on meditation.)

| ZONE | DESCRIPTION | STRESS HORMONE LEVEL | EFFECTS | BENEFITS/RISKS |
| --- | --- | --- | --- | --- |
| Red Zone | Excessive stress leading to overwhelm and reactivity. | High levels of stress hormones. | Loss of centre, increased reactivity, and difficulty coping. | Can lead to burnout and decreased mental/physical health. |
| Purple Zone | Optimal stress that keeps you motivated and centred. | Balanced 'drip feed' of hormones. | Motivated, grounded, and engaged in activities. | Enhances performance, resilience, and productivity. |
| Blue Zone | Absence of stress hormones, allowing for recovery and healing. | Minimal to no stress hormones. | Rest and relaxation, healing activation occurs. | Essential for recovery, mental clarity, and physical health. |

**A NOTE ON ALCOHOL**

Your alcohol consumption can significantly affect your prefrontal lobe's ability to function as the CEO of your brain.

### NORMAL VS NATURAL

Sometimes it's the most capable, successful women who push the limits of stress without even realising it. Constant pressure becomes the norm—especially when everyone around them is living the same way. But while this high-alert state may feel normal, it's far from natural. Without time in their Blue Zone, they remain stuck in overdrive. It can feel healthy and proactive—until the body sends a hormonal SOS that things are not OK.

The best and most desirable response to stress is to feel centred or in control without reaching your breaking point. If you do reach your breaking point, you can regain control through equanimity. (See next chapter, page 311, for more on equanimity.)

### ARE YOU THINKING YOURSELF STRESSED?

Are your thoughts racing throughout the day? Are you paying attention to the present moment? Remind yourself every day that your body is not a machine; it's a biological organism with its own wisdom. When you honour your body's needs and practise self-regulation, you can maintain a sustainable work-life balance.

### RESTING BRAIN STATE

Like your heart rate, human beings have brain waves and a resting brain state. An elevated resting brain state can signal a nervous system that's always on guard, making it difficult to relax.

### DO YOU FEEL 'WIRED BUT TIRED'?

If your nervous system is agitated, it becomes more challenging to enter the Blue Zone. To alleviate this state, prioritise spending time in the Blue Zone to lower your resting brain state.

### IT'S ALL ABOUT YOU

Your health and wellbeing should be your top priority. Known as 'me time,' this concept involves more than just good food and regular exercise. It also means managing your nervous system so that you can spend time in the Blue Zone to rest and recover.

## Think you don't have time to relax? Consider this: Do you have time to be ill?

If your health falters—physical, emotional or mental—everything else in life can start to unravel. Your family, career, finances and relationships all become harder to hold, and your hormonal balance is often the first to suffer. That's why your health and wellbeing are sacred—not a luxury, a necessity.

Self-preservation is not selfish; it's an act of love. When you're thriving, everyone around you benefits. Yet, time and again, we've seen women push through exhaustion, overriding their bodies' messages, only to end up burnt out, sick or emotionally spent.

Most are living too often in the Red or Purple Zone—high-output, high-stress states. Rarely do we spend enough time in the Blue Zone, where the body can rest, restore and repair. Without regular recovery, something will eventually break down.

We've all inherited the message that resting equals laziness. But it's time to rewrite the script: 'strategic rest is essential'. Time to simply 'be'—to laugh, nap in the sun, lie on the grass, cuddle loved ones—is what fills your tank and keeps you going.

If you're ignoring the warning signs in your body, ask yourself honestly: would you ignore a red flashing light in your car? Or would you stop, investigate, and fix the issue before it becomes worse?

Your body is no different. Both for yourself, and for your children—model a sustainable way to live.

### ARE YOU BEING HONEST WITH YOURSELF?

If you're honest with yourself, you'll know when it's time to pause. Be brave enough to feel what's underneath the pace. Your honesty is where the healing starts. When you name it, you can no longer ignore it. From there, your self-revolution begins. (Read more on this from page 309.)

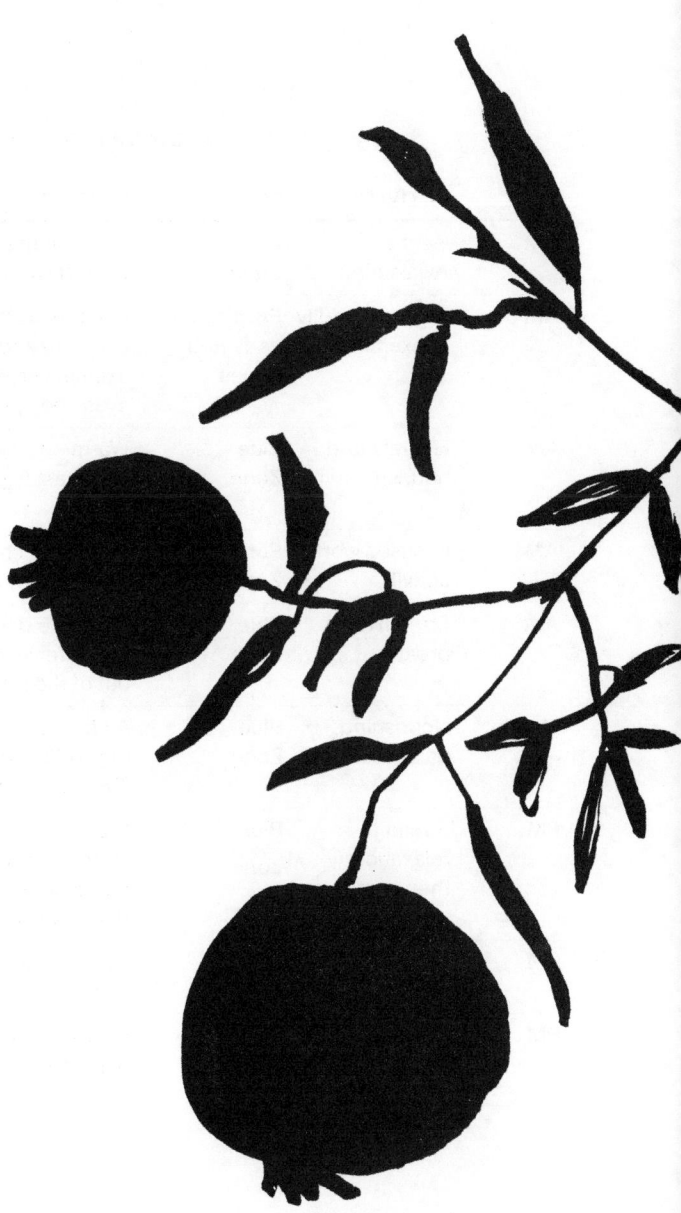

# YOUR DESTRESS TOOLKIT

**YOUR DAY IN THE ZONES**

| TIME | ACTIVITY | ZONE | DETAILS |
|---|---|---|---|
| AM | Gentle Awakening | Blue Zone | 5–10 minutes of deep breathing or guided meditation to start the day calmly. |
| AM | Move mindfully or exercise | Purple and early Red Zones | Light movement like yoga or a walk outdoors to energise and balance cortisol. Also, time for cardio exercise program. Remember to let sunlight into your eyes and spend time in nature. |
| AM | Hydrate and nourish | Blue Zone | Warm water with lemon followed by a hormone-balancing breakfast (e.g. eggs with avocado, or a green smoothie). |
| AM | Focused work/ activity | Purple Zone | Engage in challenging but enjoyable tasks to keep stress hormones at a balanced 'drip feed' level. |
| AM | Stretch and breathe | Blue Zone | 5-minute break to stand, stretch, and breathe deeply to regulate your nervous system. This will help keep you out of the Red Zone. |
| Lunch time | Nourishing, balanced meal | Blue Zone | A fibre-rich lunch with lean protein and healthy fats (e.g. grilled chicken with quinoa and vegetables). Time in nature. |
| PM | 5-minute relaxation then continue working | Blue Zone | Practise mindful breathing or step outside for fresh air to promote calm digestion. If you've been working stepping away from your desk can help you avoid the Red Zone. |
| PM | Light movement | Purple Zone | Gentle movement like walking to avoid energy slumps and regulate cortisol. |
| PM | Healthy snack | Blue Zone | Snack to balance blood sugar (e.g. a handful of nuts of hummus and crudities). |

## PSYCHOLOGICAL STRESS

| TIME | ACTIVITY | ZONE | DETAILS |
|---|---|---|---|
| PM | Creative time | Purple Zone | Low-stress creative activity (e.g. journaling, reading) to maintain balanced stress hormones. Play with the kids. Time in nature. |
| PM | Balanced, nutrient-dense dinner | Blue Zone | Magnesium-rich foods like sweet potatoes with grilled fish and spinach to support relaxation. |
| PM | Non stimulating entertainment | Blue Zone | Watching TV, listen to a podcast, read a book, time in nature or watch the sunset. |
| Evening | Unwind without screens | Blue zone | Time to put screens to bed, relaxation, meditation or deep breathing, to wind down your nervous system. |
| Bedtime | Evening ritual | Blue Zone | Calming bedtime routine (e.g. magnesium bath, shower, self-care ritual) to prepare for a restful sleep. |
| | Magnesium or herbal tea | Blue Zone | Herbal tea (e.g. Tulsi Tea) to promote deep relaxation. |
| | Sleep | Blue Zone | 7–9 hours of restorative sleep for hormonal balance and recovery. |

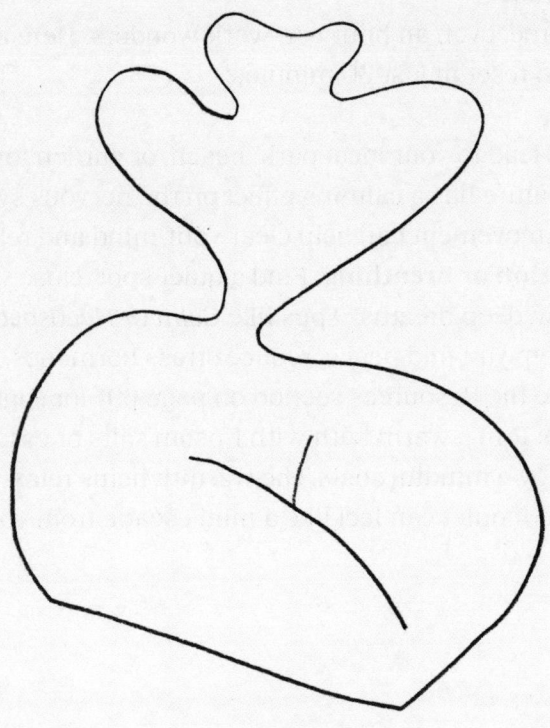

# TIME OUT FOR SELF-CARE

By now, you've likely realised the importance of taking some 'me-time'. Here, we offer a few ideas to help your body rebalance during this transition. Remember, if you break, everything around you breaks! If this feels indulgent, try reframing it as self-preservation. The kindest thing you can do for your loved ones is to take care of yourself—reassuring them that you're well now and will continue to be in the future.

Here are some practical, achievable options for time out and self-care, whether you have just an hour or a long weekend:

**1 The one-hour reset**
If you're short on time, even an hour can work wonders. Here are some simple, yet effective ways to reset in just 60 minutes:

- **A nature walk:** Head to your local park, beach, or garden for a quiet, peaceful walk. Nature has a calming effect on the nervous system, and the fresh air and movement can help clear your mind and relieve stress.
- **Mindful meditation or breathing:** Find a quiet spot, close your eyes, and focus on slow, deep breaths. Apps like *Calm* or *Headspace* offer guided meditations to help you find peace, reduce stress hormones, and reset your mental state. (See the Resources section on page 691 for suggestions.)
- **A soothing bath:** Run a warm bath with Epsom salts or essential oils, light a candle, and enjoy a mindful soak. The warmth helps relax your muscles, and this moment of quiet can feel like a mini escape from your day.

## 2  A half-day recharge

If you can find a longer block of time, such as an afternoon, here are a few ideas to rejuvenate yourself:

- **Spa at home:** Turn your home into a personal spa. Use that face mask you've been saving, do a hair treatment, and spend time pampering yourself. Taking care of your body and skin can make you feel recharged.
- **Unplug from technology:** Take a few hours to disconnect from your phone, emails, and social media. Use this time to read, journal, or sit in silence. Stepping away from the constant digital noise can be surprisingly refreshing.
- **Creative projects:** Engage in a creative activity like painting, knitting, or gardening. Creativity gives your brain a break from routine and can be a therapeutic way to relax.

## 3  The full-day retreat

When you can dedicate a full day to yourself, you have the chance to create a true retreat experience without even leaving town:

- **A day trip to a quiet spot:** If you live near a beach, lake, or forest, pack a lunch and take a solo day trip. Bring a book or journal and spend the day in nature. This change of scenery can feel like a mini vacation and is a great way to reset your stress levels.
- **Book a massage or bodywork session:** Treat yourself to a massage or acupuncture session. The physical relief combined with mental relaxation helps recharge you. Bodywork can also release built-up tension from stress.
- **Volunteer work:** Sometimes, helping others can give you a new perspective and help reset your own mind. Volunteering, even just for a day, offers a mental break from your usual responsibilities and brings fulfilment.

## 4  The long weekend escape

For the ultimate reset, take a full weekend or long weekend for yourself.

- **Staycation in a nearby hotel or Airbnb:** Sometimes, just getting out of the house for a night or two is all you need. Book a stay close by so that you're not grappling with travel and create your own peaceful getaway. Use the time to read, sleep in, take long walks and enjoy the quiet.

- **Weekend retreat at home:** Plan a weekend retreat without leaving your home. Let everyone know you're unavailable for two days, turn off devices, and immerse yourself in restful activities—long baths, meditation, journaling or sleeping in. Set the scene with soft lighting, calming music, and maybe even a schedule of planned relaxation.

### 5   Ongoing micro-breaks

Even if you can't take a full day or weekend away, incorporating regular micro-breaks into your routine can help keep stress hormones manageable:

- **Morning or evening rituals:** Create daily rituals, like enjoying a quiet cup of tea in the morning or stretching before bed. These small, consistent moments build pockets of calm into your day.
- **Lunchtime recharges:** Take your lunch break seriously! Step outside for a walk, read, or listen to music. Avoid working through your break—it's time to recharge.
- **Power naps:** If needed a 15–20-minute nap can recharge your energy, especially when stress is high. Naps are okay providing they don't interfere with your night time sleep routine.

No matter how much or how little time you can carve out, the key is prioritising yourself—even if it's just for a moment each day. These practical, easy 'time-outs' offer the relief and reset your mind and body need to stay resilient in the face of life's demands. Remember, it's not about escaping forever; it's about creating small spaces to breathe, recharge and come back stronger.

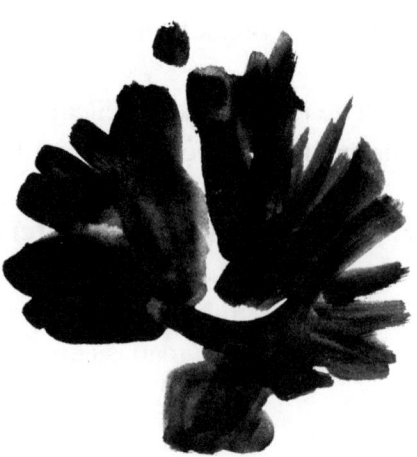

# SELF-REVOLUTION

You can't start the next chapter of your life if you keep re-reading the last one.

**MICHAEL MCMILLIAN**

### THE PAST

We are born, experience highs and lows, and develop a perspective of life based on our past. This creates the story we tell ourselves. Your story may be one of hope or of shame. We become a product of our environment and experiences. 'Become' in that sentence is key—this perspective is not who we are, it has merely shaped our view. Love, rejection, shame, happiness, and trauma all impact how our brains are wired and how we feel in the world. Unknowingly, we live today through the lens of our past, and whether positively or negatively shaped, this influences how we manage stress and uncertainty, as well as daily challenges.

> Our past is a story existing only in our minds.
> Look, analyse, understand, and forgive.
> Then, as quickly as possible, chuck it.

**MARIANNE WILLIAMSON**

### RESHAPE YOUR BRAIN

Both ancient spiritual teachings and modern neuroscience offer insight into how we can transform the narrative of our lives. The spiritual masters encouraged their students to 'wake up' and move beyond conditioned responses, while neuroscience shows us that we can literally change the structure of our brains through our thoughts and perceptions.

Positron emission tomography (PET) scans and functional MRIs reveal how different areas of the brain activate when we think in specific ways. Research shows that these thought patterns can reshape the brain, impacting what we notice and focus on in life. Whether you engage with these changes through spiritual practice or scientific understanding, the result is the same; you can rewire your brain by changing how you think and perceive the world.

This opportunity is a powerful one. You can train your brain to focus on the positives, helping you create a more balanced and fulfilling life. In essence, you can reshape your brain's wiring to create new neural pathways and reduce any negative patterns that may have developed over time. This chapter will focus on how you can embrace this opportunity for self-transformation, changing your life from the inside out.

### HOMEOSTASIS—BALANCE IN THE BODY

Homeostasis is like a tightrope walker gracefully balancing on a high wire, constantly adjusting to stay upright no matter how the wind blows. Your body operates the same way, making tiny corrections to keep everything steady and functioning. For example, when you exercise and your body heats up, it's like a gust of wind—the tightrope walker shifts their weight (you start sweating) to restore balance. This delicate act keeps critical factors like heart rate, blood pressure and things like temperature, pH, and glucose levels within a safe range, ensuring all your body's systems remain in harmony, no matter what challenges come your way.

However, stress can disrupt homeostasis. When you experience stress, your body triggers a fight-or-flight response, releasing hormones like adrenaline.

This pushes you into the Red Zone, which is designed for short-term stress but can cause health problems when activated for extended periods. Chronic stress elevates cortisol, and the constant bombardment of adrenaline makes it harder for your body to return to a balanced state, leading to issues such as high blood pressure, weakened immune function, and metabolic imbalances like disrupted blood glucose levels.

Maintaining homeostasis under psychological pressure requires effective self-regulation techniques, such as fostering mental calmness (equanimity), prioritising relaxation activities (Blue Zone), getting good sleep, and leading a balanced, healthy lifestyle.

### EQUANIMITY—BALANCE IN THE MIND

Just as homeostasis maintains physical balance within the body, equanimity serves as a crucial mechanism for balancing the mind. It refers to mental calmness and evenness of temper, particularly during challenging situations. Equanimity enables you to face psychological pressure with clarity and resilience instead of being overwhelmed by your emotions.

By promoting mental calmness and composure, equanimity helps reduce psychological pressure minimising the physiological response, like the release of adrenaline. This can prevent you from entering the Red Zone—this in turn supports physical homeostasis, keeping key bodily functions like heart rate, blood pressure, and glucose levels stable.

### UNDERSTANDING EQUANIMITY

Equanimity does not mean suppressing emotions or becoming indifferent. Rather, it is the ability to analyse situations and events as they are unfolding and choose to respond in a curious and calm manner rather than giving in to a knee-jerk mental tirade resulting in an often-unnecessary emotional reaction. This allows you to maintain a broader perspective on any unfolding situation with a sense of calm, giving you the ability to figure out the best steps to take towards resolution. It's about cultivating a balanced perspective, even when life presents both positive and negative circumstances. We can refer to this as 'maintaining your centre'.

### THE SCIENCE BEHIND EQUANIMITY

Equanimity is possible because of the brain's capacity to regulate emotional responses. The prefrontal cortex, responsible for rational thought, works to quiet the amygdala—the brain's emotional centre. This allows you to moderate pressure and emotional triggers once you have taught yourself and rewired your brain to do this. Practices such as mindfulness and meditation can strengthen the connection between these regions, enhancing your ability to maintain equanimity during stressful situations. These changes foster a mental environment where equanimity can thrive, helping you navigate life's challenges with greater stability.

Studies show that mindfulness practices can lead to structural changes in the brain, reducing both the size and reactivity of the amygdala.

## THE AMYGDALA

This is a small, almond-shaped cluster of nuclei located deep within the temporal lobe of the brain. It plays a crucial role in processing emotions, particularly those related to survival, such as fear and pleasure. The amygdala is part of the limbic system, which is responsible for our emotional responses and memory formation.

One of the primary functions of the amygdala is to detect and respond to potential threats. When you encounter a threatening situation, the amygdala quickly evaluates the sensory information and triggers the fight-or-flight.

The amygdala is also involved in forming and storing emotional memories. It helps you remember emotionally charged events more vividly than neutral ones, which can be crucial for learning from past experiences and avoiding future dangers. For example, if you have a frightening experience with a dog, your amygdala can make you more cautious around dogs in the future. When life has delivered very difficult experiences and trauma, the amygdala enlarges, on-guard continuously, and sometimes over-reacting to insignificant events; this is often referred to as 'amygdala hijack'.

Additionally, the amygdala influences social behaviour and decision-making by processing social signals like facial expressions and body language. It helps you interpret the emotions of others, which is essential for navigating complex social interactions.

Overall, the amygdala's purpose is to ensure your survival by processing emotions, detecting threats, and helping you remember significant experiences. Its ability to rapidly respond to potential dangers and encode emotional memories makes it a vital component of the brain's emotional and survival mechanisms.

# Quietening an over-reactive amygdala caused by pain and trauma is a positive step in any self-revolution project.

### REWIRING YOUR BRAIN—THE SCIENCE OF NEUROPLASTICITY

Neuroplasticity is your brain's ability to reorganise itself by forming new neural connections. This process can occur at various levels, from cellular changes involved in learning to remapping in response to injury. Neuroplasticity is driven by your experiences, thoughts, perceptions, emotions, and behaviours. When you learn something new or think in a different way, your brain creates new pathways and strengthens existing ones. Conversely, pathways that you don't use regularly can weaken or fade away.

This means that through conscious effort, you can train your brain to create positive patterns, reshaping your life's narrative and unlocking greater mental and emotional wellbeing, and fulfilment.

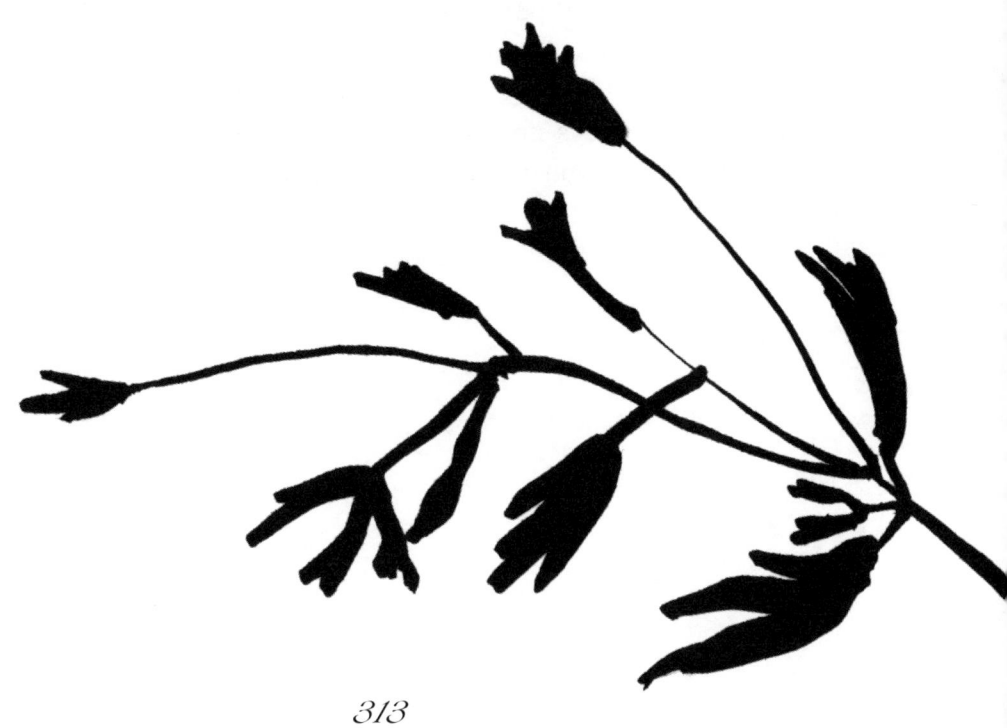

# STRESS RESILIENCE

Stress resilience is the ability to bounce back from adversity. By developing resilience, we can better maintain equanimity during difficult times. Techniques such as positive self-talk, setting realistic goals, and seeking social support can enhance our resilience.

The way you think today is shaped by your early childhood environment, societal influences, and education. Your thought processes are also influenced by both positive and negative experiences throughout your life, such as the thrill of falling in love or the challenges of dealing with trauma.

Many of us think in habitual patterns, which significantly impact the structure and function of our brains. The way your brain is wired now reflects your regular thought and perception patterns. Engaging in negative thoughts, such as rumination or self-criticism, can reinforce neural pathways associated with anxiety and depression. Conversely, positive and constructive thinking can strengthen the pathways linked to resilience and happiness. By deliberately shifting your thinking, you can foster beneficial changes in your brain's wiring.

## ACTIONS TO EMBRACE A GROWTH MINDSET

A growth mindset is the belief that abilities and intelligence can be developed through effort and learning, promoting neural growth. When you embrace your challenges and persist through setbacks, your brain forms new connections and strengthens existing ones. This mindset fosters resilience and a love of learning, enhancing your overall mental agility and cognitive wellbeing.

- **Mindfulness:** A powerful practice that involves being present and fully engaged in the moment without judgement. Research shows that regular mindfulness practice can significantly alter your brain's structure. It has been found to increase the density of grey matter in brain regions associated with learning, memory, and emotional regulation. Mindfulness is the practice of bringing your full attention to the present moment even when doing tasks and work.

- **Positive thoughts:** Enhance neural pathways related to wellbeing. By consciously acknowledging the positive experiences in your life, even the simplest ones, you reinforce the networks associated with happiness and reduce the impact of negative thinking.

> CTRL + ALT + DEL
> CONTROL YOURSELF
> ALTER YOUR THINKING
> DELETE NEGATIVITY.
> — JUST ME

- **Practice gratitude:** One of the most transformative practices you can adopt is gratitude. Regularly acknowledging and appreciating the positive aspects of your life can foster a sense of contentment and stability. Research has shown that practices like keeping a gratitude journal can help balance negative emotions and enhance overall mental wellbeing.

**CASE STUDY**
# Kate

I grew up in the 1960s with parents who seemed more focused on my mistakes than my achievements. In a desperate attempt to feel loved, I fell in love with a boy as a teenager, which led to an unplanned pregnancy. My beautiful baby girl was taken from me at birth and put up for adoption, leaving me heartbroken and filled with guilt and trauma. Years later, I was fortunate to reconnect with my daughter, and today we share a loving relationship.

Despite this, I struggled with trauma, often feeling unworthy and seeing the dark side of life. One day, a friend suggested I take a photo every day for a year of something I was grateful for and create a montage (before social media made it a trend). Months into my gratitude project, I showed her a picture of a pair of socks, explaining how they saved me from blisters on a long hike. She laughed when I told her I had learnt gratitude could come from recognising simple joys—a gorgeous sunrise, a bee on a flower, or the smile of a friend.

Many factors contribute to the extraordinary happiness I experience today, and I feel blessed. Those 365 'grateful photos' played a significant role in my inner transformation, yet the most profound change came from altering the story I told myself about my life. I now see myself as a wonderful mother, sister, and friend, believing I am worthy. This new narrative has made a tremendous difference, helping me navigate life's highs and lows with joy and gratitude.

## COGNITIVE BEHAVIOURAL THERAPY (CBT)

CBT is a powerful evidenced-based tool for rewiring your brain. It involves identifying and challenging negative thought patterns and replacing them with more positive, realistic ones. This practice not only changes the way you think, but it also modifies the underlying neural circuits. By consistently applying CBT techniques, either with a trained therapist or as a self-guided practice, you can quiet your amygdala and reshape your brain's response to stress and anxiety, promoting mental wellbeing.

- **Start your day with positive affirmations:** One of the simplest yet most effective CBT techniques is to use positive affirmations. Begin your day by repeating affirmations like, 'I am capable and strong', 'I can handle whatever comes my way and 'This is new territory, but I've got this', or 'One step at a time I will become more comfortable with the unknown'. Tell yourself 'I am worthy', 'I deserve good in my life'. Placing these statements where you can see them frequently, like on your bathroom mirror or desk, helps set a positive tone for the day and counteracts negative self-talk. Repeating these affirmations daily helps rewire your brain to focus on your strengths and potential.

- **Challenge negative thoughts:** Throughout your day, be mindful of negative thoughts. When you catch yourself thinking negatively, challenge that thought. Ask yourself, 'Is this based on fact or fear?' or 'What evidence do I have that this is true?' By questioning the validity of your negative thoughts, you can replace them with a more balanced and rational perspectives such as, 'Mistakes help me to learn, providing me with the chance to improve and gain wisdom.'

> Interpersonal experience shapes the mind as it continues to develop throughout the lifespan. Interactions with the environment, especially relationships with others, directly shape the development of the brain's structure and function.
>
> DANIEL J SIEGEL MD, NEUROPSYCHIATRIST

## CASE STUDY
# Kathleen

Kathleen, a high-powered executive, had been living in a constant state of overwhelm. Between managing a demanding career, taking care of her family, and trying to maintain some semblance of personal balance, she was burning the candle at both ends. Her energy was plummeting, and the once-driven, vibrant woman now found herself drained, short-tempered, and barely able to make it through the day. Her naturopath mentioned 'adrenal fatigue' and 'burnout', but while Kathleen recognised the symptoms, she didn't know how to fix it.

Then she stumbled across an article that explained how our thoughts physically reshape the brain—a concept that left her curious. Could her constant stress and anxiety be creating a feedback loop, wiring her brain into more negativity? And more importantly, could she reverse it?

The article introduced the idea of neuroplasticity—the brain's ability to rewire itself based on the thoughts we focus on. In that moment, Kathleen realised she wasn't powerless; she could change her brain by changing her thoughts.

But how? The first step Kathleen took was to become aware of the negative patterns running on autopilot in her mind. She noticed that her default mode was to constantly worry about what might go wrong. Whether it was work-related pressures, her kids' futures, or her own health, her thoughts were filled with 'What if?' fears. These anxious thoughts created a cycle of stress, activating her brain's alarm systems day in and day out.

With this awareness, Kathleen started to consciously disrupt the pattern. Here's how she did it:

### REPLACING 'WHAT IF?' WITH 'WHAT IS'

Instead of allowing her mind to spin into endless 'What if this project fails?' or 'What if I'm not good enough?', she began grounding herself in the present moment.

She'd ask, 'What is actually happening right now?' If she was in a meeting, she'd focus on the facts of the discussion, rather than imagining all the ways it could go wrong. This shift calmed the constant activation of her stress response, teaching her brain to focus on reality, not catastrophes.

### TURNING SELF-CRITICISM INTO SELF-COMPASSION

Kathleen noticed a constant critical voice in her head, always berating her for not doing enough or not being enough. Anytime she made a mistake, her inner dialogue was ruthless: 'How could you let that happen? You're so disorganised.' But through daily practise, she learned to stop those thoughts and replace them with compassion. When she'd slip up, she would stop, take a slow deep breath in, and tell herself, 'You're doing your best, and that's enough.' Over time, this softened her internal dialogue, by cementing new neural pathways that connected to more positive self-talk. The more she practised, the easier it became, reducing the stress hormones that resulted from her old habit of self-criticism.

### SWAPPING 'I HAVE TO' FOR 'I CHOOSE TO'

Kathleen also realised that her language around obligations was draining her energy. She often said, 'I have to finish this report' or 'I have to take the kids to soccer'. This made her feel trapped by her responsibilities, which increased her stress. She started rephrasing these thoughts with more empowering language, such as 'I choose to take my kids to soccer because I value family time'. This small shift gave her back a sense of control and made her obligations feel less burdensome.

### REPLACING WORRY WITH GRATITUDE

One of the most powerful changes Kathleen made was replacing her tendency to ruminate on future problems with gratitude for the present. Every time she caught herself worrying about what might happen, she'd pause and name three things she was grateful for in that moment. For example, during a stressful workday, instead of thinking, 'I'll never get through all of this', she'd stop and remind herself, 'I'm grateful I have a job I love, a supportive team, and the skills to handle this.' Gratitude became her go-to tool to shift her focus, reducing her stress levels almost immediately.

### PRACTISING MINDFUL PAUSES INSTEAD OF REACTING

Kathleen also noticed how reactive she had become. The smallest disruption—an unexpected email or a family request—could trigger her stress response.

Instead of reacting instantly, she began taking a few deep breaths before responding. This simple practice of creating space allowed her brain to keep her centred and regulated, giving her the clarity to respond with calm rather than panic.

### TRANSFORMING PERFECTIONISM INTO PROGRESS

Finally, Kathleen replaced perfectionism with striving for excellence. She realised that perfectionism did not tolerate any mistakes, and she had always pushed herself to meet impossibly lofty standards, which contributed to her chronic stress. She started replacing thoughts like 'This has to be perfect' with 'This is a work in progress.' She reminded herself that growth comes from action and with mistakes comes wisdom, not flawless execution. This mindset shift helped her feel more relaxed, allowing her to make progress without the weight of constant self-imposed pressure.

### REWIRING THE BRAIN

Over the months, as Kathleen practised these new thought patterns, she noticed something remarkable—she wasn't as tired anymore. Her energy started to return, and she felt more resilient in the face of daily pressure. The regular fight-or-flight Red Zone feelings she had lived with for so long began to fade, replaced by a sense of calm and control.

What was happening inside her brain was even more fascinating. Evidence from PET scans and functional MRI research show that the areas of the brain involved in positive thinking and emotional regulation become stronger and more active with time. Kathleen was potentially creating new neural pathways, allowing her brain to focus more on positivity and resilience rather than fear and stress. Kathleen's story is a powerful example of how you can actively participate in rewiring your brain. By shifting your thoughts and perceptions, whether through spiritual practices, mindfulness or clinical meditation all by using the latest insights from neuroscience, you can reshape your brain, your hormones, and your life from the inside out.

## WELLNESS ACTION PLAN
# ABC OF STRESS RESILIENCE

Kathleen's successful self-revolution was based on following a step-by-step approach to develop mental and emotional growth. This method can help rewire your brain, providing you with greater control during stressful situations and events, and leading to your ability to respond with wisdom in the face of adversity.

# A: Rewiring your brain

Rewiring your brain begins with daily practices that foster equanimity. Cultivating equanimity offers numerous benefits, including better emotional regulation, improved decision-making, and enhanced relationships. By consciously directing your thoughts and behaviours toward positive patterns, you can create lasting changes in your brain's structure and function.

The benefits extend beyond mental health—you also improve neural connections that can enhance physical health, boost immune function, and slow cognitive decline associated with ageing. Additionally, equanimity helps you regain your sense of self when faced with stress. It acts as your most powerful ally, fostering a sense of inner peace and fulfilment that contributes to your overall mental health and wellbeing. Your brain's ability to adapt and change underscores the importance of lifelong learning and mental flexibility.

- **Practise mindfulness:** Mindfulness involves paying attention to your thoughts and feelings without judgement. You can practise mindfulness throughout your daily tasks by observing your thoughts as they come and go. Spend a few moments focusing on your breath and acknowledging your thoughts. This practice helps you become more aware of your thinking patterns, reducing the power of negative thoughts.

- **Set realistic goals:** Break down larger tasks into manageable steps and celebrate your progress along the way. For example, if you're feeling overwhelmed by a work or personal project, set a goal to complete one specific part of it today. Achieving these small goals provides a sense of accomplishment and helps build momentum for tackling bigger challenges.

- **Keep a thought journal:** Essential in addiction recovery, journaling helps people transform their lives from the inside out. Through these programs, individuals begin to understand how their past has shaped their worldview and learn to become the conscious creators of a new life. A key part of this transformation is recognising how thoughts influence perception. Try tracking your thoughts and emotions daily to identify recurring patterns—especially the negative ones. Each morning, write down how you're feeling and what you expect from the day ahead. At night, reflect on any negative or positive thoughts that came up, and how you responded. This simple daily habit can reveal deep-seated patterns, improve your emotional responses, and build lasting self-awareness. Over time, journaling becomes a powerful tool for growth. It tracks your progress, reinforces your intentions, and strengthens your commitment to change.

- **Seek support:** Remember, you're not alone on this journey. Share your CBT practices with a friend or consider joining a support group. Having a support system can provide motivation and accountability, making it easier to stay committed to your daily CBT practice. By integrating these techniques into your life, you'll gradually rewire your brain, enhancing your mental resilience.

- **Embrace your emotions:** Emotions are your body's way of signalling what's been processed (and what hasn't). When you name and fully accept what you feel, emotions become easier to navigate. When confronted with a negative emotion, ask yourself, 'What am I feeling right now?' or 'What's behind this emotion?' to build emotional self-awareness. This simple practice helps you process emotions more healthily and express them authentically. With time, all feelings—pleasant or painful—can move freely through your field of awareness, allowing them to come and to go.

## NAVIGATING YOUR EMOTIONAL WAVES

Sometimes you may wake in the morning and feel emotional pain for no clear reason. There may be a constriction in your heart; a heaviness in your general disposition. It can feel overwhelming, like an uninvited dark cloud. You might think, 'OMG, here I go again. Seriously, I am not in the mood for this mood. Nor do I have the energy or the patience to deal with it!'

This overwhelming sensation can leave you feeling lost, much like an animal in pain, driven by instinct rather than reason. Your natural response might be to curl into yourself, or at times lash out at everything, including the people you love, all while catastrophising the worst-case scenarios. It can feel endless and insurmountable. However, there is another way to handle these emotions.

One way manage emotional moments is to lean into them rather than giving into the urge to push them away or get on with stuff to remain distracted.

Next time this happens, take a moment to stand, sit or lie down, close your eyes, and notice your breathing. Allow all your emotions to flood your senses. Invite them in and surrender to the feelings. Cry, shout, shake—do whatever you need to fully experience these emotions.

The trick is to hold onto these feelings rather than push them away. Embrace them fully, letting them have their way with you.

What you may notice is that somehow, they subside. Notice that the harder you try to hold on to them, the quicker they slide out of your grasp. If this happens allow these feelings to slide away.

As they slide away you simply relax rest and breathe, allowing space between waves. Watch and wait.

If the feelings return, keep your eyes closed and invite them back in. Let them have their way with you again. Try not to breathe them out or push them away. Surrender.

And notice when they subside again.

Rest and breathe.

Repeat this as often as you need until you realise that the feelings have been replaced with a sense of calm.

By practicing this mindful approach, your feelings lose the power to hold you a prisoner and you can regain both homeostasis (balance in the body) and equanimity (balance in the mind). It's like riding the waves in the ocean—you deal with each wave uniquely, sometimes diving under, sometimes jumping up with them. Yet there is always a space in between each wave, sometimes a short space and sometimes longer.

## Whatever you resist persists.

Just like waves, it's hard to dodge your emotions, try riding your emotional waves instead, and like the waves in the ocean, you may find they come and go. Eventually when the turbulence has passed you will find grace in the calm after the storm.

Whenever your life feels unrelentingly overwhelming, seek professional support always! Believe you can heal with the right guidance; millions have and so can you.

## Feelings are like children on a car trip; you can't let them drive, but you can't lock them in the boot either.

**ANONYMOUS**

- **Planning vs catastrophising:** It's important to notice the difference between critically planning to avoid failure and catastrophising about what lies ahead. Both approaches involve thinking ahead, but they have very different impacts on your mindset and overall wellbeing.

### FINDING BALANCE

The key to navigating the future effectively lies in finding a balance between critical planning and avoiding catastrophising. Through the power of equanimity, remind yourself that while it's important to anticipate challenges and prepare for them, it's equally crucial to stay grounded and not let your fears dictate your actions. By practising mindfulness and focusing on the present moment, you can prevent your mind from spiralling into negative thinking. Additionally, you can use techniques like CBT to challenge irrational thoughts and replace them with more balanced, realistic ones.

By critically planning, you equip yourself with the tools and strategies needed to handle potential obstacles. At the same time, by avoiding catastrophising, you maintain a positive and hopeful outlook, allowing yourself to move forward with confidence and resilience. This balanced approach enables you to face the future with a clear mind and an open heart, ready to embrace both the challenges and opportunities that lie ahead.

### CRITICAL PLANNING

Critical planning is a proactive, constructive way to prepare for the future. It involves assessing potential risks, considering various scenarios, and devising strategies to handle possible challenges. When you engage in critical planning, you focus on identifying realistic obstacles and creating actionable plans to overcome them. This approach empowers you to feel in control and confident about your ability to navigate the future. By thinking ahead and preparing, you can reduce the likelihood of failure and increase your chances of success. Critical planning is rooted in rational thinking and problem-solving, which helps your stay grounded and focused on solutions rather than problems.

**CATASTROPHISING**

This is a form of negative thinking where you imagine the worst possible outcomes, often blowing potential problems out of proportion. When you catastrophise, your mind races to worst-case scenarios, making you feel overwhelmed and often paralysed by fear. This type of thinking is driven by anxiety and often lacks a basis in reality. Instead of focusing on practical solutions, you get stuck in a cycle of worry and despair. Catastrophising negatively rewires your brain, drives you to the Red Zone, drains your energy and makes it difficult for you to take positive steps toward your goals. Often you can become consumed by the fear of what might go wrong.

> I have lived through some terrible things in my life, some of which actually happened!
>
> MARK TWAIN

Through these practices, you can actively rewire your brain, promote emotional resilience, and foster a healthier relationship with yourself. Your journey towards healing and personal growth will yield profound benefits, leading to a more balanced and fulfilling life.

# B: Rewrite your story

**WHAT STORY ARE YOU TELLING YOURSELF ABOUT YOUR LIFE?**
Your inner dialogue is critical to your mental and emotional wellbeing. If you have been wronged in life (and so many women have) you may be feeling helplessness. This feeling stems from a misguided belief that you have no power or control, leading you to a mindset of feeling victimised. There is no argument that trauma and pain can lead women down this path, and it can be a challenge to change your perception. Maybe you're telling yourself a story of powerlessness reinforced by a triangle of getting stuck in a victim mindset. (See graphic on page 327.) As you read the next few pages you may identify with being a victim or a rescuer, both are enabling roles that may not serve you.

> Who would you be without your story?
>
> BYRON KATIE

### RESCUER

Playing the rescuer can feel like a noble role in life—we all want to support those less fortunate than ourselves. However, balance is key. When rescuing others becomes a constant pattern, it may point to a deeper need for approval, a desire to feel needed, or reliance on external validation for self-worth.

A pain or trauma response can trigger a 'rescue mindset'—a way to feel good based on external approval. If you rely on others to feel worthy, practise equanimity and lean into a COAL state of mind (outlined later in this chapter).

### VICTIM

While it's true that you may not be able to change your circumstances or erase the suffering or trauma you have experienced in life, what you can change is how you navigate your reactions and responses to the highs and lows. This power is firmly within your control. By challenging your thinking and seeking qualified help when needed, such as booking an appointment with a mental health specialist, you can make significant strides. It's worth the effort.

Having a 'victim mindset' relies on three main elements:

1. Something happened to me that hurt me deeply (physically, psychologically, or both).
2. Someone or something did this to me (the persecutor/s), which can be many over time.
3. There are some lovely people in my life who help me (the rescuers).

#### DO YOU HAVE A VICTIM MINDSET?

This cycle can quickly and easily become a way of being in your life. You, as the victim, continually tell your story to people who are keen to help you feel better (rescuers). They offer you various ideas to feel better, help you physically and mentally, and provide support. This can go on for months, even years. They are committed to helping you out of your victim mindset and genuinely want you to be happy and healthy. However, if you don't follow their advice or act on their efforts so that they can see they are making a difference in your life, they become emotionally fatigued and often give up, thinking nothing they are doing is working. Sometimes this means they see you less often, stop listening to your story, or even cut ties on the friendship, which wounds you even more, adding them to your list of persecutors.

> **TIP**
> The truth is you are the only person who can rescue yourself. No one else can do this for you.

You may also notice that you can flip from rescuer to victim and back again. However you identify in this triangle, you are stuck in a holding pattern of emotional stagnation. There are always going to be unkind, hurtful people in life. The trick is to not let them rule how you think and perceive your life because, when you do this, you give them power over you.

Breaking free from this mindset cycle requires acknowledging your power to change your response to life's challenges. It's about stepping out of the victim and rescuer role and taking control of your narrative with a creator mindset.

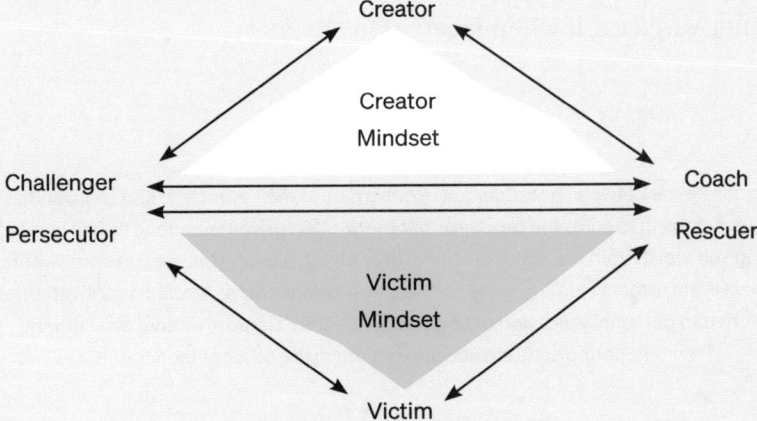

The mindset diagram above illustrates two contrasting mindset triangles. The victim mindset triangle reflects the dynamic between the rescuer, victim, and persecutor—three interdependent and interchangeable roles people may adopt in certain situations. In contrast, the 'creator mindset' focuses on facing life's challenges, coaching yourself to grow and learn, and ultimately becoming the creator of your own life journey. While we may shift between these mindsets at different times, actively moving toward a creator mindset fosters greater mental stability and enhances stress resilience.

#### THREE ACTIONS TO ADOPT A CREATOR MINDSET

A creator mindset is fundamentally different from a victim or rescuer mindset. Instead of seeing yourself as a passive participant in your life, you become the active architect of your experiences and outcomes. This shift in perspective empowers you to take charge of your narrative, enabling you to respond to challenges with resilience and equanimity.

**1   Face your challenges head on**
In the journey of life, challenges are inevitable—be they physical, mental, or emotional. They can emerge from various areas, including relationships, family, work, or business. Instead of viewing these challenges as insurmountable obstacles, acknowledge them without judgement and reframe them as valuable opportunities for growth.

**2   Coach your perspective**
Transforming your mindset from 'I can't' to 'I can' is essential for overcoming challenges. Cultivate a habit of self-coaching that encourages focus, bravery, and persistence. Remind yourself of your inherent strength and capability to navigate life's trials. This positive self-talk not only fosters resilience but also keeps you motivated even when faced with adversity.

> **TIP**
>
> The difference between a rescuer and a coach lies in their approach and motivation. A rescuer steps in to solve the problems of others, often driven by a need to feel needed, gaining self-worth from the act of rescuing. In contrast, a coach focuses on empowering oneself, and others to learn, grow and become independent. A coach's motivation isn't tied to personal validation or the outcome—they support without attachment, fostering self-reliance and growth in the other person.

**3   Be the creator of your life**
To tackle challenges effectively, embrace innovation and a willingness to learn. Develop new strategies to address problems, whether by acquiring new skills, seeking guidance from mentors, or experimenting with different approaches. Adopting a continuous learning mindset empowers you to adapt and thrive.

By adopting a creator mindset, you take control of your life and your responses to challenges. This proactive approach, coupled with equanimity, builds resilience, and empowers you to create a fulfilling and successful life. Remember, you have the power to shape your destiny. Embrace it and watch yourself thrive.

# C: Final Steps

- **Build a supportive network**

Surround yourself with positive influences that uplift and inspire you. Seek mentors, friends and support groups that encourage growth. Equally important is identifying negative influences—be it family, partners or friends. While navigating these relationships can be challenging, it's vital to prioritise your wellbeing.

> I don't walk away to teach people a lesson, I walk away because I learned mine. I choose to adjust to their absence rather than compromising my boundaries to accommodate their disrespect.
>
> ANON

- **Reflect and learn**

Take the time to reflect on your experiences. What strategies worked, and what didn't? Utilise these insights to refine your approaches, as continuous reflection enhances your resilience over time.

- **Adopt a COAL state of mind**

Renowned neuropsychiatrist Dr Daniel Siegel emphasises the importance of cultivating this acronym for improved mental and emotional wellbeing:

**OUR INTERPRETATION OF A COAL STATE OF MIND**

**Curiosity:** Fuels a sense of wonder, making us inquisitive and eager to explore new ideas. It drives us to ask questions, seek understanding, and embrace learning. It sparks persistence in solving challenges with creativity and determination.

**Openness:** Openness is about embracing diversity in thoughts, beliefs, and experiences, and respecting differences across backgrounds, and cultures. It involves actively listening to other viewpoints to genuinely understand different perspectives. Openness also means suspending judgement, avoiding premature conclusions, and being comfortable with uncertainty—accepting that it's okay not to have all the answers and embracing ambiguity rather than settling for simplistic explanations.

**Acceptance:** Acknowledging reality means facing what we can and cannot control, recognising both our strengths and limitations alongside external influences. Letting go of control allows us to focus our energy on what truly matters, while embracing imperfection reminds us that mistakes and setbacks are part of life's wisdom. Resilience helps us bounce back from adversity with courage, finding meaning and growth even in the toughest moments. Cultivating gratitude lets us appreciate life's positives amidst challenges, and self-compassion encourages kindness toward ourselves, embracing our humanity and imperfections.

> ## Surrender, practising acceptance of what you cannot change.
>
> **ANON**

**Love:** Embrace self-acceptance by fully acknowledging your flaws and strengths, treating yourself with compassion, and forgiving past mistakes as opportunities for growth. Live authentically by aligning with your values, expressing your true self, and reflecting on areas for improvement. Set healthy boundaries that protect your wellbeing, communicate your needs clearly, and prioritise decisions that honour your happiness. Practise empathy by understanding others' perspectives and feelings with an open, non-judgemental attitude, fostering genuine connections and reducing conflict. Be present, express gratitude, and nurture meaningful relationships.

> ## They must learn to hate, and if they can learn to hate, they can be taught to love, for love comes more naturally to the human heart than its opposite.
>
> **NELSON MANDELA**

By embracing Curiosity, Openness, Acceptance and Love, you foster inner peace, resilience, and balance, enhancing your wellbeing and relationships.

## PERSONAL GROWTH

Life throws curve balls and some wound deeply. Here are some gentle ways to reframe past hurts:

- **Rejection:** Embrace your uniqueness, your worth is not defined by other's opinions.

- **Abandonment:** Trust in your resilience; nurture connections that uplift and support you.

- **Betrayal:** Work on forgiveness to set yourself free, when you hold onto past hurts you wound yourself more. Let them loose, open your heart to your own beauty and vulnerability.

- **Humiliation:** Release the need for external validation, recognising inherent value within yourself.

- **Injustice:** Try to transform any adversity into growth and wisdom. What did you learn that will help you now and in the future? Tiny pieces of gold forged together build a foundation of newfound self-assurance and power.

- **Perspective:** Identify with something larger than yourself. Broaden your connection to all of life: humanity, nature and the planet. Identify with something much more enduring than a current situation, move beyond the need to cling to one particular outcome. Connect to something larger, through religion, spirituality, science, or simply history.

- **Find joy:** Something you love to do, that you do well. Your inner circle or the world needs it, and ideally, you get paid to do it.

## EMOTIONAL SELF-CARE AND STRESS RESILIENCE CHECKLIST

In this section we have been focused on self-revolution, embracing equanimity, rewiring your brain, dealing with negative thoughts and perceptions, building a creator mindset and the benefits of a COAL state of mind. The following checklist of suggestions may resonate with you to deepen your ability to be stress resilient:

- **Letting go:** Forgive yourself and others, releasing anger and resentment to restore inner peace to heal emotional wounds and move forward.

- **Mindfulness:** Be present and engage fully in each moment, listening actively and responding with love and respect.

- **Forge connections:** Build a support system through healthy relationships that provide comfort in tough times and celebration in joyful moments. Avoid toxic connections that can harm your wellbeing.

- **Gratitude:** Appreciate your achievements and express gratitude for the people in your life.

- **Encouragement:** Support yourself and others with kindness, fostering growth and connection.

- **Love:** Practise self-love and compassion daily, deepening your capacity for love and forgiveness.

- **Find purpose and meaning in your life:** To cope with uncertainty, find meaning in life, something that matters to you. The source of meaning is different for everyone, and it can change throughout life. What lights you up, makes your heart sing? Find ways to be engaged in meaningful activities, for example, art, religion, acts of service, purposeful work or personal projects.

> Love is the absence of judgement.
>
> **ANCIENT SAYING**

# Whatever you practise, you become really good at!

Being a woman is an extraordinary journey, woven with threads of resilience, intuition and boundless creativity. As women, we carry within us the ancient wisdom of the Earth, the nurturing essence of life itself. Our bodies are attuned to the rhythms of the moon, and the cycles of nature. We possess an innate strength that rises in the face of adversity and a compassionate heart that nurtures and heals. Our minds can be tapestries of dreams, visions, and untold stories waiting to unfold. Embracing our femininity in all its forms means honouring the divine energy that courses through our veins. We need to celebrate our unique power and recognise the beauty in our existence. It is in this profound recognition that we find our true essence, a force capable of transforming not only our own lives, but we can also influence the world around us. Being a woman is a spiritual dance of grace, wisdom and infinite possibility.

You are a woman. You see the world differently. You are highly intelligent and emotionally wise. You are worthy.

Refer to our Spotlight on Restorative Practices, page 372. These provide you with the keys to your resilience in the modern world, carve out time to rest, recover and heal yourself.

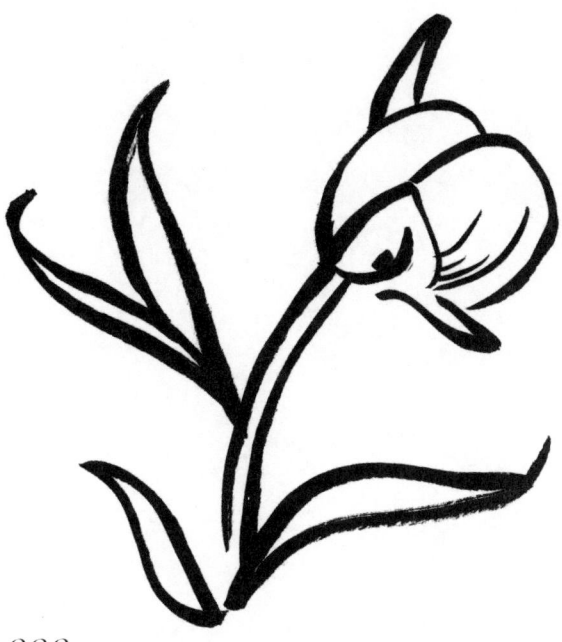

# SPOTLIGHT ON
# Adrenal Glands

In this chapter, we'll explore your adrenal glands and their profound influence your hormonal journey from puberty to the Age of Wisdom. Whether you're looking at adrenal function from a conventional or holistic perspective, understanding these glands is essential for navigating the complexities of your hormonal health.

### UNDERSTANDING YOUR ADRENALS—THE BIG PICTURE

The adrenals are part of your endocrine system, which is a network of glands responsible for creating and releasing bioactive molecules like sweat, tears, digestive juices, and hormones. Hormones are chemical messengers that coordinate various functions in your body by traveling through your blood to organs, skin, muscles, and other tissues.

## THE COMMUNICATION BETWEEN HORMONES AND CELLS

Hormones enter cells via their unique receptor. These sites on the outside of cells act like docking portals, each designed to open a specific 'door' for a particular hormone. Just as a key fits only its matching lock, hormones can only enter cells through their specialised receptor docks, triggering the exact response needed.

## WHAT YOUR ADRENAL GLANDS DO AND THE KEY HORMONES THEY PRODUCE

These peanut-sized glands, sitting on top of each kidney, are central to keeping your body in balance. Your adrenals produce a range of hormones that help regulate essential processes, including managing your energy, maintaining blood pressure and regulating fluid balance, supporting your immune system, and responding to stress. In women, the adrenals also play a crucial role in hormone regulation, especially during times of change. They produce hormones like DHEA, which can be converted into oestrogen and testosterone, stepping in to support hormonal balance as the ovaries retire in menopause. These multitaskers also ensure you stay resilient and adaptable, and are designed to enhance your survival in time of extreme danger. Adrenal hormones like adrenaline and noradrenaline are critical for regulating stress, metabolism and inflammation. Your adrenals help manage your body's response to stress, whether you're dealing with an immediate crisis or the long-term hormonal changes that come with hormonal stages like puberty, pregnancy, or menopause. Under stress, adrenal hormones assist with energy production by converting fats, proteins and carbohydrates into fuel, keeping your body powered when it needs it most.

> **THE ADRENALS THROUGH THE LENS OF DIFFERENT HEALTH PARADIGMS**
>
> You may have heard terms like 'adrenal fatigue' or even 'burnt-out adrenals,' but what does that really mean? In conventional Western medicine, adrenal glands are seen primarily through the lens of their hormonal roles—producing adrenaline, cortisol, and catecholamines (we'll unpack this shortly).
>
> Other paradigms, such as Ayurveda, Traditional Chinese Medicine (TCM), naturopathy, and Western herbal medicine, view adrenal health holistically. In Ayurveda, the adrenals are linked to 'Ojas', the vital energy supporting immunity and vitality. TCM connects adrenal function to the kidneys, focusing on balancing 'Qi' (vital energy) for endurance and life force. Naturopathy and Western herbal traditions use adaptogenic herbs like ashwagandha, rhodiola, and liquorice root to enhance the body's resilience to stress.
>
> Each of these paradigms provides valuable insights into maintaining adrenal health. Recent research highlights the benefits of integrating these approaches for women's hormonal health.

> Adaptogen herbs like withania and rhodiola reduce stress and support adrenal function—vital during hormonal shifts. Acupuncture, yoga, and meditation, rooted in TCM and Ayurveda, help balance cortisol and ease symptoms. Integrating these with conventional medicine offers a well-rounded approach to support hormonal health during perimenopause and menopause.

## THE ADRENAL HORMONE TEAM

The adrenal glands produce two main categories of hormones—your steroid hormones and your catecholamines.

### THE STEROID HORMONES

These hormones help to regulate inflammation, support immune function, balance electrolytes, and contribute to sexual development.

- **Aldosterone:** Regulates blood pressure and maintains the balance of acidity (pH) in your blood by controlling sodium and potassium levels.

- **Androgens:** Though often considered male hormones, women also produce small amounts of androgens, such as DHEA, primarily from the adrenal glands. DHEA serves as a building block for oestrogen and testosterone. It is particularly important after menopause.

- **Cortisol**: An essential hormone that, when balanced, regulates metabolism and stress response. (We cover this in detail later in this chapter.)

### THE CATECHOLAMINES: YOUR EMERGENCY RESPONSE TEAM

- **Adrenaline and noradrenaline:** These are your body's emergency responders. When you're under physical or emotional stress, these hormones are released to activate your fight-or-flight response.

- **Dopamine:** Dopamine is often thought of primarily as a neurotransmitter involved in the brain's reward system, but it is also released in smaller amounts by the adrenal glands. While adrenaline and noradrenaline prepare the body for the fight-or-flight response, dopamine helps regulate blood flow, mood, and motivation, playing a more subtle but important role in maintaining bodily functions during times of high stress. Together with your steroid hormone cortisol, these three catecholamines help manage how your body responds to stress and maintain overall homeostasis (balance).

## THE ACUTE STRESS RESPONSE—CODE RED
### ADRENALINE AND NORADRENALINE

When life is in balance, your adrenals work quietly in the background. Cortisol coordinates with your sleep and support hormones to deliver the right signals at the right time, maintaining your circadian rhythm.

The survival of the species is the number one priority for the body. The adrenals are on the front line of this priority and act as an organiser of 'who does what within the body' now there is threat of death. Historically our ancestors needed the fight-or-flight response to hunt, run from or fight any danger and survive. The sympathetic nervous system kept the adrenals on high alert in a changing environment such as in extreme cold or heat, famine, drought, war or constant threat from a nearby tribe.

The adrenals immediately prioritise safety, so processes in your regular metabolism are moved to the back burner until danger has passed. This means they quickly get your heart racing, boost your blood pressure and flood your system with glucose, giving your body a surge of energy and focus. They even help you breathe more easily by dilating your airways, making sure you're ready to take on whatever's coming your way. Essentially, they prime your entire body to handle impending doom and ensure that vital systems are prepared for action in those critical moments.

This means 'Code Red', which is why the stress survival response is your number one hormonal disrupter and health destroyer. We are repeating this for a reason—stress is not your friend!

Excess stress hormones circulating in your bloodstream too frequently or for prolonged periods can significantly impact your health. They are linked to nearly every medical condition—either as a cause, contributor, or amplifier—and can also disrupt hormonal balance. This occurs because the body prioritises survival, suppressing the parasympathetic nervous system responsible for 'rest and digest'. Without sufficient parasympathetic activation, your body struggles to heal, recover, and maintain overall wellbeing and, essentially, hormonal balance.

When the adrenals are producing surges of adrenalin too often for too long, they start producing a higher level of cortisol. This is to ensure your body:

1. Prioritises tasks.
2. Makes sure supplies are not overused to ensure they will last longer, until the danger has passed all in the service of survival.

Imagine your body asking the following questions to the 'emergency responder commander' also known as cortisol:

Q   Reproduction and production of all associated hormones?
A   Whattt ... now, let's see; run from the tiger or ovulate ... hmmm run!
Q   Fat burning?
A   No thanks, let's kill two birds with one stone; muscle needs lots of energy, so let's breakdown the muscle and use the protein for food. Then we can hang onto our greatest resource for life preservation—the fat we put into the fat cells for this very reason. We only burn fat as a last resort.
Q   Sleep?
A   No way, what if danger sneaks up on us when we are asleep? No thanks, best keep deep sleep out and only sleep lightly so we hear every movement and can run or fight for our life if needed.
Q   Convert and make oestrogen and progesterone?
A   Nope, let's keep all our ingredients like zinc to make enough stress hormones to run and fight.
Q   Immune system?
A   You're kidding me right ... let's worry about that later when we have dealt with this terrible crisis. We are in danger and may not live long enough to need our immune system!
Q   Digest food?
A   Why digest lunch when we might be lunch, later much later! We need to prioritise the blood flow to your arms and legs so we can run and fight!
Q   Produce collagen?
A   Now you are just annoying me, live with wrinkles and saggy skin–at least you will be alive.

Stress is an inevitable part of life. Hormones like adrenaline, noradrenaline, and dopamine play a vital role in helping your body respond to stress, keeping your overall hormonal balance in check. When your stress response is well-regulated, cortisol remains under control, preventing the hormonal chaos that can disrupt everything from your menstrual cycle to your energy levels. However, when stress becomes chronic and cortisol stays elevated unnecessarily, it throws hormones like oestrogen and progesterone off balance, leading to irregular periods, mood swings, and stubborn weight gain. Managing your stress response is essential for maintaining hormonal balance at every stage of life.

## WELLNESS ACTION PLAN
# REGULATE A FIGHT-OR-FLIGHT PANIC ATTACK

When adrenaline takes over, your body is primed for action—heart racing, breath quickening, and muscles tensing. This is what doctors may label a 'panic attack'. While this response is essential in emergencies, chronic or overwhelming adrenaline surges can leave you feeling jittery, anxious or exhausted. This plan focuses on immediate, practical strategies to help you regain control when adrenaline strikes, complementing your longer-term cortisol regulation plan to follow.

### IMMEDIATE STEPS TO CALM THE ADRENALINE RESPONSE

When adrenaline hijacks your calm, remind yourself that this is your body's way of protecting you—but it doesn't need to stay switched on. These strategies give you the tools to dial down the intensity in the moment and prevent future surges.

#### MOVE YOUR BODY

A few minutes of dancing, skipping, jumping on the spot or air punching in the privacy of a bathroom can dissipate adrenaline.

#### ACTIVATE THE PARASYMPATHETIC NERVOUS SYSTEM
#### (YOUR 'REST AND DIGEST' MODE)

- **Belly breathing:** Take slow, deep breaths, focusing on expanding your abdomen as you inhale for 4 seconds, holding for 4 seconds, and exhaling for 6 seconds. This signals your body to switch off the adrenaline surge.

- **Vagus nerve stimulation:** Splash your face with cold water or gargle gently —both can calm the nervous system and dampen adrenaline's effects.

### GROUND YOURSELF IN THE PRESENT MOMENT

Adrenaline often triggers a spiral of anxious thoughts. Use these techniques to regain focus:

- **Breathwork:** Practise these techniques when life is in balance, so you can activate your breath to regulate your stress response when needed. (See our breathwork options on page 384.)
- **Progressive muscle relaxation:** Tense and release muscles, starting from your toes and working upwards to discharge physical tension caused by adrenaline.

### SUPPORT A CALM BLOOD FLOW AND HEART RATE

- **Legs Up the Wall pose:** When you get home, if you feel comfortable, lie down and elevate your legs against a wall for 5 to 10 minutes to lower your heart rate and redirect blood flow.
- **Slow, rhythmic movement:** Gentle swaying or rocking motions, such as in Tai Chi or swaying side-to-side, can help calm an overstimulated system.

### REDUCE SENSORY OVERLOAD

Overstimulation exacerbates adrenaline spikes.
- Remove yourself from loud, chaotic, or crowded environments.
- Dim the lights or close your eyes for a few minutes to reduce visual stimulation.

## PREVENTIVE MEASURES FOR RECURRENT ADRENALINE SURGE PANIC ATTACK

### DAILY RELAXATION RITUALS

- See our Spotlight on Restorative Practices on page 372.

### NOURISH YOUR NERVOUS SYSTEM
- **Magnesium-rich foods:** Spinach, almonds, and a handful of pumpkin seeds can help calm your nervous system.
- **B-vitamins:** These support energy and adrenal recovery. Include whole grains, eggs and leafy greens.

### BALANCE STIMULANTS
Limit caffeine and sugar, which can exacerbate adrenaline responses. Choose herbal teas like Tulsi, chamomile or passionflower instead.

### SET BOUNDARIES ON OVERCOMMITMENT
- Prioritise time for rest and reflection each day.
- Over-scheduling and constant multitasking can trigger repeated adrenaline spikes.

### MOVE WITH INTENTION
Engage in calming physical activities like walking, Tai Chi, or light stretching, which help release pent-up adrenaline without overstimulation.

### YOUR NEXT STEPS
Revisit this Wellness Action Plan whenever you need quick, effective solutions to keep adrenaline-driven symptoms under control. If these are becoming frequent in your life, consider connecting with a stress management counsellor to learn strategies that can help to reduce your reactivity.

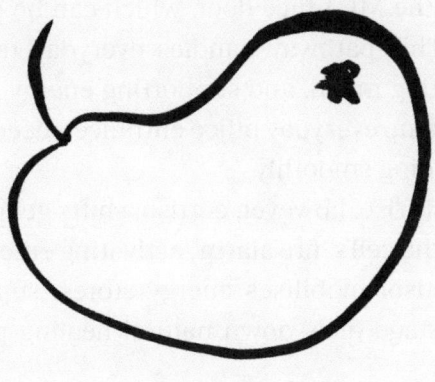

## SPOTLIGHT ON
# Cortisol

While adrenaline triggers your body's immediate fight-or-flight response, cortisol works just as diligently to support your long-term survival. Let's explore cortisol's two pivotal roles:

1   Cortisol in hormonal harmony when life is in balance
2   How cortisol shifts gears to handle the demands of a 'Code Red' stress response.

Cortisol is like a guardian with dual roles in a woman's body, managing the calm of daily life while springing into action when stress strikes. It works by entering cells through two distinct 'doors' or portals, each activating unique cellular pathways to serve different purposes.

1   **Mineralocorticoid receptors (MRs):** The entry portal office door when life is in balance.
2   **Glucocorticoid receptors (GRs):** The emergency entrance.

Under normal, low-stress conditions, cortisol takes a steady and supportive role. It enters cells through the MR office door, which can be opened by even small amounts of cortisol. This pathway handles everyday tasks like maintaining blood pressure, regulating mood, and supporting energy balance. Think of the MR office door as the calm, everyday office entrance—used regularly and quietly to keep the system running smoothly.

When stress levels rise, however, cortisol shifts gears. The GR emergency door opens, leading to the cell's 'fire alarm', activating emergency systems. Once through this door, cortisol mobilises energy stores, suppresses the immune response, and at this stage dials down natural healing processes to focus all resources on immediate survival. Interestingly, when cortisol is released slowly or in a controlled manner, 'chaperone' proteins act as gatekeepers, guarding the GR emergency door. These important proteins ensure that the GR pathway isn't activated unnecessarily, maintaining a balance between readiness and calm within the cell. However, during chronic stress, this system can become overwhelmed, leaving the GR doors unattended by the chaperone proteins making the cells constantly engaged, overwhelming the cell.

While this dual-entry system allows cortisol to balance calm and crisis, chronic stress turns the GR emergency door into a revolving gateway. Persistently high cortisol keeps this emergency pathway overactive, eventually overwhelming its capacity. Over time, this leads to exhaustion of the GR emergency system, leading to the following domino effects:

- Cortisol loses the command of the circadian rhythm.
- Chronic stress can deplete cortisol to below-normal levels, blunting its emergency response when it's needed most.
- Sleep is sacrificed.
- Cellular energy production slows.
- Stress resilience is depleted.
- Healing and repair of tissue and cells is put on hold.
- Your immune system is compromised.

This state is what naturopaths call 'adrenal exhaustion' and can be a common cause of chronic fatigue syndrome.

If you are struggling under the load of chronic stress, turn to our Spotlight on Psychological Stress on page 290 for more guidance and support.

Cultivating supportive relationships and setting boundaries helps to reduce daily stress. Over time, we can restore cortisol's essential function, *empowering* us rather than *overpowering* us.

**CORTISOL MANAGEMENT THROUGH YOUR HORMONAL JOURNEY:**

### PUBERTY

Puberty triggers a surge in oestrogen, progesterone, and testosterone, driving significant physical and emotional changes. These shifts challenge the adrenal glands to adapt to new hormonal demands and can heighten the risk of nutrient deficiencies, like zinc, which may worsen acne, mood swings, and irritability.

SOLUTIONS
- **Eat more** zinc-rich foods like seafood, lean meats, seeds, nuts, and whole grains.
- **Include** magnesium from leafy greens, avocados, and nuts.
- **Supplement** B-vitamins through whole foods or multivitamins if needed.
- **Avoid** energy drinks and caffeine to reduce adrenal overstimulation.
- **Prioritise** quality sleep.
- **Learn** relaxation techniques like yoga, meditation or breathing exercises to buffer stress.

### THE FERTILE YEARS

Monthly hormonal cycles place continuous demands on the adrenal glands, that work hard to regulate cortisol and stabilise blood sugar levels in response to the natural fluctuations of oestrogen and progesterone. Hormonal dips, particularly around menstruation, can often lead to fatigue, mood changes, and emotional lows, increasing the need for adrenal support.

SOLUTIONS
- **Boost** your intake of omega-3 fatty acids with foods like sardines, walnuts, and flaxseeds.
- **Add** antioxidants like vitamin C through citrus fruits, berries, and capsicums.
- **Support** adrenal health with magnesium from leafy greens, nuts, and seeds.
- **Limit** sugar and refined carbohydrates to stabilise blood sugar and cortisol.
- **Incorporate** stress-reducing practices such as gentle yoga, meditation, or mindful walks.
- **Prioritise** regular, balanced meals with protein and healthy fats to maintain steady energy levels.

### PERIMENOPAUSE: THE TRANSITION BEGINS

Perimenopause brings fluctuating levels of oestrogen and progesterone, creating both physical and biochemical stress on the adrenal glands. As the ovaries begin their gradual retirement, the adrenals take on a more significant role in hormone production. This shift often heightens cortisol responses, contributing to symptoms such as hot flushes, night sweats, mood changes, and increased stress sensitivity.

**SOLUTIONS**
- **Increase** protein intake with lean meats, legumes, eggs, and plant-based options.
- **Add** fibre-rich foods like vegetables, whole grains, and seeds for hormonal balance.
- **Incorporate** adaptogenic herbs like ashwagandha or rhodiola to buffer adrenal stress.
- **Limit** stimulants like caffeine and alcohol to reduce cortisol spikes.
- **Prioritise** nutrient-dense meals with plenty of vitamins and minerals.
- **Adopt** restorative practices like meditation, Tai Chi or gentle yoga to improve stress resilience.
- **Reduce exercise intensity** as this places strain on the adrenal glands in hormonal phase.

### MENOPAUSE: THE BODY'S NEW NORMAL

As oestrogen and progesterone stabilise at lower levels, the adrenal glands step in as the primary producers of these hormones, placing greater demand on the adrenal glands. This can lead to symptoms such as sleep disturbances, brain fog, and heightened stress sensitivity, making adrenal support essential for overall balance and wellbeing.

**SOLUTIONS**
- **Support** adrenal health with magnesium (from nuts, seeds, and leafy greens), vitamin C (from citrus and berries), and B5 (from avocados, mushrooms, and eggs).
- **Prioritise** low-glycaemic meals with whole grains, proteins, and healthy fats to prevent blood sugar spikes.
- **Incorporate** restorative practices like Tai Chi, breathwork or gentle stretching to calm the nervous system.
- **Limit** refined sugars and processed foods that strain adrenal function.
- **Focus** on maintaining regular sleep routines to promote recovery and balance.

### THE AGE OF WISDOM: RESILIENCE

As oestrogen levels settle into their new lower baseline, cortisol regulation becomes crucial to counter increased vulnerability to stress, inflammation and immune challenges. Supporting adrenal health helps maintain vitality and immune resilience.

**SOLUTIONS**
- **Include** omega-3-rich foods like sardines, walnuts, chia seeds and flaxseeds to reduce inflammation and support immune health.
- **Prioritise** high-quality protein sources such as lean meats, legumes, and eggs to aid tissue repair, maintain muscle mass and strengthen immunity.
- **Add** anti-inflammatory foods like turmeric, ginger, and brightly coloured vegetables to combat oxidative stress-induced damage.
- **Supplement** with zinc and vitamin D to bolster immune function and maintain energy levels.
- **Incorporate restorative activities** like yoga, Tai Chi, or stretching to improve flexibility and support recovery.
- **Practise mindfulness** through meditation, deep breathing, or relaxation exercises to calm your mind and balance cortisol.
- **Spend more time in Blue Zone activities** such as gardening, reading or creative arts. (See page 373 for more suggestions.)

### THE DOMINO EFFECT OF HIGH CORTISOL ON YOUR HORMONES

Under stress, the body diverts progesterone to fuel cortisol production, depleting progesterone levels. This imbalance reduces progesterone's ability to counterbalance oestrogen and support thyroid function, disrupting the delicate adrenal-thyroid axis.

> **TIP**
> The sacrifice of progesterone to cortisol production is one of the most significant hormonal disruptions caused by stress.

For women, this constant stress load creates additional strain by interfering with hormonal balance. Cortisol often 'hijacks' pathways shared with other critical hormones, first progesterone, then oestrogen and eventually your support hormones like testosterone.

This disruption can lead to irregular or absent menstrual cycles, intensify PMS, and amplify perimenopausal symptoms—potentially making the menopause transition a hormonal nightmare. It's as if cortisol, in trying to shield the body from stress, inadvertently crowds out the hormones that promote calm, stability and rest.

Managing stress effectively helps keep cortisol's dual roles in balance, preserving both resilience and overall wellbeing.

## WELLNESS ACTION PLAN
# CORTISOL REGULATION

When it comes to keeping cortisol in check, your lifestyle is the most powerful tool in your wellness toolkit. By focusing on balance and building habits that support your body's stress response, you can help cortisol return to its healthy, supportive role. This action plan integrates targeted strategies for hormonal harmony and complements the solutions outlined to support hormonal balance for your current hormonal stage.

### TEN CORE ACTIONS FOR CORTISOL REGULATION

1  **Incorporate Blue Zone practices:** Daily relaxation rituals are key to lowering cortisol levels and promoting resilience. (Read Spotlight on Restorative Practices on page 372 for details and techniques.)

2  **Prioritise quality sleep:** Sleep is non-negotiable for healthy cortisol rhythms. Lack of restorative sleep can cause cortisol to spike at the wrong times, wreaking havoc on your energy and mood. (See Spotlight on Sleep on page 351.)

3  **Support sleep with supplemental melatonin:** Melatonin is another casualty of stress. Take 2 to 4 mg around an hour before bedtime.

4  **Support stable blood sugar:** Balanced meals with quality protein, healthy fats, and low-glycaemic carbs are vital. (See our Wellness Action Plan for Sugar Addiction on page 436.)

5  **Nourish your adrenals:** Your adrenal glands thrive on key nutrients:

- **Vitamin C:** Found in citrus fruits, kiwi and capsicum.
- **Zinc:** Found in pumpkin seeds, seafood and legumes.
- **Magnesium:** Found in leafy greens, nuts and seeds.
- **B-vitamins:** Found in whole grains, eggs and nutritional yeast.

Tighten your boundaries around processed foods and prioritise these nutrient-rich choices. (See Spotlight on Nourishment on page 393 for inspiration.)

6  **Choose restorative movement:** Movement is crucial but needs to match your body's current needs. It is essential to avoid intense workouts, such as HIIT or marathon training, if your cortisol levels are already elevated.

7  **Book a review with your health practitioner:** Lab testing for progesterone, DHEA, thyroid hormones and nutrients such as iron, zinc and magnesium ensures that biochemical impact of nutrient deficiency or low hormones doesn't add to your stress burden.

8  **Consider a salivary cortisol assessment:** This will guide you and your practitioner to the right choices for fine tuning your stress responses. Use DUTCH testing to monitor your cortisol balance.

9  **Consider bioidentical hormone support:** During prolonged stress, consult an integrative doctor to explore bioidentical hormone options like DHEA or progesterone if testing reveals low levels. Use DUTCH testing to monitor your levels and fine-tune doses.

10  **Seek expert herbal and acupuncture support:** An experienced naturopath or Traditional Chinese Medicine (TCM) practitioner can provide tailored support. Adaptogens like withania (ashwagandha), rhodiola, and Tulsi (see page 349) have been shown to modulate the cortisol response. Acupuncture also offers proven benefits in reducing stress and rebalancing hormones.

### YOUR NEXT STEPS

This is your personalised map for cortisol regulation—start with one or two steps and build on them as you go. Balance is a journey, not a race, so focus on progress rather than perfection. For more detailed guidance on stress reduction techniques, food choices, and hormone support, Part Two of this book is filled with all the advice you need.

## SPOTLIGHT ON
# Tulsi Herbal Tea

Tulsi (*Ocimum sanctum*), known as an adaptogen, is like a trusted friend for your body when managing stress. Its active ingredients work in harmony to support your natural stress response, keeping you calm and balanced. Herbal teas with Tulsi can ease your nervous system, helping shift it into a more relaxed, restorative state—your Blue Zone of calm.

### THE SCIENCE BEHIND TULSI'S STRESS RELIEF

Also known as holy basil, Tulsi has been cherished for centuries for its medicinal and spiritual value. Its powerful phytochemicals support mood-regulating hormones and act as antioxidants, benefiting both mental and physical health. This is a list of Tulsi's active ingredients and how they work:

- **Eugenol:** One of Tulsi's key compounds, has anti-inflammatory, analgesic, and antioxidant properties. It reduces oxidative stress, calms inflammation, and helps you feel more relaxed.

- **Ocimumosides:** Unique to Tulsi, these chemicals help balance cortisol levels (your body's stress hormone) while boosting the enzymes that produce serotonin and dopamine, lifting your mood and reducing anxiety.

- **Rosmarinic acid:** A potent antioxidant that protects your cells from damage while supporting dopamine and serotonin pathways. This enhances both brain function and mood.

- **Linalool:** Also found in lavender, it has calming and sedative effects. It helps reduce anxiety by acting directly on your central nervous system, promoting relaxation and improving sleep quality.

- **Beta-caryophyllene:** Interacts with your body's natural cannabinoid system, like medicinal cannabis oil, to reduce inflammation and alleviate stress, leaving you more at ease.

- **Ursolic acid:** Providing a triple benefit—anti-inflammatory, antioxidant, and stress-soothing properties—it lowers your body's stress response by reducing inflammation and oxidative stress.

### HOW TO USE TULSI FOR STRESS RELIEF

Incorporate Tulsi into your daily routine by enjoying it as a calming herbal tea or take it in supplement form. Tulsi is a natural, holistic way to manage stress, improve mood, and support overall mental wellbeing.

Next time you enjoy Tulsi, remember it's more than just a herb—it's a powerhouse of compounds working together to reduce stress and promote a balanced, peaceful state of mind. Whether you start your day or wind down with it, Tulsi offers gentle, effective support for your wellbeing.

Note: Always consult your healthcare provider before starting any new supplement, especially if you have existing health conditions or are on medication.

## SPOTLIGHT ON
# Sleep

> It is the elixir of life, Mother Nature's best effort for immortality.
>
> Sleep is the tide that rises all the other health boats.
>
> **DR MATT WALKER**

Depriving yourself of exercise, food, or water is nothing compared to the damage one night of lost sleep can cause to your body and brain. Sleep deprivation is a global problem, yet it doesn't receive the attention it deserves from public health initiatives. The profound effects of sleep deprivation on anxiety, mental health, obesity and even suicide risk is well-documented. Yet, sleep still isn't treated as a top health priority.

The message is clear—quality sleep is crucial for maintaining hormonal balance. But when hormones are out of sync, sleep often suffers, creating a vicious cycle that's hard to break.

Nearly 50% of women do not get the recommended seven to nine hours of sleep per night. The modern world makes it increasingly difficult to rest, and it's vital that women prioritise sleep. Studies by the independent Rand Corporation show that sleep deprivation costs 2% of GDP globally. The cost to your health, however, is far more significant. If sleep has become elusive, it's time to dive into the science and explore how to reclaim restorative sleep and balance your hormones.

As Dr Matt Walker, professor of neuroscience and psychology at the University of California, Berkeley, and founder and director of the school's Centre for Human Sleep Science wisely states, 'Sleep is the single most effective thing you can do to reset your brain and body health.'

## WHY SLEEP?

Sleep is essential for detoxifying the brain, repairing muscles and organs, and resetting your health for a new day.

Did you know that sleep also helps with the following?
- Recharges your immune system, making you more resilient.
- Regulates blood sugar levels and metabolism.
- Balances hormones, including appetite and sex hormones.
- Consolidates memories, helping you learn and process the day's events.
- Reduces anxiety and promotes emotional stability by regulating neurotransmitters like serotonin and dopamine.
- Clears toxic proteins, including those linked to Alzheimer's disease.
- Increases libido—just one extra hour of sleep can boost it by 50%!

## WHAT'S STOPPING YOUR SLEEP?

There are three primary barriers to achieving good sleep:

1. **Life interference:** You may not allow yourself the time and space to rest, as modern life keeps us producing and consuming non-stop so increases your risk of exposure to sleep saboteurs. This also includes family, carer, and social commitments.
2. **Insomnia:** You might make time for sleep but struggle to fall or stay asleep.
3. **Sleep apnoea:** You may have some nose, mouth and throat physical obstructions. It's important to seek professional help for this.

In recent years, neuroscience has revealed the devastating effects of sleep deprivation, which can increase the risk of various chronic diseases.

**AS RATES OF INSOMNIA RISE, SO DO RATES OF ANXIETY!**

> **TIP**
> Netflix's CEO acknowledged that sleep is a competitor for their streaming service, saying, 'We are declaring war on sleep.'

## WHAT'S A GOOD NIGHT'S SLEEP?

A good night's sleep means falling asleep within 15 minutes of lying down, staying asleep for 7 to 8 hours, and waking up feeling refreshed without needing an alarm. Waking once or twice to use the bathroom is normal, if you fall back asleep quickly.

## ARE YOU A LARK OR OWL?

Chronotype—whether you identify as a morning 'lark' or a night 'owl'—demonstrates your sleep-wake patterns. These tendencies can change throughout your life due to hormonal shifts, such as during puberty or menopause.

- **Morningness (Lark):** Prefers an early bedtime (8–10 pm) and early rise (4–6 am).

- **Eveningness (Owl):** Prefers a late bedtime (midnight or later) and late rise (11 am or noon).

Chronotypes are not set in stone; they're influenced by genetics and environmental factors such as light exposure, work and eating patterns, and social behaviour. Chronotype variations mean that evening types sleep 2 to 3 hours later than morning types. Extreme shifts beyond this can disrupt work, school, or social life. If your 'lark' or 'owl' tendencies cause significant friction, potentially indicating a circadian rhythm sleep disorder, a change in environmental habits or a consultation with a sleep specialist can help.

Regardless of whether you're a lark or an owl, getting enough quality sleep is essential. If you go to bed at midnight, aim for the recommended 7 to 9 hours to ensure you reap the vital health benefits that sleep provides.

There is ongoing research into how chronotype might relate to evolutionary needs for a small percentage of the tribe to be responsible for night-time vigilance in ancestral societies. This research could inform future adjustments in societal schedules, such as school start times, to better align with owl sleep patterns in tweens.

# TOP FIVE CONSIDERATIONS FOR QUALITY SLEEP

Quality sleep isn't just about closing your eyes and hoping for the best—it's a finely tuned process influenced by your body's natural rhythms, environment, and habits. By understanding and addressing the following key factors, you can create the perfect conditions for restorative, uninterrupted rest.

1. Circadian rhythm
2. Blue light vs red light spectrum
3. Temperature
4. Sleep saboteurs
5. Sleep promoters

## 1. CIRCADIAN RHYTHM

Your internal circadian rhythm governs your sleep-wake cycle, heavily influenced by light exposure. Natural morning light helps align your internal clock, while exposure to blue light at night (from screens and artificial lighting) can disrupt your rhythm. Outdoor light exposure can be up to 10 times more intense than the brightest indoor lighting, leading to a stronger alignment between your internal clock and the actual time of day.

Humans are hardwired to sleep when it's dark and be productive when the sun shines. This is written into our DNA; we are daylight dwellers. Even the microscopic world within you ticks to its own biological rhythm. Your innate body clock is accurate to the second.

**SUPPORT CIRCADIAN RHYTHM**

- **Greet the morning sun**: Get sunlight into your eyes first thing in the morning for at least 10 minutes, without looking directly at the sun. This helps release serotonin, which is essential for mood regulation and converting to melatonin at night.

- **Maintaining a regular rhythm:** It is essential for your body to keep its internal clock on time. Waking up and going to bed at consistent times each day helps establish a steady sleep-wake cycle, which is critical for achieving restful sleep.

- **Quality of sleep before midnight:** Particularly valuable; it is often said that one hour of sleep before midnight is worth two hours of sleep after midnight.

- **Manage your cortisol wisely:** When cortisol rises beyond healthy levels in stress it directly impacts your ability to sleep deeply—the ancient need to keep you in a state of constant vigilance for danger. (See page 342 for more on cortisol.)

- **Nurture melatonin pathways:** Working in partnership with healthy daytime cortisol production, melatonin is the timekeeper for your sleep-wake cycle. (See page 367 on how to do this.)

## 2. BLUE LIGHT VS RED LIGHT

Managing light exposure is the number one consideration for quality sleep according to neuroscience. Avoid at all costs blue light spectrum (most artificial light) after dark. As little as 15 seconds of blue light spectrum can switch off your melatonin. When you reduce your exposure to bright artificial lights after sunset your body clock can stay on track and melatonin will be produced. This blue light toxicity is relevant from birth to Age of Wisdom.

Red light spectrum from sunset, fire and candlelight, as well as circadian lighting is the catalyst to convert your serotonin (made with exposure to morning sunlight) to melatonin for sleep. Blue light exposure can also indirectly interfere with the circadian rhythm of dopamine release, leaving you depleted of joy the next day. (See Spotlight on Dopamine on page 658.)

### HOW TO REDUCE YOUR BLUE LIGHT EXPOSURE

- **Install blue light blocking globes:** Consider installing these globes throughout your home if you're building or renovating. While they may be more expensive, they are worth the investment for your health.

- **Use red party lights:** Inexpensive red party bulbs in lamps can serve as effective red-light sources.

- **Keep salt lamps:** These can provide gentle illumination during night-time.

- **Opt for red-light book lights:** Great for reading before bed.

- **Dim your lights at night:** This helps signal your brain to produce melatonin.

- **Consider purchasing online glasses with a red lens:** Blocks out uncontrollable blue lighting.

- **Get evening sunlight:** Expose yourself to sunlight for about 10 minutes as the sun sets to provide a protective mechanism to help you deal with a small amount of blue light exposure.

- **Adjust digital devices:** Set your devices to switch to dark mode automatically at night to minimise blue light exposure.

- **Monitor app usage:** Be mindful of blue light exposure, especially for children, from apps and social media after sunset.

### 3. SETTING THE RIGHT TEMPERATURE

Keep your bedroom cool. The ideal temperature to encourage quality sleep is between 16-18°C. Your body's core temperature needs to drop by up to 1°C for you to fall asleep, and stay cool while you sleep, and then increase to wake up. An increase in temperature before morning will wake you up.

### TEMPERATURE AND SLEEP HYGIENE

- **Use your bedroom only for sleep:** Make sure your bedroom is used solely for sleeping and intimacy. Remove all electronic devices, including televisions and digital gadgets.

- **Wi-fi:** Turn off at night.
- **Prioritise natural ventilation:** Use a fan, open windows.
- **Keep your bedroom clean:** Regularly vacuum and dust to reduce irritants.
- **Invest in quality sleep essentials:**
    - Good mattress: Should last about 10 years. Consider latex or thermoregulating bed topper such as Eight Sleep.
    - Pillow: A supportive latex one lasts about five years.
    - Bed linen and sleep wear: Choose natural fibres, such as cotton.
    - Blankets and duvets: Choose materials like wool, bamboo, silk, hemp and cotton.

> **TIP**
> Body contour mattresses and pillows can increase body temperature for some people.

## 4. DECREASE SLEEP SABOTEURS

Once you have read and addressed the top three considerations for quality sleep listed above, begin to address this checklist. The saboteurs of sleep include:

- Caffeine
- Alcohol
- High sugar load before bed
- Nicotine
- Bedroom noise—including pets, and partners who snore
- Lack of physical activity during the day
- Late-night exercise
- Overhydration close to bedtime

### CAFFEINE

If you're looking for one of the biggest saboteurs of sleep, it's caffeine. Try eliminating caffeine entirely until you are sleeping soundly again. Caffeine is found in coffee, carbonated drinks and chocolate. Even cacao and cocoa contain significant amounts—around 240 mg per 100 g, equivalent to three espresso coffees.

## WHY CAFFEINE AFFECTS SLEEP

- **Caffeine:** This neurostimulator reduces your deep sleep, which is an essential part of the sleep cycle.

- **Caffeine half-life:** Caffeine has a half-life of approximately 5 to 6 hours. Several hours after consumption, about half of the caffeine remains in your system, and even 10-12 hours later, around a quarter can still linger. A caffeinated drink at midday leaves a quarter of the caffeine still in your brain at midnight.

- **Genetic factors:** Some women with specific genetic variations (SNPs) may experience a prolonged caffeine half-life of up to 36 hours—this means that your morning expresso can still be interfering with sleep into the next evening.

- **Blocking sleep signals:** Caffeine disrupts sleep regulation by blocking adenosine, a neurotransmitter crucial for regulating sleep-wake cycles. Caffeine can mask this effect, leading to a cycle of fatigue, disrupted sleep, and increased dependence on caffeine.

- **Impact on deep sleep**: Even if you believe caffeine doesn't affect your sleep, neuroscience research is clear—it hinders your ability to reach deep sleep stages, even though you may feel you had a good night's sleep, your brain did not get its requirements met. Deep sleep is essential for brain health, as this is when your body clears Alzheimer's-related toxic proteins, regulates the immune system, supports hormonal balance, enhances serotonin production, and manages metabolic pathways.

## PRACTICAL TIPS FOR REDUCING YOUR CAFFEINE INTAKE

- **Switch to decaffeinated coffee:** Choose only the Swiss water-filtered method to decaffeinate coffee, the coffee bean still has the antioxidant health benefits.
- **Limit coffee consumption:** Cap your caffeinated coffee intake to two cups per day and consume them before midday.
- **Black tea and green tea** contain caffeine (black more than green) so choose the naturally low-caffeine variety or reduce consumption after midday.
- **Moderate chocolate intake:** Limit chocolate to 20 g after midday (at most).
- **Energy drinks:** Do not consume.

### ALCOHOL

While alcohol might make you feel drowsy initially, *any* amount of alcohol will disrupt natural sleep patterns, especially REM sleep. Alcohol's effect on sleep does not stop there. Your liver ramps up its detox pathways to metabolise alcohol around 2am. If you are perimenopausal or transitioning through menopause, the impact is even greater. Alcohol detoxification can divert your liver from its crucial role in balancing hormones, making the effects on your sleep more pronounced. (See Spotlight on Alcohol on page 287.)

> **TIP**
>
> When you over-caffeinate and drink alcohol you lose both REM and DEEP sleep in your sleep cycle, depriving your body and brain of essential recovery and repair.

### SUGAR

Eating high-sugar foods at night can disrupt sleep by causing blood sugar spikes and crashes. These fluctuations trigger both insulin and cortisol release to stabilise glucose, which in turn interferes with melatonin pathways and disrupts your circadian rhythm. For tips on weaning yourself off this saboteur of sleep and general wellbeing see our Wellness Action Plan Sugar Addiction (page 436).

### NICOTINE

Although smokers may feel a brief sense of relaxation while smoking, nicotine is a powerful stimulant. It increases heart rate, boosts alertness, and disrupts the brain's ability to wind down for sleep. Additionally, nicotine withdrawal during the night can lead to restless sleep and frequent awakenings, making it a true sleep saboteur. Smoking is a key driver of most chronic diseases that impact nearly every organ system. Your health practitioner can provide support to break this habit.

### PETS

If your pet disrupts your sleep, consider keeping them out of the bedroom. While it can be challenging, your sleep is essential. Cats tend to play at night, and dogs often take over the bed.

Solution: Ask yourself honestly, 'Would you sleep better if your pets didn't share my bed?' It may take time for them to accept the new rules, so try creating a morning routine filled with love and attention instead.

**PARTNERS AND SLEEP**

If your partner snores or fidgets, it can disturb your sleep. For a good sleep, encouraging your partner to seek sleep rehabilitation may be the best solution. Sleep apnoea and other issues can prevent both of you from enjoying restorative sleep, impacting health, mood and your relationship.

> **TIP**
> One simple solution is to keep a ready supply of soft noise-cancelling wax earplugs that gently mould to the shape of your ear canal.

**BABIES AND CHILDREN**

If your sleep is interrupted by caring for a baby, try to nap during the day while they sleep. Use that time for rest rather than doing household chores. Your ability to be emotionally present for your child relies on your wellbeing. It's also worth noting that breastfeeding can provide mothers with progesterone, which helps counteract some insomnia effects.

## 5. EMBRACE SLEEP PROMOTERS

Engage in relaxing activities before bed, such as reading, stretching, or meditating. Establishing a pre-sleep routine can signal to your body that it's time to wind down.

Understanding and prioritising sleep can significantly improve your hormonal health and overall wellbeing. By making small adjustments to your routine and sleep environment, you can restore balance and reclaim the power of a good night's rest.

The following suggestions work best when combined with removing any sleep saboteurs that may be affecting your rest. Creating a regular routine is essential.

- **Dinner time:** Try to have dinner by 7pm to allow time for digestion.

- **Create a bedtime ritual:** Incorporate activities like bathing, stretching, meditating and breathwork, using soft lighting or enjoy aromatherapy oils. You might also consider sipping warm herbal tea or spending intimate time with your partner.

- **Bathing:** Have a hot shower or bath before bed to open your blood vessels and allow your core temperature to drop for you to fall asleep.

- **Aim to be in bed by 10pm:** This allows you to get the sleep you need. Early birds should calculate their bedtime to ensure they get at least seven to eight hours of sleep by counting backwards from their wake-up time.

- **Set a sleep 'Do Not Disturb' on your phone:** From 9pm to 6am, disable notifications. You can add emergency contacts so urgent matters can still reach you. Even better, leave your phone outside the bedroom while you sleep.

- **Use a soft, red-toned night-light:** If you need to use the bathroom, do so in low light to avoid waking yourself up further by exposing yourself to blue light.

> **TIP**
>
> Neuroscience suggests that your brain associates your bed with wakefulness if you spend too long awake in it, which isn't what you want. If you're awake for more than 15-20 minutes, get out of bed. Move to another room, lie on the couch, avoiding blue light.
>
> Here are other strategies to encourage sleep:
> - Maintain a comfortable temperature: Ensure you're warm or cool enough, depending on the season.
> - Engage in non-stimulating activities: Listen to calming music or pop in one ear bud on low volume and listen to a familiar audiobook (one where you know the story).
> - Consider a hot shower in the dark. This will help you cool your core temp.
> - Enjoy a caffeine-free herbal tea: Options like passionflower, Tulsi or chamomile can have a calming effect on the nervous system.
> - Don't return to bed until you yawn or feel drowsy.
> - The moment you feel sleepy, head back to bed or relax on the couch if you are happy to sleep there. Focus on your breathing, find your most comfortable position, and breathe in through your nose and out through your mouth. Slow down your exhalation to calm your nervous system and ease back into sleep. (Read more on the power of the breath on page 381).

**SLEEP SUPPORT FOODS**

What you eat significantly impacts your sleep cycle and quality. For example, pistachio nuts contain trace amounts of melatonin. Enjoying about 30 g, or a small handful, can provide a nutritious evening snack that may enhance sleep quality.

Incorporate more of the following sleep support foods into your diet: fish, oysters, chicken, turkey, pistachios, cherries, Brazil nuts, eggs, berries, dairy, tomatoes, pepitas, buckwheat, walnuts, spinach, soy, and parsley.

**HERBAL AND OTHER SLEEP AIDS**

- Hops and valerian are great starting points for supporting a good night's sleep. German research suggests that combining these herbs helps initiate and maintain natural sleep. You can source this as ReDormin, an over-the-counter purchase available in most countries.

- Other helpful herbs include ziziphus and withania, commonly found in naturopathic products (follow the recommended dosage on the container).

- Melatonin can be an effective insomnia remedy, available online, via prescription, or over the counter for those aged 55 and older. The adult dose typically ranges from 2 to 6 mg taken one to two hours before bedtime. Liquid forms may recommend 10 to 15 drops at bedtime.

- GABA may also help with sleep disturbed by anxiety, with a suggested dose of 200 mg at bedtime and an additional 100 mg if you wake up after midnight. Diaphragmatic breathing stimulates the vagus nerve causing the brain to produce GABA to self-soothe your way to relaxation.

If sleep problems persist, consult a naturopath, Traditional Chinese Medicine practitioner, integrative doctor or sleep specialist. In cases of severe insomnia, your doctor may consider prescribing short-term sleeping tablets. It's essential to continue working on your sleep solutions even if medication is needed temporarily.

**NURTURING PROGESTERONE FOR QUALITY SLEEP**

Healthy progesterone levels during the second half of your cycle act as a natural sleep aid, promoting better rest. Progesterone typically peaks between Days 18 and 22 of the menstrual cycle, playing a vital role in emotional wellbeing, creativity and memory. During the luteal phase, optimising progesterone is crucial for maintaining quality sleep. However, progesterone levels begin to decline as early as your 30s, and by perimenopause, many women are bidding farewell to its sleep-supporting benefits. (Solutions for optimising progesterone are found in your relevant hormonal stage covered in Part One.)

### PERIMENOPAUSE, MENOPAUSE, AND SLEEP

If you're navigating perimenopause or menopause, you may have noticed that sleep feels elusive, with wakefulness in the early hours, insomnia, or hot sweats disrupting your nights.

Hormonal fluctuations during this phase often bring changes to sleep patterns. Sleep research by Dr Matt Walker reveals that 30 to 40% of women report significant sleep challenges during these transitions. Combined with the sleep disturbances caused by night sweats and hot flushes, low progesterone during perimenopause and the menopause transition adds yet another challenge to achieving restful, restorative sleep.

Lower oestrogen levels can impact serotonin production, a key player in regulating sleep, while also triggering hot flushes that interrupt rest.

Here are some handy hints for managing sleep changes through hormonal transitions:

- Ensure you follow to the letter all the recommendations listed on the previous pages before you go looking for help. Please get your foundations right first.
- Tighten up boundaries on sleep saboteurs. Eliminate alcohol and caffeine until you're sleeping soundly again.
- Melatonin may help. Some studies show that medically prescribed slow-release melatonin can be effective.
- For herbal remedies, consulting a naturopath or a practitioner of Traditional Chinese Medicine can be a great first step.
- Low iron, magnesium and vitamin D can contribute to 'restless legs'. Have these nutrients checked and try an Epsom salts bath before bed or take 150 mg of magnesium phosphate at bedtime.

## IDENTIFY TRIGGERS

Pay attention to your habits on wakeful nights—there is always a reason, whether it is chronic stress, a late bedtime, dessert, an extra glass of wine, or even a full moon or loud storm. An occasional night of disturbed sleep after a celebration isn't a problem but if it becomes a regular habit, it can sabotage your hormonal health and mental wellbeing.

## NEUROSCIENCE'S TOP THREE TIPS FOR SLEEP

1 **Balance your hormones:** Bioidentical hormone replacement may be beneficial if oestrogen or progesterone are low.
2 **Meditate for 10 minutes before bed:** Apps like *Calm*, *Headspace*, or *Endel* can help.
3 **Consider Cognitive Behavioural Therapy (CBT) for insomnia:** This has scientific backing and can provide good results without side effects.

When you prioritise your natural circadian rhythm and minimise known sleep disruptors, you can reclaim quality sleep, which is worth celebrating. As you reach the Age of Wisdom, you may find that with the right support, you can sleep soundly again without medication—unless it's a super moon!

### INTERNATIONAL TRAVEL AND JET LAG

To make the most of your travels, look for apps that help minimise jet lag upon arrival. Preparing for good sleep starts a few days before your flight. Apps like *Timeshifter*, which use NASA's research, can guide you in adjusting your sleep cycles. In the future, airlines may incorporate these findings to enhance passenger comfort.

### SHIFT WORK AND SLEEP

First, a heartfelt thank you to shift workers, who often serve in emergency services and healthcare. However, shift work can significantly disrupt your natural rhythm, leading to various side effects, including increased fat gain and mental health challenges. Research suggests that shift workers may experience a higher likelihood of health-related concerns that can impact overall longevity.

> Research indicates that individuals with an evening chronotype, often referred to as 'night owls,' may experience fewer negative health impacts from shift work compared to those with a morning chronotype. This is because their natural sleep-wake preferences align more closely with the demands of non-traditional work hours.
>
> A study published in the *Journal of Epidemiology & Community Health* found that shift workers whose work schedules matched their chronotype reported better mental health outcomes than those whose schedules were misaligned with their natural preferences.

## STRATEGIES FOR MANAGING SLEEP AS A SHIFT WORKER

- **Maintain a healthy lifestyle:** Prioritise nutrition, movement, and other healthy habits.

- **Reduce alcohol and caffeine:** This supports your body in managing the demands of a disrupted schedule.

- **Create a sleep-friendly environment:** Ensure you have time in circadian sleep lighting before trying to sleep.

- **Use earplugs:** Soft, waxy earplugs can help minimise disturbances.

- **Limit afternoon naps:** Afternoon naps before work are beneficial but limit these to less than 30 minutes.

- **Try to work in a regular rhythm:** Keep your rooms as dark as possible during the day with dimmed artificial light or candlelight to simulate night.

- **Invest in blackout curtains or blinds:** Keep daylight completely out of the room where you sleep during the day.

- **Walk, move or exercise:** Before you go to work.

- **Consider a yin-style movement option:** When you have finished work to assist your nervous system to settle before you go to sleep (such as yoga, Tai Chi, Qigong, light Pilates).

- **Work on gut health:** If you experience digestive issues, consult a naturopath.

- **Talk to your GP about melatonin:** This can help regulate your sleep cycle. Aim for seven to eight hours of quality sleep in a 24-hour period.

- **Stay hydrated:** Drink plenty of water but reduce intake four hours before sleep to minimise bathroom trips.

## SLEEP HELP

If the simple strategies in the chapter are not helping you hit all your sleep goals, book a visit to a specialised sleep clinic. They can analyse your sleep patterns and use the science of sleep to help you achieve a restorative sleep.

Sleep is non-negotiable for your body. It's foundational for repair and healing, mental clarity, immune function, and emotional resilience. Prioritising sleep is essential; if you're not enjoying restful sleep, it's time to explore solutions. When you have a good night's sleep, everything is brighter and easier to handle the next day.

Read our Spotlight on Melatonin opposite. Melatonin is a multitasking hormone often thought of as just the 'sleep hormone', but it's so much more. Beyond regulating your sleep-wake cycle, melatonin supports immune function, acts as a powerful antioxidant, and even plays a key role in reproductive health and cellular repair. We explore its remarkable roles and how you can harness its full potential for optimal hormonal health.

# SPOTLIGHT ON
# Melatonin

Known traditionally as your 'sleep hormone' and for its important role as the master timekeeper of your circadian rhythm, melatonin also has an intimate relationship with your fertility hormones. This relationship is significant, influencing reproductive health through hormonal regulation, circadian rhythm maintenance, and providing antioxidant protection to cells in the ovaries and sperm. There is also evidence of a major link between melatonin levels and body weight as you transition through menopause.

Disruptions to circadian rhythms—caused by shift work or irregular sleep patterns—can impact menstrual cycles and fertility. Maintaining proper melatonin levels helps regulate circadian rhythms, supporting overall hormonal health.

### MELATONIN: NIGHT-TIME SUPPORT FOR BREAST HEALTH

Mushrooming evidence is creating excitement even in mainstream medical circles about the potential for melatonin to rival pharmaceutical drugs to improve cancer treatment outcomes.

Melatonin has powerful effects in stopping the growth of various cancers, with a special focus on breast cancer. For breast cancers that rely on oestrogen (ER-positive types), melatonin steps in, and lowers oestrogen receptor activity. It does this by working epigenetically to reduce the expression of oestrogen receptor genes in cancer cells, reducing their impetus to grow and divide.

It helps regulate the activity of nuclear receptors and the enzymes that metabolise oestrogen, ensuring that related genes function properly and oestrogen metabolises through healthy pathways.

Finally, by inhibiting 'aerobic glycolysis' (the 'food and energy source' for cancer cells), melatonin can slow down cancer cell growth, survival, and spread. It also helps to overcome resistance to cancer drugs. In essence, melatonin is not just about sleep—it's a potent ally in maintaining breast health and combating cancer.

Let's look more closely at melatonin's impact on women in their journey from puberty through to the Age of Wisdom:

### PUBERTY

Melatonin can influence the timing of puberty. Higher melatonin levels are associated with a delayed onset of puberty, while lower levels may trigger earlier puberty.

- Establish a healthy bedtime routine to supports melatonin's role in maintaining healthy sleep patterns, which are essential for growth, development, and cognitive function during adolescence.
- Incorporate more melatonin-rich foods like pistachios and cherries in your tween's diet.
- Avoid blue lights in your bedroom, use dimmers and a red spectrum book light.
- Avoid screen time in the hour before bed and encourage books instead.

### THE FERTILE YEARS

From the brain, melatonin directs the release of hormones that are critical for ovulation and the menstrual cycle including luteinising hormone (LH) and follicle-stimulating hormone (FSH).

Melatonin could be beneficial in assisted reproductive technologies, such as in vitro fertilisation (IVF). It may improve egg quality and enhance pregnancy rates in women undergoing fertility treatments. Maintaining adequate melatonin levels is important for regular menstrual cycles, fertility and overall reproductive health. Disruptions in melatonin production due to irregular sleep patterns or night shifts can negatively affect fertility and menstrual regularity.

- If you're planning a pregnancy, it may be worth reconsidering shift work to support your chances of a healthy pregnancy.

### MELATONIN AND PCOS

Women with PCOS have an altered production of melatonin that could reflect a decreased sensitivity to this hormone. Result? A disruption in the normal circadian sleep rhythm. This can lead to poor sleep, an increased risk of depression and higher stress levels that can then drive symptoms of anxiety and weight gain.

- Consider low-dose melatonin supplementation (2 mg one hour before bed).
- Establish regular sleeping patterns to support melatonin production pathways.

## PERIMENOPAUSE

As we move from the Fertile Years to perimenopause, melatonin production starts to decline, mirroring a woman's age-related declines in fertility. Supplementing melatonin in older women wishing to embark on a pregnancy has been studied for its potential to improve reproductive hormone levels and fertility outcomes.

- Supplementing melatonin during perimenopause may improve sleep quality and stabilise mood, helping to mitigate some of the disruptive symptoms associated with this phase.
- Enjoy melatonin-rich foods like pistachios as an after-dinner snack.

## MENOPAUSE

Melatonin production declines significantly during menopause, compounding the common sleep disturbances experienced in this transition. There is emerging evidence suggesting that melatonin plays a role in bone health by influencing bone remodelling and potentially protecting against osteoporosis.

- Supplementing melatonin (available over the counter for over 55s) can improve sleep quality and may offer benefits for bone health, reducing the risk of fractures and osteoporosis.

### MELATONIN AND BODY WEIGHT

Exciting research since 2021 shows a strong link between melatonin and body weight. Multiple studies in mice and rats show a reduction in weight gain, particularly in abdominal fat deposits, after mimicking menopause by removing their ovaries. Given the safety of melatonin supplementation, human studies are underway (watch this space!).

## AGE OF WISDOM

As women age, melatonin production continues to decline, often leading to poorer sleep quality and increased incidence of sleep disorders.

- Consider supplementing melatonin, 2 to 4 mg, one hour before bed.

## THE BENEFITS OF MELATONIN BEYOND SLEEP

### BRAIN HEALTH

Melatonin is also an unlikely member of your antioxidant team. Oxidative stress is a major contributor to the ageing process. Melatonin's ability to neutralise free radicals helps slow down cellular ageing and maintain youthful function in various tissues.

Melatonin supplementation through menopause and beyond can improve sleep quality, enhance overall wellbeing, and potentially offer neuroprotective benefits. Melatonin's antioxidant properties are particularly beneficial for brain health. It helps protect neurons from oxidative stress, which is implicated in neurodegenerative diseases such as Alzheimer's and Parkinson's.

### SKIN HEALTH

Topical melatonin shows promise in reversing age-related changes and damage caused by sun exposure due to its anti-inflammatory, antioxidant, DNA repair, and improve skin hydration and elasticity through collagen-stimulating properties. While more extensive clinical trials are underway, current evidence supports its potential benefits in skincare. Melatonin's added anti-inflammatory properties can help to settle inflammation underlying skin problems like eczema and acne.

---

**DR KAREN'S FACE CREAM**

Compounding pharmacists can create therapeutic skincare containing a mixture of natural bases, sun protection and powerful anti-ageing ingredients. One of my favourite prescription facial creams for older skin is a combination made up in a natural rosehip oil base, applied once or twice daily:

Vitamin C 10%
Niacinamide (vitamin B3) 5%
Melatonin 0.2%

**TIP**

For some women I'll add topical oestriol (E3) 0.05% and tretinoin (retinol, vitamin A) 0.04% to their mix for extra anti-ageing support.

### THE INTIMATE RELATIONSHIP BETWEEN MELATONIN AND SEROTONIN

Like most other hormones, melatonin is recycled from a worthy precursor: serotonin, our mood stability hormone. Deep within your brain, old serotonin is concentrated and metabolised to molecules of melatonin in two easy steps (you already know how to do this—it's written into your genetic code!).

**Melatonin**                                    **Serotonin**

The nutrients needed as co-factors for this magic to happen are our B-vitamins, along with magnesium and zinc. The following multitasking foods help streamline your nutrient intake while supporting your melatonin pathway effectively:

- **Chickpeas:** High in vitamin B6, folate (B9), magnesium and zinc.
- **Pumpkin seeds:** Rich in magnesium and zinc.
- **Spinach:** A source of folate (B9), magnesium and vitamin B6.
- **Cashews:** Contain magnesium and zinc.
- **Eggs:** Provide vitamins B6, B12 and folate (B9).
- **Sardines:** Contains vitamins B6, B12, magnesium and zinc

### FOODS THAT FEED SLEEP—PLANT SOURCES OF MELATONIN

Nature's gifts include tiny bursts of natural melatonin from plant sources. Pistachio nuts are one of the richest plant sources of melatonin. An after-dinner snack may augment your natural melatonin levels. Cherries, black and red grapes, goji berries and walnuts are also natural sources of melatonin. Be creative and try a combination of these healthy sleep foods as an after-dinner treat.

Throughout a woman's life, melatonin plays a crucial role in regulating sleep, reproductive and skin health, mood, and overall wellbeing. Its decline with age underscores the importance of maintaining adequate melatonin levels through lifestyle choices or supplementation, especially during the critical transitional phases of perimenopause and menopause.

## SPOTLIGHT ON
# Restorative Practices

Our natural state as a human female is one of calm and relaxation. However, the demands of the modern world often pull us into hypervigilance, overstimulation, and relentless pressure, pushing us into a state of fight-or-flight. This survival mode, though meant to be temporary, has become so familiar that many of us now consider it our 'normal'.

In this section, we focus on reclaiming your natural state by activating the parasympathetic nervous system (Blue Zone) more often—intermittently throughout your day and big chunks during your weeks. This part of the nervous system is the cornerstone of rest, recovery, hormonal balance and healing. You'll discover practical tools and methods to weave into your daily routine, supporting physical, emotional and mental balance. Together, we will delve into the neuroscience of meditation, the transformative power of breathwork, the wisdom of ancient healing practices, and the restorative magic of creative arts.

These restorative practices are not just essential for managing stress; they are foundational for achieving hormonal harmony and overall wellbeing. Let this chapter serve as a guide to reconnecting with your innate calm self and restore your vitality.

# ACTIVATING YOUR BLUE ZONE

Spending time in the 'rest and digest' arm of your nervous system—technically referred to as the parasympathetic arm and what we call your Blue Zone—is essential for balancing hormones, supporting healing and rejuvenation, and promoting overall wellbeing. This state fosters relaxation and restoration, helping counteract the stress-induced fight-or-flight response and guiding your body back to a state of healing and homeostasis.

However, peak productivity requires accessing what we call the Purple Zone—technically activating the sympathetic nervous system, while maintaining the ability to regulate the flow of adrenaline and cortisol. To function at your best personally and professionally, regular intervals where you dip into your parasympathetic Blue Zone throughout the day is crucial. These intentional Blue Zone moments, help you to balance your nervous system between Blue and Purple Zones each day, which will help prevent an elevation of cortisol to catabolic levels, as well as restore any elevated cortisol to normal healthy levels over time.

While dipping into your Blue Zone during your day is important, it is also essential that you prioritise longer sessions in your Blue Zone along with quality sleep to ensure your recovery and healing. This chapter is your personal guide to prioritising deep rest in your life, your strategic guide to healing, recharging and resilience.

> Women need real moments of solitude
> and self-reflection to balance out how much
> of ourselves we give away.
>
> **BARBARA DE ANGELIS**

In our fast-paced, often stressful world, finding ways to relax and rejuvenate is essential. We have outlined some ideas for you to consider so find what works best for you. The more often you activate your Blue Zone, the easier it is for your body to move between your sympathetic and para-sympathetic nervous system. Ideally, you should be able to do this at any moment of the day. Simply notice when you feel any pressure mount, pause for a moment and dip into your Blue Zone to help you to maintain balance in your nervous system.

There are many powerful methods to use that we have outlined here. So, take some take time to review and figure out what can work for you. The idea is to use some of the methods to create chunks of time in your Blue Zone, other methods are ways you can dip into your Blue Zone for 30 seconds or a few minutes.

We offer many methods, so be curious and think outside the square. Even if you don't see yourself as artistic, we encourage you to explore your creative potential through art, music, or other expression. These activities activate your Blue Zone, ease stress, and support overall wellbeing.

## BREATHWORK, MINDFULNESS AND MEDITATION

The neuroscience research into breathing techniques and meditation show extraordinary benefits beyond Blue Zone activation. We provide a deeper dive into these powerful tools on pages 382 and 386.

## IMMERSING YOURSELF IN NATURE

Nature has a profound ability to calm the mind and body. Spending time in green spaces, near water bodies, or simply in fresh air can significantly lower stress levels.

- **Forest bathing (Shinrin-Yoku):** This is a Japanese practice which involves immersing yourself in a forest environment (or in our part of the world— bush), mindfully engaging your senses with the sights, sounds and smells of the woods, forest or bush.

- **Being by water:** Whether it's a beach, lake or river, being near water has a soothing effect on the mind. The rhythmic sound of waves and the expansive views can help reduce anxiety and promote relaxation.

- **Gardening:** Engaging in gentle gardening activities, such as planting seeds or watering, allows you to connect with nature, providing a sense of accomplishment and tranquillity.

> Taking care of yourself doesn't mean me first,
> it means me too.
>
> L R KNOST

## SPA TREATMENTS AND MASSAGE THERAPY

Spa treatments and massages are excellent for activating your Blue Zone, as they reduce muscle tension, promote circulation, and encourage relaxation.

- **Swedish massage:** This gentle relaxation massage technique uses long, flowing strokes to relax the entire body. It is an excellent way to reduce your cortisol levels.

- **Aromatherapy:** Using essential oils such as Tulsi, lavender or chamomile can enhance relaxation and promote a sense of calm when used during a massage or in a home diffuser.

- **Hot stone massage:** The heat from the stones can help relax muscles, improve circulation, and soothe your nervous system.

## GEOTHERMAL BATHING

Geothermal baths and hydrotherapy treatments have been used for centuries to promote healing and relaxation.

- **Hot springs:** Soaking in natural hot springs rich in minerals can alleviate muscle pain, improve skin health and promote deep relaxation.

- **Mineral baths:** Magnesium, boron and manganese can be absorbed through the skin, assisting the relaxation response.

- **Contrast bathing:** Alternating between hot and cold water immersions can stimulate circulation and boost the immune system while promoting deep relaxation after you have finished the cycles. To activate your Blue Zone, finish your last cycle with hot, then take some time to relax for at least 20 minutes.

- **Float therapy:** Floating in a sensory deprivation tank filled with Epsom salt water can reduce stress and improve both sleep and mental clarity.

## YOGA AND QIGONG

- **Yoga:** Poses such as Child's Pose, Legs Up the Wall, and Savasana are particularly effective for inducing relaxation.

- **Restorative yoga:** As the name implies, restorative yoga is extraordinarily good at replenishing your nervous system and is great for adrenal fatigue. Find a class and go regularly.

- **Yoga Nidra**: We strongly recommend this guided meditation practice, highly beneficial for restoring adrenal fatigue and supporting sleep.

- **Qigong:** With origins in Traditional Chinese Medicine, this gentle yet powerful practice involves slow, deliberate movements and deep breathing. It restores Qi (universal energy, lifeforce) in your body helps to reduce stress, improve balance, and enhance overall wellbeing.

## GENTLE MOVEMENT

Light physical activity can help activate Blue Zoning by reducing stress hormones and promoting relaxation.

- **Stretching:** Gentle stretching exercises can relieve muscle tension and promote a sense of wellbeing. You can also do some gentle stretches when you are in water.

## NUTRITION AND HYDRATION

Proper nutrition and hydration play a crucial role in supporting Blue Zoning and overall health.

- **Hydration:** Staying well-hydrated helps maintain optimal bodily functions and reduces stress.

- **Balanced diet:** Consuming a diet rich in fruits, vegetables, whole grains and lean proteins supports overall health and can help reduce stress.

- **Herbal teas:** Teas such as Tulsi, chamomile, peppermint and valerian root have calming properties that can support your relaxation response.

## CREATING A RELAXING ENVIRONMENT

Your surroundings can significantly impact your stress levels and ability to relax.

- **Decluttering:** A clean and organised space can reduce stress and promote a sense of calm.

- **Ambient lighting:** Soft, warm lighting such as candle or fire light can create a relaxing atmosphere.

- **Soothing sounds:** Listening to calming music or nature sounds can help switch off your stress response.

## SHORT DIPS INTO BLUE ZONING DURING A BUSY DAY

Even during a hectic day, you can take brief moments to activate your Blue Zone and promote relaxation in intervals which helps to improve your ability to remain centred.

- **Intentional breathing at red lights:** When stopped at a red light, take a few deep, intentional breaths to calm your mind and reduce stress. (Also try while picking up the kids from school.)

- **Mindful moments in line:** While waiting in line, practise mindful breathing or do a quick body scan to release tension.

- **Breathing exercises on the toilet:** Use your bathroom breaks as an opportunity to practise deep-breathing exercises and reset your mind.

- **Gratitude pause:** Take a moment to reflect on something you're grateful for, which can instantly shift your mindset and promote relaxation.

- **Micro-meditations:** Spend 1 to 2 minutes focusing on your breath or a calming image, even amidst a busy schedule.

> I am working on myself, for myself.
>
> **LAUREN GLEISBERG**

### ART, MUSIC, CREATIVITY, AND BLUE ZONING: A PATH TO INNER PEACE

Creating art is more than just a hobby; it's a therapeutic process that engages the mind and body in a way that promotes relaxation and reduces stress.

- **Mindful drawing and painting:** When you focus on drawing or painting, your mind shifts away from worries and anxieties. The repetitive motions and immersion in the creative process can lower your cortisol levels.

- **Colouring:** Adult colouring books have gained popularity for their ability to promote relaxation. The act of colouring intricate patterns can induce a meditative state, allowing you to unwind and de-stress.

- **Sculpting and crafting:** Working with clay, wood or other materials requires concentration and tactile engagement. This hands-on creativity can be incredibly grounding and calming.

- **Music and Blue Zoning:** Music has a profound impact on our emotions and can be a powerful tool for inducing relaxation and activating Blue Zone.

- **Listening to music:** Certain types of music, such as classical, relaxation, chanting or nature sounds, can soothe the mind and body. Listening to your favourite calming tunes can slow your heart rate, lower blood pressure and reduce stress.

- **Playing an instrument:** Engaging in the physical act of playing an instrument such as a guitar or piano is a mindfulness activity. The focus and repetition involved in playing music can promote a sense of calm.

- **Singing and chanting:** Vocal expression, whether through singing or chanting, has been shown to reduce stress and enhance mood. The vibrations and breath control involved in these activities stimulate the vagus nerve, a key player in activating your Blue Zone.

### CREATIVITY AND BLUE ZONING

Beyond traditional art and music, various forms of creative expression can help you enter a state of relaxation and balance.

- **Writing and journaling:** Expressing your thoughts and emotions through writing can be therapeutic. Journaling allows you to process your experiences, release pent-up emotions, and gain clarity—all of which can activate your Blue Zone.

### INTEGRATING CREATIVITY INTO YOUR DAILY ROUTINE

Integrating creativity doesn't have to be time-consuming. Here are some simple ways to engage your creativity throughout your day:

- **Morning pages:** Start your day with a few minutes of free writing. This practice, known as 'Morning Pages', allows you to clear your mind and set a positive tone for the day.

- **Music breaks:** Take short breaks during your day to listen to calming music. Close your eyes, breathe deeply, and let the music wash over you.

- **Doodle and sketch:** Keep a small notebook with you and doodle or sketch during downtime, such as waiting for an appointment or during a break at work. This can be a quick way to engage your creative mind and activate your Blue Zone.

- **Mindful cooking:** Approach meal preparation as a creative and mindful activity. Pay attention to the colours, smells and textures of the ingredients, and enjoy the process of creating a nourishing meal.

By engaging in any of these Blue Zone activities, you can tap into a deeper sense of relaxation and balance, reducing stress and promoting a healthier, happier life. Whether you choose breathwork, meditation or time in nature, relax and enjoy life. Maybe you enjoy the more expressive way through painting, playing an instrument, writing, or cooking? Allow yourself the freedom to explore your creative potential and enjoy the many benefits it brings. Embrace it all as a vital part of your daily routine, calling these moments 'strategic rest'! Experience the profound impact Blue Zoning can have on your mind, body and spirit.

> If you don't pick a day to relax,
> your body will pick it for you.
>
> **KIM MALONE**

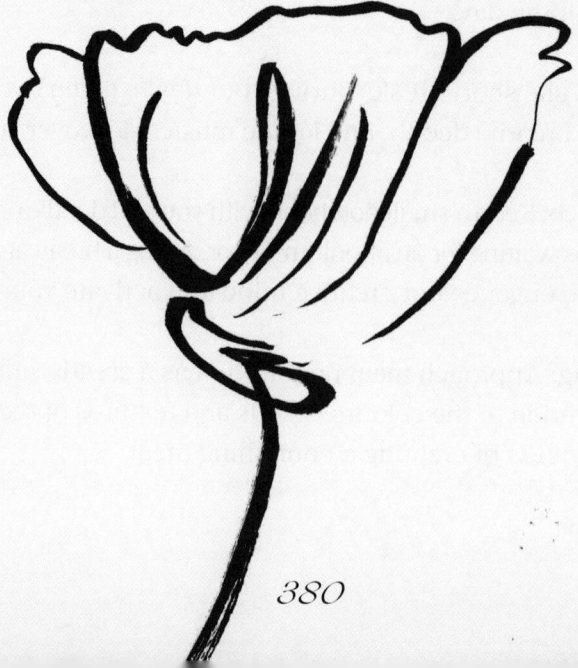

RESTORATIVE

# THE BREATH

> Just a single thought can change
> your breathing pattern.
>
> ILSE MIDDENDORF

From the moment you take your first breath until the moment you take your last, this essential element for life has enormous influence on your mind and body. When observed, your breath can give focus to the mind, slow your heart rate, reduce blood pressure, and bring internal quiet and stillness into focus.

The ancient and traditional healing systems such as Ayurveda (from which yoga is derived) have known the significance of the breath and its patterns for centuries. Yoga is the home of focused breathing. It teaches you to breathe in challenging poses and this learning can be transferred to your daily life. By learning to notice and focus on your breathing whenever you feel self-doubt, pressured or notice your body's stress response, you can change your physiology by changing the depth, rhythm, and pace of your breathing.

Paying attention to, and changing, your breathing pattern is a powerful way to manually, override your nervous system. This can allow you to see more clearly and have an enhanced capacity to respond to life rather than become triggered and reactive in life.

> Breathe, darling, this is just a chapter,
> not your whole story.
>
> SC LOURIE

Breath is free and is constantly with you; you simply need to remember and pay attention to your inhalation and exhalation.

On a consciousness level, breath connects us all. Every intake of breath is an acceptance of life—you breathe in a gas that is given by plants and trees. Every time you breathe out, you're letting go, and the gas you exhale is essential for the life of plants and trees. In this simple way, we are all connected.

## Breathe with the trees.
**MR WONG**

This cycle of giving and receiving has been present for centuries and will continue long after your lifetime. Yet many of us can go through life, lost in thought, disconnected from the essence of who we are.

Noticing when you are shallow breathing and then actively changing to belly breathing (explained later in this chapter) will help you calm down and move to parts of your brain that have more solutions and a better decision-making ability.

Qigong, Pilates and yoga are some of the activities you can engage in to learn greater breath control.

## Fear is excitement without breath.
**ROBERT HELLER**

### DAY-TO-DAY BREATHING

- Begin every day by being aware of your breath.
- Being aware of your breath will give you focus.
- Set an intention for your day—be mindful to pay attention to your breath each moment and remind yourself to regulate your breathing whenever you become challenged or busy.
- Throughout your day, notice your breathing.
- A faster pace of breath will be required in a spin class, a slower deeper pace in a massage.
- A quiet walk will allow you to notice your breathing while walking in nature.
- You may notice how much is missed when you walk and talk with others. Try to take walks on your own and reflect on how beautiful it is to be in nature.
- Be silent and listen to the rhythm of your own breathing. Feel gratitude or awareness of being alive on a brand-new day.
- You can practise your breathing wherever you are, whatever you are doing. This is the beauty and simplicity of the breath.
- Simply pay more attention to your breathing in different situations in life.
- In challenging moments, try to deepen your breathing and slow its pace.

- If you wake in the middle of the night, rather than thinking, planning, and organising, bring your awareness to focus on deep belly breathing. This induces the body to relax. With the mind engaged on the breath you will naturally fall back asleep.

## Our health and wellbeing are dependent on many elements; however, breath is the unsung HERO. Learning how to relax is as simple as breathing in and breathing out.

## Why not practise right now?

### CYCLIC BREATHING

#### BENEFITS

Cyclic breathing, or resonant breathing, has been validated by the research at Stanford University. The practice helps to stabilise heart rate and blood pressure, leading to improved cardiovascular health, reduced anxiety, and better emotional regulation. By activating the parasympathetic nervous system (your Blue Zone), cyclic breathing can significantly reduce stress and anxiety, promoting a sense of calm and wellbeing. Additionally, regular practise of cyclic breathing has been shown to improve focus, enhance emotional regulation, and boost overall mental clarity.

#### RESEARCH CYCLIC BREATHING: INSIGHTS FROM STANFORD UNIVERSITY

Cyclic breathing is a technique that balances breath rhythm, promoting relaxation and overall wellbeing. This balanced activation helps in reducing your stress response, lowers heart rate, and enhances your mental clarity. The researchers discovered that maintaining a steady, slow breath rate can lead to significant reductions in cortisol levels, thereby promoting a state of calm and wellbeing. They suggested this is a valid non-pharmacological option for anxiety. Just five minutes a day had a significant impact on the participants to reduce stress.

**HOW TO PRACTICE CYCLIC BREATHING**

In cyclic breathing, the breath is paced at a frequency of around 5 to 6 breaths per minute, a rhythm that is naturally soothing.

- Sit (or lie down) in a comfortable position with your back straight and shoulders relaxed.

- Inhale through your nose until you fill your lungs—pause and notice you can continue to inhale while allowing your abdomen to expand.

- Exhale slowly and completely through your mouth, allowing your abdomen to expand, focus on making your outward breath longer than your two inward breaths.

- Aim to breathe at a pace of 5 to 6 breaths per minute. This means each breath cycle (inhalation and exhalation) should take about 10 to 12 seconds. You can use a timer or a breathing app to maintain this rhythm.

- Inhale and exhale smoothly avoid any sudden stops or starts.

- Focus on making the transition between inhaling and exhaling as seamless as possible.

- Continue this rhythmic breathing for several minutes, gradually extending the practice as you become more comfortable.

- Aim for at least 5 to 10 minutes to experience the full benefits.

- Practise this anytime in your day, sitting or standing:
    - When you feel under pressure.
    - When you are losing your centre.
    - When you know something can easily trigger you.

- As you breathe, concentrate on the sensation of the air entering and leaving your body. This focus can help anchor you in the present moment and further reduce stress and anxiety.

### DIAPHRAGMATIC BREATHING

Also known as 'belly breathing', this technique involves inhaling deeply through your nose, allowing your abdomen to expand, and exhaling slowly through your mouth. This type of breathing activates your Blue Zone and promotes relaxation.

### 4-7-8 BREATHING

Inhale through your nose for a count of 4, hold your breath for a count of 7, and exhale through your mouth for a count of 8. This method can quickly reduce stress and anxiety.

### ALTERNATE NOSTRIL BREATHING

This yoga breathing technique (pranayama) involves closing one nostril while inhaling through the other, then switching nostrils for the exhale. It balances the nervous system and calms the mind.

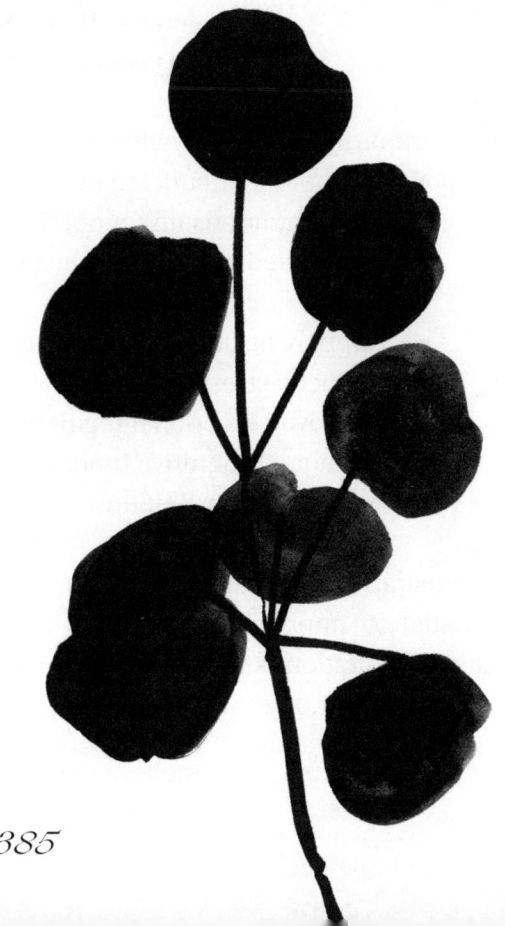

# WHY MEDITATION IS A MUST

The quieter you become, the more you can hear.

**ANON**

If you are seeking a way to feel calm more often and feel more in control of your life, that also improves your perspective and rational thinking, the answer is meditation.

Once primarily associated with spirituality, this ancient practice has emerged as a powerful tool for enhancing mental and physical wellbeing. Now grounded in both ancient traditions and modern science, meditation offers a wide range of benefits supported by neuroscience research including;

- Supporting structural and functional changes in your brain
- Reduced stress
- Improved emotional regulation
- Enhanced cognitive function
- A tool in the prevention of dementia

By integrating meditation into your daily life, you can tap into its profound potential to improve your mental clarity, emotional wellbeing, and overall health. Meditation is free of charge, with no side effects, and only takes 10–20 minutes of your day.

## BEYOND SPIRITUALITY

Today, it is widely used in clinical settings to treat a variety of physical and mental health conditions. For example, mindfulness-based stress reduction (MBSR) and mindfulness-based cognitive therapy (MBCT) are evidence-based programs that use meditation to help individuals manage chronic pain, anxiety, and depression. These programs have been shown to be extremely effective in reducing symptoms and improving quality of life for patients with a vast range of health conditions.

Also used in educational and workplace settings to enhance wellbeing and performance, schools and universities are incorporating mindfulness programs to help students manage stress and improve focus. More increasingly as the research floods into the masses, companies use meditation as part of employee wellness initiatives to reduce burnout and enhance productivity.

Athletes and coaches are recognising the benefits of meditation for enhancing mental toughness, improving focus, and promoting recovery in sport. Meditation helps athletes develop greater resilience and maintain peak performance under pressure.

## MEDITATION BENEFITS YOU

Neuroscience research shows a regular meditation practice can lead to significant changes in both the structure and function of your brain. One of the most well-documented findings is the increase in grey matter density in regions associated with memory, learning, and emotional regulation. A study led by Dr Sara Lazar at Harvard University found that just eight weeks of mindfulness meditation can increase cortical thickness in the hippocampus, a region crucial for learning and memory, and in areas associated with emotional regulation, such as the prefrontal cortex (often referred to as the CEO of the brain).

Meditation enhances connectivity between different regions in your brain, particularly those involved in attention and executive function. What is super exciting is experienced meditators have more control over mind-wandering and mind chatter, which is an essential skill in a fast-paced world. Imagine what benefits you could gain from having improved cognitive control and a greater ability to manage any distracting thoughts and challenging emotions. This heightened state of mindfulness can improve cognitive performance and reduce the tendency for you to ruminate on past or future events, providing a more balanced and focused mental state.

Altering patterns of your brain wave activity, studies using electroencephalography (EEG) have found that meditation is associated with increased alpha and theta wave activity, which are linked to relaxation and a state of wakeful rest. These changes in brain wave activity shows that meditation can offer you a state of calm alertness, enhancing your mental clarity and emotional stability.

If you are not running to your meditation app or cushion yet, in relation to balancing your hormones, know that meditation is one of the most powerful stress reduction tools available to you with evidence-based results!

Regular meditation practice down-regulates your sympathetic nervous system which can lead to lower levels of cortisol, thereby reducing the overall impact of stress. (See page 342 for more information on cortisol.)

The increased activity in the networks built by your brain during meditation are associated with greater emotional resilience and an improved ability to manage negative emotions such as anxiety and depression.

A study published in *JAMA Internal Medicine* found that mindfulness meditation can be as effective as antidepressant medications for treating symptoms of anxiety and depression, highlighting its potential as a non-pharmacological intervention for mental health.

In addition to emotional benefits your practice will deliver, meditation also enhances your cognitive function.

One study found that participants who completed an eight-week mindfulness meditation course demonstrated significant improvements in their ability to sustain attention on a task, showing that meditation can enhance cognitive control and focus.

#### MEDITATION SLOWS THE AGEING OF YOUR BRAIN

The graphic opposite highlights regions of the brain affected by ageing, shown in white. Interestingly, scans of meditators show significantly less white, suggesting they experience better preservation of healthy brain regions as they age.

## When the world grew loud and uncertain, she turned inward—not to escape, but to remember. In the quiet of her own being, she cultivated the steadiness no one else could give her.

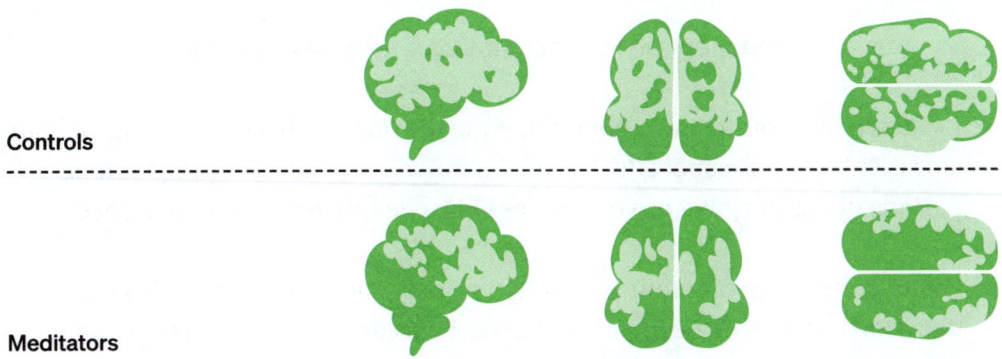

**Controls**

**Meditators**

## HOW TO MEDITATE

Meditation is the process of allowing yourself to become still, and to observe your thoughts without judgement.

As the world becomes faster and louder, meditation is a way to maintain your centre under pressure—to find the eye of your life storms, rather than getting pulled into rumination and catastrophising.

There are many different styles of meditation. Each style offers you unique benefits and can be tailored to suit your individual needs.

### SITTING MEDITATION: FINDING STILLNESS AND FOCUS

Sitting meditation is one of the most traditional and widely practised forms of meditation. It involves you sitting in a comfortable and stable position, such as cross-legged on the floor or in a chair, with your back straight and your hands resting on your knees or in your lap. The aim is for you to maintain a still posture that supports alertness and allows for prolonged focus without any physical discomfort.

There are various techniques within sitting meditation.

- Mindfulness meditation involves you focusing on the present moment, often by observing your breath or bodily sensations.

- Concentrative meditation requires you to focus on a single point, such as a mantra or a visual object, to help you cultivate deep concentration.

Sitting meditation helps you to develop mindfulness, improves your concentration, and promotes your emotional regulation. It is particularly effective for calming your mind and enhancing your self-awareness.

### LYING MEDITATION: RELAXATION AND AWARENESS

- Lie down in a comfortable position, typically on your back with arms at your sides. This style is especially beneficial for you if you find sitting for long periods uncomfortable or you are seeking a deeply relaxing experience.

- Focus on relaxing different parts of your body, moving attention from the toes slowly up to the head or vice versa. This can be done with or without guided audio instructions.

- Yoga Nidra, or 'yogic sleep', is a popular form of lying meditation that induces deep relaxation and is said to be as restorative as several hours of sleep. Very popular with neuroscience, the podcast *Huberman Lab* created non-sleep deep rest (NSDR) based on Yoga Nidra.

- In guided imagery, visualise calming and peaceful scenes, such as a beach or forest, to reduce stress and activate Blue Zoning.

Lying meditation is excellent for reducing stress and tension, promoting relaxation, and improving your sleep quality. It can help increase your body awareness and alleviate any physical discomfort you may experience.

### LOVING-KINDNESS MEDITATION

This form of meditation involves directing positive thoughts and well-wishes towards yourself and others, fostering a sense of peace and connection.

### TEA CEREMONIES

When traditional tea ceremonies are practised by a master you will experience profound stillness and silence. In Australia we highly recommend Byron Bay-based Cloud Hidden Tea. They travel to capital cities.

### WALKING MEDITATION: MOVEMENT AND MINDFULNESS

Walking meditation integrates the benefits of physical movement with mindfulness practice. It is often practised in a quiet, open space where you can walk slowly and with intention, paying close attention to each step you take and the sensations in your body.

- There are different ways to practise walking meditation. A simple approach is to focus on the sensation of your feet touching the ground with each step, noticing the weight transference from heel to toe and what parts of your body tense to help these steps and what parts relax to allow you to walk each step. Ideally coordinate your breath with the movement. Breathe in, step, breathe out as you take your next step. Slow your steps to the rate of your breath and vice versa.

- Qigong is also a form of moving meditation.

- Silent walks focus on being in nature and your breathing, letting thoughts come and go without thinking and planning.

Walking meditation helps you to ground your mind in the present moment, improves your concentration, and increases your awareness of your bodily sensations. It is particularly beneficial if you find it challenging to sit or lie still for extended periods.

### BREATHING MEDITATION: CENTRE AND CALM YOURSELF

Breathing meditation, also known as 'breath awareness' (or pranayama in yoga), centres on your breath as the primary focus of your attention. This style can be practised in various positions, including sitting, lying or even standing, making it highly versatile and accessible. There are several methods:

- Deep diaphragmatic breathing, where the breath is drawn deep into the belly.

- Alternate nostril breathing, which involves you inhaling through one nostril and exhaling through the other, place your finger/thumb on the opposite nostril as you change from one to the other.

- Mindful breathing involves you observing the natural rhythm of the breath without attempting to control it, simply noticing how you inhale and exhale.

Breathing meditation is effective for calming your mind and reducing anxiety, and a very effective way to help you manage stress. It helps you improve respiratory function and can increase your body's oxygen intake, promoting overall vitality. People with asthma find this very supportive to reduce their symptoms and offer a way to calm themselves when having an asthma attack.

**WHICH ONE WORKS FOR YOU?**
Find a style that suits you. You may like to join a meditation group or choose an app to assist you on this journey. When you first begin your meditation practice, start slowly and approach it with curiosity, rather than expectation.

> Distractions are everywhere. Notice what takes your attention, acknowledge it and then let it go.
>
> **HEADSPACE** APP

**DURATION**
It can be a good idea to set aside 10 minutes of your day to meditate. You can build from there as you will find it easier the more patient you become with your practise.

Each style of meditation offers unique advantages and can be tailored to meet your diverse needs and preferences. Whether you prefer the stillness of sitting meditation, the relaxation of lying meditation, the movement of walking meditation, or the focus of breathing meditation, integrating these practices into your daily routine can lead to profound improvements in your mental, emotional, and physical wellbeing. And, by exploring and experimenting with different styles, you can discover the meditation practice that best supports your journey toward greater mindfulness and holistic health.

SPOTLIGHT ON

# Nourishment

Maintaining hormonal balance and a stable mood isn't just about managing stress or getting enough sleep—it's also deeply connected to the foods we eat every day. Our hormones play a crucial role in regulating everything from energy levels and mood to digestion and reproductive health. By making mindful, nutritious choices, we can support our body's natural hormonal processes and promote emotional wellbeing. The following Core Food Principles for mood and hormonal health are designed to guide you towards foods and habits that nourish your body, reduce inflammation, and create a foundation for lasting hormonal harmony.

## LESSONS FROM THE BLUE ZONES

As you may have read in previous chapters, the concept of Blue Zones refers to regions of the world where people have followed lifestyle habits that lead to significantly longer and healthier lives. These regions include Okinawa in Japan, Sardinia in Italy, the Nicoya Peninsula of Costa Rica, the island of Ikaria in Greece, and the predominantly Seventh-day Adventist community in Loma Linda, California (USA). While each Blue Zone has its unique dietary practices, several common elements emerge across all these longevity hotspots.

Studies on women's health in Blue Zones show impressive results on improved fertility and reduced hormonally connected disease. Their food philosophies have a common foundation: all Blue Zones build their nutrition on plant-based food. Are you experiencing a little push back from this suggestion? What about the beautiful aroma of a perfectly grilled steak, or oven-baked chicken, you ask? The good news is that 'plant-based' does not mean 'plant-exclusive'. All Blue Zones include modest amounts of animal products—the difference is that:

## The hero of the meal is the vegetable family, not the protein.

Our experience within the health, lifestyle retreat, and medical arenas are based on similar concepts that provide irrefutable proof that the foundation of a long and healthy life span is not found in any one supplement, drug or doctor's office, but in a clean, plant-based diet. This chapter will guide you through our Ten Core Food Principles, and why adopting these for you and your loved ones may be the best investment in hormonal harmony and wellbeing that exists.

Although navigating the complex landscape of hormonal health can be challenging, the right nutrition can make a world of difference. Our Core Food Principles are tailored to support women's hormonal balance and mood regulation, providing a solid foundation for overall wellbeing.

## Pay your farmer, not your pharmacist.

**KELLY LEVEQUE**

NOURISHMENT

# IDEAL FOOD PYRAMID

The Mediterranean Diet is backed by solid research. We love this modern food pyramid, which is recommended by *Journal of the American College of Cardiology* (JACC) to prevent and treat cardiovascular disease.

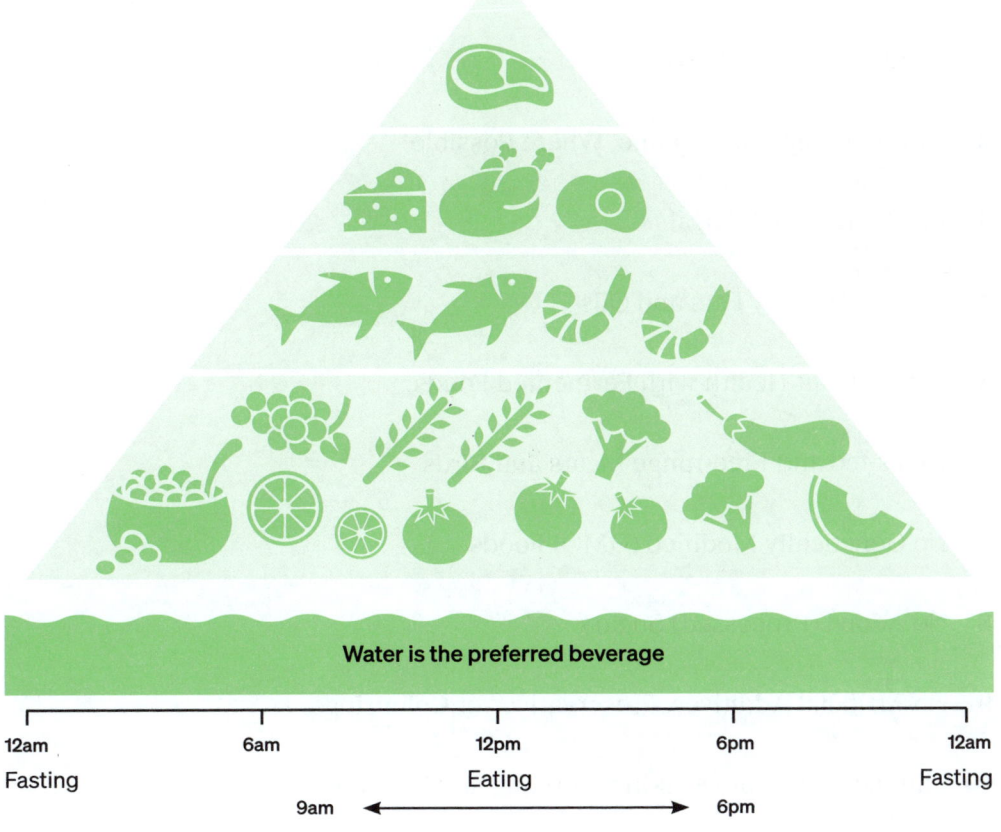

Is it coronary disease or culinary disease?

DR CALDWELL B ESSELSTYN JR

YOUR HORMONAL HEALTH PILLARS

# OUR TEN CORE FOOD PRINCIPLES

1. Plant-based, Whole Foods

2. Always Clean and Organic, Where Possible

3. Fresh, Seasonal, Local

4. Choose Healthy Fats and Oils

5. Support Gut Health with Fermented Foods

6. Grass-fed and Free-range Meats and Birds

7. No Genetically Modified (GMO) Foods

8. No Added (Processed) Sugars

9. No Artificial Additives, Preservatives or Colourings

10. Filtered Water for Drinking, Cooking and Washing

## Eat less from a box and more from the earth

ASHA ABBYKOON

The following section unpacks each of the Ten Core Food Principles to help you understand how they support long-term health and hormonal balance.

### 1   PLANT-BASED, WHOLE FOODS
Whole, plant-based foods are integral to a hormone-friendly diet. They are rich in essential nutrients, fibre and antioxidants that support hormonal balance and mental wellbeing. In the following sections, we'll dive into the specific benefits of nuts, seeds, leafy greens, grains and legumes, and how they contribute to hormonal health.

### 2   ALWAYS CLEAN AND ORGANIC, WHERE POSSIBLE
Organic foods are free from pesticides and synthetic chemicals that can disrupt your endocrine system. By choosing organic, you reduce your exposure to hormone-disrupting toxins. We'll explore why organic choices matter and how to bio-hack your way to clean food if organic is not an option for you.

### 3   FRESH, SEASONAL, LOCAL
Eating fresh, seasonal and local produce ensures you get the most nutrient-dense foods, which are crucial for supporting hormonal health. Applying this core principle ensures that that your food will always deliver and exceed your body's need for antioxidant support.

### 4   CHOOSE HEALTHY FATS AND OILS
Healthy fats are vital for hormone production. Foods like avocados, olive oil, and coconut oil provide the building blocks for your hormones. In the sections ahead, we'll explore the types of fats that benefit hormonal health and those that don't.

### 5   SUPPORT GUT HEALTH WITH FERMENTED FOODS
A healthy gut is foundational to hormonal health. Fermented foods like yoghurt, kefir, sauerkraut and kimchi are rich in probiotics, supporting a healthy gut microbiome. We'll delve into the connection between gut health and hormones, providing practical tips for incorporating fermented foods into your diet.

### 6   GRASS-FED AND FREE-RANGE MEATS AND BIRDS
Grass-fed and free-range meats are superior in omega-3 fatty acids, essential for reducing inflammation and supporting brain health. The following pages will explain the importance of these meat sources and how they can positively impact your hormonal and mood health.

## 7   NO GENETICALLY MODIFIED (GMO) FOODS

GMO foods can contain residues of herbicides like glyphosate, which is linked to hormonal disruption. Avoiding GMOs helps protect your endocrine system. We'll discuss the impacts of GMOs on health and how to identify and avoid them.

## 8   NO ADDED (PROCESSED) SUGARS

Processed sugars disrupt mood hormones like dopamine and cause blood sugar fluctuations, impacting insulin and oestrogen balance. These imbalances lead to mood swings and energy crashes.

## 9   NO ARTIFICIAL ADDITIVES, PRESERVATIVES OR COLOURINGS

Artificial additives and preservatives can interfere with hormone function and negatively impact mood. We'll investigate further in this chapter why these substances are harmful and how to choose whole, unprocessed foods.

## 10   FILTERED WATER FOR DRINKING, COOKING AND WASHING

Using filtered water helps reduce exposure to contaminants like PFAS, which can disrupt hormonal balance. Clean water is essential for maintaining hydrated cells, healthy hormones and a stable mood.

Let's explore these further.

# 1.
# PLANT-BASED WHOLE FOODS

> Came from a plant, eat it;
> was made in a plant, don't.
>
> **MICHAEL POLLAN**

We invite you to explore the transformative power of plant-based foods and discover how they can enhance your hormonal and overall wellbeing. A plant-based diet serves as the cornerstone of an anti-inflammatory wellness approach, providing your body with essential nutrients, fibre, and bioactive compounds that work to reduce inflammation, balance hormones, and support optimal health.

Rich in antioxidants, vitamins, and minerals, plant-based foods help combat oxidative stress—a key driver of chronic disease and hormonal imbalances. By focusing on vegetables, fruits, whole grains, legumes, nuts and seeds, you can create a dietary foundation that supports every stage of your hormonal journey, from the vibrant shifts of puberty and fertility to the transitions of perimenopause and menopause.

**EMBRACE THESE FOUR FOOD GROUPS:**
- Leafy vegetables, including the cruciferous family
- Starchy carbs and grains for B-vitamins and fibre
- Legumes for longevity
- Phytoestrogens for healthy oestrogen balance

## LEAFY AND FLORAL CARBOHYDRATES: NUTRITIONAL POWERHOUSES FOR HORMONAL HEALTH

When we talk about plant-based carbs that support hormonal wellbeing, it helps to divide them into two key categories: leafy carbs and floral carbs. These are the vegetables and salad greens that come straight from the garden—fresh, fibre-rich, and full of nutrients your hormones love.

Leafy carbs include tender greens like rocket (arugula), kale, collard greens, mustard greens, and watercress. They're mostly made of water and fibre but also deliver magnesium, folate and a whole suite of B-vitamins that support hormone regulation, DNA repair and inflammatory balance.

Floral carbs, on the other hand, are vegetables we eat from the flowering parts of the plant. Think broccoli, cauliflower, cabbage, Brussels sprouts, bok choy, turnips, radishes and even wasabi. Many of these are crunchier and denser—but no less important for your hormones.

Now here's where it gets interesting: some of these vegetables are both leafy and cruciferous, like rocket, kale and mustard greens. Others are floral and cruciferous, like broccoli, Brussels sprouts and cauliflower. It's not their shape that makes them cruciferous—it's their phytochemical content.

Cruciferous vegetables contain natural compounds like glucosinolates, which support healthy oestrogen metabolism and detoxification in the liver. That's why they're considered essential for hormone balance at every stage of life. Your cruciferous all-stars include:

- Rocket (arugula)
- Broccoli
- Brussels sprouts
- Bok choy
- Cabbage
- Cauliflower
- Collard and mustard greens
- Radish
- Kale
- Turnips
- Watercress
- Wasabi

We recommend you eat 1 serve of cruciferous vegetables every day. Whether leafy or floral, these veggies are hormonal multitaskers—nourishing your cells, clearing excess oestrogen, and calming inflammation from the inside out. They are low in calories, high in volume, and rich in water and antioxidants. This makes them ideal for managing body fat, staying hydrated, and reducing inflammation to support immune health.

### SULFORAPHANE: A MULTI-BENEFIT POWERHOUSE

Sulforaphane, a standout compound in broccoli, is a potent antioxidant and detoxifier with wide-ranging health benefits. It reduces inflammation, combats oxidative stress, and supports the body's natural detoxification processes, lowering the risk of certain cancers.

#### METABOLIC HEALTH BENEFITS

Research shows sulforaphane improves insulin sensitivity and lowers fasting blood glucose levels, making it particularly beneficial for individuals with insulin resistance or Type 2 diabetes. A study published in *Science Translational Medicine* found that sulforaphane significantly reduced fasting blood glucose levels in people with Type 2 diabetes.

#### BRAIN HEALTH SUPPORT

With neuroprotective properties, sulforaphane reduces brain inflammation and may lower the risk of neurodegenerative diseases like Alzheimer's and Parkinson's.

#### HORMONAL HEALTH AND OESTROGEN REGULATION

Sulforaphane aids hormonal balance by supporting detoxification enzymes and antioxidant activity. It helps metabolise oestrogen into safer forms, protecting breast tissue from oestrogen dominance-related risks such as PMS, weight gain, and breast cancer. Additionally, it protects egg cells in the ovaries from oxidative damage—a promising breakthrough in medical research.

## STARCHY AND GRAIN CARBOHYDRATES

The starchy and grain group of carbs are great value, packed with fibre, vitamins and minerals and an essential part of a daily diet—these contain a little more sugar than the leafy carbs but provide valuable resources for your gut microbiome.

We struggle to understand why some diets exclude these for weight reduction. The promoters of these diets are not understanding or considering the long-term impact on your hormonal balance and convince you this is the only way to lose body fat. Beware!

Root vegetables such as sweet potato and turnips shine here, along with grains like brown rice and quinoa. Turnips are an underrated member of your plant-based food family—the green turnip tops are part of the cruciferous family and will sing to your hormones!

### TIP

Starchy carbs earned a bad reputation in the 1990s as a major culprit behind weight gain. However, the real issue lies not in natural starchy carbs themselves, but in highly processed foods made from them. When these processed foods are removed from your diet, your body's natural biochemistry can return to its healthy rhythm, highlighting that human intervention—through food processing—was the real problem, not the carbs in their natural state.

### FIBRE AND OESTROGEN EXCRETION

The fibre in carbohydrate foods is a major player in hormonal health. Dietary fibre aids in the excretion of excess oestrogen from your body. When fibre binds to oestrogen in the digestive tract, it aids in its elimination by preventing the hormone from being reabsorbed into the bloodstream. This process is essential for maintaining balanced hormone levels and reducing the risk of oestrogen dominance. (Read more about your gut-hormone connection on page 424.)

### YOUR DAILY CARBOHYDRATE GOALS

- Leafy carbs = unlimited enjoyment! The general rule with leafy carbohydrates is simple: eat as much as you want. Their low-calorie, high-nutrient profile means you can enjoy them freely without worrying about overindulgence. Incorporating a variety of leafy greens into your diet ensures you receive a broad spectrum of nutrients, all working together to support your hormonal health and overall wellbeing.
- Eat one cup of cruciferous vegetables each day.
- Include Brussels sprouts and/or broccoli three times a week.
- Eat one or two serves of root vegetables (with skin on for the fibre) each day, for example:
    - Half cup of cooked sweet potato, turnips or beets
    - One medium sized carrot
- Eat two to three servings of whole grains per day. A serving could be:
    - Half cup of cooked brown rice, quinoa, barley, or other whole grains
    - One slice of whole-grain sourdough bread
    - Half cup of cooked oatmeal

### LEGUMES FOR LONGEVITY

Many women avoid legumes, yet they are vital for gut health, providing unique fibre essential for a thriving microbiome. This fibre supports gut bacteria linked to brain health, playing a key role in preventing dementia.

Legumes, including beans, lentils, and peas, are a rare combination of carbohydrates and proteins. They are an excellent plant-based protein source, particularly valuable for vegetarians and vegans. While they offer essential amino acids, pairing them with other vegetable proteins such as tofu and nuts can create a complete amino acid profile.

Rich in complex carbohydrates, legumes provide lasting energy and fibre that benefits gut health, supports oestrogen metabolism, and helps regulate blood sugar.

- Eat one or two serves of legumes each day
  - Half cup of cooked beans, lentils, peas or chickpeas
  - Quarter cup of hummus or other legume-based spread

### FOLATE (VITAMIN B9)—AN HONOURABLE MENTION

Folate is a superstar for women's health, as it's crucial for keeping hormones balanced, supporting fertility and a healthy pregnancy. It plays a key role in making and repairing DNA, which is vital for cell growth and division. This is a key player in keeping your cervix and uterus healthy and low levels can drive endometriosis and adenomyosis (see page 517 for Spotlight on Uterine Care). It also multitasks in mood hormone production and regulation, keeping you cognitively balanced. Getting enough folate through your diet is a smart move for overall health, happiness and wellbeing.

#### FOLIC ACID IS NOT FOLATE

While both folate and folic acid fulfill the same vitamin B9 role, they differ in source, absorption and metabolism.

**Folate is the natural form of vitamin B9** found in leafy greens, fruits, beans and whole grains. It is absorbed more slowly and undergoes natural chemical conversions in the small intestine before entering the bloodstream and liver.

**Folic acid, the synthetic version of vitamin B9,** is found in supplements and fortified foods like cereals and breads. It is rapidly absorbed and sent to the liver, where it must be converted into the active form. This conversion can be slow, leading to an accumulation of synthetic folic acid in the blood.

High levels of synthetic folic acid have been linked to bowel cancer, cognitive decline in those deficient in vitamin B12, and weakened immune function. These risks are not associated with plant-based folate from whole foods.

During times of increased folate demand, such as pregnancy, careful supplementation with folic acid can help meet needs, but balance is essential. Folate works closely with vitamin B12 in many biochemical processes, so both must always be adequately supported.

**Natural is always best**—plant-based folate poses no known risks and should be prioritised over synthetic alternatives.

> # When diet is wrong, medicine is of no use.
> # When diet is correct, medicine is of no need.
> ### AYURVEDIC PROVERB

### PHYTOESTROGENS:
### A PHYTOCHEMICAL SHIELD OF PROTECTION FOR YOUR BREASTS

Phytoestrogens, naturally occurring compounds found in plant-based foods, offer a powerful shield of protection for your breasts. These plant-derived chemicals mimic the effects of oestrogen in the body (in a good way) helping to balance hormone levels and reducing the risk of hormone-related cancers, including breast cancer.

Foods rich in phytoestrogens have been shown to have protective effects by binding to oestrogen receptors on your cells and modulating your body's oestrogen activity. This not only helps in maintaining hormonal health, it also counteracts the harmful effects of excess oestrogen that can promote the growth of cancer cells. Incorporating a diet rich in phytoestrogens provides a natural, dietary approach to bolster breast health and overall hormonal balance.

### PHYTOESTROGEN FOODS, A GIFT FROM NATURE TO YOU

Include at least two serves from the list below everyday into your diet:

- Soy products: Tofu, tempeh, edamame, miso, soy milk (one serve = one cup)
- Nuts, almonds, walnuts (one serve = 30 g)
- Seeds: Flaxseed, sesame, sunflower (one serve = 20 g)
- Legumes: chickpeas, lentils, beans (one serve = ½ cup)
- Whole grains: Oats and barley (one serve = ½ cup)
- Wheatgerm (one serve = 10 g)
- Fruits: Apples, plums, berries, peaches, pomegranates (one serve is one whole piece of fruit)
- Vegetables: Carrots, alfalfa sprouts, sweet potato—skin on (one serve = ½ cup)
- Herbs: Use freely or source as teas such as red clover (great for supporting bone density, too) fennel, anise, liquorice root, garlic, parsley

# 2.
# ALWAYS CLEAN AND ORGANIC, WHERE POSSIBLE

*The diet is a bank account:
good food choices are good investments.*

**BETHENNY FRANKEL**

### THE CASE FOR CHOOSING ORGANIC FOODS

Organic food has become increasingly popular, and for good reason. Grown without synthetic pesticides, fertilisers or GMOs, organic produce offers several evidence-based benefits, particularly in reducing pesticide exposure. Studies consistently show that organic produce contains significantly fewer pesticide residues. A systematic review in *Environmental Health Perspectives* found that people who eat organic foods have lower levels of pesticide metabolites in their urine, indicating reduced exposure.

### HIGHER NUTRIENT DENSITY

Organic fruits and vegetables may be more nutrient-dense. A meta-analysis in the *British Journal of Nutrition* reported that organic crops have higher concentrations of antioxidants, which are crucial for overall health.

### REDUCED ENDOCRINE DISRUPTION

Pesticides like organophosphates are endocrine disruptors, which can impact hormone balance. Eating organic food reduces exposure to these chemicals, helping lower the risk of hormonal imbalances and related health issues.

### NEUROPROTECTIVE EFFECTS

Lowering pesticide exposure through organic food may protect brain health. An *Environmental Research* article shows that children with higher pesticide exposure are at greater risk of developmental and behavioural issues.

### ENVIRONMENTAL BENEFITS

Organic farming promotes soil health, reduces pollution, and supports biodiversity. These practices benefit ecosystems and contribute indirectly to human wellbeing.

> **DRAMATIC GLYPHOSATE REDUCTION**
>
> Switching to organic foods can significantly lower glyphosate exposure. A study in *Environmental Research* found that participants who switched to an organic diet reduced glyphosate levels in their bodies by up to 70% within just one week.

While it might not always be possible to choose organic for every item, prioritising organic options over the most pesticide-laden produce can make a significant difference.

### WHEN ORGANIC FOOD IS NOT AN OPTION

Eating organic produce is best for your health and wellbeing. However, organic produce may not always be accessible or affordable. Even if you buy organic produce, it is still important to wash everything thoroughly to remove any bacteria.

These are a few ways to wash and clean your fruit and vegetables:

- **Water rinse:** If you rinse under water, ensure that you thoroughly scrub your fruit and vegetables. As most pesticides are oil based (to ensure they don't wash away in the rain) water alone will not effectively remove them. Ideally, you should be using filtered water; however, even rinsing with filtered water is not the most effective way to remove pesticides and bacteria from your produce.

- **Baking soda wash:** Soak your produce in water with baking soda using 1 teaspoon of baking soda to 2 cups of cold water. When mixed with water, it causes the water to become alkaline. Certain classes of pesticides are not stable at an alkaline pH, so can break down, ready to be washed away.

- **Vinegar wash:** Soaking in vinegar has also been shown to remove some of the residue of a few pesticides, however it can leave a taste behind. It works by the vinegar's acetic acid breaking down certain pesticides, so they can be washed away.

A few home washing methods online suggest washing your produce in both baking soda and vinegar. Individually they do have some cleaning properties, but as baking soda is a base, and vinegar is an acid, one neutralises the other when mixed (creating sodium acetate). If you want to get the best result from each of these methods, use them separately.

- **Electrolysis soak:** By far the best investment is to use a produce purifier, such as Crop DeTox, which uses electrolysis to remove up to 99% of pesticides and bacteria from your fruit and vegetables. Produce purifiers work by splitting water into hydrogen gas and oxygen gas. The hydrogen gas causes the water to become alkaline, breaking down the oil-based pesticides so they can be washed away. The oxygen gas, hypochlorous acid (HOCl), is the same germicide our white blood cells produce to destroy pathogens, effectively disinfecting the produce.

Of all these options, we highly recommend the electrolysis soak. It's the one we use and trust. For a produce purifier that has been lab-tested to prove its results and is available in Australia, purchase one from Crop DeTox (www.cropdetox.com). Thanks to our wellness warrior and innovator of Crop DeTox, Marnie Calli, for her contribution to our campaign for clean, affordable food, and for sharing her IVF journey with readers (see page 106).

# 3.
# FRESH, SEASONAL, LOCAL FOOD

> Maybe we should stop asking why real food is so expensive and start asking why processed food is so cheap.
>
> **FOOD MATTERS**

Vitamins needed for human health and hormonal pathway support start to decay from the moment your food leaves its connection with the earth. This Core Food Principle keeps the nutrient density and quality of your produce at the highest possible level. Fresh food maximises the antioxidant capacity of each mouthful. Keeping food local avoids the pitfalls of nutrient decay through time delays from farm to your kitchen. Long distance travel also puts fresh produce at risk of heat and light exposure that can change the phytochemicals in your produce.

The journey of your favourite plant-based foods from farm to table is quite the adventure, but it's not without its pitfalls—especially when it comes to maintaining their antioxidant levels. Antioxidants are molecules that protect your cells from damage—they can degrade during transportation. Let's dive into why this happens and what it means for your diet.

### THE ANTIOXIDANT HIGHWAY: FROM FARM TO TABLE

Antioxidants are sensitive to various environmental factors. When plant-based foods are harvested, their journey involves multiple steps: from the farm to the processing facility, then onto trucks, planes, or ships, and finally to your local supermarket. Each stage exposes these foods to conditions that can reduce their antioxidant and vitamin content.

**FACTORS CONTRIBUTING TO ANTIOXIDANT DEGRADATION:**

- **Temperature:** Antioxidants are highly sensitive to temperature fluctuations. During transportation, especially over long distances, foods can be exposed to varying temperatures. Heat accelerates the degradation of antioxidants, while improper cooling can lead to the same fate. Maintaining a consistent and optimal temperature is crucial.

- **Light:** Certain antioxidants, such as vitamins A and C, are photolabile, meaning their antioxidant effect degrades when exposed to light. Long-distance transport often means prolonged exposure to light, especially in transparent packaging.

- **Oxidation:** The very process antioxidants are supposed to combat—oxidation—can occur during transport. When plant-based foods are exposed to oxygen in the air, reactions can degrade antioxidants, leaving less in the food for your body to use.

- **Time delay:** The longer the transit time, the greater the potential for antioxidant degradation. Freshly harvested produce has the highest levels of antioxidants, which is why you should only eat food in season and from your country. Ideally, grow as much of your own produce as possible, or buy from your local farmer's market or farm gate.

- **Physical damage to the food:** Handling and transportation can cause physical damage to plant-based foods. Bruising and cutting increase surface area exposure to air and light, accelerating antioxidant loss.

- **Impact on nutritional value:** The reduction in antioxidant levels means that by the time these foods reach your table, they might not pack the same nutritional punch as when they were first harvested. This is particularly concerning for food-based antioxidants like vitamin C, carotenoids, and flavonoids, which are known for their health benefits.

## STRATEGIES TO PRESERVE ANTIOXIDANTS

- Whenever possible, buy locally sourced produce. Shorter transportation distances mean fewer opportunities for antioxidant degradation. Plus, supporting local farmers is always a bonus!

- Build a relationship with your local greengrocer and fruit and vegetable supplier—let them know how important time delay is for you.

- Once you've purchased your plant-based foods, store them properly. Refrigeration slows down the degradation process. Keep them in dark, cool places to protect them from light and heat.

- Try to consume your plant-based foods as soon as possible after purchase. The fresher they are, the higher their antioxidant content.

- If you live remotely or in countries where winter excludes a lot of fresh foods, choose frozen foods frozen. Surprisingly, frozen fruits and vegetables often retain more antioxidants than fresh ones that have been transported over long distances. Freezing locks in the nutrients at their peak.

- Ideally, try growing your own leafy greens and herbs in pots, and sprouts (mung bean/sunflower etc) in your kitchen.

## YOUR B-TEAM VITAMINS

Prioritising food that is fresh, seasonal and locally grown gives you the best chance of maximising your B-Team! From the tumultuous time of puberty to the Age of Wisdom, B-group vitamins play a pivotal role in your wellbeing. They're not just about boosting energy or keeping your metabolism in check; they're deeply intertwined with your hormonal health and mood.

Exposure to heat, light and air during transport and storage can lead to the breakdown of sensitive B-vitamins, particularly vitamins B1 (thiamine), B2 (riboflavin), and B6 (pyridoxine). The use of preservatives and processing methods to extend shelf life can further reduce the levels of these essential vitamins. By choosing fresh, local produce you minimise these nutrient losses, ensuring you receive the full spectrum of B-vitamins necessary for maintaining hormonal health.

Throughout a woman's hormonal journey, there are specific times when the need for B-vitamins increases, or your ability to extract them from your diet may be sabotaged. Being aware of these changes can keep you ahead of the pack.

By choosing fresh, local produce you minimise these nutrient losses, ensuring you receive the full spectrum of B-vitamins necessary for maintaining hormonal health.

We will later cover how to ensure you keep your B-team healthy. The most significant consequences of B-vitamin deficiencies in women are:

- **Vitamin B1 (thiamine):** Essential for accessing ATP, the cell's energy source, from carbohydrates. Deficiency is common with poor diets and high alcohol intake.

- **Vitamin B2 (riboflavin):** Supports thyroid function, fertility hormones, and adrenal health, especially during stress.

- **Vitamin B3 (niacin):** Vital for skin health, particularly in repairing sun-damaged skin and maintaining DNA integrity.

- **Vitamin B6:** Alcohol lowers absorption and active conversion, and increases excretion—a triple impact on this nutrient essential for mood-regulating neurotransmitters like serotonin, dopamine, and GABA.

- **Vitamin B9 (folate):** Critical for pregnancy, and you may be at risk of deficiency with restrictive diets.

- **Vitamin B12:** Absorption declines with age, particularly during the Age of Wisdom, increasing the need for supplementation.

## B-VITAMINS THROUGH YOUR HORMONAL JOURNEY

### PUBERTY

During puberty, the body's rapid growth and hormonal shifts require increased levels of B-vitamins to support energy production, brain development, and emotional stability. That grumpy pubertal teenager need not take all the blame for their attitude. Vitamin B6 is crucial to make your mood hormones. Stress, poor diet, and the onset of menstruation can deplete B-vitamins, making it essential to consume a balanced diet. It's worthwhile taking a good look at your young girl's diet—talk to a naturopath about supplementing the gaps.

### THE FERTILE YEARS

B-vitamins continue to support energy levels, mental clarity, and hormonal balance, which are crucial for menstrual health and fertility. Vitamin B12 and folate are particularly important for cell division and preventing anaemia. Oral contraceptives can reduce B-vitamin levels, so if you are on the Pill, have your folate checked and make sure to increase folate-rich foods—you'll find a list later in this chapter.

Pregnancy dramatically increases the need for B-vitamins, especially folate (vitamin B9), which is vital for preventing neural tube defects in the developing baby. B6 helps alleviate morning sickness, while B12 supports red blood cell production and prevents anaemia. Poor dietary choices and morning sickness can hinder B vitamin absorption, making supplementation the right choice to support a health mother and baby.

### PERIMENOPAUSE

As women enter perimenopause, hormonal fluctuations can lead to symptoms like fatigue, mood swings and brain fog. B-vitamins, particularly B6 and B12, help manage these symptoms by supporting neurotransmitter function and energy metabolism.

### MENOPAUSE

As women approach menopause, the body's ability to absorb B-vitamins can decrease, just as the demand for them rises to help manage symptoms like fatigue, mood swings and cognitive changes. Additionally, periods of high stress, chronic illness or the use of certain medications can further deplete B-vitamin stores.

Vitamin B3 (niacin) starts to shine as a skin support nutrient that reduces the risk of solar damage and skin cancers. Audit your diet for B-vitamin intake during menopause and check B12 levels with your health practitioner.

### THE AGE OF WISDOM

As we enter the period-free era of the Age of Wisdom, the risk of iron deficiency wanes, replaced with the challenge of maintaining optimal B-vitamin levels. The body's ability to absorb B-vitamins, particularly B12, decreases with age.

Iron deficiency anaemia may be replaced with a macrocytic anaemia due to vitamin B12 deficiency. Identify potential gaps in B-vitamin levels to support heart and brain health, energy levels and mental clarity. If you are on prescribed medications, check with your doctor for any possible dominos that may lead to nutritional deficiencies.

## Most heart medications and all medication prescribed for stomach ulcers and gastric acid reflux will deplete vitamins and minerals.

### CHECKLIST FOR B-VITAMIN DEFICIENCY

- Are you frequently feeling tired or fatigued without an obvious reason?
- Do you experience frequent mood swings or feel unusually irritable?
- Have you noticed memory problems or difficulty concentrating?
- Do you have a vegetarian, vegan or Paleo diet?
- Do you avoid carbohydrates and grains like bread and cereals?
- Are you taking birth control pills or other medications regularly?
- Do you consume alcohol frequently or in large amounts?
- Are you experiencing frequent headaches or migraines?
- Do you have a chronic illness, such as diabetes or coeliac disease?
- Have you recently been under a lot of stress?
- Do you have digestive issues, such as frequent stomach problems or poor absorption?
- Do you have skin problems, like dryness or cracks at the corners of your mouth?
- Have you noticed numbness or tingling in your hands or feet?
- Are you over the age of 60?

Answering yes to any of these questions indicates you are vulnerable and may not hit optimal B-vitamin levels. As the 'more is not better' rule applies to B-vitamins as well, best to check in with your health practitioner to guarantee you hit your sweet spot with your B-Team.

## HOW TO MONITOR YOUR B-TEAM

Some B-Vitamins are trickier to test for in mainstream laboratory tests. The following are the important lab tests that you can use to monitor your B-Team:

- **Full blood count:** If red blood cells are larger than normal this may indicate a low Vitamin B12 or folate.

- **Serum B12 and serum folate:** It's best to sit in the top half of the given reference range on your lab results. Your naturopath can also help here. Testing for your other important B-vitamins is possible through laboratories that work alongside naturopaths and integrative doctors.

## WHERE TO FIND YOUR B-TEAM:

- **Whole grains**: Brown rice, oats, barley, quinoa
    - Vitamin B1 (thiamine), B2 (riboflavin), B3 (niacin), B5 (pantothenic acid), B6 (pyridoxine), B9 (folate)

- **Meat**: Beef, pork, chicken, turkey
    - Vitamins B1, B2, B3, B5, B6, B7 (biotin), B12

- **Oily fish**: Sardines and mackerel:
    - Vitamins B2, B3, B6, B7, B12

- **Yoghurt and cheese**:
    - Vitamin B2, B5, B7, B12

- **Eggs:**
    - Vitamins B2, B5, B7, B12

- **Legumes**: Lentils, beans, chickpeas, peas
    - Vitamins B1, B2, B3, B5, B6, B9 (folate)

- **Leafy greens:** Spinach, kale, Swiss chard, broccoli:
    - Vitamins B2, B9 (folate)

- **Nuts and seeds**:
  - Vitamins B1, B2, B3, B5, B6, B7

- **Avocados**:
  - Vitamins B5, B6, B9 (folate)

- **Nutritional yeast** has a nutty, cheesy flavour that can complement the taste of many smoothies. It contains good amounts of all B-Vitamins from B1 to B12 and is an ideal addition to any smoothie.

## B-Team Smoothie

**INGREDIENTS**

1 banana
1 cup English spinach leaves
1 cup nut or oat milk (or any milk of your choice)
1 tablespoon nutritional yeast
1 tablespoon almond butter (or any nut butter)
1 teaspoon honey or maple syrup (optional, for sweetness)
½ teaspoon vanilla extract (optional)
Ice cubes (optional, for a colder smoothie)

**INSTRUCTIONS:**

**Blend the greens:** Place the spinach in a blender with the milk. Blend until smooth. Add the remaining ingredients, plus ice cubes for a cold thicker consistency.

**Serve:** Pour the smoothie into a glass and enjoy.

**EXTRA TIP**

Top with ½ teaspoon of cinnamon to add a power punch of calcium to your day!

# 4.
# CHOOSE HEALTHY FATS AND OILS

## When you're hungry, your body is asking for nutrients, not just calories.

Critical nutrients to include come from healthy fats and oils. They are essential to achieve a balanced diet and play a crucial role in both overall health and hormonal harmony. Eating the right balance of fats each day should not be difficult. Our ancestors naturally consumed foods that provided the ideal balance for wellbeing.

It's time to let go of the low-fat messages you've heard throughout life. Eating 'whole' fats is essential for hormonal balance and overall wellness. To simplify, let's explore the three main fat families:
- Polyunsaturated fats (PUFAs): omega-3, omega-6, and ALA (alpha linolenic acid)
- Monounsaturated fats: Olive oil
- Saturated fats: Coconut oil, butter, ghee and animal fats

### POLYUNSATURATED FATTY ACIDS (PUFAs)

PUFAs, especially omega-3s, are vital for women's hormonal health. Natural sources of PUFAs provide proven benefits, particularly for breast health. However, processed foods high in omega-6 oils have disrupted the delicate balance of dietary oils needed for essential body functions. To balance the scale, reduce processed foods and increase intake of omega-3s.

**OMEGA-3 PUFAS**
Fish oil supplements are often marketed for their EPA (eicosapentaenoic acid) and DHA (docosahexaenoic acid) content. Both are essential for cognitive function,

vision and inflammation control. DHA supports brain and eye health, while EPA reduces the risk of chronic diseases like heart disease and arthritis. Together, they enhance cardiovascular health, support brain function, and improve mood.

**OMEGA-3 OCEAN-SOURCED**

To ensure a sustainable and healthy intake of omega-3s

- **Mackerel:** Small varieties like 'school mackerel' are rich in omega-3s and can provide more than your daily requirement in one serving.
- **Sardines:** Fresh or canned, sardines are an inexpensive, convenient source of omega-3s.
- **Prawns, crab and shrimp:** Look for non-farmed sustainably sourced options from clean oceans.
- **Herring and anchovies:** Both oily fish are packed with omega-3s, popular in European and Mediterranean cuisines. Canned fish is quite cheap and a wonderful option.

### WHAT ABOUT SALMON?

Salmon is a popular source of omega-3s, but its farming practices raise health and environmental concerns. Farmed salmon is often treated with antibiotics, synthetic chemicals, and artificial colorants to replicate the natural pink hue of wild salmon. These practices can harm both human health and ecosystems.

Salmon farming's environmental impact includes overcrowded pens, water pollution, and the spread of disease to wild populations. While wild-caught salmon is a healthier and more sustainable choice, overfishing has placed significant pressure on wild stocks.

### FISH FARMING IN AUSTRALIA

In Australia and New Zealand, regulations mandate that farmed fish are free of antibiotics before sale. However, chemicals like formalin and synthetic colorants, such as canthaxanthin, remain a concern. Canthaxanthin has been linked to eye health issues, leading to tighter restrictions in some countries. For a detailed overview, refer to the *Final Report: Registration of Aquaculture Chemicals* (FRDC Project 96/314) to make informed choices about farmed fish consumption.

**PLANT-BASED AND SUSTAINABLE OMEGA-3 SOURCES**

Choosing the following omega-3 sources supports both your health and the environment.

- **Chia seeds:** A plant-based source of omega-3s, perfect for smoothies, yoghurt, or oatmeal.
- **Walnuts:** A good source of ALA, the plant-based omega-3 fatty acid.
- **Flaxseeds:** Ground flaxseeds can boost omega-3 intake when added to baked goods or smoothies. Buy whole seeds and store them in the fridge, grinding them just before use to preserve their antioxidant capacity.
- **Hemp seeds:** Perfect for salads or protein shakes. Store similarly to flaxseeds.
- **Algal oil:** Great for vegetarians and vegans needing to increase Omega-3 intake.
- **Seaweed:** Seaweed and microalgae offer small amounts of EPA and DHA.

These alternatives provide essential fatty acids without the downsides of industrial salmon farming. Choosing sustainable omega-3 sources supports both your health and the environment.

### HEALTHY OMEGA-6 FOODS

Here are some of the best plant-based choices for omega-6 foods:

- **Nuts and seeds:** good source of healthy fats, protein, fibre, and essential vitamins and minerals like vitamin E, magnesium, and zinc.

- **Walnuts:** A great source of both omega-3 and omega-6 fatty acids, helping to maintain a better balance.

- **Sunflower seeds:** Rich in omega-6 fatty acids, these provide vitamin E, which is an antioxidant.

- **Pumpkin seeds:** Offer a good dose of omega-6s along with other essential nutrients like magnesium.

- **Vegetable oils:** rich in healthy fats, including monounsaturated and polyunsaturated fats, and provide essential nutrients like vitamin E and omega-3 fatty acids.

- **Avocado and macadamia oils:** Similar to olive oil, these oils are rich in monounsaturated fats and contain omega-6 fatty acids in moderation.

- **Olive oil:** Contains a small amount of omega-6 fatty acids and is a healthier option compared to other vegetable oils (more on this on page 420).

> **THE PROBLEM WITH OMEGA-6 PUFAS**
>
> In the 1950s, processed foods shifted diets from health-focused to profit-driven, introducing omega-6-rich oils like sunflower, safflower, and canola. These solvent-extracted oils became staples in margarine and processed foods, disrupting the natural balance of fats.
>
> A healthy diet balances omega-3s, which are anti-inflammatory, and omega-6s, which support inflammation in moderation. Today's omega-6-heavy diets contribute to chronic inflammation, increasing the risk of heart disease, diabetes, and hormone-related cancers.
>
> Restoring balance is key. Choosing the whole, natural foods we have listed and reducing processed options supports hormonal health and reduces the risk of inflammation-driven diseases.

- **Whole grains**:
  - **Oats:** Provide omega-6 fatty acids along with fibre and essential nutrients.
  - **Quinoa:** Contains omega-6 fatty acids and is a complete protein source, offering a good balance of amino acids.

- **Legumes**
  - **Chickpeas:** Offer omega-6 fatty acids and are high in protein and fibre.
  - **Lentils:** Another good source of omega-6s, also rich in protein and fibre.

**STRATEGIES FOR MAINTAINING A HEALTHY OMEGA BALANCE**

- **Limit processed foods:** Avoid processed and fast foods, which are often high in unhealthy omega-6 fatty acids from refined vegetable oils.

- **Balance with omega-3s:** Ensure adequate intake of omega-3-rich foods like fatty fish, flaxseeds, chia seeds, and walnuts to counterbalance omega-6 intake.

- **Choose whole foods:** Opt for whole, minimally processed foods to maintain a healthier omega balance and overall diet quality.

**ALA (ALPHA LINOLENIC ACID) POLYUNSATURATED FAT**

ALA (alpha linolenic acid) is an essential fat that your body cannot produce, so it must come from your diet. It supports cell health, reduces inflammation, and promotes heart and brain health.

ALA has a unique benefit: your body can convert it into DHA and EPA (key omega-3 fatty acids). While this is helpful when your omega-3 intake is low, it's important not to skimp on ALA, as it plays a vital role in long-term cell health.

Women who consume omega-rich diets experience benefits beyond basic maintenance, such as improved hormonal balance. Omega-3s help reduce PMS and menopausal symptoms, supporting overall hormonal health. Understanding where to find ALA can help you make better dietary choices for long-term wellbeing.

### TOP SOURCES OF ALA

- **Walnuts:** Great for brain health, enjoy as a snack or add to salads and baked goods.
- **Flaxseeds and flaxseed oil:** One of the richest ALA sources. Add ground flaxseeds to smoothies, oatmeal or baked goods. Use flaxseed oil in dressings.
- **Chia seeds:** Packed with ALA, they're easy to add to yoghurt, oatmeal, or smoothies, or use to make chia pudding.
- **Pumpkin and hemp seeds:** Sprinkle on salads, yoghurt, or smoothies. Can also be used in baking.
- **Soy products:** Tofu and tempeh are versatile sources of ALA and support breast health due to their phytoestrogens.
- **Perilla oil:** Commonly used in Asian cuisine, perilla oil is another ALA-rich option.

## MONOUNSATURATED FATS

### OLIVE OIL IS THE STAR OF THIS SHOW

Olive oil is the star of the monounsaturated fats category, with its key component, oleic acid, offering potent health benefits. While not classified as 'essential', monounsaturated fats are crucial for reducing inflammation that contributes to chronic diseases.

Incorporating olive oil into your diet can significantly improve health outcomes—according to the *Journal of the American Cardiology Association* (2022) just one tablespoon a day has been shown to reduce:

- Cancer deaths by 17%
- Respiratory deaths by 18%
- Heart disease deaths by 19%
- Neurological disease deaths by 30%
- Deaths from other diseases by 8% to 34%

### BREAST CANCER PROTECTION

A study from the PREDIMED trial found that women following a Mediterranean diet with extra virgin olive oil had a 68% lower risk of developing breast cancer. The protective power comes from olive oil's monounsaturated fats and polyphenols, which reduce inflammation and oxidative stress—key factors in cancer development.

### HOW TO INCORPORATE OLIVE OIL

Invest in high-quality, extra virgin olive oil for the best health benefits. Here's how to add it to your diet:

- **Smoothies:** Add a tablespoon for a nutrient boost.
- **Salad dressing:** Combine with lemon juice or vinegar for a fresh, homemade dressing.
- **Drizzle over veggies:** Enhance taste and increase vitamin absorption.
- **Bread dip:** Swap butter for olive oil with herbs.
- **Marinate proteins:** Use olive oil with herbs and spices to flavour meats or tofu.

### COOKING WITH OLIVE OIL

For low-heat cooking (under 180°C), olive oil retains its health benefits, although when raw and uncooked you maximise its antioxidant value.

> **TIP**
> For higher temperatures, use oils like ghee, avocado, macadamia, or coconut oil, as olive oil can break down, lose its nutritional value and become a de-natured unhealthy fat.

## SATURATED FATS IN MODERATION

Saturated fats, though not essential like omega-3 and omega-6 PUFAs, play a role in hormone production and cell structure. Found in animal products, ghee, butter, and coconut oil, these fats can be beneficial when consumed in moderation.

### GHEE

With a high smoke point (250°C), ghee is excellent for high-heat cooking. It contains butyrate, a fatty acid that supports gut health, and is rich in fat-soluble vitamins (A, E, and K2). Ghee is also suitable for those with lactose intolerance, as it is low in lactose and casein.

## BUTTER

Butter is rich in healthy fats, including CLA (conjugated linoleic acid), which has anti-inflammatory properties. It can be used for low-heat cooking and baking and provides vitamins A, D, E and K2. Butter's lactose content is low, making it tolerable for many people with sensitivities.

### THE GREAT MARGARINE HEALTH CON—BUTTER IS PROVEN TO BE BETTER!

Margarine, once marketed as a healthier alternative to butter, is made from hydrogenated vegetable oils high in omega-6 fatty acids. This shift disrupted the balance between omega-3 and omega-6 in our diets, promoting inflammation. Starting in the 1950s, margarine was aggressively promoted as heart-healthy, while butter was demonised.

However, research by Chris Ramsden revealed the cardiovascular risks of replacing natural oils like butter with omega-6-rich margarines, such as those made from safflower oil. Ramsden re-examined studies from 1966 and found that results were manipulated to focus on cholesterol reduction while ignoring the marked increased risk of heart disease in the omega-6 group. His findings revealed that while margarine reduced cholesterol levels, it paradoxically increased the risk of heart disease. Ironically, the greatest risk of dying from heart disease was observed in those whose cholesterol levels dropped the most due to omega-6 consumption.

The shift toward processed foods and omega-6-rich oils has contributed to chronic inflammation and related diseases. Ramsden's research highlights the need to prioritise natural, minimally processed foods like butter and olive oil to support heart health.

### TIP

Steer clear of vegetable oils like sunflower, safflower, soybean, peanut, and canola oil because these oils promote inflammation in your body!

## COCONUT OIL

Coconut oil has gained popularity in recent years, praised for its unique flavour and potential health benefits. However, like any food, it comes with both advantages and disadvantages. It's a safe oil for sautés and pan-fried dishes, adding flavour to Asian cuisines, but has the same smoke point as olive oil so keep the temperature down when using this oil.

### TIP

Avocado oil has the highest smoking point at 270°C.

In addition, lauric acid in coconut oil has antimicrobial effects, which can help fight certain bacteria, viruses, and fungi, making it potentially beneficial for maintaining oral and skin health when used topically. Despite its high calorie content, the lauric acid may help with weight management by increasing feelings of fullness and boosting calorie burning.

**NUTS AND SEEDS**

If you have been paying attention to our Core Food Principle Number 4, you'll have noticed that nuts and seeds play a starring role in providing a perfect balance of your polyunsaturated fats (omega-3 and omega-6, along with ALA). They are tiny packages of anti-inflammatory goodness. Their role in health extends beyond their anti-inflammatory power—nuts and seeds provide the currency with which you pay your cellular housekeepers to clean the daily rubbish out of every cell of your body.

All body cells require these daily housekeeping helpers to clear the accumulation of reactive oxygen species (ROS), commonly known as free radicals. ROS are inflammatory by-products of healthy cell function that need to be neutralised and removed daily to prevent cell damage—the cell can rust from the inside out if not cleaned of these oxidative devils.

Recommended daily serves:

**Seeds:** ½ cup of mixed seeds daily (flaxseeds, chia, sunflower, sesame, pumpkin).

**Nuts:** 30–60 g of varied nuts daily. Include walnuts for brain health, and Brazil nuts for selenium (1 to 2 per day).

**IMPORTANT!**

While omega-3 and healthy omega-6 fatty acids are the primary essential fats, a balanced diet should include a variety of fats to support overall health. This includes monounsaturated and saturated fats, each contributing uniquely to your body's overall wellness. That said, the take home message from this Core Food Principle is that olive oil is liquid gold for your health!

# 5. SUPPORT GUT HEALTH WITH FERMENTED FOODS

### GUT HEALTH AND HORMONAL BALANCE: A KEY CONNECTION

Your gut health plays a crucial role in maintaining balanced hormones, especially oestrogen. The gut microbiota—the community of microbes in your intestines—regulates hormones like oestrogen, steroid hormones, and cytokines, which are vital for many bodily functions, including breast cancer prevention.

### PATHWAYS TO HORMONAL BALANCE

The gut influences hormones through two main pathways:

1. **Food-based:** Certain foods, like those with phytoestrogens, are metabolised by gut bacteria into compounds that help balance hormones.

2. **The oestrobolome:** A special group of gut bacteria regulates oestrogen excretion, preventing reabsorption and helping mitigate oestrogen dominance.

### THE OESTROBOLOME: YOUR GUT'S HORMONE HELPER

The oestrobolome is a collection of gut bacteria that metabolise and influence oestrogen levels. These bacteria produce enzymes that break down oestrogen, maintaining hormonal balance and overall health.

### GUT HEALTH AND OTHER HORMONES

Besides oestrogen, gut bacteria affect hormones like leptin and insulin, which regulate appetite and metabolism. They also impact progesterone and testosterone, further supporting hormonal balance.

**THE GUT-HORMONE CONNECTION**

Lower oestrogen levels, especially during menopause, are linked to an increase in gut permeability, that naturopaths call 'leaky gut'. The significant drop in oestrogen in the menopause transition can alter the gut microbiome and increase gut permeability. This can lead to more frequent digestive issues and a higher risk of inflammation-related conditions, including inflammatory bowel diseases like ulcerative colitis and Crohn's disease.

**THE GUT-BRAIN AXIS**

The gut-brain axis is a communication network between the gut and brain, influencing mood hormones like dopamine and serotonin. Maintaining gut health can boost both mental and physical health, highlighting the importance of a holistic approach to wellbeing.

**FEED YOUR GUT WELL**

Incorporating probiotics, prebiotics, fibre, and fermented foods, staying hydrated, exercising, and managing stress are key strategies for supporting gut health. A resilient, well-nourished gut helps you maintain balance throughout your hormonal journey.

## SUPPORT YOUR GUT WITH DIET
## FERMENTED FOOD—THE GUT HEALTH ESSENTIALS

Fermented foods are packed with beneficial elements that work to support the quality of your microbiome—this in turn supports an efficient digestive tract from your mouth all the way through to the other end.

The key players in fermented foods are probiotics, beneficial bacteria and yeasts that help to balance all the bacteria in your gut, promoting a healthy microbiome. Incorporating fermented foods like yoghurt, kefir, sauerkraut, kimchi, and kombucha into your diet can make a big difference in how your digestive system feels and functions, helping you feel your best.

The magic of fermented foods comes with its other qualities—they also contain prebiotics, which are the natural complex sugars and non-digestible fibres that specifically feed and stimulate the growth of beneficial gut bacteria. This helps your microbiome thrive and do their job even better.

These foods continue to ferment in your gut—this helps to break down your food and enhances nutrient absorption, making it easier for your body to get the nutrients it needs.

These foods contain high levels of B-vitamins and vitamin K, which are crucial for overall health and bone care. They also multitask on your behalf to maintain the right acidity balance in your gut, creating an environment where good bacteria can flourish.

- A diet rich in fibre and prebiotics such as berries, onions, garlic and legumes, supports a healthy microbiome, helping balance hormones and improving digestive function.

- Fermented foods like yoghurt, kefir, sauerkraut, kimchi, and kombucha provide probiotics and prebiotics, aiding nutrient absorption and maintaining gut acidity for a thriving microbiome.

> **BOOSTING YOUR GUT HEALTH**
>
> Dr Marc Cohen explains that oxymels are vinegar syrups blended with honey, and their use dates back 2500 years to Hippocrates, the father of medicine. It was later used by Avicenna during the Persian Empire. With over 1200 recipes once in use, recent research is now confirming their health benefits. Modern oxymels can be made by combining Kombucha or apple cider vinegar with herbs and high-quality manuka honey. Extremely Alive produces oxymels using certified manuka honey, organic Kombucha vinegar infused with diverse microbial species, herbs, roots, fruits, flowers, and fungi. These oxymels balance the sourness of vinegar, the sweetness of honey, and the bitterness of herbs to create complex, delicious flavours. They can be taken straight, like a dessert wine, or mixed with water, nut milks, or spirits for refreshing beverages and cocktails that double as an amazing food for your gut. (www.extremelyalive.com.au)

Throughout all these stages, maintaining a healthy gut is about balance and listening to your body. Incorporating probiotics and prebiotics into your diet, staying hydrated, exercising regularly, and managing stress are foundational to supporting your gut health.

Remember, your gut is resilient and adaptable. By nurturing it, you're supporting your digestive health and your overall wellbeing. So, embrace each stage of your hormonal journey with confidence, knowing that a healthy gut is your steadfast ally. Remember to take good care of your gut through these simple strategies, include fermented foods and fibre in your diet every day.

# 6.
# GRASS-FED, FREE-RANGE MEAT AND BIRDS

### ANIMAL PROTEINS

If you eat meat or chicken, it's best to choose grass-fed, free-range and organically raised options. Just like humans, animals thrive when they live in their natural environments, eating what nature intended. Picture a cow grazing on grass in a spacious paddock, roaming freely with its herd, and living in sunshine and rain—cows are designed to live in nature, experiencing minimal stress. This promotes the animal's wellbeing and also results in healthier, more nutritious meat for you.

Animals raised in confined spaces and fed grains or unnatural foods often become fatter and more stressed. Stress compromises their immune systems, making them more susceptible to infections, which often leads to the use of antibiotics. These antibiotics, along with pesticides and chemicals, can be stored in the animal's fat cells, potentially entering your diet. To reduce exposure to these harmful substances, it's best to avoid grain-fed meats.

Look for meat labelled as 'grass-fed' and 'pasture-raised' throughout the animal's life. This guarantees a higher level of omega-3 fats, promotes better animal welfare, and upholds ethical farming standards. The same applies to chickens and eggs—free-range, pasture-raised options ensure a healthier and more humane choice.

# 7.
# SAY NO TO GMO FOODS

**GENETICALLY MODIFIED FOODS: A GROWING CONCERN**
As authors deeply invested in the intersection of health and sustainability, we approach the topic of genetically modified organisms (GMOs) with cautious concern. While GMOs have been heralded for their potential to address food shortages and improve crop resilience, the long-term effects on human health and the environment remain uncertain. Emerging research suggests that altering the genetic makeup of our food may have unintended consequences, such as disruptions to gut health or unanticipated allergenic responses. Equally troubling are the environmental risks, including the loss of biodiversity and the unintended spread of genetically modified traits to wild species. These complexities urge us to adopt a balanced perspective, advocating for transparency, rigorous research, and a commitment to precaution as we navigate this critical area of food science.

Genetically modified foods have raised concerns among experts in genetics, science, and food safety. Despite this, organisations like Commonwealth Scientific and Industrial Research Organisation (CSIRO) in Australia and food standards bodies in New Zealand and the UK approved GMO foods in the late 1990s, without long-term safety studies. Dr Judy Carman, medical doctor with a PhD in biochemistry and a former Chief Scientist at CSIRO, protested this decision, citing the lack of research on human health impacts. Her warnings were ignored, and GMO farming was introduced in Australia—a country that had the potential to avoid GMO crop contamination seen elsewhere.

In protest, Dr Carman left CSIRO and now serves as an Associate Professor of Biochemistry at Flinders University and Director of the Institute of Health and Environmental Research. As a respected epidemiologist, Dr Carman has continued to raise concerns about GMOs, particularly following her study on pigs fed GMO diets. She found that pigs on a GMO diet had significantly higher rates of severe stomach inflammation and, in female pigs, an enlarged uterus—a potential warning for women's health.

Dr Carman's findings have fuelled ongoing debates about the potential health risks of GMOs, including a possible connection to conditions like endometriosis. While this research is still developing, there is growing concern about GMOs' effects on hormonal balance. Dr Carman advises caution, suggesting that consumers avoid GMOs until more conclusive research is available.

Her work has sparked interest in the broader scientific community, with researchers like Dr Maarten Stapper also voicing concerns about GMOs. Formerly a principal research scientist at CSIRO, Dr Stapper has raised doubts about the environmental and health impacts of GMO farming, advocating for more sustainable agricultural practices.

For more information, you can explore Dr Carman's research at GMOJudyCarman.org.

Like many new human interventions, the full impact of GMOs on human health may not become evident until later generations. Emerging concerns highlighted by credible research from experts in the field of GMOs warrant serious consideration. Until these concerns are thoroughly addressed and resolved, it is prudent to avoid GMOs as a precautionary measure to safeguard long-term health.

# 8.
# NO ADDED (PROCESSED) SUGARS

The fruit family of carbohydrates is a powerhouse for both hormonal and overall wellness. These foods in their natural form are rich in antioxidants and provide food for our gut microbiome. This directly impacts oestrogen balance through the part of our gut microbiome called the oestrobolome, a specialised team of microbes support hormonal balance (see page 424).

Unfortunately, when profit took priority over health, we altered the nutritional balance of food, leading to hormonal imbalances and mood swings that contribute to chronic diseases. By embracing the natural benefits of fruits and berries in moderation, we can reclaim our health and vitality. This Core Principle encourages eliminating processed and added sugars from your diet, reserving them for occasional celebrations, not part of a healthy diet.

## PROCESSED AND ADDED SUGARS

> **TIP**
> When reading food labels, remember that four grams of sugar equals one teaspoon.

Despite being categorised as carbohydrates, processed sugars are harmful to our health. These processed carbs, found in high-sugar foods, thrive on causing hormonal havoc and lead to both short- and long-term issues, triggering cravings for more.

First, high-sugar foods stimulate the brain's dopamine receptors, flooding the system and making you crave more. This is why it's hard to stop at just one chocolate biscuit. Second, processed carbs cause a rapid spike in insulin and blood sugar levels, followed by a crash when insulin kicks in. This cycle of highs and lows keeps your body craving more sugar, eventually disrupting insulin communication with your cells.

## YOUR DIET SPEAKS TO YOUR GENES

For over 15% of women, Type 2 diabetes is a reality, especially for those who are genetically predisposed. Epigenetically your diet plays a crucial role in whether this condition develops, particularly in women with PCOS, who are more vulnerable to diabetes during pregnancy and at a younger age.

Processed foods are stripped of the essential nutrients your body needs. Even when manufacturers try to add nutrients, it's never in the same form or balance as nature intended. The result? Empty calories that disrupt the glucose-insulin pathway and contribute to obesity and chronic diseases.

## ARE YOU ADDICTED TO SUGAR?

If you feel you have a sugar problem, you're not alone. Here we explore one of the basic saboteurs of wellness, and the driver of one of our most challenging chronic diseases, Type 2 diabetes. For some women, addressing this issue could be the missing link on the journey to cultivating more natural energy.

## SUGARY QUIZ

Take our quick test to find out if you rely too much on sugar.

### DO YOU:

- Feel the need to eat every couple of hours?
- Find that you're unable to concentrate mid-morning?
- Need a sugary snack for extra energy around 3pm?
- Get 'hangry' between meals or around 5pm?
- Feel shaky or dizzy if you haven't eaten for a couple of hours?
- Feel energised, or conversely exhausted, after a meal?
- Rely on caffeine or sugar to power you through your day?

If you've answered 'Yes' to two or more of these, we suggest you look at detoxifying your diet to eliminate sugar. This chapter will hopefully motivate you to look at your relationship with sugar through a different lens and help you make changes in your day to break the habit of sugar addiction.

**CASE STUDY | DR KAREN**

# Kate
## More of a good thing

I will always remember looking out into my waiting room and glancing at a new patient next in line for a consultation with me. The striking thing about Kate was her unusual bright orange complexion. My thoughts went immediately to high-dose vitamin A supplemention, and this was one of the first questions I asked as I took her health history. Her reply to 'Do you take any vitamin or supplements?' was met with a resounding, 'No, I have an excellent diet and feel well.'

As she was vegetarian, I suggested we check nutrients like iron and vitamin B12 to ensure her needs were being met by her diet. I also ordered a vitamin A blood check to satisfy my curiosity.

Her results came across my desk, and her Vitamin A levels were the highest I had ever seen in my career to date, and since. On her follow-up appointment I pointed out the obvious red flag on vitamin A and asked her to go over her diet in detail. She hesitated, and then replied, 'Well, it could be the carrots ...'

On further questioning this young woman was eating around two kilograms of carrots daily (organic, she was quick to point out!). It took a little longer to figure out the reason for this unhealthy obsession with an otherwise good food choice.

She was unconsciously treating hypoglycaemia symptoms (low blood sugar) by constantly nibbling on carrots through the day to feed her sugar addiction. Her reasoning was that it provided a healthier choice than cakes and lollies.

Once she understood the biochemistry of her wild blood sugar fluctuations, and the risk of a toxic level of vitamin A, Kate was able to find a more balanced way of dealing with her sugar cravings with the help of a nutritionist.

It was the only time in my professional career where I have seen a nutrient at dangerously high levels due solely to food sources.

To understand why sugar is now one of the most significant saboteurs of wellness let's go back and look at how the human-food relationship has changed over the past 30 years. Remember, even though we live in the 21$^{st}$ century, we are biochemically primitive bodies in a modern world. Though our ancient bodies are designed to process natural sugars from fruits and berries, today's processed sugars are a different story.

### KEY FACTS ABOUT SUGAR

One of the most dramatic dietary shifts in recent decades is the rise of high-fructose corn syrup (HFCS) in processed foods. Made from corn syrup, HFCS is cheap, addictive and nothing like the natural fructose in fruit—where it's wrapped in fibre and comes with nutritional backup.

By contrast, HFCS is a metabolic troublemaker. Regular table sugar, or sucrose, breaks down into glucose and fructose. But when you add table sugar to the extra HFCS in breakfast cereals, soft drinks and fast food, you create a perfect storm.

Here's what matters: fructose as a food additive is often marketed as a 'natural sugar', but don't be fooled. Unlike glucose, which can be metabolised by nearly every cell in the body, added fructose dumps the entire load on the liver. It behaves more like alcohol, demanding liver time and leaving behind metabolic chaos. It has been linked to diabetes, heart disease, cancer, fatty liver and even high blood pressure in children. The demands on your liver from HFCS impacts hormones. It has a domino effect on the delicate balance of oestrogen hormonal pathways, and the removal of toxins and chemicals from your body.

### THE PLEASURE PATHWAY OF SUGAR

The receptors that control the release of dopamine into the blood are also activated by other non-hormone substances that are very familiar to us: nicotine, heroin, codeine, caffeine, alcohol, and of course sugar—often referred to as 'sweet poison'.

So, we have sugar in a position to control the release of a powerful mood-altering hormone, dopamine. The release of this hormone is what makes nicotine, heroin, caffeine and alcohol so hard to resist. The same applies to sugar. However, sugar is a universally available and socially acceptable dopamine stimulator and drug of addiction. From a marketing perspective, this is an ideal product for profit.

The story gets a little complicated by biochemistry here. The constant bombardment of the receptor site for dopamine by sugar over time results in a depletion of the dopamine stores. The ONLY way to feel that good again is to continually batter the cells in the midbrain with more ... sugar.

We develop an increased urgency about the next sugar hit, whether that be a biscuit, cake, caramel latte or jellybean. This goes way beyond what we need for nourishment or to satisfy hunger. Understanding how the sugar demon operates is an essential next step in your journey to hormonal balance.

**DETOXING FROM SUGAR**

Cutting out sugar can cause withdrawal symptoms like headaches, fatigue, or nausea. If symptoms become severe, nibble on fresh berries or nuts for relief. Managing sugar addiction involves balancing stress, movement and blood sugar levels to avoid sugar highs and lows.

> For those with Type 2 diabetes or a family history of diabetes, stabilising blood sugar is essential.
>
> You can monitor your progress with blood tests for the following:
> - **HbA1C:** Aim for 6 or less.
> - **Uric acid:** Keep levels below 0.3 mmol/L or 5.0 mg/dL.
> - **Bicarbonate levels:** Aim for 30–32 mmol/L to maintain an alkaline system.

## ALCOHOL AND SUGAR

Alcohol's effect on blood sugar varies depending on the type, amount, and individual metabolic responses influenced by genetic detox pathways.

Sugary alcoholic drinks like cocktails, sweet wines, and liqueurs can cause a rapid spike in blood sugar due to added sugars. Beer, while less sugary, contains carbohydrates that also raise blood sugar, though more gradually.

In contrast, pure spirits like vodka, gin, and whiskey have minimal immediate impact on blood sugar as they contain no carbohydrates. However, alcohol can still indirectly affect blood sugar regulation.

Notably, alcohol can initially raise blood sugar but may cause a delayed drop several hours later, especially in people with diabetes. This happens because alcohol interferes with the liver's ability to release glucose into the bloodstream.

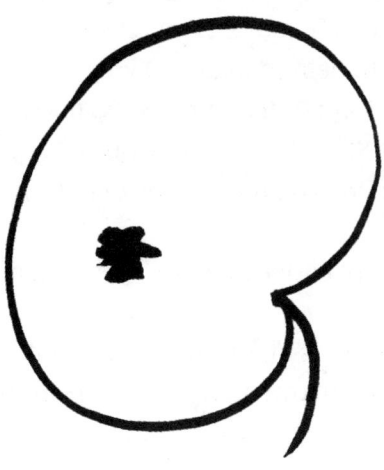

## WELLNESS ACTION PLAN
# SUGAR ADDICTION

- Identify triggers: Journal cravings to spot patterns.
- Reduce gradually: Avoid going cold turkey to ease withdrawal.
- Choose healthier snacks: Opt for fruit, nuts, seeds or dark chocolate (70% cocoa).
- Food shopping: Avoid shopping hungry.
- Read labels: Watch for hidden sugars in processed foods.
- Include protein and fibre in meals: This helps keep you full and stabilises blood sugar.
- Avoid alcohol for four weeks: Alcohol quickly breaks down into sugar.
- Add cinnamon to your meals. It helps regulate blood sugar levels and curb cravings.
- Magnesium: Cravings can sometimes be due to a deficiency (see page 465 for symptoms).
- Herbs and supplements: Consider chromium for insulin sensitivity or L-glutamine to reduce cravings.
- Herbal teas: Peppermint, chamomile or liquorice root can help reduce cravings and soothe the digestive system.
- Regular physical activity: Walking, yoga or workouts can reduce stress and improve mood, decreasing sugar cravings.
- Incorporate daily movement. Increase your daily steps, take a quick walk in nature to help manage cravings.
- Stay hydrated: Sometimes thirst is mistaken for hunger.
- Mindful eating: Slow down and savour your food to recognise fullness.
- Manage stress: Practise meditation or deep breathing to keep cravings in check.
- Get enough sleep: Fatigue can increase sugar cravings.

Breaking a sugar addiction is a journey, but with mindful eating, healthy substitutes and lifestyle adjustments, you can overcome cravings and enjoy a more balanced diet.

# 9.
# NO ARTIFICIAL ADDITIVES

**PRESERVATIVES AND COLOURINGS**

The addition of flavour additives, preservatives and colourings does nothing to enhance the nutritional value of your food. These synthetic substances are commonly added to processed foods to enhance flavour, extend shelf life, and improve appearance. However, while they may make food look and taste more appealing, they can significantly alter the natural composition of food for the worse and lead to various health issues.

Artificial additives, preservatives and colourings can drastically change the natural state of food. Many natural nutrients are lost during the processing of food to which additives are added. Vitamins and minerals can be destroyed or diminished in the manufacturing process of processed foods, reducing their overall nutritional value.

The introduction of synthetic chemicals into food can disrupt its natural composition. Foods that would otherwise be wholesome and nutritious can become laden with chemicals that the body must work to metabolise and eliminate.

Artificial flavourings and texturisers change the natural taste and feel of food, leading to a dependency on artificially enhanced flavours, making natural foods seem less appealing in comparison. MSG (monosodium glutamate) added to the Chinese takeaway food of the 1980s and 90s was a perfect example.

Preservatives extend the shelf life of food but at the expense of introducing potentially harmful substances. While this can be convenient, it often means consuming chemicals that your body doesn't need and that can accumulate in your body over time. Applying the Core Food Principle Number 2 (sourcing local produce) overcomes the need for preservatives in your food.

## THE HEALTH CONSEQUENCES

### ALLERGIES AND INTOLERANCES

The inclusion of artificial additives, preservatives, and colourings in the diet has been linked to various health problems, including allergies and intolerances. Many people have allergic reactions or intolerances to artificial additives, with symptoms ranging from mild (headaches, digestive issues) to severe (anaphylaxis). Common culprits include sulphites, food dyes, and certain preservatives like sodium benzoate. Some artificial colourings and preservatives can contribute to behavioural problems in children, such as hyperactivity and attention deficits. This has led to increased scrutiny and calls for the removal of these additives from children's foods.

### DISRUPTION OF YOUR GUT HEALTH

Artificial additives can disrupt the natural balance of gut bacteria, dominoing into a disruption of your gut microbiome and creating day-to-day symptoms like digestive issues such as bloating, gas, diarrhoea and reflux. For some individuals, these substances can exacerbate conditions like irritable bowel syndrome (IBS). Some preservatives and additives have been linked to more serious long-term health issues. For instance, certain artificial colourings have been associated with an increased risk of cancer, and high consumption of preservatives has been linked to metabolic disorders. Constant exposure to artificial additives can overburden the immune system. The body must continually work to detoxify and eliminate these foreign substances, which can weaken immune responses over time and increase susceptibility to illness.

### LINKS TO CANCER

You might come across statements like, 'There is no evidence that this synthetic chemical causes cancer.' But here's the key question: Are we actually looking deeply enough?

From a scientific perspective, it's important to understand that a lack of evidence showing harm is not the same as evidence of safety. In many cases, long-term, independent studies simply haven't been done. So, when you hear 'no evidence of harm', it may just mean we don't yet have enough information—not that the substance is safe.

> **OUR TRAVELLING SAUSAGES**
>
> The preservative butylated hydroxytoluene (BHT) is commonly used in meats and sausages to preserve the colour, and prevent bacterial growth and food poisoning. Banned or heavily regulated in most countries due to its potential health risks, including its link to cancer, Dr Karen read with disbelief one of the arguments used by the Food Safety regulator on allowing the continued use of this preservative in Australian sausages because 'our sausages have to travel so much further to get to the middle of such a big country.' So, if you live in the city you also get a dose of this preservative.
>
> The safety of this preservative, along with sodium nitrite, continues to be a subject of ongoing debate. We suggest that while government safety bodies argue the point, steer clear of processed meats and sausages, unless labelled additive-free.

## EMULSIFIERS

Common additives in processed foods like ice cream, mayonnaise, sauces and baked goods, emulsifiers help blend oil and water and improve shelf life. However, growing research suggests they may come at a cost to gut health. While regulatory bodies classify them as safe, several emulsifiers, including polysorbate 80 and carboxymethylcellulose, have been shown in animal studies to disrupt the delicate gut microbiome and weaken the integrity of the gut wall.

The gut wall is more than a digestive lining—it's a dynamic, one-cell-thick barrier designed to let nutrients in while keeping harmful substances out. Emulsifiers can damage this barrier by thinning the protective mucus layer and encouraging the growth of pro-inflammatory microbes. This creates microscopic gaps in the gut lining, a phenomenon known as increased gut permeability—or 'leaky gut'.

Once compromised, the gut wall may allow toxins, bacteria and undigested food to enter the bloodstream, triggering low-grade inflammation throughout the body. Over time, this kind of chronic inflammation has been linked to a rise in metabolic disorders, cardiovascular disease, autoimmune conditions and flare-ups in inflammatory bowel disease.

While human research is still emerging, early findings suggest that protecting gut wall integrity is a cornerstone of overall health—making it wise to limit emulsifier-rich processed foods where possible.

**TAKE HOME MESSAGE: GOVERNMENT LEGISLATION
MAY NOT LOOK AFTER YOUR CELLULAR HEALTH!**

Be vigilant about reading food labels. If you see a long list of unpronounceable ingredients, it's a sign that the food contains artificial additives.

Use this checklist to keep your meals free from unwanted additives:

- Prioritise fresh fruits, vegetables, whole grains and lean proteins. These foods are naturally free from artificial additives and are packed with essential nutrients.

- Prepare meals at home where you can ensure that your food is free from unnecessary additives and preservatives.

- Choose organic foods. Organic farming standards restrict the use of synthetic substances, making organic foods a healthier choice.

- Look for products that promote clean or 'free from' labels. Many companies now highlight their commitment to using natural ingredients and avoiding artificial additives.

- Use BPA-free storage containers. Choose glass as the best chemical-free option.

- Embrace the principle of 'No Added Anything'.

This Core Food Principle not only supports better nutrition but also reduces the risk of adverse health effects associated with synthetic substances. Embrace natural foods and enjoy the benefits of a cleaner, natural diet.

# 10.
# FILTERED WATER FOR DRINKING, COOKING AND WASHING

Water is an essential part of our lives, used for drinking, as well as cooking, washing and bathing. Ensuring the quality of the water we use daily is crucial for wellbeing. However, tap water can contain various contaminants that pose risks to our health. The chemical family called PFAS was introduced in the last century. These nasties are now found across the world (thanks to the industrial explosion in our lifetime) in our natural environment, oceans, our water supply, and very sadly within our community. While getting rid of PFAS completely is currently impossible (let's hope future generations find a solution), by mindfully filtering water we can reduce them and ensure that the water we consume and use is as clean and safe as possible.

### TAP WATER CONTAMINANTS

Chlorine is commonly added to municipal water to kill harmful bacteria, effectively reducing waterborne diseases. However, it can react with organic matter to form harmful by-products called trihalomethanes (THMs), which are linked to cancer and other health issues. Chlorine may also cause skin irritation and respiratory problems in sensitive individuals.

Tap water may contain additional contaminants, including heavy metals like lead and mercury, pesticides, pharmaceuticals, and microorganisms. Lead, which can leach from ageing pipes, poses serious health risks, particularly for children.

### PFAS (PER- AND POLYFLUOROALKYL SUBSTANCES)

PFAS are a group of man-made chemicals that have been used in various industrial and consumer products, including non-stick cookware, water-repellent clothing, and firefighting foams. These substances are highly persistent in the environment and human body, earning them the nickname 'forever chemicals'. PFAS can contaminate drinking water supplies and have been linked to cancer, liver damage, and hormone disruption.

### SOLUTIONS FOR ENSURING CLEAN WATER

A good water filtration system can effectively reduce these contaminants and ensure safer water for your household. Consider the following solutions:

- Install a high-quality water filter to remove these contaminants. We recommend a system manufactured by Beautiful Water Systems (www.beautifulwater.co). (See Spotlight on Managing Toxins on page 478 for more details.)

- Regularly replace filter cartridges to maintain the efficiency of your filtration system.

- Test your water periodically to monitor the presence of contaminants and ensure your filtration system is working effectively.

- Place a filtration system on the water supply coming into the house so all taps, showers and baths are free of the nasties, and you can drink form every tap.

Keeping safe from water-borne contaminants is a long-term project. You may not feel the benefits of this Core Food Principle immediately, but your older body will thank you one day.

SPOTLIGHT ON
# Vitamins and Minerals

### HYPE OR HELP?

In this chapter, you'll find out everything you need to know about what you need according to your current life stage. We'll focus on multivitamins, vitamin D, iron and zinc. Don't forget to take the time to answer the quizzes in each supplement chapter to learn more about what your body may need at this time.

### AVOID FALLING FOR MARKETING HYPE

It's easy to get caught up in the marketing of supplements, antioxidants, and pills that claim to promote longevity. Supplement companies often bombard us with promises of their products being the cure-all for your ailments or the secret to living to 100. However, the truth is far more complex. The push to take supplements is largely driven by our desire for a quick fix that can cure chronic disease and extend life.

### DO YOU NEED A MULTIVITAMIN?

Whether it's a scientific study or a celebrity endorsement, the marketing behind supplements can be persuasive. But before investing in a product, it's important to dig deeper and see if it's right for your unique needs. Here's a checklist to help guide you in making informed decisions about supplements.

## QUESTIONS TO CONSIDER BEFORE SUPPLEMENTING

1 **Are you experiencing any symptoms or discomfort?**
   Although it's tempting to self-prescribe, always consult your healthcare provider to rule out serious conditions. If no underlying issues are found, you can address imbalances with the right supplement while staying in touch with your health team.

2 **Have you had tests that show a deficiency in a specific nutrient?**
   If testing reveals a nutrient deficiency, it may be time to assess your diet. Work with your health practitioner to get to the root cause of the problem.

3 **Is your gut healthy enough to absorb nutrients from food?**
   Even the best diet won't help if your gut isn't absorbing nutrients. Poor gut health can hinder absorption, so working with an experienced naturopath can be invaluable.

4 **Do you have a condition that requires a higher nutrient dose?**
   In some cases, higher doses of specific nutrients can be beneficial, but the general rule is that more is not always better. The goal is to find your 'sweet spot' for nutrient intake. For example, if you're optimising vitamin D for multiple sclerosis, aim for the top 10% of the optimal reference range, rather than settling for average.

5 **Do you have biochemical or genetic barriers to nutrient absorption?**
   Genetic variants (SNPs) and chronic conditions like kidney disease can affect how your body absorbs and uses nutrients. Epigenetics offers new ways to support these challenges and boost nutrient efficiency. (Read more in Spotlight on Epigenetics on page 269.)

Improving gut health and addressing nutritional gaps takes time. If challenges arise, consult your healthcare provider to identify deficiencies and create an action plan with supplements to bridge gaps while continuing to focus on overall nourishment.

# Vitamin D

Vitamin D, often called the 'sunshine vitamin', is vital for overall health, particularly in maintaining hormonal balance and supporting bone and breast health. Acting as a master regulator, vitamin D helps manage calcium levels in the bloodstream, keeping bones strong and resilient. This is especially important for women, as it reduces the risk of osteoporosis, a common concern during and after menopause.

Beyond bone health, vitamin D plays a crucial role in hormonal balance. It influences the production and function of hormones that regulate mood, weight, and menstrual cycles. Research also suggests that adequate vitamin D levels can promote breast health by modulating cell growth and immune function, potentially lowering the risk of breast cancer.

Achieving optimal vitamin D levels through safe sun exposure, diet, and supplements can be transformative for women, laying the foundation for a vibrant, hormonally balanced life from puberty to menopause and beyond.

## WHERE TO START

Cholesterol, often referred to as the 'grandmother' of all sex hormones, is essential for producing both male and female hormones. Adding to its importance, cholesterol also serves as a building block for the body's production of vitamin D:

- Sunlight acts on cholesterol stored in the skin's epidermis, triggering a series of chemical reactions that convert cholesterol into pre-vitamin D.

- Pre-vitamin D is then transported to the liver, and later to the kidneys, for further conversion into its active form, and then transported into cells through their unique docking sites (vitamin D receptors).

## VITAMIN D RECEPTORS (VDRs) AND CELLULAR HEALTH

Vitamin D binds to specific receptors, known as vitamin D Receptors (VDRs), which guide it to the epigenetic layer within your cells' nuclei. Here, it plays a critical role in regulating cellular functions by instructing genes to perform their tasks. VDRs are found in many types of cells, including those in blood vessels, skin, bones, heart, muscles, fat, brain, gut, liver, kidneys, thyroid and breasts.

In our Spotlights on Bone, Brain, Thyroid, and Breast Care, vitamin D is highlighted as an essential factor in maintaining health and wellbeing within these vital organs.

> **DARKER SKIN AND VITAMIN D**
>
> People with darker skin need to work harder to maintain optimal vitamin D levels, as their skin produces less vitamin D from sun exposure. On the plus side, darker skin is more resilient to the sun and can tolerate longer periods of sunlight safely.

## THE ESSENTIAL ROLE OF VITAMIN D IN WOMEN'S HEALTH

Vitamin D plays a vital role in maintaining overall health and hormonal balance. It supports thyroid function, which impacts nearly every aspect of your body's biochemistry. Throughout a woman's life, vitamin D's focus shifts to meet changing hormonal and physiological needs—from puberty to menopause.

### PUBERTY

Puberty is a period of rapid growth and hormonal changes. Vitamin D is crucial for peak bone mass development during this time, ensuring lifelong strong bones by aiding calcium absorption. It also helps balance hormones related to growth and menstrual cycles, supporting girls through this transformative phase.

### THE FERTILE YEARS

During the Fertile Years, vitamin D enhances fertility by regulating menstrual cycles and ovarian function. It supports healthy pregnancy outcomes by strengthening the immune system, ensuring both mother and baby thrive. Additionally, adequate vitamin D levels help maintain strong bones, supporting overall wellbeing and an active lifestyle.

### PERIMENOPAUSE

During perimenopause, vitamin D helps manage declining oestrogen levels by preventing osteoporosis, maintaining bone density, and supporting brain health to stabilise mood swings. It also regulates the internal clock, improving sleep and easing the menopause transition. Research from 2024 recommends maintaining a minimum level of 100 nmol/L for breast health, with up to 130 nmol/L offering even better long-term results.

## MENOPAUSE

During menopause, vitamin D is crucial in preventing accelerated bone loss and fractures, which become more common as oestrogen levels drop. Women entering menopause with vitamin D levels below 80 nmol/L are at a higher risk of rapid bone density loss compared to those with optimal levels. With the added challenges of interrupted sleep from hot flushes and stress that can weaken the immune system, maintaining adequate vitamin D levels helps boost immunity, ward off infections, and support overall health.

## THE AGE OF WISDOM

For women aged over 60, vitamin D is crucial for reducing falls and fractures by maintaining bone and muscle strength. It supports heart health as the risk of heart disease increases, enhances muscle function to preserve mobility and boosts immune resilience. For those with pre-diabetes, keeping levels above 125 nmol/L can improve your chances of avoiding the disease, supporting vitality and independence in later years.

### BALANCING VITAMIN D AND HEART HEALTH

Aggressively lowering cholesterol to reduce heart disease risk can interfere with the production of fertility hormones like oestrogen, testosterone, progesterone and vitamin D. While cholesterol management is important, it's essential to balance this with the body's need for cholesterol in hormone and vitamin D synthesis. Research shows that optimal vitamin D levels can help lower cholesterol, while a deficiency increases the risk of heart attack and stroke.

### WELLNESS ACTION PLAN TO HIT YOUR VITAMIN D SWEET SPOT

- Check your blood vitamin D levels: This could be one of the most important steps for your overall wellness. Aim for a result between 100 to 150 nmol/L.

- Incorporate vitamin D-rich foods: Include foods like sardines, herring, liver, eggs, organ meats (kidneys, liver, brains), cod liver oil, dandelion and alfalfa greens, parsley, and mushrooms in your diet to naturally boost vitamin D.

### MUSHROOMS: YOUR VITAMIN D SUPERFOODS

Certain mushrooms naturally contain vitamin D when exposed to sunlight or UV light. To boost their vitamin D content, leave your mushrooms in the sun (midday sun is ideal, with gills side up) for an hour before refrigerating.

**VITAMIN D CONTENT IN SUN-EXPOSED MUSHROOMS (PER 100 GRAMS):**

- Wild Maitake mushrooms: 28 micrograms
- Chanterelle mushrooms: 5 micrograms
- Shiitake mushrooms (dried): 4 micrograms
- Field mushrooms (sunbaked for 1 hour): 8 micrograms.

**COMPARISON TO ANIMAL-BASED VITAMIN D FOODS (PER 100 GRAMS):**

- Cod liver oil: 35 micrograms
- Sardines: 5 micrograms
- Wild-caught salmon: 25 micrograms.

**BOOSTING VITAMIN D NATURALLY**

- Sun exposure: Enjoy early morning sunshine on as much skin as possible but remember sunscreen blocks vitamin D production.

- Supplementation: If your vitamin D levels are below 50 nmol/L, a daily dose of 7000 IU of vitamin D3 for 3 months is safe. To maintain optimal levels (100–150 nmol/L), you may need 1000 to 4000 IU of vitamin D3 daily through safe sun exposure, food sources, or supplements.

## VITAMIN D: YOUR QUESTIONS ANSWERED

### DOES SUNSCREEN AFFECT VITAMIN D PRODUCTION?

Yes, research shows that sunscreens with SPF higher than 16 can reduce vitamin D production. Most sunscreens on the market today are SPF 30 or higher, but there have been no studies on how much, if any, vitamin D production is possible with these high UVB blockers when used as directed.

A safe approach is to assess your current vitamin D levels, use sunscreen sensibly to avoid skin damage, include more vitamin D-rich foods in your diet, and supplement as needed to maintain optimal levels.

### HOW CAN I INCREASE MY VITAMIN D LEVELS?

Genetic variations in vitamin D pathways may reduce your ability to produce and transport vitamin D effectively. If high-dose supplements aren't working, consider switching to Calcifediol (1,25-vitamin D), which bypasses liver processing and goes straight to the kidneys, potentially leading to faster absorption in your cells.

# Iron

### IRON: A CRUCIAL MULTITASKER

Iron is a cornerstone nutrient for women's health, powering over 200 processes in the body.

Key functions of iron include:

- **Oxygen transport**: Essential for red blood cells to deliver oxygen to your body.
- **Energy production**: Fuels the energy-making processes within your cells.
- **DNA repair**: Helps maintain healthy cells by supporting DNA repair.
- **Immune support**: Boosts the activity of immune cells that fight infections.
- **Brain health**: Supports the production of mood hormones and the brain's protective myelin sheath.
- **Hormone balance**: Helps produce thyroid hormones and oestrogen.
- **Detoxification**: Powers enzymes like catalase that reduce harmful chemicals in the body.

Iron deficiency disrupts these functions, leading to fatigue, poor focus, hormonal issues, lowered immunity, and risks of depression or other health problems. Women are especially at risk due to menstruation, pregnancy and inadequate diet. Sadly, iron deficiency is the most common nutritional deficiency worldwide.

### MEDICAL RESEARCH ON WOMEN

Historically, women have been underrepresented in medical research, largely due to biases that favoured male physiology as the 'default', overlooking the unique aspects of female biology, particularly reproductive cycles. This exclusion has created gaps in our understanding of women's health.

Happily, the IronFEMME Study, launched in July 2020, examines how iron metabolism and exercise impact women across reproductive stages, including those in their Fertile Years on birth control, and postmenopausal. It explores the links between iron, hormones, and physical activity.

**WHAT DOES IRON DEFICIENCY FEEL LIKE?**

Here are the top signs and symptoms of iron deficiency:

- Exhaustion
- Pale skin
- Shortness of breath on exertion
- Muscle ache
- Rapid pulse and heart palpitations
- Chest pains
- Headaches and dizziness
- Increased anxiety
- Brain fog—poor memory and concentration
- More frequent infections

Unusual symptoms of low iron:

- Anxiety and depression
- Craving non-food items like ice or dirt (pica)
- Sore or swollen tongue (glossitis)
- Cold hands and feet
- Cold intolerance (feeling cold even in warm climates)
- Restless legs
- Spoon-shaped or brittle nails
- Tinnitus (ringing or buzzing in the ears)

If you recognise any of these symptoms, complete the following Iron Health Audit. This will help identify any biochemical, dietary, or lifestyle factors that may increase your risk of iron deficiency.

# IRON HEALTH AUDIT: DO YOU NEED MORE IRON?

## IRON IN: QUESTIONS ABOUT IRON INTAKE AND ABSORPTION

### DIET

- ○ Are you primarily vegetarian or vegan?
- ○ Do you follow a diet such as Paleo that restricts complex carbohydrates?
- ○ Is your diet low in iron-rich foods like red meat, leafy greens, and beans? (See page 460 for a list of top iron-rich foods.)

### GUT HEALTH

- ○ Have you been diagnosed with conditions that affect iron absorption, like coeliac disease or inflammatory bowel diseases (for example, ulcerative colitis or Crohn's disease)? It may be time for a specialist review to ensure these conditions are under control.

- ○ Have you had gastric bypass surgery? This can limit iron absorption by reducing the time nutrients spend in the upper digestive tract.

- ○ Do you experience frequent diarrhoea, constipation, or bloating, which could suggest a gut health issue?

### MEDICATIONS AND SUPPLEMENTS THAT BLOCK IRON ABSORPTION

- ○ Are you taking any of the following medications?
  - ○ Antacids
  - ○ Certain antibiotics (long-term use for asthma or bronchitis)
  - ○ Anti-ulcer medications (proton pump inhibitors)

Check with your healthcare provider if any of your medications might interfere with iron absorption.

- Are you taking supplements that could lower iron absorption? Some supplements can compete with iron for absorption or bind with it in the gut:
    - Calcium supplements: Compete for absorption in the intestines.
    - Magnesium supplements: Also competes with iron.
    - Zinc supplements: High doses can inhibit iron absorption.
    - Phosphates: Found in multivitamins and other supplements

## IRON OUT:
## UNDERSTANDING BLOOD LOSS AND IRON DEFICIENCY

### BLOOD LOSS FROM MENSTRUAL CYCLES

- Do you experience heavy menstrual periods that might be contributing to low iron?
- Are your periods more frequent or closer together than usual?

### OTHER CAUSES OF BLOOD LOSS

- Blood loss from gastrointestinal, kidney, or bladder problems
- Have you noticed any signs of gastrointestinal bleeding, such as black or tarry stools, or blood in your stool or urine?
- Do you have bleeding haemorrhoids?
- Have you had any recent surgeries or injuries that may have caused significant blood loss?
- Are you taking nonsteroidal anti-inflammatory drugs (NSAIDs) like ibuprofen or aspirin, which might cause microscopic bleeding in the stomach? If so, talk to your healthcare provider about possible side effects that could lead to blood loss.
- Have you tested positive for any bleeding disorders that could affect your iron levels?
- Do you have a history of uterine fibroids or gastrointestinal ulcers that could be causing chronic blood loss?
- Do you frequently get nosebleeds? While they may seem minor, frequent nosebleeds can significantly deplete your iron stores over time.
- Do you regularly donate blood?

If you answered 'Yes' to any of these questions, it's important to discuss them with your healthcare provider. They can help identify the root causes of your low iron and guide you towards the right treatment.

### PREGNANCY CONSIDERATIONS

A recent pregnancy can leave women with low iron levels. Be sure to discuss this at your postnatal check-up to ensure your iron needs are being met.

### IRON AND CANCER

Women who have recently been diagnosed with cancer may develop iron deficiency. Cancer cells grow and multiply quickly, using up more iron than normal cells. This increased demand can drain the body's iron stores, leading to deficiency.

### CHRONIC DISEASE AND IRON

Chronic diseases, including cancer and its treatments, can trigger inflammation that affects how your body handles iron. Inflammation can block access to stored iron, resulting in what's called 'anaemia of chronic disease'—a condition where your body has iron, but it can't effectively use it.

## LET'S UNPACK IRON DEFICIENCY

### IRON DEFICIENCY VS ANAEMIA

Many people get confused between iron deficiency and anaemia, but they are not the same. Iron deficiency is the first stage, leading to a reduction in the oxygen-carrying capacity of your blood before it progresses to anaemia.

New red blood cells need iron to mature properly. Once they mature, they carry oxygen from your lungs to every cell in your body. If there isn't enough iron, these cells can't mature correctly, leading to a lower level of haemoglobin, the protein that binds oxygen.

As iron deficiency progresses, red blood cells shrink in size, becoming 'microcytic' (smaller than usual). These smaller cells are less efficient at delivering oxygen to your cells.

Anaemia happens when iron levels drop even further, preventing red blood cells from surviving to maturity. This leads to a significant reduction in red blood cells, and as a result, a formal diagnosis of anaemia is made when the red blood cell count, and haemoglobin levels fall below normal.

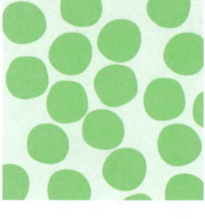

**NORMAL BLOOD FILM**

Plenty of plump, iron-rich red blood cells.

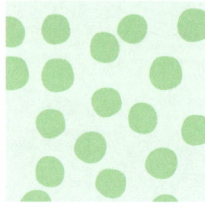

**IRON DEFICIENCY**

Same number of cells, but smaller in size due to low iron, losing some oxygen-carrying capacity.

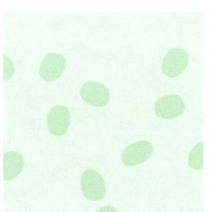

**IRON DEFICIENCY (ANAEMIA)**

Loss of red blood cells—less in number and much smaller again, with limited oxygen-carrying capacity.

#### TESTING FOR IRON DEFICIENCY

To get an accurate picture of your iron stores, timing matters. For menstruating women, blood tests for iron are most revealing when performed just after your period ends (around Day 8 of your cycle). This is when iron levels are typically at their lowest due to recent blood loss, making your results more likely to align with how you're feeling. If you're not menstruating, blood can be drawn at any time.

#### KEEPING TRACK OF YOUR LAB RESULTS

It's a great idea to keep your past lab results for iron, vitamins B12 and D, and zinc handy. Tracking changes over time reveals where you've been, where you are now, and where you should aim to be. Subtle shifts toward the high or low ends of the reference range can be early warning signs of an imbalance. By catching these trends early, you can adjust your diet and optimise bowel health to prevent complications from abnormal iron levels.

### UNDERSTANDING IRON IN YOUR BODY

Iron from food must be converted into a usable form called ferritin before your body can put it to work. This means you could feel extremely tired from a severe iron deficiency, even if your raw iron (serum iron) levels seem normal or high.

Many women with iron-deficiency anaemia go about their daily lives unaware of how depleted they are—until stress, illness, or pregnancy highlights the full impact of anaemia. To put it in perspective, the same degree of anaemia caused by acute blood loss would often require hospitalisation and possibly a blood transfusion!

It's also possible to be severely iron deficient even if your doctor tells you your iron is 'normal'. Standard blood tests don't always show how much usable iron is stored in your red cells and tissues. Iron deficiency affects more than 100 biochemical processes in the body, so it's essential to assess all aspects of your iron studies. Even slightly low levels in these tests can signal an imbalance that needs attention.

#### KEY IRON TESTS

To fully assess your iron status, you'll need the following four tests:

1 **Serum iron**: This measures the raw iron absorbed from food, showing how much circulating iron is in your blood now.

2. **Total iron-binding capacity (TIBC)**: TIBC shows how much iron your body can bind. In iron deficiency, this capacity increases as your body tries to grab onto any available iron.

3. **Transferrin saturation**: Transferrin is your iron transport protein within your red cells. This test measures the percentage of transferrin (a protein in your blood) that is saturated with iron. Simply put, it shows how much of your red blood cells are filled with iron, reflecting how much oxygen they can deliver to your tissues.

4. **Serum ferritin**: This measures your body's usable iron reserves. Most ferritin is stored in the liver, where it regulates iron levels in your blood and helps maintain balance.

#### INTERPRETING YOUR IRON RESULTS FOR OPTIMAL HEALTH:

Now that you have your results, the next step is understanding them. The goal is to hit the *optimal* range—not too low, not too high. More iron isn't always better; in fact, excess iron can be inflammatory. Stay within the upper limit of the reference range and never supplement beyond optimal levels.

### SPECIAL CONSIDERATIONS

#### CHRONIC DISEASE AND IRON STUDIES

If you've been diagnosed with a chronic illness, interpreting your iron results can be more complicated. In these cases, work with your healthcare provider to fully understand what your results mean.

### BREAKING DOWN THE IRON TESTS

#### SERUM IRON

If your serum iron is low or trending toward the lower end of the range, it may indicate a problem with how your body is absorbing iron from food. If your ferritin is still within the normal range, this might seem reassuring, but ongoing issues with iron absorption will eventually affect your ferritin stores. Some clues that all is not well could include:

- A diet low in iron.
- Gut health issues that block iron absorption.
- High levels of hepcidin, a liver protein that inhibits iron absorption (often linked to low-carb diets—see page 458).

If your serum iron is low but your ferritin is still in the optimal range, consider working on your diet and gut health before turning to iron supplements. Your adequate ferritin levels give you time to address the root causes of iron absorption issues.

### TOTAL IRON-BINDING CAPACITY (TIBC)

This measures how much iron your body *could* bind if it were available. In iron deficiency, TIBC is often high, as your body is ready to grab onto any available iron.

### TRANSFERRIN SATURATION

This tells you how much of your transferrin is carrying iron. A higher saturation means more oxygen can be delivered to your cells. The optimal range for transferrin saturation is 33% to 45%.

### NOTE FOR ATHLETES

Endurance athletes should aim for a transferrin saturation level above 34% to optimise performance. Levels below this can limit oxygen delivery to muscles, reducing your ability to perform at peak levels.

### TOO MUCH IRON

On the flip side, if your transferrin saturation is over 50%, it may indicate overuse of iron supplements or a genetic condition like haemochromatosis, which causes your body to absorb and store too much iron. Excess iron can damage organs like the liver and pancreas, and even lead to diabetes.

### SERUM FERRITIN

The standard reference range for ferritin is between 16 and 320 micrograms per litre of blood. However, true wellness is found within a narrower range.

Optimal Range: 50–180 micrograms per litre.

Staying within this range ensures you have enough iron to meet your body's needs and provides a buffer for heavier menstrual periods without tipping into deficiency.

## DRILLING DOWN INTO THE COMMON CAUSES OF LOW IRON

- **Restrictive diets:** Vegetarians typically have serum ferritin levels about half those of meat-eaters, making it harder to maintain optimal iron stores for energy and detoxification. While plant-based diets offer health benefits, strict vegans face an even higher risk of iron deficiency and should also monitor nutrients like vitamins B2, B3, B12 and D, iodine, zinc, omega-3 fats and calcium.

**Solution:** Explore Core Food Principles (page 399) for suggestions on plant-based nutrient sources. For example, adding nutritional yeast to a smoothie of dark leafy greens and dates can boost your iron intake.

- **Paleo and Atkins diets:** Even high-protein diets like Paleo can cause low iron stores due to elevated hepcidin, a hormone that blocks iron absorption when carbohydrates are limited. Athletes on low-carb diets may experience reduced muscle oxygenation and performance. In such cases, increasing quality carbs and considering intravenous iron may be needed to address the deficiency.

- **Heavy or frequent periods:** Iron deficiency can lead to heavy periods, which in turn can worsen iron deficiency—a vicious cycle. The stress on your body from low iron can affect progesterone production, causing oestrogen dominance and heavier bleeding in subsequent cycles.

- **Blood donations:** Before donating blood, the quick screening test checks haemoglobin levels to ensure you're not anaemic (the cut-off is usually 12 g/dL). However, you can still be iron-deficient even if your haemoglobin passes this test. Regular donors should have their full iron levels checked annually to avoid deficiency.

**Solution:** If you have a rare blood type, discuss how to maintain healthy iron levels with your healthcare provider, especially if you have heavy periods or other signs of low iron.

- **Medications linked to iron deficiency:** Some medications can reduce iron levels in two ways:
  - Iron Binders: Drugs like tamoxifen, anti-ulcer medications, and antacids bind to iron in the gut, preventing absorption.
  - NSAIDs (like aspirin and Nurofen) and anticoagulants can cause gut inflammation and microscopic bleeding, leading to iron loss. If you experience upper abdominal pain or notice black, tarry stools, seek medical attention as this could indicate serious bleeding from ulcers or other causes.

- **Bowel diseases and iron deficiency:** Low ferritin and iron deficiency anaemia should always be investigated for more serious conditions. These include:
  - Inflammatory bowel diseases (for example, Crohn's or ulcerative colitis)
  - Diverticulitis (inflamed pouches in the colon that cause bleeding)
  - H. Pylori (a stomach infection causing ulcers that hinder healing)
  - Coeliac disease (which affects iron absorption)

In some cases, an intravenous iron infusion may be the best treatment option.

### PREGNANCY

Starting pregnancy with low iron levels can make it difficult to maintain healthy iron as the pregnancy progresses. A gentle iron supplement throughout pregnancy can help keep your levels steady, especially if your iron stores are low at the outset.

### IRON SUPPORT WELLNESS ACTION PLAN

Iron deficiency isn't just about taking supplements. It's crucial to understand and address the root cause for long-term health.

Start by consulting your doctor to rule out serious conditions and then work with a naturopath for a holistic approach to reaching optimal iron levels.

If heavy or frequent periods are the cause, focus on restoring hormonal balance. Naturopathic remedies, such as herbal support, can help balance your body's biochemical pathways. Additionally, review your Iron Audit results to identify factors that may be blocking iron absorption, such as calcium, magnesium, zinc, or high-fibre intake.

### SUPPORTING GUT HEALTH

Improving gut health can also aid iron absorption. Include probiotics or fermented foods like yoghurt and sauerkraut in your diet to support a healthy microbiome. (For more tips, see Core Food Principles on page 424.)

### OPTIMISING YOUR DIET FOR IRON

To improve iron absorption, include iron-rich foods along with complex carbohydrates and vitamin C. Animal-based iron is generally better absorbed, but high-quality plant sources can also be effective with the right combination of nutrients.

> **TIP**
> To maximise absorption, take calcium and iron supplements at least two hours apart. For even better results, take calcium with low-iron meals.

Choose a variety of foods from this list:

**PLANT AND ANIMAL-BASED IRON-RICH FOODS**

| ANIMAL-BASED IRON-RICH FOODS | IRON CONTENT (MG) | PLANT-BASED IRON-RICH FOODS | IRON CONTENT (MG) |
| --- | --- | --- | --- |
| Beef liver (85g) | 4.1 | Cooked spinach (1 cup) | 6.4 |
| Oysters (85g) | 7.8 | Lentils (1 cup, cooked) | 6.6 |
| Sardines (85g) | 2.5 | Tofu (½ cup) | 3.4 |
| Chicken liver (85g) | 7.2 | Quinoa (1 cup, cooked) | 2.8 |
| Turkey (dark meat, 85g) | 2.3 | Pumpkin seeds (30 g) | 2.5 |
| Beef (chuck, lean, 85g) | 2.1 | Edamame (1 cup, cooked) | 2.3 |
| Pork (85g) | 0.9 | Chickpeas (1 cup, cooked) | 2.1 |
| Chicken breast (85g) | 0.9 | Black beans (1 cup, cooked) | 3.6 |
| Eggs (1 large) | 0.6 | Potato (1 medium, baked with skin) | 1.9 |

If your iron stores are not severely depleted, oral iron supplements can be a good option. The same principles apply as with food—combining iron supplements with vitamin C-rich foods enhances absorption. Some iron tablets even come with added vitamin C for this reason.

> **TIP**
>
> To further boost iron absorption and haemoglobin levels, you can combine iron with the herb **withania** (ashwagandha). Aim for a daily dose of around 2000 mg of dried root, which contains approximately 200 mg of withania extract.

For women with significant iron deficiency or iron-deficiency anaemia, an intravenous iron infusion, known as Ferinject in Australia, New Zealand, and the UK, can be life changing. Before 2010, iron infusions carried a higher risk of severe allergic reactions and required hospital supervision. Today, Ferinject has made the process much safer and more accessible, with most GP clinics able to provide it. While mild side effects like headaches, dizziness, flushing, or nausea can occur during the infusion, they usually pass quickly, and serious reactions are rare.

Regular follow-ups with your healthcare practitioner are essential to monitor progress and set clear iron level goals.

### IRON'S ROLE THROUGHOUT A WOMAN'S LIFE

Maintaining optimal iron levels helps you sustain energy, prevent fatigue, and improve overall wellbeing at every stage of your life.

#### PUBERTY

During puberty, rapid growth and increased activity require more iron. Focus on iron-rich foods, combined with vitamin C for better absorption. Oral iron supplements may help if stores are low, along with withania (ashwagandha) to boost haemoglobin levels.

#### THE FERTILE YEARS

Heavy or frequent periods can drain iron stores. Monitor your levels regularly and consider oral iron or iron infusions like Ferinject if deficiency is significant. Combining iron with vitamin C and paying attention to hormonal balance can help prevent the vicious cycle of low iron and heavy bleeding.

Pregnancy puts significant strain on iron levels, and replenishing these stores during the postnatal period can be challenging with the additional demands of motherhood. As you age, your body's biochemical efficiency slows, and dietary choices may further impact iron levels.

#### PERIMENOPAUSE

Fluctuating hormones may impact iron absorption and stores. Iron supplements, along with a well-balanced diet rich in iron and vitamin C, can support energy and overall wellbeing as your body transitions.

#### MENOPAUSE

Though periods stop, iron remains crucial for maintaining energy, immune function, and cognitive health. Keep up with iron levels, especially if your diet changes or you face gut-related absorption issues.

#### THE AGE OF WISDOM

With ageing, the body's efficiency in absorbing nutrients slows. Ensure dietary choices support optimal iron levels and consider gentle supplementation if needed. Iron helps maintain vitality, cognitive function, and immune support in these later years.

# Magnesium and Calcium

**THE YIN AND YANG OF THE MINERAL WORLD**
Calcium and magnesium have a delicate balance, like yin and yang. Too much or too little of either can lead to hormonal and health issues for women. When these minerals are out of sync, your body signals imbalance with unmistakable symptoms.

Magnesium and calcium work together to ensure smooth muscle function. Calcium contracts your muscles, while magnesium relaxes them. This partnership allows efficient movement. For example, when you flex your biceps, calcium contracts the muscle while magnesium relaxes the triceps, preventing opposing muscles from working against each other. If this balance breaks down, muscle cramps and spasms are the result.

This calcium-magnesium balance also plays a vital role in regulating blood pressure. Calcium constricts blood vessels, raising blood pressure, while magnesium relaxes them, lowering pressure. Both need to work together for cardiovascular health. If calcium dominates, blood pressure rises.

## CASE STUDY
# Dr Karen
## Lesson on magnesium in blood pressure regulation

Back in the 1980s, during my postgraduate obstetrics training at a rural hospital, I learned an unforgettable lesson about magnesium's role in blood pressure regulation. I was fortunate to be mentored by three brilliant, outside-the-box thinkers who brought common sense and innovation to their obstetrics practice. One of my key tasks was to meet ambulances transferring emergency obstetrics patients to our unit, often for pregnancy-induced hypertension (then called pre-eclampsia)—a serious late-pregnancy complication.

My job was to administer a sublingual antihypertensive drug the moment the patient was unloaded. If her blood pressure didn't stabilise by the time we reached the hospital lift, I had a magnesium infusion ready to go by the time we hit the 5th-floor antenatal ward. The specialist's words stayed with me: 'Karen, we try the drug first because protocol demands it—but the drug rarely works. Magnesium always helps and never harms mother or baby.'

At the time, the only definitive solution for pre-eclampsia was delivering the baby. Fast forward 30 years, and magnesium sulphate infusion is now the gold-standard treatment in obstetrics units for preventing and controlling seizures in severe pre-eclampsia, reducing life-threatening complications. It is now also used in preterm deliveries for foetal neuroprotection, significantly lowering the risk of cerebral palsy.

## MAGNESIUM—THE NEGLECTED NUTRIENT

Magnesium often goes unnoticed until muscle cramps appear, by which time a deficiency may have existed for months. As the body's second most abundant mineral after calcium, magnesium is essential for over 400 biochemical processes, including energy production, DNA repair, cardiovascular health, and blood pressure regulation. Yet, studies show over 40% of people may have suboptimal levels without realising it. Ironically, many heart and blood pressure medications, as well as proton pump inhibitors (used for ulcers) can further deplete magnesium.

### ATHLETES AND MAGNESIUM

Athletes benefit greatly from magnesium. Within just one week, magnesium supplements can reduce inflammation, ease muscle soreness, and improve blood glucose regulation after exercise.

The usual dose is 300–400 mg/day—best taken as Magnesium bisglycinate—this form of magnesium is highly absorbable, gentle on the stomach, and ideal for athletes needing support for muscle recovery, energy production and stress reduction, with minimal risk of gastrointestinal upset.

Endurance athletes may require slightly higher amounts due to increased magnesium loss through sweat and urine, particularly during intense training or competitions. For heavy training loads, up to 600 mg/day may be appropriate under professional supervision.

## MAGNESIUM THROUGH HORMONAL STAGES

### PUBERTY

Teenagers often miss out on magnesium due to poor dietary choices (like processed foods and sugary drinks). Encourage magnesium-rich snacks like nuts, seeds, and whole foods to make up for what's lost in refined grains.

### THE FERTILE YEARS

Busy lifestyles, poor dietary choices, and high-intensity exercise can deplete magnesium. Exercise increases the need for magnesium but also leads to higher excretion through sweat and urine. Women who overdo aerobic exercise may risk deficiency.

### PERIMENOPAUSE

Stress during perimenopause burns through magnesium stores, and alcohol consumption further depletes it. The result is difficulty absorbing magnesium from food, leading to greater deficiency.

### MENOPAUSE

Magnesium is essential for bone health, helping to absorb calcium and form new bone. A magnesium deficiency during menopause can accelerate bone loss and increase fracture risk. Additionally, taking a magnesium supplement at bedtime (75 to 150 mg) supports better sleep, mood, and bone health.

### THE AGE OF WISDOM

Magnesium is key for eye health and cataract prevention as we age. It also supports cancer resilience and plays an important role in maintaining healthy vitamin D levels, which is essential for overall wellbeing.

> **TIRED? COULD IT BE LOW MAGNESIUM?**
>
> It's not surprising to see that studies have shown magnesium injections improved chronic fatigue symptoms in 80% of patients, while those given a placebo saw no change.
>
> **DR KAREN'S NOTE**
>
> Magnesium supplements are not created equal. It's best to avoid supermarket brands and opt for practitioner-recommended products. Look for magnesium in forms like glycinate, chloride, or phosphate, which are better absorbed by the body. A daily dose of 250–300 mg is ideal, though some women with deficiency symptoms may need a higher dose. Always confirm this with a blood test measuring red cell magnesium before increasing supplementation.

### A CHECK FOR MAGNESIUM DEFICIENCY

The following symptoms may indicate a significant magnesium deficiency:

- Muscle and general fatigue
- Muscle twitching or cramping
- Muscle weakness
- Tight muscles (especially in the head, neck, and shoulders)
- Shooting pains in the head or neck
- Nausea and loss of appetite
- Irregular heartbeats or palpitations
- Numbness or tingling (especially around the mouth or extremities)
- Higher-than-usual blood pressure

Blood serum magnesium levels are unreliable—that said, a low result is significant; the more accurate test is red cell magnesium, which measures magnesium stored within your red blood cells.

### UNDERSTANDING YOUR MAGNESIUM LEVELS

The standard reference range for red cell magnesium is 4.20 mg/dL to 6.70 mg/dL. A 2020 study of European postmenopausal women showed that 70% had magnesium levels below 4.20 mg/dL. By contrast, optimal magnesium levels for athletes are typically around 6.5 mg/dL or higher.

### WHERE TO FIND MAGNESIUM

Start by improving your diet with magnesium-rich foods like pumpkin and sunflower seeds, Brazil nuts, almonds, cashews, spinach, oatmeal, bananas, avocado, and dark chocolate. However, due to modern farming and food processing, our food is often less magnesium-rich than in the past. Gut health also plays a role, as even the best diet can be ineffective if magnesium isn't absorbed properly.

Magnesium is a safe and cost-effective supplement, but it's important not to overdo it. Excessive supplementation can crowd out other important nutrients and raise breast cancer risk. Stick to practitioner-recommended brands and forms like glycinate, chloride, or phosphate, with a daily dose of 250-300 mg. For severe deficiencies, consult a doctor for appropriate dosing.

### TRANSDERMAL MAGNESIUM

If oral supplements cause gut issues, magnesium oil is a great alternative since magnesium is well absorbed through the skin. Just be careful not to overuse it, as skin absorption is efficient. For a more relaxing option, try an Epsom salts bath—the magnesium sulphate in the salts is quickly absorbed through the skin, and even a 20-minute soak can boost your magnesium levels.

**CASE STUDY | DR KAREN**

# Sue
## Too much of a good thing

Sue was a sought-after massage therapist specialising in female athletes. Knowing the importance of magnesium for muscle health, she replaced her usual massage oils with magnesium oil, and her clients loved the results. However, three months later, Sue came to me with brain fog and muscle weakness so severe she had cancelled her clients for the month. Being insightful, she had already linked her symptoms to the magnesium oil.

Her clinical exam revealed a heart rate of 52 beats per minute, a concerning sign of magnesium toxicity. While her ECG was otherwise normal, her red cell magnesium level was alarmingly high at 7.2 mg/dL. Since she had stopped using the oils a week earlier, I advised rest and plenty of hydration to help her kidneys clear the excess magnesium. At her six-week follow-up, Sue's symptoms had completely resolved, and her energy was back, though she sadly had to return to her traditional massage oils.

## POTASSIUM AND MAGNESIUM: THE DYNAMIC DUO

If you're struggling to maintain good magnesium levels, low potassium might be the issue. These minerals work together in your body. Diuretics, often prescribed for blood pressure, can deplete potassium and trigger magnesium excretion.

> **INTRAVENOUS MAGNESIUM—A QUICK FIX FOR SEVERE DEFICIENCY**
>
> For severe magnesium deficiency, intravenous magnesium is an option. I've used this in my practice for over a decade. A quick 15–30-minute infusion of 2.5 g of magnesium sulphate is safe and highly effective at boosting magnesium levels—and yes, I even indulge in it once or twice a year for a burst of relaxation!

## ALL ABOUT CALCIUM

Calcium is a powerhouse mineral for women's health, essential for strong, resilient bones and vital for heart function, nerve signalling, and muscle contractions. It works in synergy with magnesium during muscle function—calcium triggers muscle contraction, while magnesium ensures relaxation, maintaining balance and preventing cramps.

When dietary calcium is insufficient, the body 'borrows' it from bones to maintain essential functions like muscle contractions and nerve signalling. This process is regulated by the parathyroid hormone (PTH), which releases calcium from your bones into the bloodstream when levels drop. Over time, frequent borrowing without adequate calcium replacement can weaken bones, increasing the risk of osteoporosis and fractures.

Both too little and too much calcium can cause issues. Inadequate intake leaves bones vulnerable, while excessive supplementation, especially without balancing nutrients like magnesium or vitamin D, can lead to kidney stones or artery calcification. Achieving the right balance is key to unlocking calcium's full benefits for lifelong health.

## THE CALCIUM AND MAGNESIUM PARTNERSHIP

High-dose calcium supplements can cause your body to excrete magnesium more quickly. This calcium-magnesium imbalance is one reason long-term use of high-dose calcium supplements has been linked to coronary artery disease and heart attacks. Aim for balance rather than excess and get calcium primarily from your diet, unless advised by your health practitioner.

## WHERE TO FIND CALCIUM

### FOODS FOR A CALCIUM-RICH DIET WITH A MAGNESIUM BALANCE

**DAIRY**
- Yoghurt: Perfect for breakfast.
- Cheese: Cheddar and mozzarella are great choices.

**VEGETABLES**
- Swiss chard
- Mustard greens (look for these at your farmer's market)
- Kale
- Spinach
- Bok choy
- Broccoli: Load your plate with this antioxidant, magnesium, and calcium powerhouse.

**NUTS AND SEEDS**
- Almonds: Add to cereal or enjoy as a snack.
- Pumpkin and sesame seeds: Ideal for homemade snacks
- Chia seeds: Make a simple dessert by simmering with fruit and water, then cooling overnight.

**PROTEIN FOODS (RICH IN CALCIUM AND MAGNESIUM)**
- Sardines
- Salmon (with bones)
- Black beans
- Green beans
- Edamame
- Lentils
- Tofu
- Fruits
- Oranges
- Figs
- Kiwi
- Whole Grains
- Quinoa: A nutritious alternative to rice.
- Oats: Pair with yoghurt or milk for a calcium-rich start to your day.

**OTHER FOODS**
- Tahini (sesame paste)
- Dark chocolate (a delicious source of magnesium!)

## CALCIUM AND MAGNESIUM—A LIFELINE

### PUBERTY

Calcium supports bone and brain development during puberty. It's essential for forming strong teeth, healthy bones, and neural pathways that are critical for learning and memory. A calcium deficiency during this stage can increase the risk of fractures and future osteoporosis.

### THE FERTILE YEARS

Low calcium impacts bone density starting in your 30s, and athletes should be particularly mindful of this. Studies show that consuming calcium-rich foods before intense training can reduce bone breakdown. During pregnancy and breastfeeding, calcium needs rise by 20%. A prenatal dietary audit can help ensure adequate calcium and magnesium intake to support both mother and baby.

### PERIMENOPAUSE

Low calcium in perimenopause increases the risk of mood swings and anxiety. It also contributes to the first signs of tooth and gum disease. This stage is a crucial time to meet your daily calcium needs.

### MENOPAUSE

Bone health becomes the primary focus. Calcium, in conjunction with magnesium, helps regulate hot flushes by controlling blood vessel dilation and relaxation. A balanced intake of these minerals is key during menopause.

### THE AGE OF WISDOM

Calcium continues to play an important role in mood, bone, and cardiovascular health. At this stage, your total calcium needs increase to 1,200 mg per day (note that this includes what you consume in your *daily diet*!). However, absorption declines with age, especially with lower oestrogen levels and the use of medications that affect calcium uptake. Your doctor will be happy to measure calcium and, if indicated, its partner hormone PTH (the parathyroid hormone) that regulates the movement of calcium within your body.

> **SPECIAL CONSIDERATIONS**
>
> If you have a medical condition that disrupts calcium levels, like cancer, kidney disease, parathyroid issues, or bowel disease, always follow your doctor's advice on calcium intake.

### DO YOU NEED A CALCIUM SUPPLEMENT?

If you have been recommended calcium to support bone density, or in preparation for pregnancy keep daily calcium supplements well below 1000 mg, unless advised by your GP or obstetrician; make sure to include magnesium with your daily calcium tablet in a 2 to 1 ratio (that means 500 mg magnesium for 1000 mg of calcium). Be aware that good levels of vitamin D and magnesium are much more likely to support bone density than calcium alone, particularly if you exceed optimal levels.

### WHAT THIS MEANS FOR YOU

Aim for calcium-rich foods (see list on page 469) and pair them with vitamin D for optimal absorption, and magnesium for balance. Calcium is not just about strong bones; it's about overall vitality, hormonal harmony and resilience.

# Zinc

### ZINC: ESSENTIAL FOR HORMONAL HARMONY, FERTILITY AND MOOD

Zinc is a mineral, just like iron and calcium, and plays a key role in over 3000 biochemical pathways. Low zinc levels can lead to more frequent viral respiratory infections, especially during the winter months, but its benefits go far beyond fighting colds.

### THE QUEEN OF GENES

Vitamin D may be the 'king' of genetic wellness, but zinc is the 'queen.' It's involved in over 300 genetic and biochemical pathways that support women's health. Zinc is crucial for adrenal function, helping produce stress hormones and the building blocks necessary for fertility.

## Over 2 billion people worldwide are zinc-deficient.

Zinc is essential for producing stomach acid, and low stomach acid (often caused by anti-ulcer or anti-reflux drugs) can reduce zinc absorption, creating a cycle of chronic deficiency and poor digestion.

### ZINC THROUGH YOUR HORMONAL STAGES

#### PUBERTY

Zinc is vital for skin health, and low levels can contribute to acne and breakouts during adolescence. Other signs of deficiency include mouth ulcers or cracks in the corners of the lips. Zinc also plays an early role in breast development and continues to support breast health throughout life.

A gentle zinc supplement, like zinc gluconate (around 15 mg, taken with food to prevent nausea), can prevent problem mouth ulcers and support healthy hair, skin and nails.

### THE FERTILE YEARS

Zinc is crucial for immune function, especially as women are more likely to develop autoimmune diseases during their Fertile Years. Zinc deficiency can increase the risk of autoimmunity, and babies born to zinc-deficient mothers are more likely to experience acid reflux.

Zinc also plays a critical role in maintaining a healthy menstrual cycle, fertility, and egg quality. It supports the production of follicle stimulating hormone (FSH) and luteinising hormone (LH), which regulate oestrogen and progesterone. During fertilisation, zinc triggers the 'zinc spark', which activates the egg and helps prevent multiple sperm from penetrating.

Zinc deficiency can lead to irregular cycles, infertility, miscarriage, and complications during pregnancy such as slow foetal growth, premature delivery, and postpartum bleeding.

> **FERTILITY PRESCRIPTION:**
>
> Have your zinc levels checked by your Health practitioner and consider taking 15 to 30 mg of supplemental zinc picinolate for immune support ahead of winter. If planning pregnancy, optimise zinc by increasing zinc-rich foods like oysters and supplement to support egg quality.

### PERIMENOPAUSE

As hormonal stress increases during perimenopause, your body's ability to absorb zinc decreases, especially if you're taking medications for ulcers or reflux. Oestrogen dominance, common during this time, can cause the body to absorb more copper, further depleting zinc. Zinc is essential for producing serotonin, the mood hormone, and its deficiency can affect both mood and sleep, as serotonin converts into melatonin, which regulates sleep cycles.

To help protect from autoimmune activation optimise your zinc by supporting gut health and supplement with zinc picinolate 15-30 mg daily with food.

### MENOPAUSE

Zinc plays a role in preventing hair loss, maintaining skin health, and supporting nail strength, which can become issues during menopause. Optimal zinc levels also help bolster immunity, reducing vulnerability to seasonal infections.

Now is the time to prioritise cognitive support—have zinc levels checked and supplement with zinc gluconate for extra brain help (both zinc and gluconate protect your brain).

## THE AGE OF WISDOM

As we age, the immune system becomes more fragile. A combination of vitamin D and zinc works best to support immune health. Zinc also remains crucial for maintaining healthy sleep cycles and mood by supporting the production of mood hormones like serotonin.

Zinc becomes super important here to support your immune system and continue to nourish your brain—have levels checked and supplement with zinc gluconate 15 to 30 mg daily to optimise levels.

> **ZINC AND BREAST CANCER**
>
> There is an inverse relationship between zinc intake and breast cancer risk—lower zinc levels increase the risk, particularly in 'triple-negative' breast cancer, which has fewer treatment options. Remember, more zinc isn't better; aim for the right balance. (Read more about breast cancer on page 578.)

**If you follow a vegan, vegetarian or Ornish diet you have an increased risk of zinc deficiency. Consider a supplement if you struggle to meet your zinc needs through diet alone.**

## WELLNESS ACTION PLAN
# ZINC

### CORRECTING ZINC DEFICIENCY

Keep in mind that reference ranges for zinc levels can vary depending on the laboratory, as they are based on population averages. To check your zinc status, visit a naturopath for a simple zinc tally test or ask your doctor for a blood test.

For optimal health, aim for a serum zinc level between 14 to 28 µmol/L, regardless of where you live. When you receive your test results, ask for your exact number. If you fall outside this range, consider supplementation.

Zinc gluconate or zinc picolinate are good forms to start with, as they are less likely to cause nausea. Begin with 15 mg daily after meals, and if tolerated, you can gradually increase the dose to 50 mg to correct the deficiency.

Increase the following zinc-rich foods (listed in order of their zinc content):

**SEAFOOD**
- Oysters
- Mussels
- Crab and lobster
- Sardines

**MEAT**
- Beef (especially beef liver)
- Turkey
- Chicken
- Pork

**VEGETABLES**
- Spinach
- Brussels sprouts
- Mushrooms (especially shiitake)

**NUTS AND SEEDS**
- Pumpkin seeds
- Sunflower seeds
- Sesame seeds
- Hemp seeds
- Cashews, almonds, hazelnuts, peanuts
- Brazil nuts and walnuts

**LEGUMES AND GRAINS**

- Chickpeas (garbanzo beans)
- Lentils
- Quinoa

**DAIRY**

- Greek yoghurt
- Cheese (especially Swiss, gouda, and cheddar)

**OTHER**

- Cocoa powder (unsweetened)
- Wheat germ
- Eggs

Monitor your levels with the support of a qualified naturopath or integrative doctor, checking your levels 6 to 8 weeks after beginning zinc supplementation.

## THE ZINC-COPPER PARTNERSHIP

If you're struggling to maintain good zinc levels despite supplementation, copper overload could be the culprit. Copper is an essential mineral, but too much can block zinc absorption and disrupt other essential biochemical pathways. This imbalance may even begin at birth, as copper can pass through the placenta, creating a zinc deficiency in newborns, leading to issues like gastric reflux or colic.

### SIGNS OF COPPER OVERLOAD

- Fatigue
- Menstrual disorders
- Heavy periods
- PMS
- Infertility
- Depression
- Anxiety
- Migraines
- Allergies
- Childhood learning disorders

## CAUSES OF COPPER OVERLOAD:

Copper overload can result from the use of copper cookware, copper plumbing, and herbicide sprays (like copper sulphate) on vegetables and in the water supply. Even taking the oral contraceptive pill (the Pill) can contribute to this issue. Since copper is a trace mineral essential for human health, it is allowed as a pesticide spray on organic produce. To reduce dietary copper, soak vegetables and remove outer leaves from leafy greens.

## HOW TO DO A COPPER 'DUMP'

Supporting gut health is vital because a strong microbiome helps move unwanted metals out through the bowel.

Staying well-hydrated helps the kidneys flush excess copper more easily, keeping detox pathways flowing smoothly.

Ensure a healthy zinc intake, as zinc competes with copper for absorption and encourages balance.

Certain foods act as natural copper chelators, helping to eliminate excess copper from the body:

- Parsley, garlic, and coriander bind with copper and support elimination.
- Molybdenum-rich foods (for example, beans, peas, broccoli and cabbage) help the liver remove copper.
- Selenium-rich foods, like Brazil nuts, also help regulate copper levels.

## SPOTLIGHT ON
# Managing Toxins

Imagine going about your day—sipping from a plastic water bottle or applying your favourite face lotion—unaware of the invisible culprits that might be disrupting your hormones. These culprits are endocrine disrupting chemicals (EDCs) that mimic or block hormonal signals, impacting fertility, mood, immune function and increasing the risk of breast cancer, endometriosis and thyroid disorders.

### HORMONAL HIJACKERS:

#### THE TOP THREE ENDOCRINE-DISRUPTING CHEMICALS (EDCs) YOU NEED TO AVOID

1. **Xenoestrogens:** Mimic oestrogen, contributing to oestrogen dominance.
2. **Adrenal disruptors:** Affect cortisol and adrenal health (corticosteroid disruptors).
3. **General endocrine disruptors:** Affect thyroid, insulin and other hormonal pathways.

## XENOESTROGENS

Xenoestrogens are man-made compounds that interfere with the body's natural oestrogen signals, which are crucial for hormonal balance, fertility and cellular health. Xenoestrogen chemical burden is a common cause of oestrogen dominance symptoms and can result in a range of health issues, including mood swings, increased risks of breast cancer, endometriosis, and other hormonal imbalances.

These chemicals are persistent and accumulate in body tissues, dissolving into fat cells and making them hard to eliminate.

### WHERE ARE THESE CHEMICALS FOUND?

Xenoestrogens are commonly found in everyday items like:
- Plastics (the bisphenol family, especially bisphenol A or BPA)
- Skincare products (phthalates and parabens)
- Herbicides (atrazine)

### EFFECTS OF XENOESTROGENS

The impact of xenoestrogens can range from mild to severe. They add a layer of complexity to hormonal imbalance like oestrogen dominance that won't show up on standard medical testing. (See a list of oestrogen dominance symptoms on page 125.) In wildlife, they've been shown to cause hormonal disruptions like the masculinisation or feminisation of fish. This serves as a warning for their potential harm to human health.

---

**FROM SHARON K**

In the 1990s, I was already warning women about the dangers of plastics leaching xenoestrogens, long before BPA became widely recognised. I urged women not to microwave food in plastic or put hot food into plastic containers. I was especially concerned about plastic baby bottles, urging mothers to use glass instead. Thankfully, awareness has grown, and BPA-free products are now more common. Still, there's often a significant lag between scientific discoveries, public health messages, and eventual legislation.

> **FACT ALERT: THE SHRINKING PENISES OF FLORIDA ALLIGATORS**
>
> Research by Dr Louis Guillette in the 1980s found that exposure to EDCs caused male alligators in Florida to develop smaller penises and female alligators to prematurely lose their egg follicles. If EDCs can cause reproductive harm to alligators, imagine what they might be doing to humans!

### THE BISPHENOL FAMILY OF XENOESTROGENS

Products marked with recycle number 7 often contain BPA or similar chemicals. Though BPA is now banned in many baby bottles and food containers, other chemicals in the bisphenol family persist in everyday products like thermal paper used for EFTPOS receipts. Even BPA-free plastics may still contain harmful chemicals.

**STRATEGIES TO MINIMISE EXPOSURE TO BPAs**

- Choose BPA-free drink bottle like stainless steel or glass.
- Keep contact with EFTPOS receipts to a minimum or wash your hands after contact.
- Buy BPA-free cans. Most food cans have an internal lining to protect the metal from the food's acidity.

### TAMPON TOXINS

Throughout your life, you may use over 11,000 tampons or pads, placing them in intimate contact with your body. This allows chemicals to leach into your bloodstream, disrupting your hormones and vaginal microbiome. Xenoestrogens, like phthalates, phenols and parabens that can impact fertility and hormone balance, are commonly found in these products.

**STRATEGIES TO MINIMISE EXPOSURE:**

- Choose pads and tampons made from natural, non-bleached materials.
- Consider switching to menstrual cups made from 100% medical-grade silicone. These reusable options are cost-effective, eco-friendly and safe for swimming or exercising.
- Explore period underwear, which is becoming increasingly popular, especially with teens.

## ADRENAL DISRUPTORS

Exposure to these chemicals has a significant health cost. These EDCs are found in pesticide residue on non-organic food and in areas where these chemicals are used. Farming communities are at higher risk of exposure.

Limit exposure to corticosteroid disruptors by choosing organic produce to avoid pesticide residues like organophosphates and glyphosate. When organic is not an option, turn to page 406 for advice on how to keep your clean non-organic food pesticide free.

### PFAFS: OUR NEW TOXIC CHALLENGE

Per- and polyfluoroalkyl substances (PFAS), known as 'forever chemicals,' are found in stain-resistant fabrics, non-stick cookware, food packaging, cosmetics, and firefighting foam. They persist in the environment for thousands of years and are linked to developmental issues, reproductive problems, cancers, weakened immunity, high cholesterol, thyroid disorders, obesity, and asthma.

### THE CURRENT PFAS SITUATION ACROSS THE WORLD

The global awareness surrounding the dangers of PFAS is steadily growing. Governments and regulatory bodies are beginning to act, but the approach varies from country to country.

### NEW ZEALAND: LEADING THE CHARGE

New Zealand is setting an example by becoming one of the first countries in the world to ban PFAS in cosmetic products. From 2026 onwards, the import or manufacture of any cosmetics containing PFAS will be strictly prohibited. By June 2028, any remaining PFAS-containing cosmetic products must be disposed of, demonstrating the country's proactive stance in safeguarding public health and the environment.

### AUSTRALIA: PHASING OUT BUT NOT BANNING

While Australia has not yet implemented a nationwide ban on all PFAS, the government is taking steps to manage and limit their use. The focus has been on phasing out PFAS in specific products like firefighting foams, a major source of environmental contamination. Australia is also developing national environmental management plans, showing a commitment to protecting both your health and the environment from the impact of these harmful chemicals.

## UK: GROWING CALLS FOR STRICTER REGULATIONS

PFAS haven't been banned outright in the UK yet but the push for change is growing. Government bodies and advocacy groups are calling for stricter regulations and potential future bans on PFAS in consumer products. Regional efforts are also underway to limit exposure, highlighting the increasing concern about the health risks posed by these persistent chemicals.

### PFAS IN OUR DRINKING WATER

In April 2024, *The Sydney Morning Herald* reported alarming levels of PFAS in the water supplies of towns and cities across Australia. Local councils are now working to find ways to remove this hormone disruptor from their communities. Similarly, in the United States, the Environmental Protection Agency (EPA) has launched significant efforts to clean up widespread PFAS contamination. Strict regulations have been introduced to restrict the ongoing use of PFAS, with new laws enforcing action against polluters.

### CAN YOU FILTER PFAS OUT AT HOME?

When we first started learning about the health impacts of PFAS we felt deeply frustrated and worried. The more we uncovered, the more we realised just how pervasive these chemicals are, and how limited our options seemed in protecting ourselves and our families from these invisible toxins.

PFAS molecules are incredibly small, often in the nanometre range. To give you an idea, one nanometre is one-thousandth of a micron, which means even the largest PFAS molecules are much smaller than the pores of the 3-micron filter we used in our own homes. Like many people, we assumed a high-quality water filter would offer some level of protection, but it became clear that PFAS can easily slip through these standard filters.

We soon realised that specialised filtration methods—such as activated carbon, ion exchange resins, or high-pressure membranes like reverse osmosis—are required to capture particles as small as PFAS molecules. This knowledge left us feeling even more anxious. How could we safeguard our water supply at home?

Thankfully, Sharon reached out to our friend and colleague, Professor Marc Cohen, who has been researching this problem for years. As both a medical doctor and researcher, Marc was alarmed by the health risks associated with PFAS and took action. His passion led him to develop an advanced water filtration system called Beautiful Water, designed to tackle not only PFAS but a wide range of other contaminants.

Marc's Beautiful Water systems use advanced filtration techniques, including mechanical and electric absorption, ion exchange, and activated carbon with bacteriostatic silver, to remove a wide range of contaminants. These include heavy metals, pesticides, PFAS, pharmaceuticals, VOCs, microplastics, and other endocrine disruptors, as well as chlorine and its by-products.

With countertop, under-sink, and whole-house options, Beautiful Water has brought us peace of mind. Knowing our family's water is safe feels like such a relief. After all, if you don't use a filter, your body becomes one—and drinking less poison is always a good idea.

For more information on how to protect your water, visit BeautifulWater.co.

## WELLNESS ACTION PLAN
# REDUCE YOUR EXPOSURE TO ALL EDCs

Minimising your exposure to harmful EDCs requires a thoughtful approach to everyday choices. Use this plan to take proactive steps and incorporate helpful tools to support a healthier environment for you and your family.

### REDUCE EXPOSURE TO EDCs

- **Embrace organics:** Choose organic produce to avoid pesticide residues that act as xenoestrogens. Opt for sustainably raised protein sources, such as pasture-raised meat and wild-caught fish, as factory-farmed animals are often exposed to EDCs.

- **Embrace naturals:** Use natural cleaning and personal care items. Look for products labelled 'phthalate-free' or 'fragrance-free' to avoid concealed EDCs.

- **Purify your water:** Invest in a high-calibre water filtration system to eliminate contaminants, including EDCs, from your shower, kitchen and drinking water.

- **Support natural detox pathways**: While 'forever chemicals' persist in the environment, supporting detox pathways can lessen their impact.

- **Exercise caution with packaging:** Avoid supermarket food wrapped in packaging, especially plastics.

- **Choose whole foods**: Prioritise minimally processed foods over packaged ones to reduce exposure to additives and preservatives that may contain EDCs.

- **Sidestep hormone-altering plastics:** Choose glass, ceramic, or stainless-steel containers for food and beverage storage. Never heat food in plastic containers.

- **Inspect cosmetic labels:** Carefully check personal care product labels and avoid those with parabens, phthalates or other known EDCs.

- **Mind your home environment:** Limit exposure to EDCs in household items like flame retardants in furniture and carpets by selecting non-toxic alternatives.

- **Be a conscious shopper:** Stay informed about potential sources of EDCs and make conscious decisions to minimise exposure in your daily routines.

Consider these resources to help reduce your exposure to PFAS and other harmful chemicals:

- *Detox Me* **(app)**: Created by the Silent Spring Institute, this app provides tips to reduce exposure to harmful chemicals like PFAS. It covers personal care, food packaging, and household cleaners, with a barcode scanner to identify safer products.

- *EWG Skin Deep* **(website and app)**: This database rates cosmetics and personal care products for PFAS and other harmful chemicals, helping you make safer choices.

- *Yuka* **(app)**: A user-friendly barcode scanner for food, cosmetics, and personal care items, offering overall scores and healthier alternatives.

- *Clearya* **(website and app)**: Flags toxic chemicals like PFAS in cosmetics, skincare, and household products and integrates with online shopping to suggest safer options.

## ADVOCATE FOR CHANGE

Support policies and regulations aimed at reducing the prevalence of EDCs in consumer goods and promoting safer alternatives for both human health and the environment.

## SPOTLIGHT ON
# Movement and Exercise

What's the difference between movement and exercise? We need to find the right balance of the two for hormonal harmony. And we need to balance intense Yang exercises with restorative Yin exercises. Both movement and exercise have a profound influence on your overall wellbeing.

### MOVING YOUR BODY

Many women under-exercise, some over-exercise, but most simply under-move. Few find that sweet spot of balanced physical activity.

Are you an 'under-mover'?

Exercise and movement are not the same. Movement is essential for daily health, while exercise targets specific outcomes—you need a balance of both. Performing thousands of small movements throughout the day is what's most beneficial for your overall wellbeing. We know that hitting the sweet spot of moving is beneficial for your general health, we encourage you to use a tracker to meet the quota of 7000 to 10,000 steps per day.

When you exercise intensely for 30 to 60 minutes each day, you might be less active overall (perhaps not meeting your daily step quota). Surprisingly, many fitness enthusiasts assume their vigorous workout session covers all their physical activity needs. Research shows that regular movement throughout the day is far more beneficial. Small, consistent movements are key to overall wellbeing, making it essential to stay active beyond that one-hour workout.

Think of movement and exercise as two parts of the same story: movement is the baseline for health, while exercise adds targeted benefits.

- Movement—like walking a minimum of 7000-10,000 steps daily—supports fundamental health, engaging over 4000 beneficial genes.

- Exercise delivers specific outcomes (cardiovascular fitness, strength, flexibility, stability) when layered onto a day already rich in movement.

In essence, movement is a non-negotiable part of our nature, and exercise is a powerful supplement when done in balance.

### SIX SIMPLE WAYS TO INCREASE YOUR DAILY STEPS

1. Take the stairs whenever possible—view escalators and elevators as last resorts.
2. Park farther away from your destination when shopping or running errands.
3. If able, carry a basket instead of using a shopping cart (within reason).
4. Take a short walk during lunch, even if it's just around the block.
5. Make movement a priority—look for small ways to move more throughout your day.
6. Play actively with your children and pets.

### YIN AND YANG: BALANCING EXERCISE

Twenty years ago, we borrowed from Chinese philosophy to categorise exercise into two types: Yin and Yang.

- **Yang:** High-energy, intense activities like cardio, weight training, sports, or vigorous yoga (for example, Vinyasa flow or Ashtanga).

- **Yin:** Restorative, gentle activities like Tai Chi, Qigong, stretching, foam rolling, joint mobilisation, and gentle walks. Yin still provides health benefits without depleting your body or pushing your adrenals to produce an excess of stress hormones, particularly pushing cortisol to catabolic levels.

Depending on your stress levels, health and hormonal stage, you'll need to balance Yin and Yang activities. This may go against your natural inclination to either 'go hard' or only focus on the soft and slow activities. However, exercise like all elements of good health, is all about balance. The general rule is to listen carefully to your body.

**YOUR YANG AUDIT**

If you are pushing hard in your exercise routine and experience any of the following, reduce your Yang activities and replace with Yin:
- High stress
- Mood changes mid-cycle (around Day 16)
- Insomnia or waking unrefreshed
- Difficulty losing body fat despite healthy eating and exercise
- Heavy or irregular periods (especially during perimenopause)
- Anxiety, overwhelm, frequent illness or digestive issues
- Injuries, joint pain or excessive muscle soreness

**YOUR YIN AUDIT**

If you love your Yin activities and notice any of these signs, Yang exercise may benefit you:
- Loss of muscle mass, gaining body fat
- Struggling with physical endurance (for example, difficulty walking upstairs)
- Regular menstrual cycles with no heavy bleeding
- Waking refreshed and energised
- Flat or low moods
- Diagnosis of osteopenia or osteoporosis (see Spotlight on Bone Care page 612)

Yang exercise offers many benefits, and if you're not unwell, including one or two sessions a week is a great idea. If you're new to this type of exercise, start slowly and set healthy, achievable goals. Join a beginner-friendly walking or jogging group, try a dance class like Five Rhythms or Latin, or explore swimming, cycling, or gym-based resistance training. You'll be amazed at how quickly your body adapts and strengthens.

Activities like playing sports, walking the dog, or playing with kids also improve physical function. If you're recovering from an injury or dealing with physical limitations, connect with Pilates, physiotherapy, or hydrotherapy to rebuild strength and mobility in a supportive way.

### WHY OVER-EXERCISING CAN BE BAD FOR YOU

If you're a regular exerciser who loves intense cardio, it's worth reviewing our Yang audit to make sure you're not overdoing it. Exercise is a healthy stressor—it triggers stress hormones that help your body adapt and grow stronger. But when intensity piles on top of daily stress, it can tip the balance, disrupting ovulation, lowering progesterone and ultimately diminishing the benefits of exercise.

Pushing beyond your sweet spot suppresses immunity, compromises digestion and reduces your ability to absorb nutrients. Your adrenal glands become overworked and undernourished, setting the stage for chronic fatigue. Add in the build-up of lactic acid and free radicals from prolonged intensity, and oxidative stress rises—placing even more strain on your system.

### EXERCISE AND HORMONAL CHANGES

As you transition through different hormonal stages, your exercise needs change. Intense cardio, while valuable, needs careful moderation, especially during perimenopause, to support hormonal balance. Post-menopause, you can gradually reintroduce more cardio while monitoring your body's signals as fitness is key to longevity. General guidance on tailoring your routine follows in the chart provided.

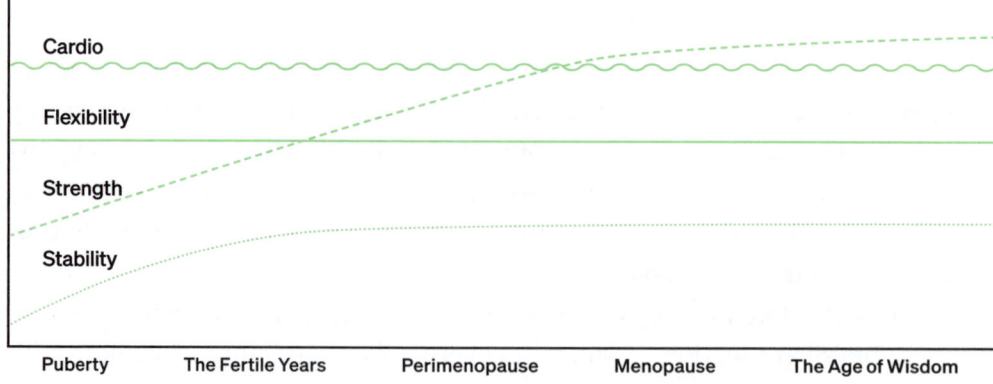

**MOVEMENT HEALTH POSSIBILITIES**

**THE THREE PRINCIPLES OF YANG EXERCISE: INTENSITY, DURATION, REGULARITY**

As you navigate your exercise routine, you'll need to adjust these three guiding principles—intensity, duration and regularity—based on changes in your menstrual cycle or sleep patterns. By balancing these principles, you can create a personalised exercise plan that supports your wellbeing and hormonal balance. This is the Goldilocks principle—not too much, not too little, just right.

**UNDERSTANDING EXERCISE INTENSITY**

Exercise intensity refers to how hard your body works during physical activity. It's key to improving cardiovascular health, muscle strength, and endurance, but it also greatly influences hormonal balance. Pushing your intensity too high when your body signals for lower intensity can disrupt your hormones and cause a cascade of issues.

**HORMONAL TIP**

If you experience any of the following symptoms, we recommend reducing your exercise intensity to low or moderate for at least three months, or until the symptoms improve:

- Irregular, heavy, or infrequent menstrual cycles
- Clots in your menstrual blood
- Mood changes mid-cycle (around Day 16)
- Insomnia or waking unrefreshed
- Gaining body fat despite healthy eating and exercise
- Anxiety or feeling overwhelmed
- Frequent colds, flu, or digestive issues
- Excessive muscle or joint pain

If symptoms return after increasing intensity, your body is telling you to slow down.

### A NOTE ON ENDURANCE TRAINING

#### DR KAREN SAYS

We advise serious caution with endurance sports (such as marathons, triathlons, or long-distance running) after your mid-30s. Overdoing endurance activities in your 30s and beyond can be detrimental to your hormones and bone density levels.

However, individuals with strong genetic lineages tracing to regions in East Africa may possess a natural aptitude for endurance training, including greater hormonal resilience and efficiency in energy metabolism.

In my experience caring for elite female endurance athletes, they peaked in their 20s but faced hormone imbalances by their mid-30s. Overtraining suppresses fertility hormones, often stopping periods, dropping oestrogen to menopausal levels and accelerating bone loss. Every one of them retired in their mid-30s, and I helped them recover after years of pushing their bodies to the limit. Each paid a price in health for the pursuit of Olympic medals.

It concerns me to see women entering perimenopause taking up marathon running or triathlons, believing it will improve their health—when it can actually worsen hormonal imbalance. In my years as an integrative doctor, I've seen many women lose their menstrual cycles or experience irregular periods with endurance training—clear signs that the ovaries and adrenals are under pressure. Ignoring these early signals can contribute to dysfunctional uterine bleeding, or even hormone-sensitive cancers. For women over 30, high-intensity exercise needs to be approached with awareness. It's not just about fitness—it's about protecting your long-term hormonal health.

#### WHY WOMEN SHOULD TRAIN DIFFERENTLY THAN MEN

Boys and men do not menstruate, allowing them to engage in moderate to high-intensity exercise more often and for longer durations. Many male trainers—and even some female trainers—overlook the delicate balance of the hormonal cycle forgetting women's bodies respond differently to exercise due to menstruation, ovaries, adrenal influences, and reproductive genes. Trying to compete with or match men in workouts can come at a hormonal cost.

Yes, your body is designed to adapt, and yes, you can push yourself, but the key question is: *What will this cost me hormonally?* Do I value a healthy womb, balanced hormones, and most importantly is my period normal and regular?

#### FOCUS ON STRENGTH

Maintaining strength is essential at any age or hormonal stage. Whenever you reduce cardio intensity for hormonal balance, prioritise resistance training through Pilates, yoga, or gym workouts. Muscles play a critical role in metabolism, blood sugar control, and hormone balance, accounting for 60% of your resting metabolic rate. Losing muscle reduces energy needs, with unused energy storing as fat, so building and maintaining muscle is vital—especially as you age.

Starting strength training before age 30 helps preserve bone density and boosts metabolism, supporting a healthy fat-to-muscle ratio. Exercises like yoga, Pilates, and weightlifting improve strength, while water-based activities or guided Pilates are great for those with physical limitations. For arthritis, strengthening muscles reduces strain on joints and improves function.

Before committing to intense programs like CrossFit, audit your hormonal health. Ask yourself these questions:

- Is my period normal and regular?
- How is my daily energy (adrenal health)?
- Are my sleep patterns consistent?

If your energy levels are low and your sleep patterns are irregular, visit a naturopath for review of your adrenal system. (See Spotlight on Adrenal Glands on page 334 for further information.) Exercise stimulates the adrenal glands, so if your system is already overstressed, it's best to opt for restorative Yin exercise until you're back on track.

## RESTORATIVE YIN MOVEMENTS

Restorative 'Yin' movements—like yoga, Qigong, Pilates rehabilitation, and walking—are essential for health and wellbeing, especially when managing muscle, bone, fat, and fluid balance. Continuous intermittent movement (CIM) throughout the day is key to long-term wellness so always aim for a minimum of 7000 steps (or the equivalent if walking is not an option for you).

To determine if you need more Yin (gentle activities like yoga, meditation, or walking) or Yang (higher intensity like spinning, boxing, or interval training), consider your current hormonal health. The balance will shift as you transition from your Fertile years into your 40s, perimenopause, and the Age of Wisdom.

## MOVEMENT AND EXERCISE OPTIONS

### WALKING

Of all the movements we do, walking is the most essential because it helps us move around and accomplish daily tasks. A semi-brisk or brisk walk each day is a great way to start reaching your step goal. However, walking mainly strengthens your legs. It doesn't help you squat or lunge nor does it significantly build your postural muscles. Most importantly, walking alone doesn't effectively maintain or regenerate bone density.

While walking is great for movement, getting out in nature, and reducing joint strain, it's not the all-rounder we need for building strength and bone health. Keep walking but complement it with resistance exercises to build muscle and maintain bone density.

### AEROBIC EXERCISE
#### EXAMPLES: WALKING, JOGGING, CYCLING, SWIMMING, DANCING

Aerobic exercise improves cardiovascular health, boosts mood, helps maintain a healthy weight, and enhances sleep quality. Be mindful not to exceed your sweet spot of aerobic training because over-exercising can increase cortisol to unhealthy levels. (See Spotlight on Adrenal Glands on page 334.)

### HIGH-INTENSITY INTERVAL TRAINING (HIIT)
#### EXAMPLES: CIRCUIT TRAINING, SPRINT INTERVALS

HIIT involves short bursts of intense activity followed by rest. It boosts cardiovascular health, metabolism and insulin sensitivity. Just 5 minutes of HIIT, three times a week, has been shown to improve cardiovascular health. HIIT is perfect when you need effective cardio without long sessions.

### STRENGTH TRAINING
#### EXAMPLES: WEIGHTLIFTING, RESISTANCE BANDS, BODYWEIGHT EXERCISES (PUSH-UPS, SQUATS, PLANK)

Strength training helps maintain muscle mass and bone density, which can decline during perimenopause. It also boosts metabolism, supports weight management, and improves overall strength and stamina. Strength training is particularly beneficial for younger women with PCOS and older women looking to maintain bone health during menopause and beyond.

### YOGA
#### EXAMPLES: HATHA YOGA, VINYASA YOGA, RESTORATIVE YOGA

Yoga improves flexibility, balance, and strength. It also reduces stress, anxiety, and depression—common symptoms during perimenopause. Certain poses can alleviate hot flushes and improve sleep. Ideally, everyone should practise some form of yoga, from restorative to more intense styles. If nothing else, try Yoga Nidra, which is highly restorative for hormonal balance, adrenal recovery and sleep improvement.

## PILATES
### EXAMPLES: MAT PILATES, REFORMER PILATES

Pilates focuses on core strength, pelvic floor health, joint mobility, flexibility, and balance. It improves posture, reduces back pain and enhances body awareness. Pilates is ideal for stress management and relaxation, and is particularly effective for recovering from injuries or surgeries.

## TAI CHI AND QIGONG
### EXAMPLES: TAI CHI FORMS, QIGONG ROUTINES

These ancient practices combine slow, deliberate movements with deep breathing and meditation. They improve balance, reduce stress, enhance mental clarity and promote overall wellbeing. Both are especially beneficial for reducing anxiety and improving sleep.

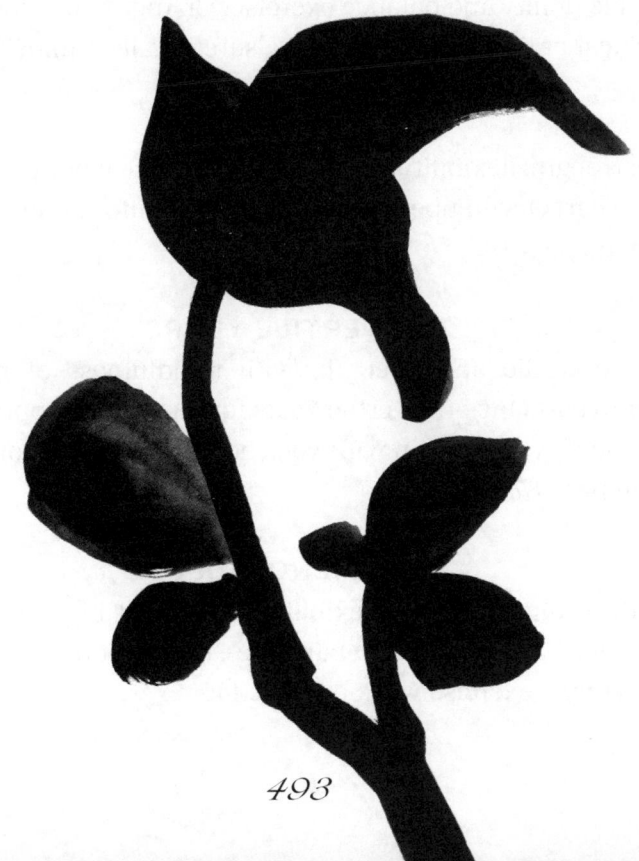

# BALANCED WEEK OF MOVEMENT AND EXERCISE

The following example balances Yang and Yin movement, while aiming to maintain hormonal balance:

**Day 1:** Cardio (moderate intensity, 30-45 minutes) + min 7000 steps
**Day 2:** Strength training (30-60 minutes) or Pilates + min 7000 steps
**Day 3:** Rest or active recovery (light stretching or Yin yoga) + min 7000 steps
**Day 4:** High-intensity interval training (15-20 minutes) + min 7000 steps
**Day 5:** Strength training (30-60 minutes) or Pilates + min 7000 steps
**Day 6:** Flexibility and balance exercises or Yoga + min 7000 steps
**Day 7:** Rest or light activity (like a leisurely walk) + min 7000 steps

### PUBERTY

Focus: Build strength, flexibility, and cardio endurance while protecting growing joints. Refer to Part One—Puberty for more specific information and an example training week on page 61.

### THE FERTILE YEARS

Focus: Balance cardio and strength, with mindfulness of menstrual cycle phases. Refer to Part One—the Fertile Years for our unique approach to exercise designed specifically to work in with your hormonal fluctuations from Day 1 to Days 28-30 on page 87.

### PERIMENOPAUSE

Focus: Prioritise joint mobility, flexibility, and avoid high-intensity cardio to support hormonal balance. Refer to Part One—Perimenopause for more specific advice and a sample exercise week on page 145.

## MENOPAUSE

Focus: Strength and flexibility while minimising intensity to avoid hormonal disruption. Refer to Part One—Menopause for a detailed outline and suggested programs for both beginners and seasoned exercisers on page 209.

## THE AGE OF WISDOM

Focus: Strength and cardiovascular fitness. Workout to improve cardiovascular fitness, a key factor in longevity. Muscle mass is critical to maintain as you age, so take up Pilates or weight training. You are never too old to begin a new exercise regime provided you go slowly and increase your intensity over time.

- Your hormones have now flatlined so increasing intensity in your cardio workouts is encouraged.

- Try to fit in 2 to 3 cardio workouts a week, ideally swimming, walking or other activities that do not put too much pressure on your joints.

- Aim to maintain range of motion in your joints and work on strength, and mobility exercises to maintain bone and muscle health.

- Yoga is the perfect exercise for life, try to engage in both restorative or Yin yoga as well as more challenging classes that encourage you to improve your balance and maintain rotation of the spine.

- Join a gym and start lifting weights, start light and increase or take up Pilates.

- If you have arthritis, it is essential to move your joints and keep your muscles strong to support damaged joints.

> **TIP**
>
> There is a sweet spot in stimulating bone density without overtaxing your joints. Exercise physiologists, physiotherapists and CHECK Trainers (Level 2 certification) are your best support crew if you require guidance. We strongly advise you seek support to ensure you:
>
> - Start correctly
> - Perform exercise with great form and technique
> - Access enough diversity to stimulate your body
> - Maintain bio-mechanical balance (avoiding injury, join and muscle pain)

## FIND YOUR BALANCE IN MOVEMENT AND EXERCISE

Remember to keep the balance in your constant movement and regular exercise. They are not merely physical activities; they are the bedrock of a healthy lifestyle that deeply influences your overall wellbeing. Stay awake to your inner drives of insecurity, weave in the various elements, we described earlier—intensity, duration, and regularity. You can craft an effective program tailored to meet your unique needs and support yourself emotionally to find the ideal hormonal balance. Whether you're a beginner embarking on your fitness journey or an advanced athlete pushing your limits, the key to success lies in your ability to adapt and understand the profound impact on your hormonal health.

> **TIP**
> The most effective exercise program is one that adheres to the Goldilocks principle—striking a perfect balance of not too much and not too little.

Remember to incorporate both Yin and Yang, ensuring a harmonious blend of exertion and recovery that is one you genuinely enjoy and can sustain over the long haul. As you continue to explore and engage in various forms of physical activity, you'll not only notice significant improvements in your physical health but also enhance mental clarity, emotional resilience, and gain a greater sense of fulfilment. Keep moving throughout your day, stay motivated with your chosen exercise routines, and celebrate the progress you make each step of the way.

# SHARON'S STORY

In my younger years, I worked in the fitness industry through the 1980s, teaching aerobics and managing gyms. By the early 1990s, I was strong, lean and one of the first personal trainers on the Gold Coast. I trained other instructors, won awards, featured in fitness magazines, and toured Australia, New Zealand, the UK, Europe and Asia to train fitness professionals.

Outwardly, I was the poster child for health and fitness. But behind the façade, I was adrenally exhausted, mentally overwhelmed, depressed and experiencing suicidal ideation. I was ashamed to show anything other than 'fitness equals health', yet I was far from well.

Today I share with all who'll listen: wellness is not what it looks like—it's not a shape or a size. Wellness is what it feels like—connected, supported from within and being your own best friend. When you look in the mirror, remember to ask, 'What is right with this?' rather than 'What is wrong with this?' We need to manage the inner bully from driving us to do too much—or not enough—especially with food and exercise.

I know firsthand the damage caused when one pillar of wellness, like fitness, is taken to extremes. My training pace tipped me into serious imbalance, physically, mentally and emotionally. It took years to restore balance in my body, mind and spirit.

Working in health retreats over the past 30 years, I've met countless women who push themselves through food, exercise, work or toxic relationships. I recognise them instantly—not with judgement. I see them as a soul sister. 'I too have walked that path. May you find peace.'

Qigong became my lifeline, alongside deep spiritual inquiry and revisiting my childhood emotional scars and conditioning. I came to understand: I am not my mind. That truth set me on a path I still walk—toward wholeness, self-love and the forgiveness I needed most—my own.

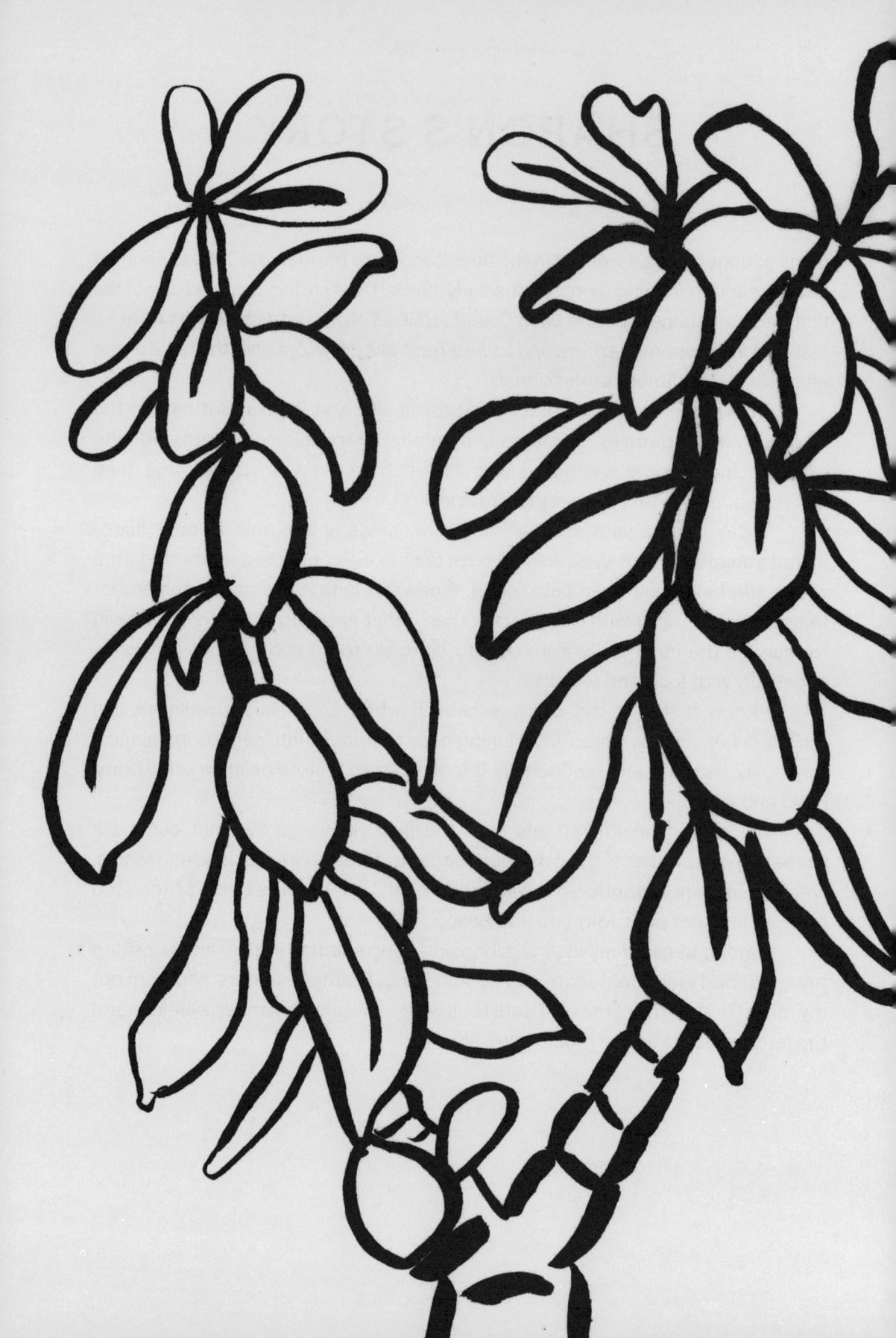

# 3. MASTERING WOMEN'S UNIQUE HEALTH CHALLENGES

Now we delve into the health challenges that commonly arise during different hormonal stages in a woman's life. From navigating endometriosis and PCOS to talking care of your female body parts.

This section addresses the key concerns many women face throughout life. We provide practical, evidence-based solutions designed to empower you to take control of your health with confidence.

Whether you're confronting a current concern or reflecting on past experiences, Part Three delivers guidance to inspire meaningful action, promote healing, and support your wellbeing for years to come.

**SPOTLIGHT ON:**

**PELVIC WELLNESS PAGE 501**
**YOUR CERVIX PAGE 511**
**UTERINE CARE PAGE 517**
**OVARIAN HEALTH PAGE 524**
**BLADDER SUPPORT PAGE 530**
**ENDOMETRIOSIS PAGE 534**
**PCOS PAGE 546**
**INSULIN RESISTANCE PAGE 564**
**BREAST CARE PAGE 569**
**LIVER CARE PAGE 592**
**THYROID PAGE 599**
**BONE CARE PAGE 612**
**BRAIN CARE PAGE 635**

## SPOTLIGHT ON
# Pelvic Wellness

### JOURNEY FROM YOUR VULVA TO VAGINA, UTERUS TO YOUR OVARIES

This chapter takes a journey through the incredible female reproductive system, from the vulva to the uterus and ovaries, to understand how to support its health. The vulva, vagina and cervix form a connected pathway, working together to support life and adapt to hormonal changes, especially during pregnancy.

Caring for your for pelvic organs is essential at every stage of life. From maintaining a healthy vaginal microbiome to meeting changing nutritional needs, preparing for these shifts helps ensure a smoother transition through life's hormonal phases.

### YOUR VULVA

The vulva, the outer lips of the vaginal entrance, acts as a guardian of the vagina. Throughout the hormonal transitions from puberty to the Age of Wisdom, your vulva may need special attention.

## CHECKLIST
## VULVAL CHANGES AND CHALLENGES
## THROUGH YOUR HORMONAL STAGES

**PUBERTY**
- Skin irritation from soaps, detergents, fabric softeners, or bath salts.
- Vaginitis: Inflammation caused by poor hygiene, irritants, or infections.
- Increased risk of STIs (sexually transmitted infections) as sexual activity begins.

**THE FERTILE YEARS**
- Greater risk of yeast infections due to hormonal changes, pregnancy, or antibiotics.
- STIs like HPV or genital herpes may appear on the inner lips of the vulva.
- Postpartum changes in vulval comfort due to trauma or scarring from childbirth.
- Changes in the vaginal microbiome, which may cause itching and irritation.

**PERIMENOPAUSE**
- Higher sensitivity to irritants and infections.
- Painful intercourse due to dryness and thinning tissues.

**MENOPAUSE**
- Thinning and drying of the vulval skin as oestrogen levels decrease.
- Lichen sclerosis: A chronic condition causing thin, white patches on the vulva.
- Irritation from urine leakage due to the loss of oestrogen support for the bladder and urethra (located near the clitoris).

**THE AGE OF WISDOM**
- Persistent dryness and thinning of vulval tissues.
- Greater vulnerability to irritation, infections, and UTIs.
- Worsening of chronic skin conditions, causing discomfort or scarring.

While these issues can arise due to hormonal changes, lifestyle factors, and ageing, they can be managed with understanding and care. By being proactive, you can avoid many of these challenges and maintain vulval health and overall wellbeing through every stage of life. A pre-emptive approach will make all the difference in staying comfortable and healthy.

## VAGINAL HEALTH

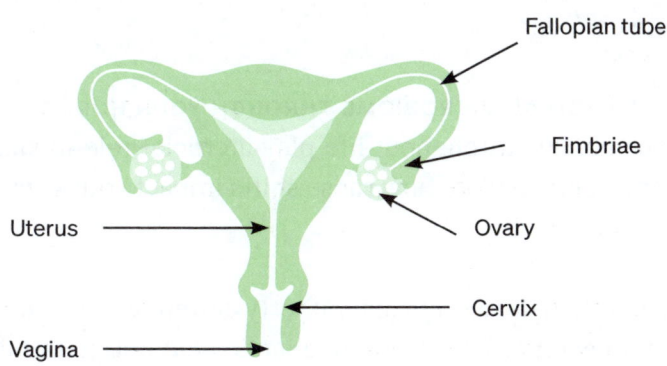

### YOUR VAGINAL MICROBIOME

The microscopic life in your vagina, known as the vaginal microbiome, works to maintain balance and protect your health. Often neglected, this diverse community of bacteria, viruses and fungi acts as a natural defence system, preventing infections like yeast infections and bacterial vaginosis while maintaining an ideal pH to support beneficial bacteria.

Hormonal fluctuations during puberty, menstruation, pregnancy, and menopause can disrupt this balance, making it vital to understand their impact on your microbiome.

Simple steps to support your microbiome:

- Eat a diet rich in probiotics and prebiotics.
- Avoid harsh soaps, douches and scented or dyed toilet paper.
- Avoid overcleaning—the inside area self-cleans. Simply wash the outside area with a small amount of mild pH-balanced soap and rinse well.
- Practicing safe sex to minimise risk of sexually transmitted infection.
- Consider strategies to support natural vaginal acidity.

### VAGINAL ODOUR: A SIGN YOUR MICROBIOME IS OUT OF BALANCE

Vaginal odour is a common concern caused by factors such as hormonal changes, infections and invasive practices such as douching. It's important to differentiate between normal variations in vaginal odour throughout your cycle and foul smells that may indicate an infection. Good hygiene practices, wearing breathable cotton underwear, and avoiding scented products can help manage odour. If the odour persists or is accompanied by other symptoms, consult your healthcare provider.

**THE VAGINAL MICROBIOME THROUGH YOUR HORMONAL JOURNEY**

Hormonal changes throughout life play a crucial role in shaping your vaginal microbiome. Let's explore how these shifts impact your vaginal health:

**PUBERTY**

Rising oestrogen levels during puberty stimulate the growth of beneficial lactobacilli bacteria, which produce lactic acid and maintain a healthy pH in the vagina.

This acidic environment prevents the overgrowth of harmful bacteria and yeast, reducing the risk of infections.

- Avoid using bubble baths, highly scented bath salts, or soaps, or female vaginal deodorant sprays as they can strip away beneficial bacteria and lead to infections like thrush or bacterial vaginosis.

**THE FERTILE YEARS**

Hormonal fluctuations during the menstrual cycle influence the vaginal microbiome.

In the follicular phase (before ovulation), rising oestrogen promotes lactobacilli growth and a healthy vaginal pH.

After ovulation, progesterone levels increase, temporarily reducing lactobacilli and slightly raising vaginal pH, which can create a more favourable environment for certain bacteria, increasing the risk of infections.

Increased vaginal discharge and irritation may occur just before menstruation and ease off after bleeding starts. Inserting a small amount of plain organic yoghurt can help rebalance the microbiome.

**PREGNANCY**

Elevated oestrogen levels during pregnancy promote the growth of lactobacilli, which help protect against infections. However, hormonal shifts can still make some women more prone to yeast infections or bacterial vaginosis.

To mitigate these risks, consider these safe daily practices:

- Wear breathable, cotton underwear to prevent moisture buildup.
- Avoid tight clothing that can create a warm, damp environment.
- Use gentle, fragrance-free cleansers and avoid douches or harsh soaps.
- Maintain a balanced diet rich in probiotics (like yoghurt) and prebiotics (like garlic or onions) to support healthy bacteria.
- Stay hydrated to help flush out toxins and maintain overall vaginal health.
- Consult your healthcare provider if you notice unusual symptoms, as early treatment is key.

**PERIMENOPAUSE**

As oestrogen levels decline, the vaginal tissue thins, glycogen production decreases, and the number of *lactobacillus* diminishes.

This can lead to fluctuating symptoms of dryness and make you more vulnerable to bacterial or yeast infections.

> **TIP**
> Applying organic coconut oil after showering can be a game changer, thanks to its hydrating and antibacterial properties.

**MENOPAUSE**

The sharp decline in oestrogen and progesterone levels during menopause alters the vaginal microbiome, resulting in fewer *lactobacillus* and a higher pH.

These changes can cause vaginal dryness, irritation, and a greater risk of infections.

Hormone Replacement Therapy (HRT) or low-dose bioidentical hormones used vaginally can help maintain a balanced vaginal microbiome and support overall vaginal health.

**THE AGE OF WISDOM**

After menopause, maintaining vaginal moisture becomes key. Before the decline in oestrogen, vaginal cells were like plump grapes; with reduced oestrogen, they become more like dried sultanas.

Hydration is essential, and options like vaginal oestrogen or organic coconut oil can help restore moisture (see page 180).

## WHEN YOUR MICROBIOME IS OUT OF BALANCE

### BACTERIAL VAGINOSIS (BV)

Bacterial vaginosis (BV) occurs when harmful anaerobic bacteria, like *Gardnerella vaginalis*, outnumber the beneficial lactobacilli. This imbalance often results in a thin, greyish-white discharge with a fishy odour, especially after sex. Other symptoms may include itching, burning during urination, and general irritation. If left untreated, BV can cause complications, especially during pregnancy, such as an increased risk of preterm labour or postpartum infections.

### STREP VAGINITIS

Group B Strep (*Streptococcus*) is a more serious vaginal infection that can pose risks to both the mother and baby during childbirth. It can infect newborns during delivery, leading to serious lung infections. Your healthcare provider will typically screen for Group B Strep during late pregnancy. Balancing your vaginal microbiome before pregnancy can help reduce the need for antibiotics at delivery.

### VAGINAL CANDIDA (THRUSH)

Thrush, caused by an overgrowth of yeast (*Candida*), can range from mild discomfort to severe irritation. Some women may experience mild symptoms, such as slight itching or a change in vaginal discharge, while others may suffer from unrelenting itching, burning and a cottage cheese-like discharge. Severe cases can extend to the vulva, causing red, inflamed skin that makes even contact with soft underwear unbearable. It's essential to manage thrush promptly to avoid these uncomfortable symptoms.

By understanding how your vaginal microbiome responds to hormonal changes and knowing the signs of imbalance, you can take steps to support your vaginal health throughout life. Whether through diet, lifestyle changes, or healthcare interventions, maintaining a balanced microbiome is key to long-term wellbeing.

## SUPPORTING YOUR MICROBIOME BY BALANCING VAGINAL PH

- **Apple cider vinegar (ACV)** Instead of applying ACV directly, add 1 to 2 cups of apple cider vinegar to a warm bath and soak for 10 to 20 minutes. Used once or twice a week, this gentle method can help maintain overall vaginal health.

- ***Lactobacillus* yoghurt for vaginal health**
  Plain, unsweetened yoghurt with live cultures of *Lactobacillus* can help maintain a healthy balance of bacteria in the vagina. Here's how to use it:
  Topical Application:
  - Wash your hands thoroughly.
  - Apply a small amount of yoghurt to the external vaginal area using a clean finger or applicator. You can also apply it internally with a clean applicator.
  - Leave it for 10 to 15 minutes, then rinse with warm water and gently pat dry.

  Yoghurt-soaked tampon:
  - Dip an unscented tampon into plain yoghurt with live cultures of *Lactobacillus*.
  - Insert the tampon and leave it in place for 1 to 2 hours (no longer).
  - Remove the tampon, rinse the vaginal area with warm water.
  - Limit yoghurt application to once or twice a week to avoid disrupting the natural balance. If irritation occurs, discontinue use and consult your healthcare provider.

### PROGESTERONE AND YOUR VAGINAL MICROBIOME

Progesterone has a complex relationship with your vaginal microbiome. During the luteal phase, progesterone increases glycogen production in vaginal cells, which acts as a prebiotic food for *Lactobacillus*, protecting against infections. However, prolonged high progesterone levels (for example, in pregnancy or from vaginal pessaries during IVF) can lead to less favourable *Lactobacillus* strains that lower vaginal acidity, promoting yeast infections like *Candida*.

Understanding these hormonal dynamics can help you manage changes in vaginal health during hormonal transitions. Good hygiene, a balanced diet, and discussing hormonal management with your healthcare provider are key steps to supporting a healthy vaginal microbiome.

WELLNESS ACTION PLAN

# VULVAL AND VAGINAL HEALTH

Your vaginal microbiome is an essential part of your reproductive health and overall wellbeing. Following the steps below to nurture this intricate ecosystem:

- **Stay hydrated:** Hydration is key. If you're dehydrated, your body prioritises vital organs like the brain, kidneys and heart over vaginal tissues, leaving them dry.

- **Avoid harsh products:** Protect your microbiome by avoiding harsh soaps, fragrances and chemical-laden laundry detergents.

- **Coconut oil for hydration:** Move your bottle of organic coconut oil from the kitchen to the bathroom. After showering, apply a little with your fingers around the vulva and as far inside as comfortable, then pat dry. Coconut oil has antibacterial, antifungal and acidic properties, making it a perfect partner for vaginal health.

- **Coconut oil for lubrication:** Coconut oil is also an excellent lubricant during sex, providing longer-lasting moisture compared to gel-based lubricants, and it's edible! This is a great option for women unable to use oestrogen due to medical reasons.

- **Vaginal oestrogen cream**: If more support is needed, your doctor can prescribe vaginal oestrogen cream, specifically estriol (E3, marketed as Ovestin in Australia, New Zealand and the UK), to support vaginal health.

> **DR KAREN'S TIP:**
>
> If you're using Ovestin cream, skip the annoying applicator! Instead, squeeze out about half a centimetre of cream directly onto your fingers after showering, two or three times a week.
>
> Apply the cream vaginally as far as you feel comfortable, then rub the remaining cream around the vulval area, including the urethra (the bladder opening near the clitoris), and sweep it down towards the areas involved during intercourse. This helps hydrate where you may experience dryness, both day-to-day and during sex. You can also use coconut oil alongside Ovestin for added hydration.

## ACTION PLAN TO ERADICATE THRUSH AND BACTERIAL VAGINOSIS

If you prefer to treat vaginal thrush or bacterial vaginosis without pharmaceuticals, follow these simple steps:

### STEP 1: BORIC ACID PESSARIES

Use 600 mg boric acid vaginal pessaries once daily for 7 to 14 days. These are available through compounding pharmacies. (Boric acid is also effective for eradicating *Strep* vaginitis, which can be problematic during late pregnancy.)

### STEP 2: RESTORE VAGINAL PH

After the pessaries, use Acigel (available over the counter at pharmacies) for 3 to 5 days to restore vaginal pH. Alternatively, you can opt for natural methods described below to rebalance your vaginal microbiome.

### DON'T FORGET YOUR PARTNER

If the infection is yeast-related (like thrush), ensure your partner is treated too. A 3-day application of antifungal cream can prevent reinfection and support healing.

By following all steps, you can support a healthy vaginal microbiome and prevent recurrence of the infection. Treating *Strep B* infection with this method, followed by microbiome care, may also help eradicate these harmful bacteria.

## FOR STUBBORN, HARD-TO-TREAT THRUSH AND BACTERIAL VAGINOSIS

If standard treatments haven't cleared the infection, especially when caused by factors like antibiotic use, try the following remedy:

**PRE-TREATMENT WITH PROGESTERONE**
Use a 3-day course of 100 mg progesterone vaginal troche once daily to help break down the protective biofilm of the yeast.

**FOLLOW THE ACTION PLAN**
Immediately follow with the boric acid and pH restoration steps outlined on the previous page.

SPOTLIGHT ON
# Your Cervix

Your cervix is the lower part of your uterus that extends into the upper end of your vagina, serving as the gateway between the two.

Before childbirth, it has the firm consistency of your nose. During labour, the cervix dilates with each contraction until it's wide enough for the baby to pass from the uterus, through the cervix, and into the vagina, where the baby's head 'crowns' at the vulva.

Regardless of whether you plan to have children, monitoring the health of your cervix is vital from your Fertile Years through to the Age of Wisdom. Routine cervical smear tests are an essential part of preventive healthcare for all women.

## CERVICAL CANCER RISK AND HPV

Research has identified certain strains of the human papilloma virus (HPV) as the leading cause of cervical cancer. HPV is a sexually transmitted wart infection, and the subtypes HPV 16 and 18 are particularly known for causing cancer. Other HPV subtypes may cause abnormal cervical smear results (CIN changes) but have an extremely low chance of developing into cervical cancer over a woman's lifetime (less than 0.02%).

HPV can be transmitted through various forms of sexual contact, not just intercourse. Even women who haven't had penetrative sex or still have an intact hymen can be at risk of HPV infection and should consider cervical screening.

## HOW IS A CERVICAL SMEAR TEST PERFORMED?

During a cervical smear examination, your healthcare provider collects a sample of cells from your cervix during a pelvic examination. A speculum is gently inserted into the vagina to access the cervix, and a small brush or spatula is used to gather cells for testing.

Results are sent to a lab, and your doctor will discuss the findings with you.

## THE CERVICAL SCREENING PROGRAM

The cervical screening program, replacing the well-known Pap smear, was introduced in Australia in 2017, followed by the UK in 2021 and later in New Zealand. This new method detects and monitors high-risk HPV subtypes, which will contribute to a further reduction in cervical cancer rates.

If your cervical smear test is negative and shows no evidence of infection with HPV subtypes 16 or 18, a repeat test every five years may be recommended. However, always follow your doctor's advice on how often to get tested, and report any unusual symptoms, regardless of the timing of your last smear.

If you're hesitant about having a cervical smear, ask your doctor about a self-collection kit. This simple, step-by-step process allows you to collect a sample in the privacy of your own home. However, if you've previously had an abnormal smear, consult your doctor about whether self-collection is suitable for you.

## THE HPV VACCINATION

The HPV vaccine, known as Gardasil 9 (or Cervarix in the UK), is recommended for 12- to 13-year-old girls and boys as part of the school vaccination program to prevent HPV infection. Discussing the risks and benefits with your family doctor is an essential step in making an informed decision about the vaccine.

For parents with children approaching this age, it's helpful to consider the following:

The HPV vaccination program was introduced in Australia in 2007, 16 years after cervical screening began. The statistics and outcomes in Australia, the UK and New Zealand are similar for comparison.

If we look at the statistics, we can see the following;

The greatest impact on reducing cervical cancer came from cervical screening (Pap smears),
- Before screening, in 1991, 14 to 15 women out of every 100,000 women developed cervical cancer.
- After screening (statistics gathered between 1991 to 2007), 9 to 10 women out of every 100,000 women developed cervical cancer, which is a significant drop!
- Statistics gathered after 2007 shows that with both screening and HPV vaccination, 7 to 8 women out of every 100,000 developed cervical cancer.

Many treatment interventions, while extremely well intentioned, also run the risk of side effects. After 17 years of use, the safety profile of this vaccination is favourably low. A 2020 *Lancet* study documented a small number of girls experiencing long-term fibromyalgia symptoms related to the vaccine (73 out of 1,000,000 girls vaccinated). When weighing up having the vaccination or not, consider:

- Some girls will be more sensitive to all treatment interventions than others.
- Some girls will be more sexually adventurous and hence at more risk of infection.

In areas where access to screening is limited or expensive, the HPV vaccination plays a significant role in reducing deaths from cervical cancer.

## WELLNESS ACTION PLAN
# CERVICAL HEALTH

Maintaining a healthy cervix starts with supporting your vaginal microbiome. A balanced, acidic vaginal environment helps prevent infections from bacteria, yeast, and viruses. As cervical cells are immersed in vaginal fluids, their health depends heavily on the balance of good bacteria.

### MINIMISE YOUR CHANCES OF EXPOSURE TO HPV INFECTION

In new relationships, it's important to avoid unprotected sex until both partners have been screened for sexually transmitted infections (STIs), including HPV, to protect yourself. This is the single most important thing you can do for the health of your cervix.

### ESSENTIAL NUTRIENTS FOR A HEALTHY CERVIX

Cervical health is essential for overall wellness, with key nutrients helping protect against infections and HPV-related changes. During recovery from abnormal smears, support any planned medical treatment with targeted nutrients, transitioning to food sources once results normalise. For long-term supplementation, monitor zinc and vitamin D levels and maintain a healthy zinc-copper balance with professional guidance.

### YOUR NUTRIENTS FOR CERVICAL HEALTH

#### SELENIUM
**Recommended dose**: 100 mcg daily

Just two organic Brazil nuts grown in selenium rich soils a day can provide your selenium needs. Backed by over 2000 studies, selenium offers proven anti-cancer benefits and is vital for cervical health and overall wellbeing.

This label corrects a misprint in dosage.

### TIP

Australian soils are low and often depleted in selenium. Source Brazil nuts grown in Brazil, Peru, Bolivia and the Amazon Basin for the highest concentration of selenium.

### ZINC

**Recommended dose**: 30 mg daily

Zinc supports immune function and helps prevent HPV infections. If supplementing, up to 60 mg daily may be recommended, but it's important to check your levels first. Include zinc-rich foods like oysters, nuts, and seeds in your diet, and monitor copper levels to maintain balance during long-term supplementation.

### VITAMIN C

**Recommended dose**: 1000 mg daily

Low vitamin C levels are associated with a tenfold increase in abnormal cervical smear results. This antioxidant plays a crucial role in cervical cell health.

### VITAMIN A

**Recommended dose:** 50,000 IU daily for 10 weeks (then maintain at 25,000 IU)

Studies show that low vitamin A levels increase the risk of cervical cancer. You can get your daily intake from orange vegetables like sweet potatoes and carrots—just 40 g of sweet potato and 20 g of shredded carrot provide all your daily needs.

### VITAMIN E

**Recommended dose**: 15 mg daily (20 mg for breastfeeding women)

This fat-soluble vitamin is essential for cell protection. A handful of sunflower seeds, pine nuts, hazelnuts or almonds in trail mix can meet your daily needs.

### VITAMIN D

**Recommended dose**: 5000 IU daily (adjust based on levels)

Start with 5000 IU until your levels reach 100 mmol/L. Maintain between 100 to 150 mmol/L and check your levels after 4 months of supplementation.

### FOLINIC ACID (VITAMIN B9)

**Recommended dose:** 0.5 mg daily

The active form of folic acid (folinic acid or MTH-folate) supports healthy cell renewal and reduces the risk of cervical cancer. Folate deficiency is linked to multiple cancers, including cervical cancer.

### RIBOFLAVIN (VITAMIN B2)

**Recommended dose:** Riboflavin is essential for hormone regulation and cell health. Nutritional yeast is a great source, with 17 mg per 100 g. Add a teaspoon to your morning smoothie or mix it into sauces for a nutritional boost.

### ANTIOXIDANT SUPPORT FOR YOUR CERVIX

You'll find antioxidant-rich foods listed on page 393 in Spotlight on Nourishment. To further boost your body's natural antioxidant defences (your internal 'housekeepers'), you can also consider using a SOD Inducer supplement. One option available online is Cell Logic Clinic Essentials GliSODin BioActive.

**Recommended dose:** 1 capsule, twice daily.

### SULFORAPHANE: A POWERFUL NUTRIENT

Sulforaphane, a powerful compound in broccoli, is backed by over 40 studies for its cancer-fighting properties, particularly against hormone-related cancers, making it a valuable addition to your wellness routine.

You can find sulforaphane online in products like Cell Logic EnduraCell BioActive.

**Recommended dose:** 1 capsule, twice daily.

Sulforaphane not only supports cancer prevention but also enhances the effectiveness of vitamin D by opening cell receptor sites, helping your body absorb this vital nutrient more efficiently.

For nutrient-rich food ideas, see our Spotlight on Nourishment on page 393. Supporting your microbiome with food sources of probiotics and prebiotics is equally important, as a healthy vaginal microbiome protects against infections and promotes overall vaginal health.

Regular check-ups with your healthcare provider or women's health nurse are key for early detection and effective management of any concerns.

By adopting these practices, you can maintain vulval, vaginal and cervical health, allowing you to thrive well into the Age of Wisdom.

## SPOTLIGHT ON
# Uterine Care

Caring for your uterus is essential to maintaining overall reproductive health. Let's look at the effect of oestrogen dominance on your uterus, fibroids and adenomyosis. Our Wellness Action Plan provides practical steps to help you nurture a healthy uterus.

### UTERUS

This remarkable organ is centre stage through your hormonal journey. The uterus, often called the 'cradle of life', provides the nurturing environment for a developing baby, Just like any other part of your body, your uterus deserves attention and care to ensure it function optimally. Understanding the importance of uterine and ovarian health and incorporating practices that support them can promote a balanced hormonal environment, enhance fertility, and improve overall wellbeing.

### THE UTERUS—A CASUALTY OF OESTROGEN DOMINANCE

While a marvel of biological engineering, the uterus can be particularly vulnerable to hormonal imbalances, especially oestrogen dominance. Although oestrogen, is crucial for the normal functioning of the uterus, when levels are too high relative to progesterone, it can lead to a variety of health issues. This hormonal imbalance can cause the uterine lining to grow excessively, leading to conditions such as fibroids and adenomyosis, which can significantly impact a woman's quality of life. This extra oestrogen messaging can come from endocrine disruptors too. (Review pages 405 and 478 for more on this.)

### FIBROIDS

Fibroids are non-cancerous growths that develop within the muscular walls of the uterus. They can vary in size and number, from tiny seedlings undetectable to the human eye to large masses that can distort and enlarge the uterus and can grow as large as a football. Women with fibroids may experience heavy menstrual bleeding, prolonged periods, pelvic pain, frequent urination, and even complications during pregnancy and labour. The exact cause of fibroids is unknown but their growth is linked to oestrogen dominance.

## ADENOMYOSIS

This condition occurs when the inner lining of the uterus, known as the endometrium, breaks through the muscular wall of the uterus. Adenomyosis can cause the uterus to become enlarged and tender, leading to severe menstrual cramps, heavy or prolonged menstrual bleeding, and chronic pelvic pain. The root cause of adenomyosis is not fully understood, but it is similar to endometriosis in that the uterine lining has worked its way from the inside of the uterus to its muscular wall, somewhere that it should not be growing! Oestrogen dominance is believed to play a significant role.

This condition often affects women in their 30s and 40s and can be particularly challenging to diagnose if the growths are tiny. Larger areas are usually detected on a pelvic ultrasound.

By the time women realise they have a problem, adenomyosis is already firmly established and will continue to create menstrual havoc.

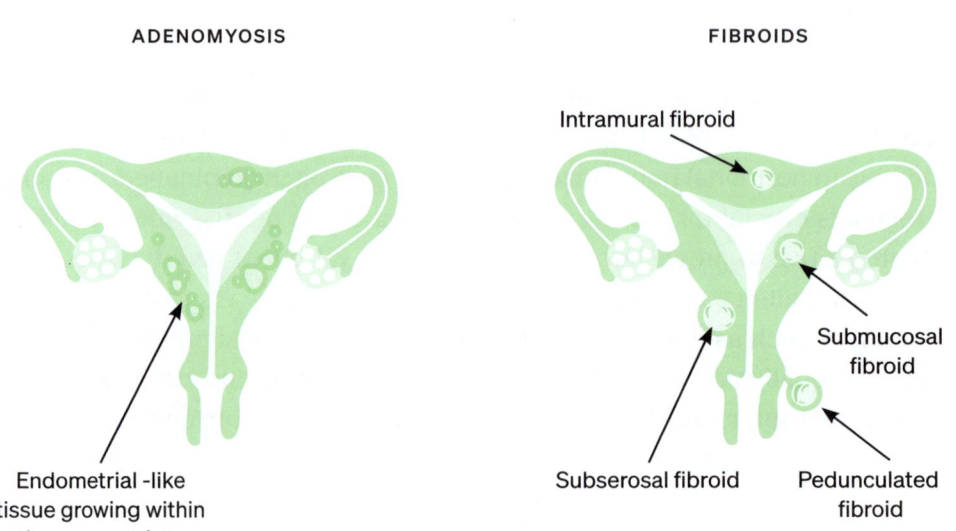

## DOES ADENOMYOSIS RUN IN FAMILIES?

While definitive genetic links have not been firmly established, having a family history of adenomyosis or related conditions, such as endometriosis or fibroids, may increase the likelihood of developing the condition.

Other factors, such as oestrogen dominance, immune system disorders, and prior uterine surgery, such as a past caesarean section, can also contribute to the risk of adenomyosis.

## SYMPTOMS OF FIBROIDS AND ADENOMYOSIS

There are a lot of symptoms that these two distinct conditions have in common, making it difficult for doctors to tell the difference. Both have the following symptoms in common:

- Heavy or prolonged periods leading to iron deficiency, anaemia and severe fatigue.
- Painful periods with pain that may worsen over time.
- Persistent dull pelvic pain: throughout the menstrual month.
- Pain during intercourse caused by uterine tenderness and inflammation.
- Enlarged uterus making the uterus feel tender or bloated.
- Abdominal pressure in the lower abdomen.
- Passing large blood clots during menstruation.
- Irregular menstrual cycles: with periods occurring more often or last longer than usual.

Large fibroids can also give your further challenges to add to this list and may include:

- Frequent urination: Pressure from large fibroids pressing against the bladder.
- Difficulty emptying the bladder: The pressure from fibroids can also make it difficult to completely empty the bladder.
- Constipation: Fibroids can press against the rectum, leading to constipation and bowel discomfort.
- Back or leg pain: If fibroids press on nerves, they can cause pain that radiates to the back or legs.

These symptoms can deeply affect your quality of life, making daily activities and relationships more difficult. It's important to consult a healthcare provider for an accurate diagnosis and appropriate treatment.

Treatment options depend on whether you are planning a pregnancy and may include hormonal therapies, pain relief, or, in severe cases, surgery.

For those planning a pregnancy, fibroids can pose additional challenges. Doctors often recommend a fibroidectomy to remove the fibroid while preserving healthy uterine muscle. However, in cases of adenomyosis, where abnormal tissue is spread throughout the uterine body, surgical options are more limited.

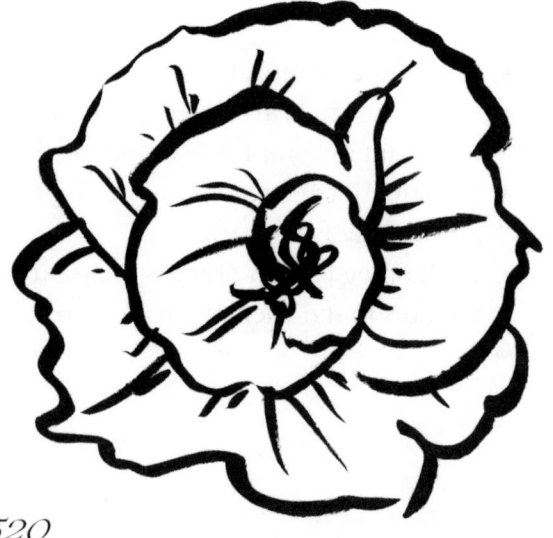

## WELLNESS ACTION PLAN
# HEALTHY UTERUS

Taking charge of your uterine health is an empowering step toward overall wellbeing. This Wellness Action Plan aims to prevent conditions like adenomyosis and fibroids while addressing oestrogen dominance, a common hormonal imbalance that impacts reproductive health. This plan promotes natural, proactive steps to balance hormones, reduce inflammation and maintain a healthy reproductive system, helping you feel your best inside and out.

### NUTRITION FOR A HEALTHY UTERUS

- **Focus on phytoestrogen-rich foods:** These support hormonal balance. (See page 404 for our Phytoestrogen Food list in Core Food Principle Number 1.)

- **Include plenty of fibre-rich options:** Beans, lentils and leafy greens bind excess oestrogen and support its elimination from the body. These foods also nourish your oestrobolome, the gut bacteria essential for oestrogen balance (learn more about the oestrobolome on page 424).

- **Include healthy fats:** Incorporate omega-3 fatty acids found in fish, flaxseeds, chia seeds and walnuts. These anti-inflammatory fats can help balance hormone levels.

- **Limit red meat and processed foods:** Reducing consumption of red meat and processed foods can decrease inflammation and lower oestrogen levels.

## LIFESTYLE CHANGES FOR A HEALTHY UTERUS

- **Reduce exposure to toxins:** Avoiding xenoestrogens found in plastics, pesticides, and personal care products is an essential investment in uterine and hormonal health. (See our Spotlight on Managing Toxins on page 478.)

- **Incorporate regular exercise:** Aim for at least 30 minutes of moderate exercise most days of the week. Exercise helps regulate weight, reduce stress and balance hormones.

- **Practise stress-reducing activities:** Chronic stress dominos into hormonal imbalances. (See Spotlight on Restorative Practices on page 372.)

- **Maintain a healthy body weight:** This can help reduce the risk of oestrogen dominance, as excess body fat can increase oestrogen production.

- **Support your liver detox pathways:** Herbs like St Mary's Thistle can help the liver metabolise and detoxify excess oestrogen. (See our Spotlight on Liver Care on page 592 for more details.)

- **Use Chaste Tree (*Vitex agnus-castus*):** This herb can help balance progesterone levels, countering the effects of oestrogen dominance.

- **Include Diindolylmethane (DIM) vegetables:** Along with sulforaphane, DIM is another phytochemical in cruciferous vegetables like broccoli and cabbage, DIM helps balance oestrogen levels.

- **Increase turmeric in your diet:** With its anti-inflammatory properties, turmeric can help reduce inflammation and support hormonal balance.

### MAKE A DATE!

Regular check-ups with your health practitioner are important. Annual check-ups can help detect any early signs of uterine health issues. Discuss any changes to the way your pelvis feels, or the pattern of your period cycle. Your menstrual cycle is a key indicator of the overall wellbeing of your uterus and your hormones. Don't ignore early signs and symptoms that could tell you things are out of balance.

### DETECT OESTROGEN DOMINANCE EARLY

If any hormonal changes start to impact the way you feel or the pattern to your period cycle check with your health practitioner. Testing for oestrogen and progesterone balance can give you an early confirmation of hormonal imbalance and give you a head start on preventing these hormonal hurdles. We cover the steps for managing oestrogen dominance from page 137 onwards.

If you are already troubled by fibroids or adenomyosis we recommend sourcing an experienced naturopath as a part of your health team to keep uterine and hormonal health at optimal levels.

From regular check-ups and mindful nutrition to stress management and exercise, taking proactive steps can make a world of difference in your reproductive health journey.

# SPOTLIGHT ON
# Ovarian Health

Maintaining healthy ovaries depends largely on supporting antioxidant pathways. Research highlights that reducing oxidative stress on ovarian cells and eggs is crucial for sustaining ovarian health throughout life.

## YOUR OVARIES IN ACTION

Your ovaries are more than tiny organs in your pelvis—they are dynamic hormonal powerhouses driving much of what makes you, you. From your first period to menopause, they lead in producing oestrogen and progesterone, orchestrating your menstrual cycle, reproductive health, mood, energy, and bone strength. They also produce small amounts of androgens, often-overlooked hormones essential for libido, muscle tone, and vitality. Think of your ovaries as conductors of a symphony, coordinating a delicate hormonal balance that influences every system in your body. Their work may be invisible, yet their effects are profound.

## OXIDATIVE STRESS AND YOUR OVARIES

Along with your breasts, your ovaries are highly vulnerable to the inflammatory effects of cellular Inflammation caused by oxidative stress. It can impact ovarian tissue and egg health in your 30s, ageing your eggs prematurely and contributing to faltering fertility and an earlier menopause. Taking steps to reduce oxidative stress may also serve as an insurance policy against unhealthy ovarian changes that could contribute to ovarian cancer. (See Spotlight on Oxidative Stress on page 273.)

## OVARIAN HEALTH AND CHALLENGES AT EACH HORMONAL STAGE

### PUBERTY

Puberty marks the ovaries' debut, as they begin producing oestrogen and progesterone to kickstart the menstrual cycle. As the ovaries adjust, irregular cycles and functional ovarian cysts may appear but are usually harmless.

### THE FERTILE YEARS

Here your ovaries are at their peak, releasing eggs and maintaining hormonal balance for fertility, vitality, and overall health. They regulate cycles and support energy, libido, and bone health. Challenges like PCOS or functional ovarian cysts can arise, but the ovaries remain resilient and adaptive. This is the time to be mindful of preventive ovarian health care—see Spotlight on Oxidative Stress page 273—your ovaries will thank you!

### PERIMENOPAUSE

As your ovaries begin their retirement, hormone production becoming erratic. This phase often brings irregular periods, and the possibility of simple ovarian cysts. While most are benign, and resolve without treatment, monitoring is important.

### MENOPAUSE

During menopause, the ovaries complete their retirement and the responsibility for hormonal support shifts to the adrenal glands. This marks a quiet time for your ovaries.

### THE AGE OF WISDOM

No longer under the ebb and flow of fertility hormones, the ovaries settle into a quiet retirement. However, for women with a silent background of oxidative stress, the risk of ovarian cancer may be higher, emphasising the need for regular check-ups, especially if you have a history of endometriosis, or family history of breast or ovarian cancer.

## OVARIAN CYSTS

Ovarian cysts are fluid-filled sacs that form on or within the ovaries, and they're surprisingly common. Most cysts are functional, meaning they develop as part of the normal menstrual cycle and typically resolve on their own without causing harm. However, some cysts, such as dermoid cysts, endometriomas, or cystadenomas, can persist and grow, occasionally leading to pain, bloating, or pressure. While most cysts are benign, complex or persistent cysts may require further evaluation to rule out malignancy, and some require surgical removal. Regular check-ups and ultrasounds are key tools in distinguishing between benign cysts and those that may require intervention—be guided by your doctor on the best management plan. To prevent recurrence after medical treatment, turn to our Wellness Action Plan for Ovarian health on page 527 for solutions.

## OVARIAN CANCER

Ovarian cancer is one of the top five causes of cancer deaths in high-income countries. Screening options remain limited, and most diagnoses occur after the cancer has spread beyond the ovaries and fallopian tubes.

While the relationship between hormones and ovarian health is complex, ovarian cancer is not typically considered oestrogen-dependent, unlike some breast cancers. Factors like genetics (for example, BRCA1 and BRCA2 mutations), family history, and reproductive history play more established roles in ovarian cancer risk.

### NEW OVARIAN CANCER TESTING AND SCREENING

In November 2024 Australian scientists announced the development of a promising blood test for improving the early detection of ovarian cancer, aimed at dramatically increasing survival rates for ovarian cancer.

Researchers at the Hudson Institute of Medical Research have identified a novel biomarker, CXCL10, which is produced early and at high levels by ovarian cancers but not in non-malignant disease. This discovery has led to a new blood test, now commercialised by Cleo Diagnostics, to improve ovarian cancer diagnosis and reduce unnecessary surgeries.

Additionally, researchers from the University of Queensland, led by Professor Carlos Salomon, are working on developing an early detection test for ovarian cancer. Their goal is to improve the five-year survival rate from 25% to over 90% when the cancer is detected early.

These developments represent a significant step forward in the fight against ovarian cancer, offering hope for earlier detection and better outcomes for women worldwide.

Meanwhile, until these tests become easily available if you are concerned about future ovarian cancer risk due to family history or endometriosis, testing for the tumour marker Cancer Antigen 125 (CA-125) may be helpful. While not always covered by Medicare, this test can serve as a useful baseline for tracking potential pelvic symptoms in the future.

## WELLNESS ACTION PLAN
# OVARIAN HEALTH

This holistic wellness plan focuses on managing oxidative stress and promoting overall ovarian health.

### REDUCE OXIDATIVE STRESS

This is the single most important thing to action for ovarian health. Refer to our Spotlight on Oxidative Stress (page 273) and apply the strategies listed to protect your breast and ovarian cells.

### REGULATE PSYCHOLOGICAL STRESS

Chronic stress can disrupt hormone production. Practise mindfulness, meditation, or yoga to keep stress hormones in check (see Spotlight on Restorative Practices on page 372).

### BALANCE HORMONES

Read through the information in Part One, relevant to your hormonal stage. Apply the Core Food Principles of Part Two to minimise the hormonal imbalances that contribute to ovarian cyst formation.

Embrace phytoestrogen-rich foods like flaxseeds. (See Core Food Principle Number 1 on page 404 for the full list.)

### AVOID ENDOCRINE DISRUPTORS

See our Wellness Action Plan to Reduce Your Exposure to All EDCs on page 483.

### HYDRATION AND HERBAL TEAS

Stay hydrated and consider herbal teas like spearmint, which can help balance hormones.

### ANTI-INFLAMMATORY DIET

See Core Food Principle Number 1 on page 399.

### SUPPORT ANTIOXIDANT PATHWAYS

- Boost antioxidant intake with foods rich in vitamins C, E, and selenium (for example, citrus fruits, nuts, seeds, spinach).

- Consider supplements like N-acetylcysteine (NAC), which may help reduce cyst formation and improve ovarian health.

### MAINTAIN BLOOD SUGAR BALANCE

- Avoid high-sugar and refined carb diets to support insulin sensitivity because insulin resistance is linked to ovarian cysts.

- Include high-fibre foods, lean proteins and healthy fats in meals to stabilise blood sugar levels.

### SUPPORT LIVER DETOXIFICATION

- The liver processes excess hormones, so keep it healthy by eating cruciferous vegetables (broccoli, kale, cauliflower) and avoiding alcohol or excessive toxins.

- Avoid caffeine and alcohol, which may exacerbate cyst-related symptoms.

### REGULAR PHYSICAL ACTIVITY

Exercise regularly to improve insulin sensitivity, reduce stress, and maintain hormonal balance. Aim for a mix of aerobic and strength-training activities.

### HERBAL SUPPORT

**Chaste Tree (*Vitex agnus-castus*)** supports hormonal balance and regulates menstrual cycles. Prescribed dose: 1000 mg taken on rising each morning.

**Withania (ashwagandha)** is an adaptogen that helps manage stress and supports hormonal health. Prescribed dose: Between 300 to 500 mg of a standardised extract, best used under guidance from your health practitioner.

## MEDICAL GUIDANCE FOR OVARIAN CYSTS

For recurring or problematic cysts, work with your healthcare provider to assess hormonal imbalances or other underlying conditions, such as PCOS or endometriosis.

Discuss the possibility of medications or treatments, such as hormonal contraceptives, if needed.

## MONITOR SYMPTOMS

Track menstrual cycles and symptoms, and consult your healthcare provider if you experience irregular periods, severe pain or unusual symptoms. By combining dietary, lifestyle, and medical strategies, you can proactively reduce the risk of ovarian cysts, support overall reproductive health, and protect your ovaries as you move through your hormonal stages.

SPOTLIGHT ON
# Bladder Support

Picture this: you're enjoying a lovely afternoon out with friends when suddenly, you feel that dreaded urge. You know the one—the need to find a bathroom fast. If this sounds familiar, you're not alone. As women journey from pregnancy to menopause and beyond, changes in bladder control can sneak up on even the most prepared among us. But don't worry—this chapter is here to help you reclaim control and put those worries to rest.

## YOUR BLADDER THROUGH YOUR HORMONAL JOURNEY

### PUBERTY AND YOUR BLADDER

During puberty, the sensitive vaginal and urethral areas are especially vulnerable to irritation. Avoid bubble baths, harsh soaps, and heavily fragranced products, as these can disrupt the natural pH balance and lead to bladder symptoms like burning or frequency. Instead, use gentle, fragrance-free cleansers and warm water to maintain hygiene and prevent discomfort.

### YOUR BLADDER DURING THE FERTILE YEARS

During the Fertile Years, bladder health can be impacted by lifestyle habits and physical changes. Irritation of the urethra during sex, consuming bladder irritants like alcohol and caffeine, and delaying trips to the bathroom due to a busy schedule can all contribute to bladder symptoms like burning or urgency. Low water intake can also lead to concentrated, acidic urine that irritates the bladder lining. Staying hydrated, urinating after sex, and limiting irritants can help maintain a healthy bladder during this stage of life.

### POSTPARTUM BLADDER CHANGES

After childbirth, many new mums notice changes in bladder control due to pregnancy and delivery stretching the pelvic floor muscles. You might experience leaks when you laugh, cough or exercise—this is known as 'stress incontinence'. It's a common postpartum issue but there are effective ways to manage it. These include activities such as Pilates that focus on pelvic floor and core strength. (See our Healthy Bladder Wellness Action Plan on page 532 for more strategies.)

### MENOPAUSE AND BLADDER CONTROL

Menopause brings significant changes, including shifts in bladder health. Lower oestrogen levels weaken pelvic floor muscles and reduce tissue hydration, making pelvic tissues more like sultanas than plump grapes. This can lead to stress incontinence, causing leaks during sneezing, laughing or exercise, and 'urge incontinence' with sudden, strong urges to urinate.

The good news? Many strategies and treatments can help.

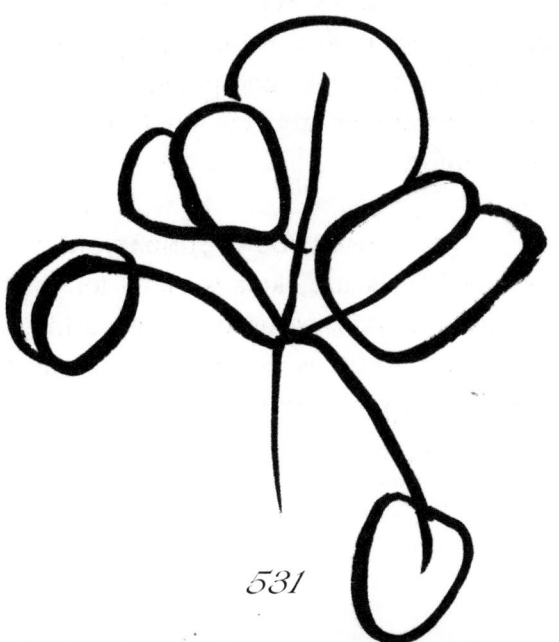

## WELLNESS ACTION PLAN
# HEALTHY BLADDER

### HYDRATION: DRINK SMART, NOT LESS

Drinking enough water is crucial, even when managing bladder control. Dehydration can irritate the bladder and cause more frequent urges. Aim for 6 to 8 glasses of filtered water daily, sipping throughout the day to stay hydrated without overwhelming your bladder.

### CUT CAFFEINE, ALCOHOL AND OTHER BLADDER IRRITANTS

To reduce bladder irritation, cut back on caffeine, alcohol and carbonated drinks. These can worsen incontinence by stimulating your bladder. Swap that second cup of coffee or fizzy drink for water or herbal tea, and your bladder will thank you.

### URINARY ALKALINISERS

Urinary alkalinisers can help reduce urine acidity, which may ease bladder irritation. Foods like bananas, melons and potatoes are naturally alkaline and can be soothing. Over-the-counter products like Ural are also available to help relieve burning or discomfort.

### STRENGTHEN YOUR FOUNDATION

Pelvic floor exercises, or Kegels, are like a workout for your bladder's support system. Simply contract the muscles used to stop urination, hold for a few seconds, then relax. Repeat 10 times, several times a day. If you're unsure of your technique, a pelvic floor physical therapist can provide guidance and use biofeedback to help you stay on track.

### TOPICAL VAGINAL OESTROGENS

Reduced oestrogen during menopause weakens pelvic muscles and tissues. Topical vaginal oestrogen creams, rings, or tablets can help rejuvenate these tissues, improving bladder control. Consult your healthcare provider to see if this treatment is right for you.

### CONSIDER VAGINAL PESSARIES

These are small, removable devices inserted into the vagina to support the bladder and other pelvic organs. They are commonly used to manage stress incontinence or pelvic organ prolapse, providing immediate relief by reducing pressure on the bladder. Pessaries come in various shapes and sizes and can be fitted by a healthcare provider to ensure comfort and effectiveness.

### SURGICAL OPTIONS

If lifestyle changes and non-invasive treatments aren't enough, surgical options are available. These range from minimally invasive procedures like urethral bulking agents to sling procedures, which provide extra support to the bladder and urethra. Surgery is typically considered when other treatments haven't worked, especially if there's significant pelvic support loss, such as a prolapse.

### THE WAVE BRILLIANCE CHAIR

The Wave Brilliance Chair offers a non-invasive, innovative solution for incontinence. Using electromagnetic waves, it strengthens pelvic floor muscles effortlessly, simulating thousands of Kegel exercises in just one session.

Each 30-minute session requires no downtime, allowing you to resume daily activities immediately. Many women notice improvements after a few sessions, with up to 80% experiencing lasting benefits after completing the treatment. Safe and effective, Wave Brilliance requires a referral from your doctor to access.

Every woman's experience with bladder control over all hormonal stages is unique. What works for one person may not be as effective for another. The key is to stay informed, explore your options and work closely with your healthcare team to find what's best for you.

And most importantly, don't lose heart. With the right approach, you can take control of your bladder health and continue enjoying life to the fullest.

So, let's raise a glass (of water, of course) to better bladder control and a confident, empowered you!

# SPOTLIGHT ON
# Endometriosis

### THE SILENT THIEF OF FERTILITY

Endometriosis has recently become a prominent topic thanks to the advocacy of women's health groups. Progress is happening, and while medical research and advancements may be slow, there are strategies available to help manage this challenging condition.

### WHAT IS ENDOMETRIOSIS?

The uterus is lined with a layer of cells called the endometrium, which is shed each month during menstruation, or as a withdrawal bleed if you are on the Pill. Endometriosis occurs when cells from the uterine lining (endometrium) grow outside the uterus, often within the pelvic cavity. Like the healthy cells lining your uterus, these rogue cells respond to hormonal changes and shed tissue and blood during menstruation. However, with no way to exit, this triggers inflammation each cycle, irritating nearby organs like the bladder, bowel, ovaries, and fallopian tubes.

Over time, this persistent inflammation can lead to adhesions, pain, and the wide range of symptoms associated with endometriosis.

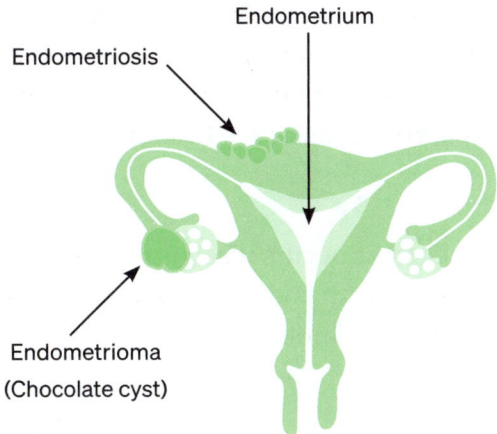

### SYMPTOMS OF ENDOMETRIOSIS

While some women remain symptom-free in the early stages, once endometriosis takes hold in the pelvis, it rarely stays silent. Period pain, which doesn't respond to simple painkillers, and other symptoms can severely impact daily life. Symptoms may include:

- Period pain unresponsive to regular painkillers
- Mid-cycle pelvic pain
- Pain during bowel movements
- Pain during sex
- Blood in urine or stool, particularly around menstruation.

Turn to page 539 for our Endometriosis Audit if you suspect you may have endometriosis.

### WHY IT HAPPENS

Endometriosis begins with your genes, influenced by hormonal imbalances, inflammatory diets, and your body's ability to manage oxidative stress. Let's break down the key contributors:

- Genetic link: Endometriosis often runs in families, but lifestyle and targeted therapies can alter gene expression and reduce risk. By understanding the epigenetic factors, you can influence how these gene variants express themselves. (see Spotlight on Epigenetics page 269.)

- Inflammation: Chronic pelvic inflammation is the primary driver of pain in endometriosis. It occurs without the typical triggers of tissue damage but inherited inflammatory gene variations can worsen symptoms. Genetic testing can help tailor treatment plans. (See Resources for gene testing options on page 691.)

- Oxidative stress: Oxidative stress occurs when free radicals damage cells, causing inflammation. Women with endometriosis often have higher oxidative stress, which worsens symptoms. (See Spotlight on Oxidative Stress on page 273.)

- Immune system dysfunction: In endometriosis, the immune system may fail to recognise the abnormal endometrial cells in the pelvic cavity. When the immune system eventually reacts, it may attack these cells, intensifying inflammation and pain.

- Hormonal imbalance: Oestrogen fuels endometriosis. These cells rely on oestrogen, and, to complicate matters, they can produce their own supply of oestrogen exacerbating the inflammation.

- Environmental toxins: Chemicals like BPA, parabens, phthalates and dioxins disrupt hormones and the immune system, increasing the risk of endometriosis. Found in common products like skincare, detergents, and plastics, these toxins are linked to the disease. (See Spotlight on Managing Toxins on page 478.)

> **TIP**
>
> Don't expect legislation to keep pace with research! Benzophenone, a common UV filter in sunscreens and skincare products, was first linked to endometriosis in 2012. Despite numerous studies confirming its harmful effects, it remains in use in Australia, New Zealand, and the UK. Environmental lobbyists have successfully banned it in coastal states of the USA and Pacific Islands due to its impact on marine ecosystems, yet it's still prevalent in personal care products elsewhere. Until more is done, avoid products containing this toxic ingredient.

## WHAT DRIVES THE DISEASE

Endometriosis begins with your genes, influenced by hormonal imbalances, inflammatory diets, and your body's ability to manage oxidative stress. Let's break down the key contributors:

- Immune system dysfunction: In endometriosis, the immune system may fail to recognise the abnormal endometrial cells in the pelvic cavity. When the immune system eventually reacts, it may attack these cells, intensifying inflammation and pain.

- Hormonal imbalance: Oestrogen fuels endometriosis. These cells rely on oestrogen, and, to complicate matters, they can produce their own supply, exacerbating the inflammation.

> **RETROGRADE MENSTRUATION**
>
> One theory suggests that menstrual blood flows backward into the pelvic cavity, seeding endometrial cells. Another theory points to embryonic cells that failed to migrate properly during foetal development. While logical, these theories don't change the approach to treatment or prevention.

## COMPLICATIONS OF ENDOMETRIOSIS

Severe pain that can persist beyond menstruation and severely disrupt daily life. Complications like 'chocolate cysts', made of congealed blood and fibrous tissue, causing bloating and pain. Over 30% of women with endometriosis experience infertility due to blocked fallopian tubes. While pregnancy often brings symptom relief, endometriosis can return postpartum. Menopause also halts symptoms as hormonal cycles stop.

## NEW RESEARCH: PROGESTERONE RECEPTOR RESISTANCE

Progesterone is a natural moderator of oestrogen, making it a potential treatment for endometriosis. However, endometriotic cells can become resistant to progesterone by reducing the sensitivity of their receptors. This forces doctors to use higher doses of synthetic progestins after surgery to prevent regrowth, as bioidentical progesterone is often too gentle to be effective. Progestins, though strong, can halt menstrual cycles, making them unsuitable for women trying to conceive. In these cases, bioidentical progesterone may help regulate the cycle and support conception. Interestingly, pregnancy can often switch off endometriosis entirely.

> **MISTAKEN IDENTITY**
>
> Endometriosis is sometimes diagnosed coincidentally during procedures for unrelated medical issues. It can mimic other conditions like spinal disc disease or cause symptoms like bowel bleeding, leading to misdiagnoses and delays in treatment. The frustration of waiting for the wrong specialist while managing pain and discomfort is common for women with undiagnosed endometriosis.

## DIAGNOSIS AND MEDICAL TREATMENT

A revolutionary new blood test, PromarkerEndo, is poised to transform how endometriosis is diagnosed. Developed in Australia by Proteomics International in collaboration with the Royal Women's Hospital and the University of Melbourne, this non-invasive test detects a unique set of 10 protein biomarkers—essentially a biological fingerprint for endometriosis. In clinical studies involving more than 800 women, PromarkerEndo achieved over 85% accuracy in detecting early-stage disease and 99.7% accuracy in severe cases. This breakthrough could drastically reduce diagnostic delays and the need for surgery.

Currently, laparoscopy under general anaesthetic remains the gold standard for both diagnosing and treating endometriosis, allowing doctors to confirm the presence of the disease and remove abnormal tissue at the same time. However, diagnosis is often delayed—sometimes for years—due to long public hospital waitlists and a widespread tendency among GPs to mislabel symptoms as ·just period pain.

When validated for routine use, PromarkerEndo offers new hope for earlier diagnosis, faster access to treatment, and a significant shift in how this often-misunderstood condition is managed.

> **TIP**
>
> Be aware of long-term risks—women treated for endometriosis during their reproductive years have up to a 90% increased risk of ovarian cancer post-menopause. (See Ovarian Health on page 524 for more information.)

### MAINSTREAM TREATMENT OPTIONS

Conventional treatments include the oral contraceptive pill (the Pill), hormonal drugs like danazol, and progestins in various forms (tablets, injections or intrauterine devices). While effective for many, these options come with risks and side effects that must be weighed against the benefits.

Sadly, many women experience symptom recurrence months or years after treatment, with some facing infertility issues due to fallopian tube blockages.

> **TIP**
> True wellness and a life free of endometriosis means putting in the hard work to address all the factors that feed the disease.

> **BE PROACTIVE ABOUT HEART HEALTH**
> The inflammatory pathways and genetic variations seen in women with endometriosis closely mirror those affecting coronary arteries. Bottom line—A diagnosis of endometriosis during your Fertile Years increases cardiovascular risk from menopause onwards. Knowing this gives you a heads up to take care of yourself, improve your nutrition, decrease your stress with meditative practices and exercise wisely.

### USE THE WAITING TIME WISELY

There's often a delay between suspecting endometriosis and confirming the diagnosis through laparoscopy. Use this waiting period to start your Wellness Action Plan, outlined in the next chapter. This plan focuses on addressing all factors contributing to your endometriosis, following a logical sequence to tackle reversible drivers. This approach will not only prepare your body for any planned surgery but also reduce the inflammation behind your symptoms.

### ENDOMETRIOSIS AUDIT

The symptom checklist on the following page can help you assess whether you're experiencing common signs of the condition. Simply tick the boxes that apply to you and share it with your healthcare provider to facilitate an open conversation about your symptoms and next steps. Clues to the presence of endometriosis can be classed in three separate categories:

1. Pelvic pain
2. Your periods
3. Fertility roadblocks

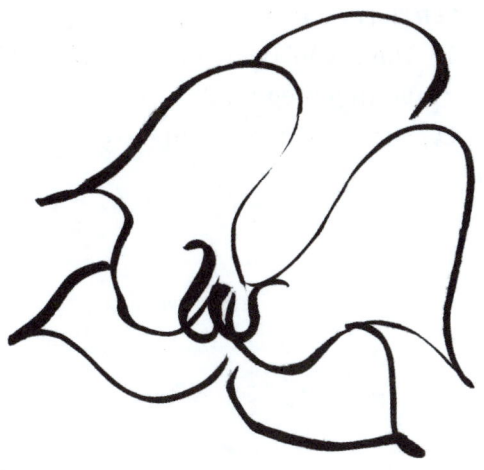

## SYMPTOM CHECKLIST

**PELVIC PAIN**
- O  Do you experience pain or discomfort in your abdomen?
- O  Do you experience pain or discomfort in your pelvic area?
- O  Pain during menstrual bleeding?
- O  Pain when urinating?
- O  Pain during bowel movements?
- O  Do you take pain medication for period cramps?
- O  Is light touch on your lower abdomen painful?
- O  Do you wear loose clothing due to bloating or pressure in the pelvic area?
- O  Do you have pain in other parts of your body, such as headaches, back or neck pain, or fibromyalgia?
- O  Does pelvic pain interfere with daily activities, work, or school?
- O  Do you experience nausea, vomiting, or fainting during period pain?
- O  Do you ever worry your pain will never improve?

**PERIODS**
- O  Do you need to change pads or tampons more than every 2 hours?
- O  Do you use both pads and tampons (or menstrual cups) together?
- O  Does your period last more than 7 days or come more often than once a month?

**COMFORT**
- O  If sexually active, do you experience pain or discomfort during or after sex?
- O  Do you avoid sex because of pain or discomfort?

**FERTILITY**
- O  Have you been diagnosed with any condition that could interfere with getting pregnant?
- O  Have you been trying to conceive for more than 6 months without success?

**NEXT STEPS**

If you answered 'Yes' to many of these questions, you may have a higher likelihood of endometriosis. While other conditions can cause similar symptoms, it's crucial to discuss your responses with your doctor. Bring a copy of this checklist to your healthcare provider to start the conversation and expedite the investigation process.

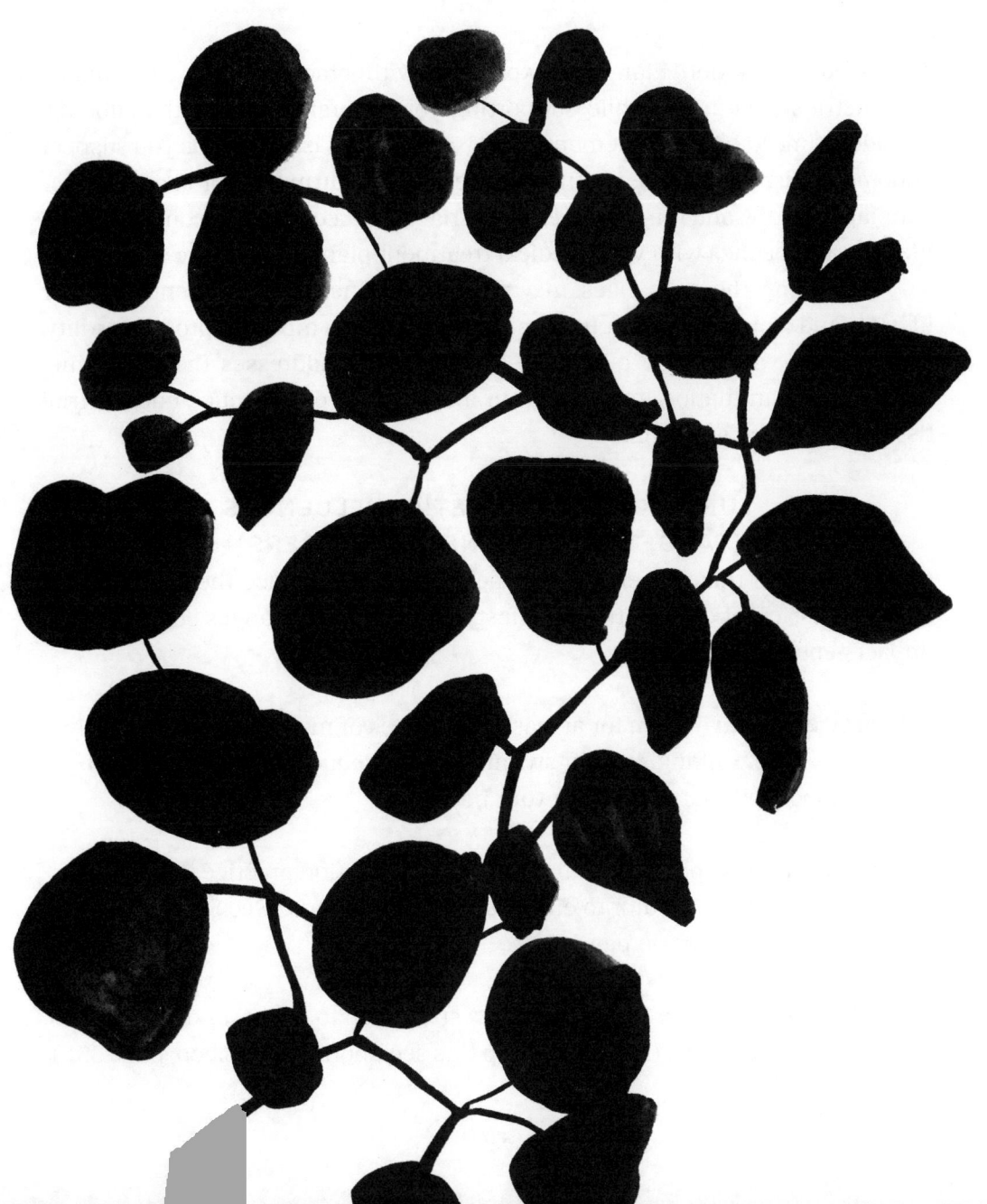

## WELLNESS ACTION PLAN
# MANAGING ENDOMETRIOSIS

This Wellness Action Plan empowers you with practical steps to manage endometriosis naturally while supporting your overall health and wellbeing. The ideal time to begin implementing these strategies is as soon as you suspect endometriosis, often while waiting for specialist confirmation or surgery. After your laparoscopy and removal of endometrial tissue, continue to combine these lifestyle approaches with your medical treatment plan for a holistic approach.

Adopting these changes may require significant adjustments to your lifestyle and diet, but the benefits can help minimise symptoms, protect fertility, and improve your overall quality of life. This plan addresses the underlying drivers of inflammation, working from a cellular level to reduce endometrial tissue growth and symptoms.

### TURNING DOWN GENETIC INFLUENCES
### (TARGETING EPIGENETIC TRIGGERS)

Research shows that epigenetic modifications can influence the development and progression of endometriosis. Lifestyle and dietary changes can positively impact gene expression.

- **Exercise regularly:** Aim for at least 30 minutes of moderate exercise daily. Activities like walking, yoga or swimming help reduce inflammation and boost mood without overtaxing your body.

- **Meditation:** Incorporate a 10-minute daily meditation practice to reduce stress, a major contributor to endometriosis symptoms. (See Spotlight on Restorative Practices on page 372.)

- **Quality sleep:** Ensure 7 to 8 hours of restful sleep to support hormone balance and recovery. (For more sleep tips see Spotlight on Sleep, page 351.)

- **Omega-3 supplements:** Start a high-quality fish oil supplement to reduce inflammation. Begin with 4000 mg twice daily for a few weeks, then reduce to 4000 mg daily as a maintenance dose.

### OXIDATIVE STRESS SOLUTIONS

Oxidative stress contributes to cellular damage in endometriosis. Follow our Wellness Action Plan to reduce oxidative stress starting on page 282.

### REDUCING INFLAMMATION

Chronic inflammation drives endometriosis. Dietary changes and supplements can help reduce inflammation.

- **Anti-inflammatory foods:** Follow our Core Food Principles starting on page 396.

- **Herbs and spices:** Add rhubarb, fennel, cinnamon and sage to your meals for their anti-inflammatory properties.

- **Supplements:** Take DIM (di-indolylmethane) or sulforaphane from broccoli or Brussels sprouts for their proven benefits in balancing hormones and reducing inflammation.

### SUPPORTING A HEALTHY IMMUNE RESPONSE

Endometriosis is influenced by immune dysfunction, so supporting your immune system is crucial.

- **Vitamin D:** Optimise your vitamin D levels with safe sun exposure and supplements. (For more on vitamin D, see page 445.)

- **Traditional Chinese Medicine (TCM):** TCM and acupuncture have shown excellent results in managing endometriosis and supporting fertility. Schedule acupuncture sessions the week before and during your period.

### TURNING DOWN OESTROGEN

High oestrogen levels exacerbate endometriosis symptoms. These strategies can help balance oestrogen levels:

- **Herbs:** Chaste Tree, Dong quai, schisandra and rhodiola can help balance hormones.

- **Progesterone:** Discuss a four-month trial of oral bioidentical progesterone with your doctor to help regulate your menstrual cycle and reduce uterine cramping. The usual dose is 200 mg taken in the luteal (second half) of your menstrual cycle.

### REDUCING TOXIC CHEMICAL EXPOSURE

Limit exposure to endocrine disruptors linked to endometriosis.

- **Organic food:** Buy organic or local, pesticide-free produce.
- **Natural skincare:** Switch to organic, toxin-free skincare products.
- **Household products:** Avoid household products with harmful chemicals like triclosan, commonly found in handwashes and some toothpastes.

### SPECIFIC SYMPTOM MANAGEMENT

- **Pelvic cramping:** Take 300 mg of magnesium around period time or enjoy a warm bath with magnesium salts.

- **Peppermint tea:** Swap coffee for peppermint tea, especially during your period, as caffeine can irritate the bladder.

## NEW DISCOVERIES:
## ENDOMETRIOSIS AND THE MICROBIOME

Recent research suggests that microbiome imbalances, including gut, oral, and vaginal flora, may play a role in endometriosis. While testing for this is still in early stages, nurturing your microbiome is an excellent preventative measure.

- **Gut care:** Start with our chapter on gut health (page 424), then explore vaginal microbiome support on page 503.

> **TIP**
>
> Your surgeon may advise you to stop taking natural products like omega-3 fish oils before surgery.

Always follow the guidance of your healthcare practitioner regarding therapies and supplements, ensuring they are tailored to your unique needs at every stage of your endometriosis management.

## SPOTLIGHT ON
# Polycystic ovary syndrome (PCOS)

PCOS is not just about the ovaries. It's a complex endocrine problem that can be addressed by understanding its roots.

This common health condition affects millions of women globally. It results from an imbalance in reproductive hormones, leading to a variety of symptoms that affect your menstrual cycle, fertility, appearance and overall health. Rather than focusing on what the ovaries are doing, a better understanding comes from viewing it as a condition rooted in cellular resistance, where cells begin to lock out hormones from their natural pathways. This imbalance creates a ripple effect, influencing how various hormones are produced and interact with each other.

Depending on whether these cellular disruptions occur in the ovaries or other areas, the symptoms and associated risks of PCOS can vary.

### THE FIRST DOMINO TO FALL

PCOS begins when a genetic sequence is activated by an environmental trigger, such as exposure to chemicals or stress. This activation occurs through the epigenetic layer of control—this is why some women experience no issues until suddenly, something shifts. For one woman, this may mean missed periods, while for another, it could be unexpected weight gain, unwanted hair growth or acne.

CASE STUDY | DR KAREN
# Mandy
## Managing PCOS naturally

My patient Mandy discovered she had PCOS in high school, and started to work with me to balance her hormones soon after. Her diagnosis came after an ovarian cyst ruptured during a flight home from a surfing trip. An ultrasound revealed the classic 'pearl necklace' of cysts, and blood tests confirmed PCOS.

Mandy didn't turn to medication; instead, she embraced a lifestyle plan that addressed the root causes of PCOS. Coming from a family of active beach lovers, she continued surfing and followed a specific movement program while navigating the stress of her final year at university. She knew that maintaining a healthy body weight was her best chance to avoid PCOS-related diabetes, which ran in her family.

With the help of a carefully tailored nutrition plan, Mandy was able to reduce her androgen (male hormone) levels by 40%—a better result than many prescribed PCOS drugs. As a result, she experienced less unwanted hair growth and had no trouble conceiving when she was ready to start a family.

## THE ORIGINS OF OUR PCOS GENE CLUSTERS— ADAPTIVE EVOLUTION

Many modern health issues, including PCOS, may have ancient roots. Our bodies still process information based on survival instincts hard-wired into our DNA from a time when life was a cycle of feast and famine, war and peace.

In ancient times, young women faced the following challenges:

- Avoiding pregnancy during dangerous periods of tribal unrest
- Conserving energy and food during shortages
- Gaining strength to survive physical threats

To meet these needs, women could activate a 'survival switch' deep in the brain that temporarily halted ovulation and reduced metabolism, allowing them to conserve energy and survive. This survival mechanism also boosted androgen levels, contributing to muscle strength, which could be lifesaving in battle.

Interestingly, higher levels of body hair, a byproduct of increased androgens, were once a desirable sign of vitality and strength. These 'warrior women' had the genetic advantage to survive and reproduce once the threat passed.

## UNDERSTANDING PCOS IN THE MODERN CONTEXT

Today, PCOS reflects the ancient survival mechanisms still embedded in our DNA. However, in our current environment, this once beneficial genetic adaptation has led to the hormonal imbalances, we associate with PCOS. These imbalances can cause:

- Irregular menstrual cycles or missed periods
- Unexplained weight gain
- Acne and oily skin
- Excessive hair growth in unwanted areas

By understanding PCOS through this evolutionary lens, we gain a better sense of why it affects so many women today and how we can use modern strategies to manage the condition effectively.

For many, the journey toward a PCOS diagnosis begins with missed periods or through findings from a pelvic ultrasound. However, it's important to note that simply having a polycystic pattern of cysts on your ovaries does not necessarily mean you will develop the full spectrum of PCOS-related risks.

Many women with ovarian cysts never experience the more serious hormonal and metabolic disruptions associated with the syndrome.

The real challenge lies in recognising and addressing the broader metabolic issues that often accompany PCOS, even in women who don't show obvious symptoms. Early diagnosis and proactive management are key to reducing the long-term effects of this condition.

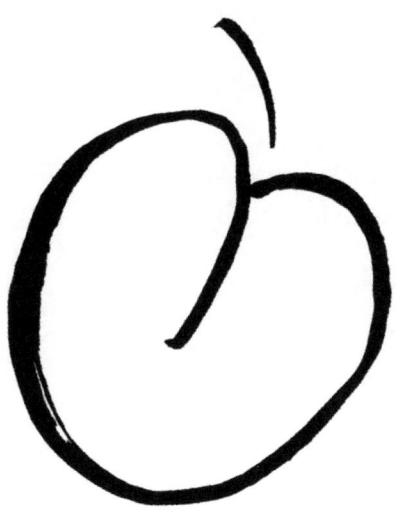

## PCOS SYMPTOM CHECKLIST

**MENSTRUAL IRREGULARITIES**
○ Do you have irregular periods, such as fewer than eight periods a year?
○ Do you usually go more than 34 days between periods?
○ Do you need to change your menstrual products more than every 4 hours?
○ Do your periods last more than 7 days?

**EXCESS ANDROGEN SYMPTOMS**
○ Have you noticed excess facial or body hair on your face, chest, or back?
○ Do you struggle with severe acne or oily skin?
○ Have you experienced thinning hair or a receding hairline?

**OVULATION PROBLEMS**
○ Are you having difficulty getting pregnant?
○ Do you suspect that you are not ovulating regularly?

**WEIGHT AND METABOLISM**
○ Have you had unexplained weight gain or found it difficult to lose weight?
○ Do you tend to gain weight around your middle/abdomen?

**SKIN CONDITIONS**
○ Have you noticed dark patches of skin, especially around your neck, groin or underarms?
○ Do you have small, skin-coloured growths (skin tags), particularly in your armpits or neck area?

**MOOD AND MENTAL HEALTH**
○ Do you often feel depressed or have mood swings?
○ Do you struggle with anxiety or irritability?

**SLEEP ISSUES**
○ Do you have problems with breathing during sleep, such as sleep apnoea?
○ Do you feel excessively sleepy during the day?

**OTHER SYMPTOMS**
○ Do you experience pelvic pain?

○ Do you often feel fatigued or unusually tired?
○ Do you frequently have headaches?

**ADDITIONAL CONSIDERATIONS**

**FAMILY HISTORY**
○ Do you have a family history of PCOS or related symptoms?

If you answered 'Yes' to more than three of these questions, it may be helpful to discuss your symptoms with a healthcare provider for a thorough evaluation and further testing.

**PCOS IN THE MODERN ERA: ANCIENT GENES IN A MODERN WORLD**
The concept that PCOS has roots in inherited survival traits offers a fascinating perspective on how ancient genetic advantages may influence modern health. The genes that helped women survive periods of scarcity and danger are now being activated by modern-day psychological stress, environmental chemicals, and an over-abundance of food.

While food is plentiful and threats to survival are different, the constant pressures of modern life—stress from work, family and being constantly connected—can trigger the same genetic responses that once helped women survive harsh environments. Over time, if left unchecked, these genes may lead to more severe complications like diabetes or increased cardiovascular risk.

Understanding these connections between our evolutionary past and modern health challenges not only deepens our understanding of PCOS but also opens the door to more effective treatments, including lifestyle changes that can help manage symptoms and prevent complications.

> **TIP**
> Even though it may take longer to fall pregnant due to a reduced number of fertile months, women with PCOS can maintain their fertility into later life. This is a genetic trade-off that has its origins in tribal survival.

While formal medical plans may focus primarily on symptom control with medications, many women with PCOS express frustration at the lack of emphasis on optimising long-term wellbeing and addressing future health risks.

Women with PCOS may face increased risks for several health issues, including:

- Insulin resistance, contributing to weight gain
- Type 2 diabetes
- Heart disease and stroke at a younger age
- Endometrial cancer, due to hormonal imbalances.

### HOW DOCTORS DIAGNOSE PCOS

A formal diagnosis of PCOS is based on meeting at least two of the following three criteria:

1. Polycystic ovaries seen on ultrasound (at least 20 follicles or unusually large ovaries)
2. Irregular or absent menstrual periods (fewer than six periods per year)
3. Excessive hair growth on the face, chest or abdomen or high male hormone levels.

If you only have polycystic ovaries on an ultrasound without the other two indicators, it is unlikely that you'll face the long-term health risks of PCOS. But if you tick at least two of these boxes, our PCOS Wellness Action Plan on page 556 can guide you toward better wellness.

## FAST FORWARD TO THE 21ST CENTURY: WHAT WENT WRONG?

Why are the same warrior genes that once ensured survival now a disadvantage in the modern world? The reasons are complex, and focusing solely on diet won't provide the best chance of avoiding the medical consequences of PCOS or thriving. Elements of these four key wellness areas have changed in the modern era to the detriment of women with PCOS:

1. Nourishment

In tribal times, we ate 'low human intervention' food, consuming the entire animal, including vitamin-rich organs like kidneys and brains. We ate whole fruits with the skins, which contain fibre—a powerful anti-inflammatory nutrient. In contrast, modern processed foods, like high-fructose corn syrup, are damaging for PCOS. For example, juicing fruits creates quick access to sugars that spike blood sugar levels, unlike eating the whole fruit, which provides a more gradual release of energy.

## 2   Movement

Our ancestors moved constantly, and this physical activity activated over 4000 beneficial genes that promote health. Today, we sit for long hours, losing the genetic advantages that regular movement provides for overall wellness, including metabolic health.

## 3   Unrelenting stress

While food is abundant today, we experience stress in ways our ancestors did not. Modern stress comes from body image pressures, financial worries, social media, and the constant demand to be 'plugged in'. Unlike the situational stress of physical survival in tribal times, today's stress is chronic and undermines health, especially in women with PCOS.

Addressing these fundamental shifts in lifestyle and environment through a holistic approach can help manage the long-term risks associated with PCOS and foster a more balanced, healthier life.

## 4   Hormone burden in PCOS

Cortisol is a crucial hormone for survival. Under normal conditions, it is gradually released throughout the day to support the circadian rhythm. In response to sudden, unexpected stress, the body perceives danger and releases an additional surge of cortisol, along with adrenaline. For women with PCOS, daily cortisol production often deviates from the ideal pattern. Research shows that women with PCOS tend to experience elevated cortisol levels, especially in the late afternoon.

In the graph below two cortisol production patterns are shown:

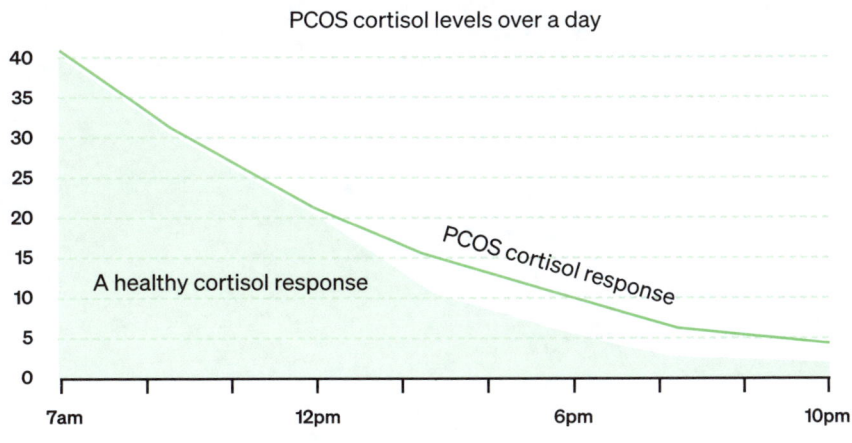

The solid green shading represents a healthy cortisol response, where cortisol levels peak in the morning and gradually decrease throughout the day.

The green line depicts the typical PCOS pattern, where cortisol levels show an upturn in the late afternoon.

This subtle but consistent increase in cortisol adds up, resulting in a higher total cortisol load over time—daily, weekly, and monthly. Even on a typical day without acute stress, this elevated cortisol burden contributes to the overall hormonal imbalance seen in women with PCOS.

### THE DOUBLE HORMONAL WHAMMY IN PCOS

Excess cortisol doesn't just stop at driving further stress—it converts into testosterone, compounding the hormonal imbalance. Women with PCOS already tend to have elevated testosterone levels, so this additional cortisol-to-testosterone conversion worsens the situation, exacerbating symptoms like weight gain, excess body hair, and irregular periods.

### CHEMICAL LOAD

For the first time in human history, we've added a chemical load to our food, chemicals like BPA, and phthalates. This places a significant burden on the livers of women with PCOS, disrupting the delicate balance of fertility hormones. The result is an overload of oestrogen messaging, undermining the calming and mood-supporting effects of progesterone.

Your body isn't broken, but in today's stressful and toxic world, the PCOS warrior genes no longer provide the survival advantage they once did. Understanding your body this way empowers you to find creative strategies to quiet these genes and avoid the challenges of being a warrior woman in the modern world.

CASE STUDY | DR KAREN

# Marie

From our first consultation, Marie was determined to regain control of her hormones. Her menstrual cycles were irregular, occurring just two or three times a year, and when they did, the flow was so heavy she had to take time off work. In her late 20s and eager to start a family with her partner Scott, Marie knew she needed to make changes.

Previous doctors had suggested the oral contraceptive pill to regulate her periods, but Marie understood this wouldn't help her achieve her goal of pregnancy before turning 30.

Her initial lab tests revealed low levels of key nutrients crucial for PCOS management: zinc, vitamin D and magnesium. Recognising this, I prescribed supplements to address these deficiencies. I advised her to aim for vitamin D levels at the high end of the reference range to best support hormonal health.

Marie's hormone panel showed classic PCOS patterns: elevated androgens (male hormones), often linked to irregular periods. However, her anti-mullerian hormone (AMH), indicating ovarian reserve, was high—reassuring her of strong fertility potential.

A lifestyle review revealed she was over-exercising, especially with excessive cardio that raised her cortisol levels. We adjusted her routine, reducing cardio and adding yoga to help her feel less stressed. Within weeks, her cortisol levels dropped, improving her sleep.

Marie also began following the nutrition recommendations in the Wellness Action Plan for PCOS (see following pages), shifting her main meal to earlier in the day. After a month, she noticed modest weight loss and increased energy.

Nine months later, Marie's cycles had become regular, with ovulation every 32 days. She started tracking ovulation and, two months before her 30th birthday, surprised me with the news of a positive home pregnancy test.

WELLNESS ACTION PLAN
# PCOS

## A. Nutritional Fundamentals

With so much confusion around the 'right' diet for PCOS—should you go vegan, keto, or low GI? The truth is, every woman with PCOS has a unique genetic and hormonal landscape, yet they all share a glitch in glucose processing. This means avoiding overwhelming your body with excessive carbohydrates, which can drive insulin resistance. Use the following nutritional steps to success:

### STEP ONE:
### CHECK YOUR ESSENTIAL PCOS NUTRIENTS

Ensure that your nutrient levels are optimal to manage PCOS symptoms more effectively. Lab tests ordered by your healthcare provider can check these levels.

Key nutrients include:

- **Vitamin D**: Aim for blood levels between 100 and 150 nmol/L. Take with a probiotic food like yoghurt or kefir for best absorption.
- **Zinc**: Optimal range is between 14 and 28 µmol/L.
- **Magnesium**: Signs of deficiency include muscle twitching, cramping, and tension, particularly in the neck and shoulders.
- **Folate**: Ensure adequate intake, especially if you've been on the Pill or restrictive diets like keto or Paleo.

#### ADD THESE PCOS WELLNESS NUTRIENTS

Some nutrients work best in combination with others, creating a synergistic effect that can improve PCOS symptoms. This combination has been shown in studies to be more effective than Metformin for regulating blood sugar and insulin levels.

- Myo-inositol (2 g)
- Chromium (40 mcg)
- L-tyrosine (0.2 mg)
- Selenium (55 mcg): Either in food form (two Brazil nuts) or as a supplement.

> **DR KAREN'S TOP 2 SUPPLEMENTS FOR PCOS WELLNESS**
>
> As a medical doctor and herbalist, I know it can be overwhelming to choose supplements for PCOS. Here are my top two essentials:
>
> - Vitamin D: If your levels are sub-optimal, take 5000 IU daily until blood levels reach 100 nmol/L. Then reduce the dose to maintain levels between 90 and 180 nmol/L. Recheck after four months.
>
> - *Lactobacillus Bifidum* probiotic: When paired with vitamin D, this combination helps regulate testosterone, reduce acne, improve mood and lower inflammation. It's a winning, risk-free duo.

## STEP TWO: WHEN TO EAT

An often overlooked but powerful tool for managing PCOS is timing your meals. Research has shown that inverting the traditional eating pattern can have profound benefits for hormone balance and overall metabolic health.

- **Substantial breakfast**: Your largest meal of the day should be breakfast. Aim for a hearty, protein-rich meal that provides sustained energy and stabilises blood sugar levels. This could include options like eggs, avocado, and whole grains. A substantial breakfast helps set the stage for balanced blood sugar and insulin levels throughout the day.

- **Moderate lunch**: Lunch should be balanced but not as heavy as breakfast. Include protein, healthy fats and fibre-rich vegetables. A moderate lunch helps maintain energy levels without overburdening your digestion or insulin pathways.

- **Small dinner**: Make your evening meal the lightest of the day. Focus on lean proteins, light vegetables, and fewer carbohydrates. By eating lighter in the evening, you avoid large insulin spikes before bed, which can support better sleep and improve hormonal regulation.

- **Snack:** If you need a snack in the evening, opt for something light like a handful of nuts or a small piece of fruit.

This simple adjustment in when you eat can yield remarkable results to improve your symptoms, support weight management and promote fertility with the added advantages of:

- **Reduced androgen levels**: Male hormone levels (androgens) can decrease by 50%, which can lead to improvements in symptoms like acne and unwanted hair growth.

- **Improved insulin sensitivity**: Insulin resistance markers drop by nearly 60%, which is a game-changer for managing blood sugar levels and weight control.

- **Hormonal balance**: In a study on the 'Big Breakfast' approach, 50% of women restored their monthly cycles and saw healthy progesterone levels return within three months.

> **TIP**
>
> For women whose lifestyle doesn't allow for a large breakfast, there are alternative strategies that can still offer similar benefits. Check out our overnight fasting approach or the Fast 800 Diet discussed on page 566. These methods offer flexibility while still focusing on managing insulin resistance and PCOS symptoms.

## STEP THREE:
## WHAT TO EAT

Choosing the right carbohydrates is essential for managing PCOS, as the condition fundamentally impacts how your body processes glucose.

### TWEAK YOUR INTAKE

The standard Western diet is heavy on carbohydrates, often accounting for 50% of daily intake. For women with PCOS, this can be problematic, especially with insulin resistance in the mix.

- **Carbs are not your friend so cap carbs at 25%**: Aim to reduce your carbohydrate intake to 25% of your total daily food intake. This means cutting back on starchy grains, and berries are your best fruits.

- **Replace with protein**: Reallocate the calories you would normally get from carbohydrates to protein sources. This adjustment helps stabilise blood sugar and contributes to lower testosterone levels, improving overall PCOS symptoms.

For a deeper dive into the importance of balancing carbohydrates and proteins, turn to our Spotlight on Insulin Resistance page 564.

If you have been diagnosed with insulin resistance (pre-diabetes) or Type 2 diabetes, you will have less wiggle room for celebratory foods that belong to the processed sugar carb family. Keep those foods as a once or twice a year celebration and your body and hormones will thank you!

## B. Movement Fundamentals for PCOS

Incorporating movement into your routine is essential for managing PCOS, especially considering our modern sedentary lifestyles. Despite being genetically wired for physical activity, many of us do not move as much as our DNA requires.

### MUSCLE-BUILDING EXERCISES

Building muscle helps manage blood sugar because muscle tissue can absorb sugar and convert it into energy without needing insulin. Resistance training is a powerful tool for PCOS because it helps improve insulin sensitivity, a common issue for women with the condition.

### HIT YOUR DAILY STEPS

Around 8000 steps per day has been shown to provide excellent health benefits. If you're already hitting or exceeding this number, keep up the good work! This regular movement helps keep blood sugar in check, reduces stress, and promotes overall health.

### INCORPORATE GENTLE MOVEMENT

Practices like Tai Chi or Qigong are excellent for managing stress. These gentle, flowing exercises promote relaxation, mental clarity, and physical health. Integrating these practices into your weekly routine will help balance hormones, reduce cortisol, and improve PCOS symptoms.

### ADDITIONAL MOVEMENT PROGRAMS

Depending on your hormonal stage, consider incorporating more movement into your routine. This could include cardio, yoga or Pilates. However, be mindful of not overtraining, as pushing beyond your body's limits can spike cortisol levels, which may hinder your progress. For more detailed guidance on finding your movement sweet spot, refer to the Spotlight on Movement on page 485.

## C. Stress Resilience Strategies

Crucial for PCOS wellness because chronic stress increases cortisol, which in turn raises androgen levels and disrupts hormonal balance. For effective stress management strategies, review our Spotlight on Psychological Stress on page 290, and Restorative Practices on page 372.

## D. Avoid Hormone-Disrupting Chemicals

Environmental pollutants exacerbate hormonal imbalances in women with PCOS. (See Spotlight on Managing Toxins on page 478.)

### BPA AND ITS IMPACT ON PCOS

Bisphenol A (BPA) is a chemical found in plastics that can impair the mitochondria—the energy-producing centre of cells—leading to weight gain and disrupting cellular function. Additionally, BPA has been shown to reduce the effectiveness of chemotherapy in killing breast cancer cells.

## BPA: AVOIDING HORMONE-DISRUPTING CHEMICALS

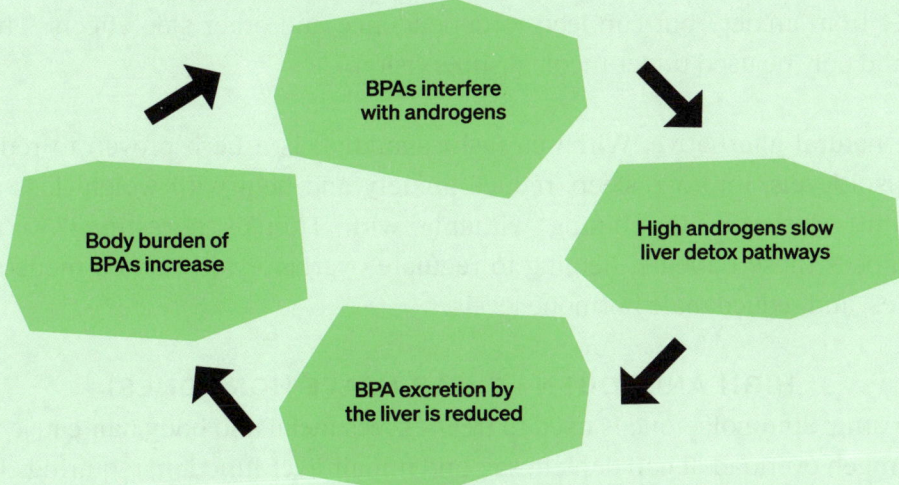

# E. Support Your Body with Proven Complementary Modalities for PCOS

### ACUPUNCTURE

A Swedish study from 2009 demonstrated that acupuncture can benefit women with PCOS. The study participants experienced normalised menstrual cycles, lower testosterone levels, and reduced waist measurements after four months of acupuncture therapy compared to a control group.

### TRADITIONAL CHINESE MEDICINE

Traditional Chinese herbal medicine has been used for centuries to treat hormonal imbalances, including PCOS. Research supports its effectiveness, often matching or surpassing pharmaceutical options, with fewer side effects.

# F. Targeted Natural Supplements Proven to Help

When managing PCOS, balancing conventional medical treatments with natural alternatives can be highly effective. Common drugs like Metformin (for insulin resistance) and Spironolactone (for androgen overload) are commonly prescribed, but there are proven natural options that can work in conjunction with or in place of these medications.

## STRESS SUPPORT

The drug: Benzodiazepines drugs like Valium and Xanax provide short-term relief from anxiety but can lead to dependence and other side effects. These should only be used under medical supervision.

The natural alternative: Withania (ashwagandha) is a herb proven to reduce cortisol levels, improve sleep, reduce anxiety and help with weight loss and insulin resistance. Combining withania with *Tribulus terrestris* (750 mg) enhances these benefits, helping to regulate ovarian cysts, restore menstrual cycles, and reduce male hormone levels.

## HIGH ANDROGEN LEVELS (MALE HORMONES)

The drug: Spironolactone is used to treat excess facial and body hair caused by androgen overload. It can deplete salt and impair liver function, requiring close monitoring, especially to avoid BPA accumulation.

The natural alternative: Both paeonia and liquorice have been proven to lower androgen levels. However, caution is advised for those with high blood pressure, as liquorice can increase blood pressure.

## GETTING PERIODS BACK ON TRACK

The drug: The oral contraceptive pill (the Pill) can prevent the development of ovarian cysts and help regulate periods, but it does not address the underlying issues of PCOS. Some pills can increase the risk of deep vein thrombosis.

The natural alternative: Optimising vitamin D levels, together with melatonin (10 mg, taken at night) can help regulate menstrual cycles and improve fertility without the side effects of the Pill.

## INSULIN RESISTANCE AND BLOOD SUGAR

The drug: Metformin is commonly used to reduce insulin resistance, aid in weight loss, and boost fertility. It is important to monitor its effects, as insulin resistance improves with dietary changes and may require adjusting medication levels.

The natural alternative: Inositol, specifically in its myo-inositol form, has been shown to be as effective as Metformin in managing insulin resistance, reducing male hormone levels, and improving egg quality. It has a strong track record of safety but may cause side effects in women with certain variants in the COMT gene (Met/Met-Allele). Gene testing can help determine if Inositol is the right option for you.

### PCOS NUTRITIONAL TARGETS

A major step in managing PCOS involves addressing nutritional imbalances. Some essential nutrients to monitor include:

- **Vitamin D:** Target blood levels between 100-150 nmol/L.
- **Zinc:** Ensure levels are between 14-28 µmol/L.
- **Magnesium:** Deficiencies can lead to muscle tension and headaches.
- **Folate:** Women on restrictive diets or the oral contraceptive pill are at higher risk of deficiency.

The following table summarises the power of nutrients to turn down the symptoms of PCOS:

| FOOD-DERIVED NUTRIENT | ANTI-INFLAMMATORY EFFECTS | MENSTRUAL REGULATION | INSULIN SENSITIVITY | ANDROGEN REDUCTION |
|---|---|---|---|---|
| Selenium | ✓ | ✓ |  | ✓ |
| Zinc | ✓ | ✓ |  | ✓ |
| Magnesium | ✓ | ✓ | ✓ |  |
| Cinnamon | ✓ | ✓ | ✓ |  |
| *Lactobacillus* | ✓ |  |  |  |
| Spearmint | ✓ | ✓ |  | ✓ |
| Omega-3 Fatty Acids | ✓ |  | ✓ | ✓ |
| Vitamin E | ✓ | ✓ |  | ✓ |
| Chromium |  |  | ✓ | ✓ |

By combining proven complementary therapies, stress resilience techniques, and natural alternatives to conventional medications, you can effectively manage PCOS and improve your quality of life.

> **TIP**
> Insulin resistance is a major consideration for your success in managing PCOS so read on for our Spotlight on this issue.

## SPOTLIGHT ON
# Insulin Resistance

Insulin resistance is a hidden disruptor of energy, weight and long-term health, with unique impacts on women due to hormonal shifts like those in PCOS, perimenopause and menopause.

### WHAT IS INSULIN RESISTANCE?

Insulin resistance occurs when your cells stop responding effectively to insulin, the hormone that regulates blood sugar, which can lead to subtle symptoms like fatigue, weight gain, and cravings. It is especially influenced by hormonal shifts such as those seen in PCOS, perimenopause, and menopause.

### SYMPTOMS OF INSULIN RESISTANCE

- Increased hunger, particularly cravings for carbohydrates or sweets
- Fatigue or low energy, especially after meals
- Difficulty losing weight, particularly around the abdominal area
- Unexplained weight gain or resistance to weight loss
- Brain fog or difficulty concentrating
- Darkened patches of skin, particularly on the neck, armpits, or groin (acanthosis nigricans)
- High blood pressure or elevated cholesterol levels
- Irregular menstrual cycles or symptoms of hormonal imbalance (for example, PCOS)
- Skin tags or small growths, particularly in areas of friction
- Frequent bloating or digestive discomfort
- Increased thirst or frequent urination

- Mood swings, irritability or anxiety
- Increased susceptibility to infections, particularly skin or urinary tract infections.

### THE RISKS OF INSULIN RESISTANCE

Over time, insulin resistance increases the risk of chronic conditions like Type 2 diabetes and heart disease, but the good news is that lifestyle factors like diet, exercise, and sleep can dramatically improve insulin sensitivity. Testing for insulin resistance, exploring the gut microbiome's role, and addressing its impact on mental health provide a comprehensive approach to managing this condition and protecting long-term health.

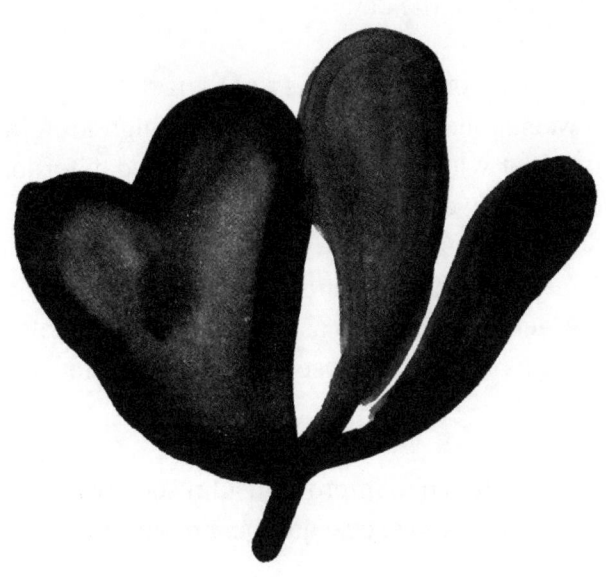

**WELLNESS ACTION PLAN**

# REVERSING INSULIN RESISTANCE

The strategies listed here are science-based and can show fast results to optimise blood and insulin balance.

### OPTIMISE MEAL TIMING

- **Overnight fast**: Aim for a 12 to 14 hour fast overnight to allow your body to reset insulin sensitivity and promote fat burning. For example, finish dinner by 7 pm and eat breakfast after 7 am.

- **Big breakfast approach**: Incorporate findings from the Israeli study that showed a protein- and fibre-rich breakfast (for example, eggs, vegetables, oats or Greek yoghurt with nuts) can improve insulin sensitivity and reduce blood sugar spikes later in the day.

### ADOPT THE FAST 800 DIET

For two days each week, follow a low-carbohydrate, high-protein, and high-fibre Mediterranean-style diet with up to 800 calories per day for long-term insulin improvement and modest weight loss over 6 to 8 weeks.

### FOCUS ON INSULIN-FRIENDLY FOODS

- Prioritise low-glycaemic foods such as non-starchy vegetables, whole grains (in moderation), lean proteins, nuts, seeds and healthy fats like olive oil and avocado.

- Magnesium has been shown to improve insulin sensitivity and is found in dark leafy greens, nuts and seeds, quinoa, brown rice and oats.

> **TIP**
>
> Around 30 g of pumpkin seeds provide 150 mg of natural magnesium.

- Avoid all highly processed sugars.

- Include insulin-sensitising foods like cinnamon, apple cider vinegar, turmeric, and omega-3-rich foods like sardines, chia seeds, walnuts, and flaxseeds.

### EXERCISE REGULARLY

Incorporate a mix of resistance training (such as weight training) and aerobic exercises (like walking, swimming) to improve glucose uptake by muscles and reduce insulin resistance.

### PRIORITISE SLEEP

Aim for 7 to 9 hours of quality sleep each night, as poor sleep worsens insulin resistance and increases hunger hormones like ghrelin. (See Spotlight on Sleep on page 351.)

### MANAGE STRESS

Practise mindfulness techniques such as yoga, meditation or deep breathing to lower cortisol levels, which can exacerbate insulin resistance. (See Spotlight on Restorative Practices on page 372.)

### SUPPORT GUT HEALTH

Include fermented foods like yoghurt, kefir, sauerkraut and kimchi to support a healthy gut microbiome, which plays a role in blood sugar regulation. (More details in Core Food Principle Number 5 on page 424.)

### MONITOR PROGRESS

Work with your doctor to monitor fasting blood glucose, HbA1c or insulin levels and adjust your action plan as needed.

### HERBS AND SUPPLEMENTS THAT HELP

- **Myo-inositol:** Available through naturopaths. Follow your practitioner's advice on dosage.

- **Vitamin D:** Crucial for proper insulin receptor function.

- **Omega-3 fatty acids:** Found in fish oil or algae supplements, omega-3s help reduce inflammation associated with insulin resistance and improve lipid profiles.

- **Berberine:** Improves insulin sensitivity, enhance glucose uptake, and reduce blood sugar levels, comparable to some pharmaceutical medications.

- **Alpha-lipoic acid (ALA):** An antioxidant that enhances insulin sensitivity and reduces oxidative stress.

- **Fenugreek:** Rich in soluble fibre and compounds that help slow glucose absorption and improve insulin sensitivity.

- **Gymnema sylvestre:** Known as the 'sugar destroyer,' this herb helps reduce sugar cravings and improve glucose metabolism.

By combining these strategies, you can tackle insulin resistance from multiple angles, giving your body the best chance to restore balance and thrive.

SPOTLIGHT ON
# Breast Care

From the hormonal surges of puberty to the fluctuating balance of perimenopause and the steadier rhythms of the Age of Wisdom, your breasts respond to hormonal changes in ways that can shape your health.

## BREAST HEALTH IN YOUR HORMONAL STAGES

Breast care starts in puberty, and continues for the rest of your hormonal journey.

### PUBERTY

During puberty, breast care is crucial, and it's important to teach young girls how to notice significant changes. Hormonal changes during this time can cause mild breast pain, known as mastalgia. Any hard, painful or persisting lumps should also be evaluated.

Educating young girls about breast self-exams can build a foundation for future breast health, helping them feel more confident and aware of their bodies.

### THE FERTILE YEARS

During your Fertile Years dietary choices can have a profound impact on breast health.

- Include cruciferous vegetables like broccoli, cauliflower, Brussels sprouts, and kale in your diet, as they support healthy oestrogen pathways.

- Antioxidant-rich foods such as berries and omega-3 fatty acids (from fatty fish, flaxseeds, chia seeds, and walnuts) offer protection by reducing inflammation and inhibiting tumour growth.

### PERIMENOPAUSE

During perimenopause, hormonal fluctuations can lead to heavy periods and iron deficiency, so make sure to incorporate iron-rich foods into your diet.

- Focus on a balanced intake of fruits, vegetables, whole fats (such as olive oil and avocado), fibre-rich foods, and soy products to support breast health.

- Moderating alcohol intake is essential during this stage, as it can exacerbate hormonal imbalances.

### MENOPAUSE

As you age, antioxidant pathways that keep breast cells healthy begin to slow.

- Ensure you're getting enough trace minerals like selenium and manganese from foods like Brazil nuts, quinoa, and seeds.

- Vitamin D is also vital for breast and bone health, so make sure your levels are optimal.

- Isoflavones, found in soy products like tofu, tempeh, and soy milk, provide mild oestrogenic effects that can help reduce hot flushes and support breast health. Including these foods in your diet during menopause can offer protective benefits against breast cancer.

### THE AGE OF WISDOM

With lower overall hormone levels, breast tissue becomes less dense but remains susceptible to oxidative damage and external influences.

- Focus on maintaining breast health through antioxidants.
- Phytoestrogens like Flaxseeds (15-30 g) actively protect breast cells.
- Regular screenings, and a lifestyle that supports cellular repair and resilience.

## WHY OXIDATIVE STRESS AND HORMONAL BALANCE MATTER

Breast tissue, with its high metabolic activity and hormonal responsiveness, is particularly vulnerable to oxidative stress. Unchecked oxidative stress can disrupt DNA, weaken cell membranes, and create an environment that increases the risk of unhealthy changes in breast tissue. (Read more in Spotlight on Oxidative Stress on page 273).

Hormonal balance is another cornerstone of breast health. When oestrogen levels are too high relative to progesterone—a state known as oestrogen dominance—breast tissue can become denser and more fibrous. This density not only increases discomfort and tenderness but is also linked to a greater risk of developing breast conditions, including cancer. Oestrogen dominance can also overstimulate the growth and division of breast cells, creating a higher likelihood of mutations during these processes.

By addressing oxidative stress and achieving hormonal harmony, you're giving your breasts the best chance to stay healthy and resilient. Taking these steps early and consistently can have a profound impact on long-term breast health. (Our Wellness Action Plan to Manage Oestrogen Dominance starts on page 143.)

## SYNTHETIC HORMONES AND YOUR BREASTS

Synthetic progestins, often used in some hormonal therapies and contraceptives, add another layer of complexity. Unlike bioidentical progesterone, which works synergistically with oestrogen to regulate breast cell growth, synthetic progestins have been shown in studies to negatively impact breast tissue, potentially increasing the risk of certain cancers. Understanding these risks highlights the importance of informed choices about hormonal support, whether you're using contraception, treating perimenopausal symptoms, or considering hormone replacement therapy (HRT).

## THE IMPORTANCE OF BREAST IMAGING

Breast imaging is a cornerstone of proactive breast health care, especially given the prevalence of breast cancer, which affects one in eight women over a lifetime. Early detection through tools like mammography, ultrasound and

MRI can identify changes in breast tissue long before they are detectable by touch, significantly improving outcomes. These technologies not only aid in diagnosing cancer at an earlier, more treatable stage but also help monitor dense or fibrocystic breasts, where visualising abnormalities can be more challenging. Regular breast imaging, tailored to your age, risk factors, and breast density, empowers you to detect potential issues early, providing both peace of mind and a vital layer of defence in your health strategy. Work closely with your trusted health practitioner to determine the most appropriate imaging options and frequency for your individual needs.

### TIP

Mammograms struggle to detect changes in fibrocystic and dense breasts so specialists are now turning to breast MRI for clarity. MRI delivers less radiation for sensitive breast tissue over your lifetime, however, is more expensive and time consuming. If available, breast ultrasound with a baseline MRI may give you more reassurance about the health of your breasts. Discuss these options with your health practitioner.

### UNDERSTANDING DENSE BREASTS

Dense breasts are characterised by a higher proportion of fibrous and glandular tissue compared to fatty tissue, which appears white on a mammogram—just like potential abnormalities—making it more challenging to detect early signs of breast cancer. Dense breast tissue is influenced by factors such as genetics, hormonal changes, oestrogen dominance, and even certain lifestyle habits. Women with dense breasts not only face difficulties in imaging they also have a higher risk of developing breast cancer. While you can't change your genetic predisposition, there are proactive steps to reduce risks. Managing oestrogen dominance through dietary and lifestyle changes—in the Wellness Action Plan for breast care—can help balance hormones and support healthier breast tissue. Regular breast imaging using ultrasound or MRI, as guided by your doctor, is crucial for staying ahead of breast problems.

### TIP

Omega-3 fatty acids support healthy breast tissue structure, calm breast inflammation and reduce the risk of abnormalities. Aim for two servings of fatty fish per week or consider a high-quality omega-3 supplement for optimal benefits.

## ALCOHOL AND BREAST HEALTH

Reducing your alcohol intake can be one of the single most important things you can do to support the lifelong health of your breasts. We cover the impact of alcohol on breast health in Spotlight on Alcohol on page 287.

> **TIP**
> Limit alcohol consumption to one standard drink per day or less. If you choose to indulge, red wine is preferable due to its antioxidant resveratrol content, which supports both breast and heart health.

## BREAST-FRIENDLY HERBS

Certain herbs and natural supplements can play a supportive role in managing dense breast tissue by helping to balance hormones, reduce inflammation, and combat oxidative stress. These include:

- DIM (Diindolylmethane): Found naturally in cruciferous vegetables, DIM supplements can support the healthy metabolism of oestrogen, reducing the effects of oestrogen dominance that can contribute to dense breast tissue.

- Chaste **Tree**: Can help offset the relative dominance of oestrogen.

- Turmeric: The active compound curcumin has anti-inflammatory and antioxidant properties that protect breast tissue from oxidative stress and support cellular health.

- Withania (ashwagandha): Supports the body's stress response, as chronic stress can disrupt hormonal balance and exacerbate breast density issues.

- Milk thistle (*Silybum marianum*): Supports liver function, helping to metabolise and eliminate excess oestrogen from the body.

> **TIP**
> A healthy liver is essential for hormonal balance and breast tissue health. (More in our Spotlight on Liver Care on page 592.)

## THE POWER OF FOOD

Never underestimate the impact of nutrient-rich foods on your breast health. The right nutrients can support biological processes, repair DNA, and maintain healthy cell walls, while inflammatory foods can harm breast cells.

> **TIP**
> Flaxseed, a powerful phytoestrogen-rich food, is excellent for supporting breast health. It also provides fibre, which promotes gut health and helps eliminate excess oestrogen from your body. Adding 1–2 tablespoons of ground flaxseeds to your daily diet is an easy and effective way to combat oestrogen dominance—
> a key contributor to dense breast tissue.

## THE BREAST MICROBIOME

In December 2022, the European Network for Breast Development and Cancer (ENBDC) highlighted an emerging area of research—the breast microbiome. While we already know the significance of the gut microbiome for overall health, more research is needed to understand the role of the breast microbiome in cancer prevention and progression. This could unlock why, in some cases, one twin may develop breast cancer while the other does not.

In the meantime, we can rely on tried-and-true strategies to maintain breast health throughout your hormonal journey. (See Our Wellness Action Plan for Breast Care to follow.)

## WELLNESS ACTION PLAN
# BREAST CARE

### A NOTE ON BREAST CANCER

The support outlined in this Wellness Action Plan can be safely used before, during, and after surgery, chemotherapy and radiotherapy. They are proven to enhance the benefits of treatment, reduce side effects, and support your long-term wellbeing. Our next chapter gives you more specific information on support after breast cancer treatment.

### NOURISHMENT

Never underestimate the impact of nutrient-rich foods on your breast health. The right nutrients can support biological processes, repair DNA, and maintain healthy cell walls, while inflammatory foods can harm breast cells.

- **Vitamin D**: Essential for cell growth and repair. Aim for optimal levels, especially during cancer treatment. (See Spotlight on Vitamins and Mineral on page 443 for guidance.)

- **Omega-3 fatty acids**: Reduce inflammation and support healthy cell membranes. Omega-3 oils have been proven to reduce breast cancer risk and improve survival rates.

- **Antioxidants**: Vitamins C and E, selenium, and beta-carotene protect breast cells from oxidative stress.

- **Fibre**: Regulates oestrogen levels, reducing breast cancer risk. A high-fibre diet from fruits, vegetables and whole grains is essential.

- **Folate**: Vital for DNA repair. Women on the contraceptive pill may need additional folate, as the Pill can interfere with absorption.

- **Iodine**: Critical for thyroid function and breast health. Source from foods like sushi wraps or seaweed snacks rather than supplements as too much iodine can affect thyroid health.

- **Phytoestrogens**: Found in soy and flaxseeds, these plant-based compounds help regulate hormone levels and protect against breast cancer.

- **Choline**: Particularly important after menopause, choline-rich foods like eggs, liver and peanuts are essential for breast health.

## MOVEMENT STRATEGIES

- Physical activity is a key factor in breast cancer prevention and recovery. Aim for at least 150 minutes per week of aerobic and strength training exercises. Even a brisk 20-minute daily walk can reduce cancer recurrence by 24%.

- Add resistance training to support muscle and overall health. Exercise physiologists can help develop a plan tailored to your needs, especially during treatment.

## SOCIAL CONNECTION AND STRESS MANAGEMENT

- Make time for family, friends, and hobbies. Social connection is just as vital for breast health as diet and exercise.

- Adopt a meditation practice, whether through apps like *Calm* or *Endel* or by taking a peaceful walk in nature followed by quiet reflection. Meditation has been shown to reduce stress, improve emotional wellbeing, and support recovery.

## WELLNESS ACTION PLAN CHECKLIST FOR BREAST CARE

○ **Lab tests**: Check vitamin D levels (100-150 nmol/L), iodine (120-220 µg/L), B12 (for vegans or those with autoimmune conditions), iron, zinc and magnesium. Supplement if needed.

○ **Diet audit**: Ensure your diet includes nutrient-dense foods, fibre, phytoestrogens, and choline-rich foods (especially in menopause).

○ **Omega-3**: Consider a high-quality omega-3 supplement (3000-6000 mg daily) to enhance treatment results and reduce inflammation.

○ **Sulforaphane**: This compound, found in cruciferous vegetables, has cancer-preventive properties. A supplement may further inhibit cancer stem cells and improve chemotherapy results.

○ **Melatonin**: Used by integrative oncologists in higher doses (around 20 mg), melatonin can provide additional support during treatment.

○ **Biobran (Ribraxx)**: A combination of shitake mushroom and rice bran, Biobran has shown improved long-term survival in cancer patients. (See page 590 for more information on Biobran.)

○ **Alcohol**: Limit alcohol to three drinks per week. Red wine is preferable due to its resveratrol content.

○ **Caffeine**: Limit to one or two cups of coffee before midday. If sleep quality is poor, consider cutting caffeine altogether.

Every small step you take toward a healthier lifestyle positively impacts your breast health. From nourishing your body with the right foods to incorporating regular exercise and staying on top of medical screenings, you now have the tools to support your breast health and overall wellbeing. Embrace these changes with confidence, knowing your commitment to self-care is your best defence against breast cancer.

# BREAST CANCER

This chapter is dedicated to empowering you with the knowledge and strategies needed to navigate the complex and challenging journey of breast cancer. Alongside the information here, Part Two Spotlights provide additional insights to support your wellbeing.

### THE GROWING NUMBERS: AN OPPORTUNITY FOR ACTION

Although the increase in breast cancer diagnoses may seem overwhelming, it also sheds light on the power of modern medicine and public health efforts. The rise in cases has been met with advances in:

**Early detection**: Enhanced screening techniques such as mammograms, ultrasounds, and MRIs allow for the identification of breast cancer in its earlier stages, leading to improved outcomes. Be proactive in knowing your body and reporting any unusual changes to your healthcare provider.

**Personalised treatment plans**: The advent of targeted therapies, hormone treatments, and immunotherapies has allowed doctors to tailor treatments to each individual's cancer type and genetic makeup.

> Breast cancer is the most common cancer diagnosed in Australian women.

## WHEN CANCER IS SUSPECTED

Upon receiving a cancer diagnosis, it's common to seek answers online. The explosion of this information is both a blessing and a curse for women. Full of products that promise to cure ailments ranging from cancer to ingrown toenails. Researching meaningful and reliable information requires a reasonable amount of medical knowledge and caution, these are hard skills to muster when you are working from a space of fear, after receiving the news of a breast cancer diagnosis. Beware—it's essential to approach all claims with scepticism, as many lack scientific backing and may even interfere with conventional treatments. Here are some important guidelines to help you through this challenging time:

## WHEN YOU FIND ADDITIONAL INFORMATION OR PRODUCTS THAT INTEREST YOU

- **Check with your healthcare provider**: Before trying any supplement or product, consult your doctor to ensure it is safe and compatible with your treatment.

- **Seek professional advice**: A nutritionist or naturopath can provide valuable insight into supporting your body with the right nourishment, ensuring you are physically prepared for surgery and other treatments.

- **Stick to reputable sources** such as:

    - Medical websites like Cancer Council, Breast Cancer Network Australia (BCNA) Macmillan Cancer Support (UK)
    - Peer-reviewed studies or journals recommended by your healthcare team
    - Information provided by your oncologist or surgeon.

- Avoid forums or websites that make exaggerated claims or suggest extreme treatment alternatives without evidence.

## HOLISTIC CANCER CARE

Unfortunately, the current conventional medical system prevents specialists from providing access to holistic information and this is unlikely to change any time soon. This leaves many women searching for alternative perspectives on their treatment options.

While traditional cancer treatments like surgery, chemotherapy, and radiation therapy are essential and often lifesaving, holistic care can complement this approach. A focus on nutrition, stress management, and overall wellness may improve recovery and enhance your health. After completing acute treatments, incorporating our Wellness Action Plan for Breast Care (page 575) can guide you towards a healthier, cancer-free future.

> **TIP**
>
> When you ask your doctor or specialist (from any medical field), 'Should I eat a particular diet?' and they respond something like, 'Eat whatever you like, it won't make a difference', note that they are not up to date with the explosion of research in nutritional medicine. Without exception, the right diet will make a difference!

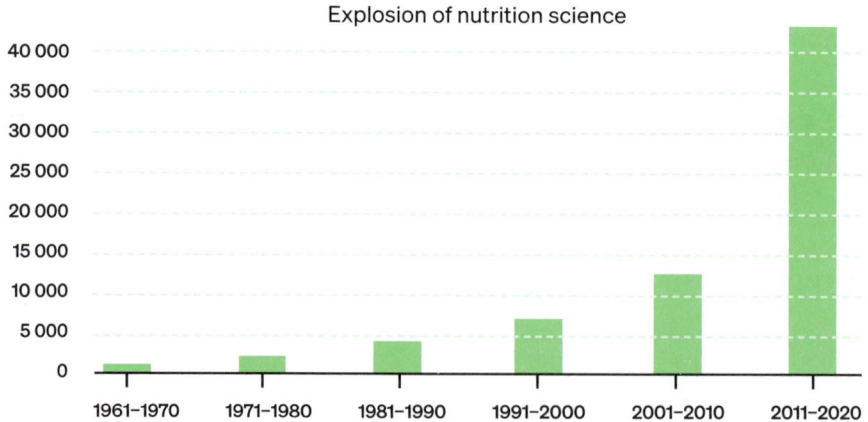

This graph reflects the explosion of research papers across all medical specialities from 1961 to 2020. From 2011 to 2020 there were over 40,000 papers published compared to a total of 5000 in the previous 50 years.

### HOW TO NAVIGATE A BREAST CANCER DIAGNOSIS

When first confronted with the news of a breast cancer diagnosis, feelings of fear, shock, and uncertainty are natural. Here are some tips for coping:

**BUILD YOUR SUPPORT TEAM:**

Having a network of trusted medical and supportive professionals is crucial. This team should include:

- Your oncologist or surgeon
- Your trusted local doctor
- A nutritionist or naturopath to support your overall health and wellness
- A therapist or counsellor to help you navigate the emotional journey
- Family members or friends for emotional and practical support

**MANAGING STRESS AND ANXIETY**

Stay present and focus on now. Getting extremely stressed from anticipating worst-case scenarios or dwelling on events that may never happen can make difficult news feel even more overwhelming. Of course, It's natural to feel daunted by the journey ahead but worrying about treatments that haven't been decided increases your stress response and right now you need to help your body to heal by activating the parasympathetic nervous system. This can be very challenging so here are some steps to help:

- Try to focus on immediate practical steps—such as scheduling consultations, undergoing further tests or preparing for surgery.

- Keep your focus on improving your diet, gentle movement and exercise, and removing stressful events as much as possible, try to take some time off work to navigate your current health challenge.

- Concerns about future treatments can wait until you and your support team have more information.

- For strategies on managing stress and supporting emotional wellbeing, see our Spotlight on Psychological Stress beginning on page 290.

- Ensure to thoroughly read our Spotlight on Restorative Practices on page 372. Engaging in these practices everyday will assist you physically, mentally and emotionally and can provide an anchor for you to lean on through this turbulent time.

- Take time to process: give yourself time to absorb the diagnosis and avoid making rushed decisions. Surgery is often the first step in treatment, and the detailed results from the pathology will give you more information about the cancer, which can guide future treatment decisions.

- Read Spotlight on Alcohol on page 287.

### GIVE YOURSELF TIME TO CONSIDER BIG DECISIONS

A breast cancer diagnosis is typically confirmed via a biopsy. Some women, however, may opt to skip this step and proceed directly to a lumpectomy if the suspicious area is small. It's essential to have a frank discussion with your GP at this time, as your preferences may influence your choice of surgeon and oncologist.

Should the lump be confirmed as cancer, you don't have to make decisions about chemotherapy or radiation therapy immediately. Often, surgery comes first, followed by a thorough review of pathology results, take each step, one day at a time. This extra time allows you to discuss treatment options in-depth with your medical team, family and friends, armed with more information to make confident, informed decisions. In some cases, radiotherapy may be offered before surgery, depending on the size of the tumour and your circumstances. For women with early-stage breast cancer, a surgeon might recommend a lumpectomy after consulting with your oncology team.

### CHOOSING YOUR MEDICAL TEAM

The first step after a breast cancer diagnosis is recruiting your medical support team. If you have a strong relationship with your GP, their recommendation—often based on feedback from other patients and knowledge of a specialist's expertise—is a great starting point. Friends or family who have gone through similar experiences may also have helpful suggestions.

> **DR KAREN SAYS**
>
> I place a lot of weight on specialists who come highly recommended by nursing staff and allied health professionals. They witness the bedside manner, medical expertise, and clinical outcomes behind the scenes. In my experience, nurses consistently provide an accurate 'report card' for specialists. When it comes to breast surgeons, clinical expertise and low complication rates are what really matter.
>
> If chemotherapy is planned, you'll spend more time with your oncologist, so it's important to have a comfortable, supportive, and open relationship. If the first meeting with your chosen oncologist doesn't feel right, don't hesitate to seek a second opinion. YOU are the most important person in your medical team, and there's no room for egos.

## CASE STUDY | DR KAREN
# Jill
## A broken therapeutic relationship

Jill had successfully navigated conventional breast cancer treatment and was nearly 12 months post-chemotherapy when she came to see me for a referral renewal to her oncologist. She started with a matter-of-fact attitude, detailing how she managed the challenges of the past year. She had been balancing chronic pain from radiation burns with the desire to avoid pain medications that caused unpleasant side effects.

When I asked her about her specialist, she burst into tears. 'I know he's a good oncologist, but every time I see him, he criticises me for using natural therapies to manage my pain. I feel like I'm a failure,' she said.

Jill explained that in the days leading up to each appointment, she couldn't sleep and even experienced panic attacks on the way to see him. I suggested that her anxiety might stem from reliving the trauma of her cancer treatment, but Jill said it was more than that. 'When I mention my natural remedies, he shuts me down and says he won't treat me if I keep using them.'

Jill had been taking a natural product called PEA (palmitoyl ethanol amide), which had significantly reduced her pain. PEA is well-researched, safe and effective for nerve-related pain, and it had transformed Jill's life. I asked if she would consider changing oncologists, but she hesitated, 'I don't want to upset him. I think it would make him angry.'

I suggested seeing a psychologist for stress management. Jill readily agreed, and after a few visits, she returned, feeling more positive. She asked for a referral to a new oncologist known for being open to discussions about natural therapies. It was heartening to see her confidently prioritising her own needs rather than fearing the ego and judgement of a medical specialist.

## UNDERSTANDING THE PATHOLOGY REPORT

After surgery or biopsy, a tissue diagnosis helps the oncology team plan treatment. This diagnosis assesses the cancer's response to hormones, such as oestrogen and progesterone, and is reported as ER positive or negative, and PR positive or negative. Another receptor analysed is the HER2 receptor status, which can indicate whether the cancer is more aggressive and may respond better to targeted therapies.

## MAKING IMPORTANT DECISIONS

When making decisions about treatment, it's essential to have all the information you need. Some women prefer to be fully informed, while others rely on their medical team to guide them. Both approaches are valid, but make sure your team aligns with your needs.

## ASKING FOR HELP

Talk to your healthcare team about how you're coping. It can be helpful to speak with a counsellor from a breast cancer support group, many of whom are cancer survivors themselves. These support services often offer practical advice, like using cold caps during chemotherapy to reduce hair loss.

## FOR YOUR SUPPORT PEOPLE TO READ

If you are supporting someone with a breast cancer diagnosis, it's important to have conversations about the need for them to become 'self-centred' as they navigate this challenging journey. Many women are natural caregivers, often prioritising their needs of others. However, during cancer treatment, they must shift that focus inward.

Being self-centred in this context isn't selfish; it's about recognising that their wellbeing is paramount which is self-care. This shift is vital for enduring and recovering from all treatments. By prioritising self-care, women can better manage the side effects of treatment, reduce stress, and improve their quality of life.

## SELF-CARE

If you've been diagnosed with breast cancer, embracing self-care means:

- Prioritising health appointments and treatments: Attend all appointments and follow your treatment plan.

- Delegate household tasks: Ask loved ones and friends for help to conserve your energy.

- Listening to your body: Recognise when you need rest, nutrition, or exercise. Don't push yourself beyond your limits; allow yourself time to recover.

- Surround yourself with positivity: Engage in activities that bring you joy.

- Nutrition: Eat a balanced, nutrient-rich diet to support your immune system and overall health.

- Stay active: As recommended by your healthcare provider.

- Setting boundaries: Ensure your needs are met first. It's okay to say no to additional responsibilities and take time off work.

> **TIP**
> Putting yourself first during this time is a vital part of your healing process.

> **THE POWER OF A SIMPLE SEED**
> Animal studies showed that 30 g of flaxseeds daily, combined with the oestrogen-blocking medication Tamoxifen reduced breast cancer tumour size more than Tamoxifen alone. Additionally, women who regularly include flaxseeds in their diet have a lower incidence of breast cancer.

### ORGANIC FOOD AND BREAST CANCER RISK

Although not enough high-quality studies have conclusively linked organic food consumption with a reduced risk of breast cancer, what we do know points toward caution. Conventionally farmed foods often carry higher pesticide residues, including organophosphates and glyphosate, an ingredient in common home herbicides freely used around the garden! Research has raised concerns about these chemicals due to their potential to disrupt hormonal functions. For instance, glyphosate has been shown in some lab studies to promote the growth of hormone-sensitive breast cancer cells under specific conditions.

Additionally, an Ethiopian study also highlighted a significant connection between organophosphate exposure and breast cancer in Ethiopian women.

> **TIP**
>
> With all these clues, based on current science the safer option is to choose organic where possible. This seems like a practical approach while the science catches up to common sense. When organic choices are limited, focus on low-pesticide foods to reduce exposure. (See Core Food Principle Number 2 on page 405 for more tips on clean food.)

## NAVIGATING CHEMOTHERAPY WITH OMEGA-3 SUPPLEMENTS

Omega-3 PUFA supplements are a safe and powerful addition to conventional cancer treatments, promoting a more manageable and supportive recovery:

- Omega-3s have been shown to minimise chemo side effects help reduce pain, improve appetite, and decrease weight loss during chemotherapy.

- They reduce the risk of cancer recurrence: they play a role in reducing cancer cell proliferation and inflammation, improving overall survival rates.

- Research has shown that omega-3 PUFA supplementation, when used alongside chemotherapy and radiotherapy, can significantly enhance treatment outcomes by reducing tumour growth.

## MAKING HEALTHIER DIETARY CHOICES

### EXCLUDE FROM YOUR DIET:

**Sugar:** Added sugar and processed foods are demons that can sabotage a healthy recovery from cancer.

> **TIP**
>
> To avoid temptation when faced with sugary treats, always have a healthy alternative snack handy to temper that sugar craving, and remember:
>
> Nothing tastes as good as healthy feels.

**Alcohol:** As your body focuses on healing, avoid anything that puts an extra inflammatory load on your system. Alcohol breaks down to both sugar and a chemical called acetaldehyde; neither are good for your recovery process.

### INCLUDE PHYTOESTROGEN FOODS

Historically, women with breast cancer were advised to avoid phytoestrogen-rich foods, such as soy, due to their oestrogen-like properties. However, there is now abundant evidence on the benefits of natural therapies and food-based supplements like phytoestrogens for women who have a history of breast cancer. This benefit extends to those women who have an oestrogen sensitive (ER-positive) type of breast cancer. It's important to consult your health care team to tailor your diet to your specific needs and recovery plan.

This well-rounded approach to nutrition, coupled with your medical treatment, can greatly support your recovery and long-term health.

## TAMOXIFEN

It's a proven fact that oestrogen-modulating drugs, like Tamoxifen, reduce the risk of recurrent breast cancer and significantly improve long-term survival rates.

The Early Breast Cancer Trialists' Collaborative Group, based in Oxford, UK, found that women with ER-positive breast cancer who take Tamoxifen have a five-year survival rate of 76%, compared to 67% for those who did not take the drug.

### NEW RESEARCH ON TAMOXIFEN

As of February 2024, a new meta-analysis, co-directed by researchers from the Johns Hopkins Kimmel Cancer Centre, has reinforced the effectiveness of tamoxifen in extending survival for women with ER-positive breast cancer. This study further strengthens the case for using tamoxifen as a key treatment in reducing recurrence and improving survival rates.

### THE POWER OF NUTRIENTS IN BREAST CARE

Nutrients and lifestyle interventions can offer complementary support alongside conventional hormone treatments like tamoxifen.

Research collaboration with Australia, Denmark, England and Norway showed:

> **Women with ER-positive breast cancer who have a high isoflavone diet (at least 60 mg of isoflavones per day) have a five-year survival rate of about 84%, compared to 67% for those with a low isoflavone intake.**

Dr Karen says, 'Although it wasn't clarified in the published summaries of the research, I took a deep dive into the full journal article and found that around 75% of women with oestrogen positive breast cancer in the studies were also taking Tamoxifen. This study highlights the power of choosing the best of both worlds unless intolerable side effects limit choices.'

> **TIP**
>
> This study also reassures women who suffer the unbearable side effects of oestrogen-blocking drugs that impact their daily lives, who decide to stop taking the medication and lean into nutritional support. In these situations, it's even more crucial to embrace nutritional and lifestyle options that have been shown to boost survival after a breast cancer diagnosis.

## MOVEMENT AND EXERCISE DURING CHEMOTHERAPY— THE FACTS

The fatigue and brain fog (referred to in the business as 'chemo brain') is the collateral damage of chemotherapy's killing effect on the faster growing cancer cells. As counter-intuitive as it may sound, gathering a little strength for exercise can help you with the day-to-day side effects of chemo.

Staying active despite your symptoms is powerfully motivating when you consider the research. These findings come from long-term studies tracking physical activity and survival outcomes in women following a breast cancer diagnosis.

- Exercise acts as a potent 'metabolic shield', helping to prevent cancer progression by improving immune function, regulating hormones, enhancing circulation, reducing inflammation, and supporting a healthy weight.

- Exercising during acute breast cancer treatment improves survival chances by 55%.

- Women who maintain regular exercise after treatment see an even more impressive 68% increase in survival rates compared to those who remain inactive.

- Even though it may be the last thing you feel like when you are in the middle of chemotherapy, working with an exercise physiologist as part of your medical team can be particularly helpful.

- Personalised exercise plans have been shown to reduce fatigue, improve mental health, and enhance clinical outcomes.

- Aim for 20 to 30 minutes of activity five to six times a week, totalling around 150 minutes.

- Activities can include strength training, brisk walking, gardening or water-based exercises.

- On days when rest feels necessary, be kind to yourself and consult your exercise team.

- Even five minutes of outdoor movement can make a significant difference in how you feel.

> **TIP**
> A 2022 study revealed an astounding 73% reduction in cancer recurrence risk with just 30 minutes of exercise twice weekly. Try to commit to this as a minimum weekly goal.

## SULFORAPHANE: A SUPPLEMENT WORTH ITS WEIGHT IN GOLD

Sulforaphane, a compound found in broccoli sprouts, is emerging as a valuable supplement in the fight against breast cancer. In more aggressive forms, like triple-negative breast cancer, concentrated extracts of sulforaphane have been shown to inhibit breast cancer stem cells, which are responsible for cancer recurrence. Additionally, it can enhance chemotherapy's effectiveness by making cancer cells more susceptible to treatment. Consider using a high-quality sulforaphane supplement like Cell-Logic's EnduraCell products, available over the counter in Australia, New Zealand and the UK. Follow the prescribed dose on the package.

## BIOBRAN/RIBRAXX:
## (MGN-3) SUPPORTING YOUR IMMUNE SYSTEM NATURALLY

Biobran, also known as Ribraxx in Australia and New Zealand, is a natural compound derived from rice bran. Its active ingredient, arabinoxylan, is enzymatically modified using extracts from shiitake mushrooms, which enhances its absorption and activity in the body. What makes Biobran unique is its ability to support your immune system by boosting the activity of natural killer (NK) cells—key players in your body's defence against abnormal cells, including cancer cells. While it's not a cure for breast cancer, Biobran is often considered as a supportive option in integrative care, working alongside conventional treatments to strengthen your body's natural defences. This is considered a dietary supplement. Check with your healthcare provider to see if it's the right choice for you.

Advantages:
- Used for two decades by Swiss Oncology Clinics with impressive outcomes
- Well-researched to improve breast cancer outcomes
- No significant side effects
- Boosts immunity during chemotherapy

Drawback:
- Cost is approximately $5 per day

## MOVING FORWARD AFTER BREAST CANCER TREATMENT

Navigating breast cancer treatment is an emotional journey, remember that you are stronger than you realise. Lean on your loved ones and healthcare team for support—they are your pillars of strength. Celebrate each small victory, acknowledging your resilience and courage. Let hope and positivity guide you through, knowing that every step forward is a testament to your strength.

While the road may be challenging, it is also a reflection of your unwavering spirit and determination. Trust in yourself, cherish moments of joy, and look toward the bright future ahead. You are not just surviving; you are thriving!

> **SELF-REFLECTION—DR KAREN**
>
> In more than 30 years of caring for women with breast cancer, I've observed two distinct attitudes that emerge after a diagnosis. Some women, determined not to let cancer disrupt their lives, declare war on their illness. They push through, refusing to change their routines or slow down, often unintentionally feeding the enemy through the stress and inflammation this approach can cause. These are the patients I worry about most.
>
> On the other hand, some women view their diagnosis as a wake-up call, almost seeing cancer as a kind of teacher. These women take time to reflect on their lives, considering what might have contributed to their diagnosis, and embrace the opportunity to live with more awareness, finding more gratitude and joy in everyday moments. They become more mindful of their choices—what they eat, how they spend their time, and how they express love to those around them. They seem to accept what comes with a sense of peace and openness.
>
> These women's bodies often respond better to treatment, perhaps because, rather than waging a war from within, they are nurturing themselves from the inside out. This gentle, reflective approach seems to transform their healing journey, and I can't help but notice how their calm, inward care influences their recovery.

Our Spotlight on Breast Care (page 569) is suitable for all women, including those transitioning from breast cancer treatment. Remember, you are not alone on this journey—there are many women who have walked this path, and if you seek support there is a network of care, compassion, and strength willing to help you. However, you need to be your own best friend on this journey and ensure you take compassionate care of yourself.

# SPOTLIGHT ON
# Liver Care

The liver is a central player in maintaining overall health by detoxifying the blood, producing vital proteins, regulating blood clotting and aiding digestion through bile production.

For women, the liver holds particular importance due to its key role in hormone metabolism and regulation. Throughout the different stages of life, the liver processes and balances hormones such as oestrogen and progesterone, helping to keep hormonal fluctuations in check. The liver's ability to function even under significant stress makes it vital for sustaining hormonal wellbeing.

## THE LIVER THROUGH YOUR HORMONAL JOURNEY

### PUBERTY

During puberty, the liver is responsible for managing the dramatic hormonal changes that mark the transition from childhood to adolescence. It helps to regulate the menstrual cycle and mitigate common puberty-related issues like acne and mood swings. Additionally, the liver detoxifies various chemicals, including medications such as oral contraceptives, and drugs prescribed for acne.

## THE FERTILE YEARS

As you enter your Fertile Years, the liver continues to support hormonal balance by breaking down and removing excess hormones such as oestrogen produced during the menstrual cycle. This function is essential for preventing hormonal imbalances, which could lead to conditions like premenstrual syndrome (PMS) or endometriosis. The liver also aids in storing and releasing essential nutrients like iron and vitamin B12, helping to maintain the energy and stamina needed for daily activities and, potentially, pregnancy.

## PERIMENOPAUSE

Hormonal fluctuations become more pronounced during perimenopause as the body prepares for menopause. The liver's role in metabolising hormones is critical during this stage, helping to alleviate symptoms such as hot flushes, night sweats, and mood swings. Efficient liver function can also assist with weight management and reduce the risk of metabolic disorders that may arise from these hormonal shifts. However, the liver may become vulnerable to conditions like fatty liver, often a sign of excessive stress on the organ due to an inflammatory diet, insulin resistance or a lack of antioxidants to counter rising cellular stress.

## MENOPAUSE

As you transition into menopause and oestrogen levels naturally decline, your liver metabolises any remaining hormones, including those provided by hormone replacement therapy (HRT). At this stage, the liver's workload may increase, juggling hormone metabolism alongside its ongoing task of detoxifying substances like alcohol. When faced with competing priorities, your liver will always choose to eliminate harmful aldehydes from alcohol first, leading to those unwelcome night-time hot flushes after a glass of wine.

## THE AGE OF WISDOM

In this phase of life, the liver contributes to bone health by metabolising vitamin D, which is crucial for preventing osteoporosis. By continuing to support digestion and nutrient absorption through bile production, the liver ensures that women entering the Age of Wisdom can maintain good nutritional status, essential for longevity and overall wellbeing. With the increasing likelihood of prescribed medications as we age, the liver's workload may increase, often at the cost of its own cellular health as it works harder to process daily doses of drugs.

## OPTIMAL LIVER FUNCTION: WHAT YOU NEED TO KNOW

Healthy liver cells act like incredible toxic waste recycling centres, using enzymes to detoxify the body. Ideally, these enzymes stay contained within the liver cells. However, when liver cells are damaged, the cell walls break, and enzymes are released into the bloodstream. If a blood test shows elevated liver enzyme levels, it indicates damage—the higher the enzyme levels, the greater the damage to the liver.

In a perfect world, liver enzyme levels in the blood would be zero, but it's inevitable that some liver cells will get damaged as they perform their essential detoxification work. If you're on medication, you may always have some degree of liver stress, making it even more important to support optimal liver function.

## KEY LIVER ENZYMES TO WATCH

The liver enzymes routinely measured in blood tests for liver disease include:

- GGT (Gamma-glutamyl transpeptidase)
- AST (Aspartate transaminase)
- ALT (Alanine transaminase)
- ALP (Alkaline phosphatase)
- LD (Lactate dehydrogenase)

Of these enzymes, AST and GGT are the most significant indicators of liver health and will rise early in liver damage. ALP reflects the health of the bile ducts and gall bladder. When the liver experiences significant damage, all enzyme levels will start to rise.

> **TIP**
> Just because your liver function tests come back 'within normal limits' doesn't necessarily mean your liver is working at its best.

## WHEN THE LIVER STARTS TO STRUGGLE

It's common for liver enzyme levels to rise during viral infections, but this usually settles down once you're well again. To get an accurate picture of your liver health, it's best to have blood tests done when you're healthy, as this provides a true baseline of your liver's condition.

Before a formal diagnosis of liver disease, your liver might begin struggling to keep up with its detoxification duties, resulting in a variety of symptoms, such as:

- Mental sluggishness
- Fatigue
- Symptoms of oestrogen dominance
- Menstrual cycle changes
- Acne
- Irritability
- Fluid retention
- Dark circles under the eyes
- Sleep disturbances (especially waking between 2-3 am)
- Bad breath
- Coated tongue
- Excess wind or flatulence

### INTERPRETING YOUR RESULTS

If you've had liver function tests, now's the time to take a closer look at your results. What's considered 'optimal' for liver enzyme levels? A good rule of thumb is to calculate the midpoint of the reference range provided and aim for your results to fall below that midpoint.

Lower enzyme levels indicate a healthier liver. If you have past test results, use them to track changes over time. Consider recording this information in a health journal to monitor your progress as you implement strategies to support liver health. Keeping a record of your liver function provides a valuable baseline for assessing improvements and maintaining optimal wellness.

### LIVER FUNCTION TEST RESULTS TEMPLATE

| LIVER ENZYME | RANGE (U/L) | IDEAL LESS THAN: | YOUR BASELINE RESULTS | FOLLOW-UP |
|---|---|---|---|---|
| AST | 0–41 | 20 | | |
| ALT | 0–45 | 22 | | |
| GGT | 0–45 | 22 | | |
| ALP | 30–115 | 85 | | |
| LD | 80–250 | 170 | | |

## FATTY LIVER DISEASE

Fatty liver is medically referred to as non-alcoholic fatty liver disease (NAFLD). Recently, there has been a shift among medical professionals to rename it metabolic associated fatty liver disease (MAFLD). This new terminology emphasises the role of metabolic factors—such as obesity, insulin resistance and Type 2 diabetes—in the development of the condition. The change aims to more accurately reflect that fatty liver disease is often linked to metabolic health issues rather than alcohol consumption. Fatty liver occurs when fat builds up within liver tissue, surrounding cells where it doesn't belong. This condition is often identified after blood tests show elevated liver enzyme levels, but it can be tricky to detect. More than half of women with polycystic ovary syndrome (PCOS) are affected by fatty liver. However, up to 80% of women with fatty liver will still have normal liver function test results, meaning the condition may go unnoticed for years. The more reliable way to diagnose fatty liver is with a liver ultrasound.

Recent research points to high body weight and insulin resistance as primary drivers of fatty liver in individuals who don't drink excessively. If your liver function tests show elevated enzyme levels, it's crucial to consult your doctor to rule out serious causes of liver inflammation. Once other concerns are ruled out, the following plan can help guide you in improving your liver health and lowering those enzyme levels.

### DR KAREN

While fatty liver is often considered irreversible, I have seen significant improvements—and even normalisation of liver function tests—with natural support, lifestyle changes and targeted herbal treatments. Early intervention is key, as untreated fatty liver can progress to fibrosis or cirrhosis, even in those who don't consume alcohol.

## WELLNESS ACTION PLAN
# LIVER SUPPORT

### LIVER HELP

There are several natural remedies, and lifestyle changes you can consider:

- **St Mary's Thistle (silymarin extract)**: Try Legalon from Flordis (one tablet twice daily). This herb is also available as a liquid herbal extract from naturopaths.

- **Turmeric**: Add turmeric to your meals—just a little helps, but more is even better! You may also consider taking a turmeric/curcumin extract (500mg twice daily).

- **Stop alcohol**: Take a minimum four-week break from alcohol. If your liver function tests are out of range, consider stopping altogether, except for the occasional celebration.

- **Limit alcohol**: Reevaluate your long-term relationship with alcohol and aim to cap intake at three standard drinks per week.

- **Dandelion root tea**: Incorporate this into your routine for added liver support.

- **N-acetyl cysteine (NAC)**: For those with medically challenged liver function, consider a six-week course of NAC (2 g twice daily). Avoid if you have a history of kidney stones.

- **Increase cruciferous vegetables**: Add more broccoli, Brussel sprouts and leafy greens to your diet to support detoxification.

- **Choline-rich foods**: Ensure you're eating foods rich in choline, such as eggs, grains, cereals, and legumes.

- **Sulforaphane**: Derived from activated broccoli sprout powder, try CELL-LOGIC EnduraCell BioActive Caps (2-4 per day, providing 1400-2800 mg daily, taken twice daily).

- **Herbal support**: Experienced herbalists and naturopaths can create a tailored liver support blend based on your individual health history. We also recommend Liver Love made by Bio Blends by Dr Libby.

- **Manage insulin resistance:** See our Spotlight on Insulin Resistance on page 564.

## SUPPORTING LIVER HEALTH THROUGHOUT YOUR HORMONAL JOURNEY

As you navigate the stages of your hormonal journey—from puberty to the Age of Wisdom—supporting your liver becomes increasingly important. Your diet, removing toxins, regular physical activity, managing stress, and ensuring adequate sleep all help support liver function by promoting overall metabolic balance. Supplements and herbs such as milk thistle, turmeric, and dandelion root can provide additional assistance, but be sure to consult your healthcare provider before adding them to your regimen.

As you enter the Age of Wisdom, continuing these practices will help maintain optimal liver function, which plays a crucial role in hormone regulation and overall wellbeing throughout the rest of your life.

# SPOTLIGHT ON
# Thyroid

### THYROID AND PROGESTERONE: MARRIED FOR LIFE
#### NOTE: THIS CHAPTER IS VERY, VERY IMPORTANT!

When it comes to thyroid health in a woman's hormonal journey, it's crucial to highlight the vital partnership between the thyroid and another key hormone: progesterone. Together, these hormones can mean the difference between vibrant energy and hormonal wellness or the daily struggle of feeling out of sync.

### YOUR THYROID: THE BODY'S THERMOSTAT

The thyroid gland, a small butterfly-shaped structure in the front of your neck, just below the Adam's apple, is central to your body's energy regulation. It produces two key hormones, T3 (triiodothyronine) and T4 (thyroxine), that communicate with your brain to maintain hormonal balance. To be well, your body must convert T4 into the active form T3.

## WHAT DOES YOUR THYROID DO?

The thyroid is your body's energy powerhouse, controlling metabolism, heart rate, body temperature, and digestive efficiency. It's also deeply involved in menstrual cycles, cholesterol regulation, bowel movements and skin hydration—playing a role in almost every system that keeps you feeling vibrant.

A healthy thyroid is key to mental clarity and mood stability. When it isn't functioning optimally, symptoms like fatigue, weight fluctuations, mood swings, and disrupted menstrual cycles can surface.

## THYROID-BRAIN COMMUNICATION

The thyroid and brain maintain a constant dialogue. The pituitary gland releases thyroid stimulating hormone (TSH) to signal the thyroid to produce T3 and T4. This feedback loop ensures balance: when T4 levels rise, TSH decreases; when T4 drops, TSH increases to boost production.

This balance is why TSH levels are often the focus of thyroid function tests. High TSH can indicate low T4 levels (hypothyroidism), while low TSH suggests hyperthyroidism (overactive thyroid).

Symptoms of an underactive thyroid in women (hypothyroidism):

- Unexplained weight gain or difficulty losing weight
- Persistent tiredness or lack of energy
- Increased sensitivity to cold
- Dry, coarse skin and brittle hair or hair loss
- Constipation
- Irregular, heavy or more frequent periods
- Muscle weakness, cramps, or aches
- Low mood, depression, or lethargy
- Memory or concentration difficulties
- A hoarse or raspy voice
- High cholesterol that doesn't respond to diet or medication
- Swelling or puffiness in the face, especially around the eyes
- Joint stiffness, swelling or pain.

Common symptoms of an overactive thyroid in women (hyperthyroidism):

- Unexplained weight loss despite an increased appetite
- Rapid heartbeat or palpitations
- Excessive sweating and heat sensitivity
- Anxiety, nervousness or irritability
- Slight shaking, particularly in hands and fingers
- Irregular or lighter menstrual periods
- Muscle weakness, especially in the thighs and upper arms
- Fatigue and sleep disturbances
- More frequent bowel movements or diarrhoea
- Thin or brittle hair
- Bulging eyes, dryness, irritation, or vision issues
- Noticeable swelling at the base of the neck (goitre).

Understanding the role of the thyroid in your overall health is a critical part of maintaining hormonal balance. Not only is the thyroid gland in constant communication with your brain to ensure that metabolic support is 'just right', but healthy thyroid function also depends on a balanced dose of both oestrogen and progesterone. It's not surprising, then, that there are key moments in a woman's hormonal journey when the perfect balance of your thyroid can be disrupted.

## THE ROCKY MARRIAGE OF THYROID AND PROGESTERONE THROUGHOUT YOUR HORMONAL JOURNEY

Thyroid and progesterone have a deeply intertwined relationship. From puberty to the Age of Wisdom, at every stage, there's a new twist that can make you stop and wonder, 'What's happening to my body now?!'

## PUBERTY

Remember those teenage years when everything seemed to be changing at once? Well, your thyroid remembers too. The surge in oestrogen and a sluggish start to progesterone can disrupt thyroid function. Oestrogen increases thyroid-binding globulin (TBG), a protein that carries thyroid hormones, reducing the availability of free thyroid hormones and causing fluctuations in thyroid balance.

For some girls, these changes may trigger autoimmune activity, like Graves' disease that causes an overactive thyroid, as the immune system responds to the hormonal shifts.

Girls can develop Graves' disease as young as 10 years old, particularly during puberty when hormonal fluctuations are at their peak. This then means a lifelong monitoring of thyroid health. If your child is diagnosed, it's best to consult with a paediatrician for proper management.

> **WHAT'S AUTOIMMUNE DISEASE?**
>
> Autoimmune diseases occur when your immune system, which usually protects you from infections, mistakenly attacks healthy cells. These diseases can be influenced by genetics and often run in families, presenting as an 'autoimmune cluster' in your family history.
>
> Epigenetic triggers such as stress, infections, certain foods (like gluten), environmental exposures and hormones—can activate these unhelpful genes, acting as catalysts in the autoimmune process.

## THE FERTILE YEARS

In your 20s and 30s, your thyroid is working overtime to support everything from menstrual cycles to pregnancies, or even the effects of birth control—all of which impact thyroid function.

Your menstrual cycle relies on steady thyroid hormone production. Too little thyroid hormone can lead to heavy or irregular periods, while too much can cause lighter or absent periods. During pregnancy, the demand for thyroid hormones increases to support both your metabolic health and your baby's development.

> **AN UNWELCOME BABY GIFT: POSTNATAL THYROIDITIS**
>
> Pregnancy brings changes that suppress autoimmune diseases (a gift during pregnancy), but after childbirth, your immune system reverts, sometimes triggering postpartum thyroiditis. This condition presents in two phases:
>
> 1. The overactive (hyperthyroid) phase: Occurs within the first few months after delivery, making you feel anxious, irritable or even experience weight loss and heart palpitations.
>
> 2. The underactive (hypothyroid) phase: Several months later, you might swing to the opposite extreme, feeling sluggish, gaining weight, and becoming more prone to depression. In most cases, this phase resolves on its own, however some women may require temporary thyroid hormone therapy.
>
> To make a full recovery, it's essential to check thyroid and iron levels, as iron deficiency can slow down recovery. Nourishing the thyroid with proper care is key to bouncing back. (More on this in the Wellness Action Plan to follow.)

### PERIMENOPAUSE

Perimenopause, often marked by fluctuating oestrogen and progesterone, can wreak havoc on thyroid function. As progesterone levels drop, you're more prone to developing thyroid issues. Autoimmune thyroid conditions may also flare up during this time.

### MENOPAUSE

With menopause comes a significant drop in oestrogen and progesterone, impacting thyroid function, causing fatigue, weight gain, and constipation. Although related to a slowing of thyroid support for your metabolism, this may not show up on standard thyroid testing.

### THE AGE OF WISDOM

As you enter your 60s and beyond, the decline in oestrogen can trigger thyroid issues like Hashimoto's thyroiditis, an autoimmune condition that slows thyroid function. Regular thyroid checks become important to monitor any changes.

### PROGESTERONE AND THYROID: A CRUCIAL PARTNERSHIP

If you've ever ticked all the boxes for an underactive thyroid—fatigue, weight gain, mood changes—only to have your doctor tell you your thyroid tests are normal, you're not alone. This often happens because mainstream medicine tends to overlook the intricate relationship between progesterone and thyroid hormones. Understanding this connection is key to addressing symptoms that don't show up in standard lab results.

Here's how these hormones interact:

1. **Progesterone enhances thyroid sensitivity**: When progesterone levels are optimal, your body can better utilise thyroid hormones.

2. **Progesterone lowers thyroid-binding globulin (TBG)**: Your oestrogen boosts the production of TBG. When thyroid hormone is attached to TBG it becomes inactive and can't enter the cell. Progesterone comes along and lowers the total amount of TBG in your blood releasing your thyroid hormone, now able to enter cells and be active.

3. **Progesterone supports thyroid hormone production**: It increases the efficiency of an enzyme crucial for making thyroid hormones T3 and T4.

## WHY MOST DOCTORS MISS PERIMENOPAUSE-RELATED THYROID ISSUES

There are three main reasons why your thyroid may not work well.

### 1  Loss of progesterone support

Traditional tests like TSH may not capture thyroid inefficiency (a blocked thyroid messaging) caused by a loss of progesterone support, especially moving into perimenopause and beyond. This leaves many women with untreated symptoms and no clear answers. Understanding this connection is essential to uncovering the real cause of those 'normal' test results that don't match how you feel.

The good news? Your body likely needs progesterone rather than thyroid medication; however, this understanding is not yet mainstream. This is why keeping records of your thyroid test results can be a lifesaver.

### 2  The screening test is faulty

Standard thyroid tests for TSH (Thyroid Stimulating Hormone) often miss subtle issues. By perimenopause, even small shifts within the 'normal' range can cause symptoms of an underactive thyroid. While the diagnostic range for an underactive thyroid is typically above 4.5 mIU/L, the wellness 'sweet spot' for some women is when their TSH sits below 2 mIU/L.

> **TIP**
>
> Focussing on outcomes rather than numbers on a page will go a long way toward helping women get support for their underlying thyroid dysfunction. If you've struggled to get proper treatment, point your doctor to research published in the *Canadian Medical Association Journal*. They recommend treating women with TSH levels higher than 2.0 mIU/L as potentially hypothyroid.

### 3   You may have a high level of reverse T3

Reverse T3 (rT3) is like the 'mirror image' of the active thyroid hormone T3. While T3 keeps your metabolism running efficiently, rT3 acts more like a brake, slowing things down. This happens because rT3 is biologically inactive—it blocks the T3 docking site (receptor) on the cell membrane and it can't stimulate your cells the way T3 does.

When your body is under stress, sick or lacking nutrients, you will often convert more T4 (the thyroid hormone precursor) into reverse T3 instead of active T3. This shift is your body's way of conserving energy and is a cortisol-driven response during survival times. However, if rT3 levels stay too high for too long, it can disrupt your thyroid function and leave you feeling tired, sluggish or struggling with other low thyroid symptoms.

> **TIP**
>
> The remedy for high reverse T3 is stress management—the herb withania can also help to reduce cortisol.

The body thrives on balance—too much or too little thyroid hormone can have consequences. Prolonged elevated thyroid hormone levels, even slightly above normal, can strain the heart, so caution is called for—so is common sense and a knowledge of basic biochemistry.

CASE STUDY | DR KAREN

# Monica

## A thyroid health journey and the importance of a health journal

Monica had always been diligent about tracking her health, especially her thyroid—a habit a encouraged by her mother, who was diagnosed with an underactive thyroid after menopause. When Monica came to see me at 48, she suspected menopause was on the horizon and wanted guidance on her shifting hormones. Her dedication to journaling, which she started at 16 after a routine thyroid check, gave us insights into the connection between progesterone and thyroid health. Here are some highlights from her journal.

### THYROID JOURNAL

#### JOURNAL ENTRY 1988: AGE 16—TSH 0.7
Feeling well, general check-up.

'Mum had me go to the doctor today for my results from my thyroid check-up. She says I should keep track of how I feel, especially because both she and Grandma had thyroid problems later in life. The doctor said everything looks fine.'

Dr Karen's comment: This was Monica's baseline TSH level during her teenage years—a healthy 0.7 mIU/L, reflecting optimal thyroid function. Monica's thyroid is running efficiently, and her hormones are balanced.

#### 1992: AGE 20—TSH 2.7
Feeling tired, hormones crazy. Uni life is so stressful!

Dr Karen's comment: Monica's TSH levels rose to 2.7, reflecting a thyroid under strain. The stress of a fast-paced lifestyle had clearly taken a toll. While still within the medical 'normal' range, this was a noticeable shift from her healthier baseline. A drop in progesterone levels further affected her overall wellbeing.

### 2001: AGE 29—TSH 1.8
Prenatal check—been looking after myself

Dr Karen's comment: Monica was now preparing for pregnancy, having embraced lifestyle changes to reduce stress and prioritise self-care. Her TSH levels had decreased, signalling that her thyroid was functioning more efficiently. With her body aligning for conception, her commitment to healthier habits was clearly paying off.

### 2002: AGE 30—TSH 1.9
Pregnant—only three months to go!

Dr Karen's comment: At this stage, Monica's balanced fertility hormones supported her thyroid, keeping her TSH levels stable throughout pregnancy. While not as low as in her teenage years, her results showed good thyroid function, with progesterone and thyroid hormones working in harmony again.

### JANUARY 2003: TSH 0.02
My neck is sore! Doc says it's thyroiditis

Dr Karen's comment: Monica was diagnosed with postnatal thyroiditis, a common autoimmune condition following childbirth. Her TSH levels plummeted to 0.02, indicating hyperthyroidism (overactive thyroid).

### MARCH 2003: TSH 4.9
What's happening—baby brain? Can't get out of bed?

Dr Karen's comment: Monica's thyroid swung to the opposite extreme, now showing hypothyroidism (underactive thyroid). With a TSH level of 4.9, her body was struggling, leading to fatigue, sluggishness, and amplifying the effects of the notorious baby brain.

### JULY 2003: TSH 2.4
Feeling better—back to normal

Dr Karen's comment: After the turbulent postpartum phase, Monica's thyroid stabilised at a TSH of 2.4. Though higher than her teenage levels, this became her new 'normal'. Over the next decade, her TSH fluctuated a little, often mirroring the stressful periods in her life.

**MAY 2018: AGE 46—TSH 4.8**
Wow—Doc says underactive thyroid. Hope the meds help!

'Today I met with Dr Karen to check my hormones, as I think menopause is just around the corner. I've also been monitoring my thyroid due to low energy and mood changes. Dr Karen recommended further testing for thyroid and progesterone levels. I'm so grateful for my journal—it's helped me spot patterns and advocate for my health.'

Dr Karen's comment: By 46, Monica was navigating the challenges of perimenopause. Her progesterone levels had dropped significantly, straining the balance between her hormones and thyroid. Her TSH levels signalled a thyroid under stress, further impacted by the hormonal turbulence of perimenopause.

**REFLECTION ON MONICA'S JOURNEY**

Monica's story underscores the power of keeping a health journal. By tracking her symptoms, thyroid function, and hormonal changes over the years, her journal identified subtle shifts in her thyroid health, and its delicate connection with progesterone. From early warning signs in her twenties to the impacts of pregnancy, postnatal thyroiditis, and perimenopause, her journal provided invaluable insights that allowed her to proactively manage her health.

Monica's DUTCH hormone test showed nearly non-existent progesterone levels. (See page 168 for details on this method of assessing your hormones.) She started bioidentical progesterone troches (lozenges) and noticed significant improvements in body weight, mood and libido.

For women, especially those with a family history of thyroid or hormonal imbalances, maintaining a health journal is a vital tool. It helps establish a baseline, monitor fluctuations over time, and provides essential information for you and your healthcare provider to make informed decisions. Monica's proactive approach highlights how this simple practice can support balance and wellbeing through every stage of life.

## WELLNESS ACTION PLAN
# THYROID SUPPORT

Monica's journey had a happy ending, these are the steps we took to support her thyroid.

### THYROID ULTRASOUND IMAGING
#### ULTRASOUND IS THE BEST WAY TO VIEW YOUR THYROID

This checks the health of your thyroid gland, helping you and your doctor to formulate a thyroid support plan.

### TIP

If you're taking thyroid hormone replacement but not feeling the benefits, and your ultrasound shows mostly healthy thyroid tissue (like Monica's), low progesterone might be the missing piece. With optimal progesterone and stress management support, it may be possible to reduce or even stop thyroid medication, under the supervision of your doctor.

### LAB TESTING

Check for these thyroid-supporting nutrients:
- Vitamin D
- Zinc
- Iron stores (iron is essential to convert T4 into the active hormone T3)
- Morning urinary iodine test

Full thyroid panel:
- T3, T4, TSH
- Consider testing for Reverse T3: The cost for this is around $80
- Fertility hormones: Progesterone and oestrogen. Have bloods done between Days 18 and 21 in puberty and the Fertile Years, and at any time if you are in menopause or beyond.

## CONSIDER BIOIDENTICAL PROGESTERONE

If your thyroid blood test is within the range, connect with a practitioner skilled in prescribing this treatment. Alternatively, your GP may be happy to write a script of Prometrium, the pharmacy form of bioidentical progesterone.

If you are still having periods, your doctor may prescribe 200 mg of progesterone for the last two weeks of your cycle—an experienced doctor can guide you here and tweak your dose. If you are in menopause or beyond then 100 mg per day from the 7th day to the end of each calendar month is a good starting dose.

## DIET TWEAKS

### THYROID SUPPORT FOODS

- Whole fats like avocados and olive oil to reduce inflammation
- Seafood and complex grains to support B-vitamin intake
- Zinc-rich foods like oysters to address her low zinc levels
- Brazil nuts to provide selenium, which is essential for thyroid function
- Tulsi herbal tea (see more about Tulsi on page 349)
- Nuts and seeds for magnesium and manganese

### SUPPLEMENTS

Supplement these nutrients if low on testing or diet review:
- Vitamin D: for an optimal range of 100-150 mmol/L
- Omega-3 oils: four capsules a day (2000 mg morning and evening) to reduce inflammation

> **TIP**
> Seaweed-based food can help optimise iodine. Avoid these foods if you have a history of Graves or an overactive thyroid.

### HERBAL SUPPORT

- Withania (ashwagandha) to reduce cortisol, improves sleep.

## POSTSCRIPT: BE THE KEEPER OF YOUR HEALTH STORY

After following her Wellness Action Plan for eight weeks, Monica was able to stop her thyroid medication. Six weeks later, her TSH had settled at a healthier 2.0. More importantly, her energy returned, her sleep improved, and her abdominal fat began to decrease.

> **TIP**
>
> Keeping a health journal is recommended—ask your doctor for your results, they belong to you and understanding them can empower you to take control of your health, unless there are significant mental health issues that would be triggered by your results, and that is an exceeding rare situation).

# If you request your lab results and face resistance, it might be time to find a different doctor to join your medical support team.

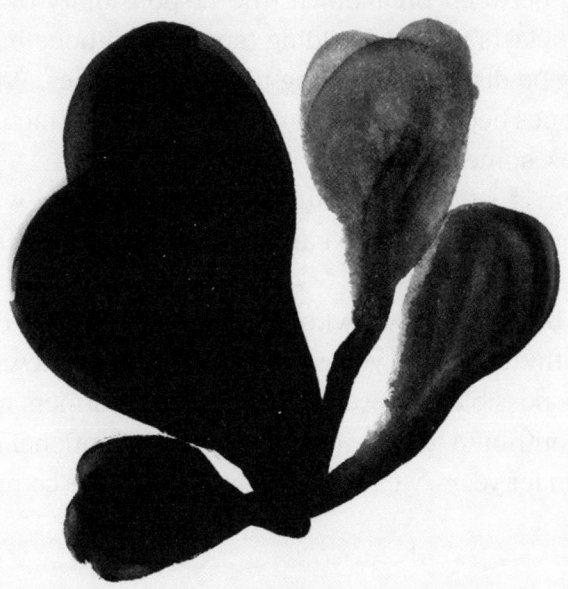

# SPOTLIGHT ON
# Bone Care

**WHY BONE DENSITY MATTERS**

Your bones are living tissue, constantly being broken down and rebuilt. As you age, the balance between breakdown (the responsibility of specialised bone cells called 'osteoclasts') and rebuilding (specialised bone-builder cells called 'osteoblasts') can be disrupted, leading to thinning bones. When bone density decreases, the bones become weaker and more prone to fractures, especially in areas like the hips, spine and wrists.

The problem is osteoporosis often progresses silently, without symptoms, until a fracture occurs. That's why early detection and proactive management are critical.

Have you been diagnosed with low bone density? Or perhaps you want to maintain healthy bones as you age? First, the good news: osteoporosis is reversible! Yes, it's possible, however it requires a commitment to piecing together the factors that contribute to bone health. While conventional medicine focused mainly on calcium for years, we now know it's much more complex than that.

## WHAT IS OSTEOPOROSIS?

Understanding the terms doctors use when discussing low bone density is key to tackling the condition. There are three main terms used to describe the strength of your bones:

- **Low bone density**: This is a general term that might be mentioned after an X-ray done for another reason (like an injury or chest X-ray), where the radiologist comments that the bones appear translucent, indicating low bone density. This clue suggests you should pursue a DEXA bone density scan to assess the health of your bones.

- **Osteopenia**: This term describes bone density results that aren't optimal for your age and increase the risk of future fractures, but don't meet the criteria for full-blown osteoporosis.

- **Osteoporosis**: This is a more severe diagnosis indicating that bone density has decreased significantly, putting you at a higher risk for fractures. It is diagnosed based on a DEXA scan, which measures bone density and generates two key scores:

    - **Z-score**: Compares your bone density to women of your own age.
    - **T-score**: Compares your bone density to that of a healthy 20-year-old woman.

The sliding scale of these scores helps determine if you have healthy bones, osteopenia or osteoporosis.

## MOVING BEYOND CALCIUM

Strong bones rely on more than just calcium intake—these key factors all play a role:

- **Vitamin D** helps your body absorb and use calcium effectively.
- **Magnesium** activates vitamin D and supports bone formation.
- **Vitamin K2** directs calcium into bones and away from arteries.
- **Protein** supports bone structure and repair.
- **Weight-bearing exercise** stimulates bone growth and strength.

Together, these factors reduce the risk of fractures and osteoporosis.

## OSTEOPOROSIS

This is a diagnosis based solely on your DEXA bone density T-score, which we will explain soon. In general terms, osteoporosis is a loss of the support mineral matrix of bone which results in a brittleness and increased risk of fracture.

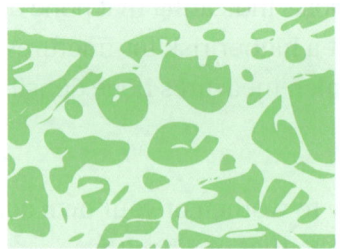

**NORMAL BONE WITH STRONG MATRIX**

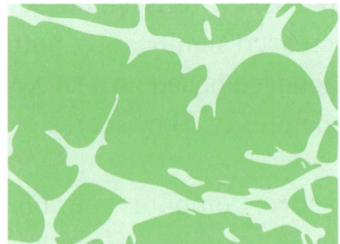

**OSTEOPOROTIC BONE**

## INTERPRETING YOUR DEXA BONE DENSITY RESULTS

When you receive your results, it's important to understand that the data is based on statistics and uses a mathematical sliding scale to evaluate your bone health. The results help assess your current bone density, estimate your future risk of fractures, and establish a baseline for monitoring changes over time.

## UNDERSTANDING THE T-SCORE

Your T-score is the key figure in your bone density report. It compares your bone density to that of a healthy 20-year-old woman, who is considered to have peak bone health. This comparison generates your T-score, which helps determine where you stand on the bone health spectrum:

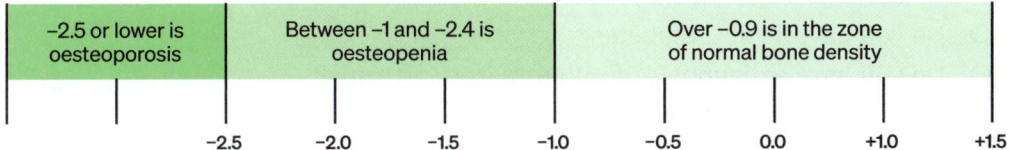

- Normal Bone Density: T-score of -1.0 or higher.
- Osteopenia (low bone density): T-score between -1.0 and -2.5.
- Osteoporosis: T-score of -2.5 or lower.

While osteoporosis is officially diagnosed when your T-score hits -2.5 or worse, it's important to note that even a T-score of -2.4 puts you at a high risk of fractures and suggests you're on the path to osteoporosis. In such cases, early intervention is crucial to prevent further bone loss and reduce the risk of fractures.

**WHY YOUR RESULTS MATTER**

Understanding your T-score helps you gauge your bone health and take steps to either maintain or improve it. Whether you're managing osteopenia or osteoporosis, proactive treatment can make a significant difference in preserving bone density and preventing fractures. Regular monitoring through DEXA or Echolight scans (more on this technology soon) will allow you and your healthcare provider to track progress and adjust your treatment plan accordingly.

**OSTEOPOROSIS RISK CHECKLIST**

Use this checklist to assess your risk of osteoporosis. Tick any risk factors that apply to you.
- ○ Have you experienced early menopause (before age 45)?
- ○ Have your periods disappeared for six months or more (excluding pregnancy)?
- ○ Do you have a history of anorexia?
- ○ Have you been told that you have low testosterone?
- ○ Do you smoke?
- ○ Do you walk less than 4000 steps per day on average?
- ○ Do you engage in endurance sports (triathlons, marathons, long-distance biking)?
- ○ Is most of your week spent indoors?
- ○ Have you ever been diagnosed with low vitamin D levels?
- ○ Check your blood test results for vitamin D and tick if your result was less than 80 units (nmol/L).
- ○ Have you lost more than 4 cm in height since your 20s?

- ○ Do you have Type 2 diabetes?
- ○ Do you have a diagnosis of inflammatory arthritis?
- ○ Are you a night-shift worker?
- ○ Do you have regularly disrupted sleep?
- ○ Have you been diagnosed with Graves' disease of the thyroid or thyroid cancer?
- ○ Have you had an overactive parathyroid gland (hyperparathyroidism)?
- ○ Do you have high cortisol levels (from chronic stress or conditions like Cushing's disease)?
- ○ Have you had chemotherapy?
- ○ Do you have muscle disease (myositis, myopathies, dystrophies)?
- ○ Do you have inflammatory bowel disease (Crohn's disease, ulcerative colitis) or coeliac disease?
- ○ Do you suffer from asthma or COPD?
- ○ Do you have darker skin pigment (which reduces access to vitamin D from sunlight)?
- ○ Have you had prolonged use of glucocorticoid (cortisone) medications for asthma or inflammatory conditions?
- ○ Do you have neurological conditions (Parkinson's disease, multiple sclerosis)?
- ○ Do you have chronic kidney or liver disease?
- ○ Are you nutrient deficient, especially in vitamin D, magnesium, calcium or trace minerals?
- ○ Do you drink carbonated cola beverages (for example, Pepsi, Coca-Cola)?
- ○ Do you drink more than two caffeinated beverages daily?
- ○ Do you take any of the following medications long-term?
  - Immune suppressants for autoimmune disorders
  - Long-term use of sleep medication, especially diazepam and zolpidem
  - Hormone blockers used in treating endometriosis or breast cancer
  - Some antidiabetic drugs (glitazones)
  - Drugs used in mental health treatment that raise prolactin hormone levels
  - Anticonvulsants for epilepsy
  - Proton pump inhibitors for gastric reflux or ulcers

**NEXT STEPS**

If you checked one or more boxes, consider sharing this self-assessment with your doctor. Taking proactive steps can help address any reversible causes of low bone density, improving your long-term bone health.

CASE STUDY | DR KAREN

# Susan
## Osteoporosis

Susan was a 39-year-old gym enthusiast, particularly fond of her weight training sessions. Like many, she believed that weight training was the key to building strong bones. However, one day, during a modest bench press session, she felt a sharp, stabbing pain shoot through her chest and back. She dropped the weights, gasping in pain, and collapsed to the floor, drenched in sweat. Her trainer immediately called an ambulance, suspecting a heart attack.

When paramedics arrived, they too thought she was experiencing a heart attack and rushed her to the coronary care unit. After a thorough cardiac workup, including blood tests, a cardiogram, and continuous heart and blood pressure monitoring, everything came back normal. The doctors even remarked that she was one of the fittest patients they'd seen in coronary care.

But the real issue came to light with a simple X-ray, revealing an osteoporotic fracture in her thoracic spine, located between her shoulder blades. This diagnosis, usually associated with the elderly, left Susan stunned. Discharged with pain medication and bisphosphonates, Susan was told by her doctor that genetics were likely to blame.

Susan couldn't understand how this had happened. She was young, active, didn't smoke, had regular periods, exercised more than most, and ate a healthy diet. The mystery of her fracture remained unsolved—until four years later, when she attended one of my workshops.

I was discussing the role of stomach acid in calcium absorption and how certain medications, particularly proton pump inhibitors (PPIs) like Somac, Nexium and Losec, can reduce stomach acid and lead to poor calcium absorption over time, increasing the risk of low bone density. At that moment, Susan had a revelation. She exclaimed, 'You've got to be kidding me?!'

She then shared her story. At 19, after a stressful year at university, Susan was diagnosed with gastritis. Her doctor prescribed a PPI drug to reduce stomach acid and prevent potential complications like cancer. She took the medication daily, feeling much better and able to enjoy meals and drinks without pain. And she kept taking it—for 20 years.

What Susan didn't know was that by suppressing her stomach acid, the medication had been blocking calcium absorption from her diet. As a result, her body had been pulling calcium from her bones to compensate, leading to her eventual fracture.

After learning this, Susan immediately stopped taking the stomach meds. Two years later, her bone density had improved significantly, and she was off all medications.

### DR KAREN

I first learned about this link between PPIs and bone fractures from a 2006 article in the *Journal of the American Medical Association* (JAMA). To this day, many medical professionals remain sceptical of this connection, but the research continues to support that long-term use of these medications can be a significant cause of bone fractures in both older men and women.

## MEDICAL CONDITIONS

If you have a medical condition like inflammatory bowel disease (such as Crohn's disease or ulcerative colitis), thyroid issues, coeliac disease or a history of anorexia, you are at an increased risk for bone fractures. Children who have been treated with large doses of inhaled or oral cortisone (prednisone) for asthma may need screening as young adults to detect early osteoporosis.

## PROGESTERONE

Women in their late 30s and early 40s often experience a drop in progesterone levels well before menopause. Progesterone plays a role in slowing the recycling of old bones, helping preserve bone density. A premature decrease in progesterone during perimenopause can accelerate bone loss.

## OESTROGEN

Early menopause is another risk factor. Oestrogen supports bone-building during a woman's pre-menopausal years, and a significant drop in oestrogen during menopause slows bone metabolism. Women who experience absent periods for six months or more, or those who use synthetic progestin contraceptives, are also at higher risk for osteoporosis as they age.

> **TIP**
> A DEXA bone density scan is recommended after five years of progestin use, and this may be eligible for a government rebate under female hypogonadism for more than six months before the age of 45.

## DIET

A poor diet, especially one high in fast foods, lacks the essential nutrients for maintaining strong bones. Consuming carbonated drinks, especially cola, can disrupt calcium-phosphorus balance, increasing the risk of osteoporosis.

## OVER-EXERCISING

Professional female athletes and women who engage in excessive exercise (four or more intense sessions per week) are at risk for osteoporosis later in life due to two main factors:

- Overtraining leads to high levels of cortisol, a hormone that breaks down tissue, including collagen, muscle, and bone.
- Overtraining can result in the loss of menstrual periods and female hormone support.

### BE AWARE

A delay in osteoporosis diagnosis often stems from a lack of awareness about risk factors. While many associate brittle bones with the elderly, bone loss begins in our 30s and accelerates after menopause. Younger people, particularly those with risk factors, can also develop osteoporosis.

Osteoporosis can drastically impact your quality of life, leading to physical changes like a thoracic spine curve (commonly known as a 'Dowager's Hump') and pain from fractures. In younger individuals, fractures often occur in the spine and can cause chronic pain, while older adults are more prone to hip fractures, which can be life-threatening. Wrist fractures are also common due to falling on an outstretched hand, which is why strong muscles are crucial— not only for improving bone density but also for preventing falls.

### IF IN DOUBT, SCAN

If you're concerned about osteoporosis, a baseline bone density scan can provide important motivation for making lifestyle changes. While government rebates may not always apply, a private DEXA scan typically costs around $250 to $300.

All women should consider a bone density assessment around menopause or earlier if they have risk factors for osteoporosis. Men with risk factors, such as low testosterone or long-term use of reflux medications, should also consider a DEXA scan.

### LOW BONE DENSITY—WHAT NOW?

Whether you've been diagnosed with low bone density or want to maintain healthy bones, review the list of risk factors (page 615) and minimise them where possible. This may involve working with your healthcare provider to review your medications or implementing tighter boundaries to support bone health.

Bone health is a dynamic process. To maintain good bone density, especially as you age, your body needs to replenish bone at the same rate it's being broken down. If you've been diagnosed with osteoporosis, replenishing bone faster than it's lost is essential.

CASE STUDY | DR KAREN

# Judith

## Supporting Bone Health

Judith, a woman in her mid-50s, came to me seeking advice on wellness after officially entering menopause. I congratulated her on her transition into the Age of Wisdom. She was in good health, active and had grown up in the cool regions of New Zealand's South Island before moving to Australia in her 30s. She had passed all her regular women's health checks—her breast imaging and Pap smears had always been normal.

During our consultation, I suggested a baseline bone density scan (DEXA) and blood tests, including vitamin D levels.

### RESULTS AND ACTION PLAN

Judith's DEXA scan revealed a worryingly low bone density score. Her T-score was -2.4—not yet osteoporosis, but close. Her Z-score, which compares her bone density to the average for her age, was -1.6. Her vitamin D levels were also below optimal, at 69 nmol/L.

We discussed her bonehealth management plan, reviewing the risks and benefits of pharmaceutical drugs for osteoporosis. Unfortunately, Judith didn't qualify for reduced-cost pharmaceuticals as she hadn't sustained two bone fractures or reached the T-score threshold of -2.5 for an official osteoporosis diagnosis. Due to financial limitations, she opted against drug therapy.

The only major risk factor we identified was her vitamin D deficiency. I advised her to aim for vitamin D levels between 100 and 150 nmol/L and gave her a list of vitamin D-rich foods, alongside starting her on supplements.

## EXPLORING ALTERNATIVE THERAPIES

Judith and I also reviewed the potential of herbal therapies, dietary adjustments, and bioidentical hormones. She declined formal hormone replacement therapy (HRT), concerned about the potential link between oestrogen and breast cancer due to a friend's diagnosis.

Instead, she was interested in red clover, a botanical that research shows can significantly improve bone density in just six months—rivalling the effects of oestrogen therapy, but without increasing breast cancer risk.

## MONITORING PROGRESS

'We agreed it was important to monitor her bone health closely. One tool I've used for over 20 years is a urine test measuring bone fragments to assess bone breakdown. We chose the N-telopeptide test, which offers early confirmation of improvements in bone breakdown rates within four months—well before a follow-up DEXA scan would be possible.'

Judith committed to our Wellness Action Plan for Bone Support (more details on page 627).

## JUDITH'S PLAN

- Dietary changes to ensure she met all nutritional needs for bone health.
- Optimising her vitamin D levels, aiming for 100–150 nmol/L.
- Taking red clover extract (80 mg daily).
- Weight training four days per week, focusing on both upper and lower body strength.

## POSITIVE RESULTS

Four months later, Judith's N-telopeptide test showed a 50% reduction in urinary bone fragments, indicating less bone breakdown. Her follow-up DEXA scan at the 12-month mark showed an improved T-score for the first time since her diagnosis.

Ten years on, as she enters her Age of Wisdom, Judith continues to thrive, feeling fit, strong, and—importantly—has dodged any bone fractures since her initial diagnosis.

> **TIP**
> Even though an early menopause promotes an extra risk for your bones, the sad fact is that for women menopause is the most common risk factor for low bone density.

## MEDICATION OPTIONS FOR LOW BONE DENSITY

Making informed decisions about treatment for low bone density is crucial, especially when aiming for prevention rather than addressing an established medical condition. Two main drug categories are used to support a diagnosis of osteopenia and osteoporosis:

- Bisphosphonates
- Denosumab, a monoclonal antibody drug.

### BISPHOSPHONATES

Common brands: Fosamax, Aclasta, and Didronel (Australia, New Zealand, UK). Initially popular in the 1990s, bisphosphonates slow bone resorption, improving DEXA T-scores. However, concerns about long-term side effects have reduced their use.

### LONG-TERM RISKS

- **Brittle bones and atypical fractures:** Prolonged use may lead to brittle, less elastic bones, causing atypical hip fractures, even without falls, which are difficult to treat.

- **Osteonecrosis of the jaw:** A rare but serious condition where the jawbone decays, often after three or more years of use.

- **Other side effects:** Nausea, vomiting, and a heart condition called atrial fibrillation.

- **2020 findings:** Studies revealed higher rates of hip fractures in women using bisphosphonates for more than five years, despite better T-scores. Current guidelines recommend limiting use to no more than five years.

### LEGAL CONCERNS

Ongoing U.S. legal proceedings allege inadequate warnings about atypical fracture risks. A Supreme Court ruling is expected in 2025.

How much benefit can you expect from 10 years on bisphosphonate drugs? These are the conclusions of the 2022 Cochrane review which assessed the effectiveness of bisphosphonates in preventing fractures among postmenopausal women with osteoporosis.

The review found that over a 10-year period, the number needed to treat (NNT) to prevent one hip fracture was approximately 100. This means that 100 women would need to be treated with bisphosphonates for 10 years to prevent one hip fracture in the group.

In other words, 99% of women will achieve no benefit by taking the drug for a decade The decision to use bisphosphonates depends on individual factors like age, bone density, and fracture history—in collaboration with your doctor, their benefit must be weighed against overall fracture risk.

### DENOSUMAB

Denosumab (brand names—Prolia, Xgeva and Wyost): A monoclonal antibody, slows down bone resorption, which in turn improves bone density scores on DEXA scans. However, there are concerns about long-term use.

### BENEFITS

- **Results:** This drug does a better job of reducing vertebral fractures:
  - treating 21 post-menopausal women for three years prevents one vertebral fracture.

- **Convenience:** A quickly administered six-monthly injection at the doctor's clinic.

### LONG TERM RISKS

- **Atypical fractures:** These can occur in the absence of trauma, like falls (as with bisphosphonates).
- **Osteonecrosis of the jaw:** Decay of the jawbone (as with bisphosphonates).
- **Low blood calcium levels:** If undetected, this accelerates bone loss.
- **immune suppression:** Increasing the risk of infection.
- **Indefinite use:** Accelerated bone loss and rapids fractures may occur if stopped. This can only be mitigated by changing over to the bisphosphonate family.

## THE REAL STORY OF BONE STRENGTH: WHY FLEXIBILITY MATTERS

Until recently, assessing your risk of future fractures has relied solely on DEXA bone density testing. When we think about bone health, we often focus on density. Here's the twist: strong bones aren't just about density; they're about flexibility too. Imagine a tree in a storm—if it's too rigid, it snaps, but if it's flexible, it bends and withstands the pressure. Your bones work the same way.

> **TIP**
>
> This is where things get tricky with osteoporosis. Many treatments focus on making bones more dense but have a side effect: they can leave bones brittle—more likely to break under stress. The scans we've traditionally relied on, like the DEXA scan, only measure bone density. They don't tell us how flexible or truly resilient your bones are.

## ECHOLIGHT SCANNING: A NEW WAY TO LOOK AT YOUR BONES

Over the past five years another testing modality for low bone density has come to the forefront in both clinical and research areas, one that is rewriting the story of bone health. This technology is called radiofrequency echographic multi spectrometry (REMS), or Echolight scanning.

This acts like a detective that uncovers what's really happening in your bones. It uses ultrasound—not X-rays—to examine both the density and quality of your bones. By analysing signals from your spine and hip, it offers a clearer picture of your fracture risk. Here's the best part: it's completely radiation-free and non-invasive.

### WHAT MAKES ECHOLIGHT SCANNING SPECIAL?

- **Accuracy**: Studies show that REMS is just as precise as DEXA for measuring bone density.

- **Predicted bone loss**: REMS doesn't just measure; it predicts.
  - In one study, it forecasted fractures up to five years in advance, making it a powerful tool for women wanting to stay ahead of bone loss.

- **Bone quality assesment**: Unlike traditional scans, REMS assesses your bone quality, the factor that tells us whether your bones are tough and flexible, or rigid and vulnerable.

**WHY THIS MATTERS**

If you've been on osteoporosis medication—or are considering it—you know the focus is often on boosting density. But many treatments don't address bone flexibility, and that's where fractures happen. Echolight scanning helps bridge this gap, giving you and your doctor a more complete understanding of your bone health so you can make smarter, more informed decisions. If you have recently been diagnosed with low bone density, then the extra information gained from Echolight can help you make decisions about treatment options.

**BONE DENSITY SUPPORT TEAM**

Bone density is a priority consideration when weighing up the benefits of commencing or continuing with Hormone Replacement Therapy (HRT). Although oestrogen is your primary bone support hormone, progesterone and testosterone also play a role.

It's essential to discuss with your doctor whether HRT or mainstream medication is the right long-term strategy for bone density support. If you're not keen on medication, proven natural therapies—combined with a nutrient-rich diet, targeted supplements and regular resistance training—can improve bone strength and restore youthful resilience to your bones. Even if you opt for mainstream medical treatments like pharmaceuticals, combining them with the strategies in our Wellness Action Plan for Bone Care that follows will yield better results.

**BORON**

Boron has been used for decades to ensure that racehorses have the best nutrition available to prevent bone injury. Veterinarians have long known that Australian soil is deficient in this essential bone nutrient. Unfortunately, most doctors appear to be unaware of this fact.

It is not recommended that women take unregulated amounts of boron as it can be toxic in large doses. Up to 3 mg per day is the safe recommended dose if taken via supplements.

## WELLNESS ACTION PLAN
# BONE CARE

Use the following ten steps to support strong and resilient bones using a combination of evidence-based strategies, including nutrition, movement, stress management and sleep. (For further insights, see Part Two Spotlights.)

### 1. VITAMIN D ASSESSMENT

- Check vitamin D levels—aim for 100-150 nmol/L for optimal bone support.
- Supplement if sun exposure and diet are insufficient (see Spotlight on Vitamins and Minerals on page 443 for more details on doses and the best form of vitamin D to take).
- Monitor vitamin D levels periodically (annually once target levels are achieved).
- Include vitamin D-rich foods like sun-fortified mushrooms, oily fish, and egg yolks.
- Sensible sun exposure (short bursts) can improve levels naturally.
- If you have low bone density, your health practitioner can check calcium and parathyroid hormones (PTH) levels for medical causes of low bone density.

> **TIP**
> Entering menopause with a vitamin D score less than 80 nmol/L has been shown to accelerate bone loss and increased the risk of osteoporosis and bone fractures.

### 2. ESSENTIAL NUTRIENT PARTNERSHIPS

- Vitamin K2 (dose 100 to 200 μg): Works with vitamin D to support bones.
- Calcium and magnesium: Maintain a 2:1 calcium-to-magnesium ratio for strong bones and muscle function. (Read more on page 462.)
- Trace minerals: Zinc, manganese, phosphorus, silica and boron play vital roles in bone health. Find food sources of these minerals starting on page 283.

> **TIP**
>
> If you prefer to get your boron from food, try enriching your home-grown produce. Simply mix 1 teaspoon of borax powder (found in the laundry aisle) with 1 litre of water and use it to water your plants, like alfalfa or bean sprouts on your windowsill. This creates boron-rich soil, allowing your plants to provide a safe, natural source of boron. Just a heads-up—don't drink the boron water directly. Let nature work its magic to deliver the right amount!

### 3. AVOID DIETARY BONE SABOTEURS

- Avoid cola-based sodas: Phosphoric acid harms bones.
- Limit caffeine to two drinks daily to avoid calcium loss. Ensure calcium intake offsets caffeine effects.

### 4. HERBS AND BOTANICALS

- Evidence supports herbs for bone health. (See our comprehensive table on page 630 for more details.)
- Consult with your health practitioner to ensure compatibility with other treatments or medications.

### 5. CORTISOL: HEALTHY LEVELS

Chronic stress accelerates bone breakdown so avoid high evening cortisol levels through proper sleep hygiene and stress management techniques. (See our Cortisol Reduction Wellness Action Plan on page 347.)

### 6. SLEEP AND BONE HEALTH

- Bone repair peaks at night, especially around 4 am.
- Prioritise sleep hygiene and consider melatonin supplementation (1 to 3 mg nightly) if sleep is disrupted.

### 7. MOVE FOR YOUR BONES

Engaging in the right type of exercise is crucial for maintaining and improving bone density and strength. According to Professor Belinda Beck, an expert in exercise physiology and osteoporosis, targeted weight-bearing and resistance exercises are key to building stronger bones.

- Targeted resistance training: Weightlifting and high-impact exercises, under professional supervision, can significantly improve bone density and reduce fracture risk.

- Supervised programs: Seek guidance from exercise physiologists or physiotherapists experienced in bone health to ensure safety and effectiveness.

### 8. REGULAR MONITORING

- Follow your health practitioner's advice for interval scanning.
- Consider an Echolight scan, which evaluates both bone density and flexibility.

### 9. ALCOHOL AND BONE HEALTH

Limit alcohol—more than three drinks per day significantly increases your risk of hip fractures. (Can we assume this may be partly due to increased falls associated with a bottle of bubbles? Ha ha).

### 10. HORMONAL SUPPORT

- Oestrogen and progesterone: Hormonal replacement therapy (HRT) slows post-menopausal bone loss.
- Testosterone: Plays a key role in bone density. Seek medical advice for tailored dosing.
- Natural progesterone may be an option if oestrogen therapy isn't suitable for you.
- Melatonin dose of 1 to 3 mg one hour before bed has a dual action to improve bone density by stimulating osteoblast activity (bone-building cells) and suppressing osteoclasts (cells that break down bone).

## HERBS AND BOTANICALS

Your Bone Health Wellness Action Plan incorporates a variety of herbs and botanicals that are backed by strong historical use and varying levels of clinical evidence. You'll find a concise summary of these botanicals on the following page, along with their evidence ratings, breast safety and recommended doses.

## HERBAL OPTIONS FOR BONE HEALTH

| | EVIDENCE | BREAST SAFE | DOSE | CLINICAL OUTCOMES |
|---|---|---|---|---|
| Red Clover (*Trifolium pratense*) | Strong | Yes | 80–150 mg of isoflavones daily | Improved bone mineral density (BMD), increased bone formation markers (osteocalcin, urinary DPYD, and N-telopeptides). |
| Soy (*Glycine max*) | Strong | Yes (may reduce breast cancer risk) | 40–110 mg of isoflavones daily | Similar to Red Clover, improves BMD and bone formation markers. |
| Black Cohosh (*Actaea racemosa*) | Medium | Yes | 40 mg daily. Caution: Rare liver inflammation; report symptoms like nausea, yellowing of the skin or dark urine. | Increases bone formation markers (osteocalcin, alkaline phosphatase). |
| Devil's Claw (*Harpagophytum procumbens*) | Strong | Yes | 600–1200 mg daily | Improves BMD, reduces bone resorption markers. |
| Veldt Grape (*Cissus quadrangularis*) | Strong | Yes | 600 mg daily | Improves BMD, decreases bone turnover markers. |
| Dried Plums (*Prunus domesticus*) | Strong | Yes | 50–100 g daily | Increases BMD, reduces bone breakdown markers. |
| Horsetail Herb (*Equisetum arvense*) | Medium | Yes | 270 mg of silica daily | Improves BMD, boosts bone formation markers. |
| Licorice (*Glycyrrhiza glabra*) | Medium | Yes | 75–150 mg glycyrrhizin daily | Increases BMD, reduces bone breakdown markers. |
| Grape Seed Extract (*Vitis vinifera*) | Medium | Yes | 150–300 mg daily | Reduces bone breakdown markers (urinary DPYD). |
| Alfalfa (*Medicago sativa*) | Traditional | Yes | 5–10 g daily | Nutrient-rich in phytoestrogens, calcium, and magnesium, and improves BMD. |

**IMPORTANT REMINDERS**

- Personalisation: You don't need to take all the herbs listed—focus on a few based on your needs and goals. Connect with a naturopath for advice on herbal tonics that include combination herbs suitable for your needs.

- Monitor interactions: Herbal remedies are potent, so be mindful of any potential herb-drug interactions. Always consult with your healthcare provider before adding these to your regimen.

By incorporating these herbs into your Bone Health Wellness Action Plan, alongside a nutritious diet, regular exercise, and lifestyle adjustments, you can significantly enhance your bone health. Keep track of your progress and consider adding or adjusting herbs based on your body's needs.

> **RED CLOVER EXTRACT AND BONE DENSITY— COMPARING APPLES TO ORANGES**
>
> A 2018 study confirmed previous research that this natural bone support was as effective as Hormone (Oestrogen) Replacement Therapy at supporting healthy bone density through menopause and beyond.

## HOW TO EXERCISE FOR BONE DENSITY

Let's go straight to the expert and look at the recommendations of Australian Professor Belinda Beck. Professor Beck who has a PhD in exercise physiology, is currently running a prospective study on the effectiveness of prevention of osteoporosis for Australians over the age of 45 years. She is an internationally respected researcher and practitioner in the exercise component of osteoporosis.

- Her research conclusions revolve around evidence that those who maintain good movement practice from their youth through to older age, maintain boss mass and dodge the osteoporosis bullet.

- She has had extensive hands-on experience of creating exercise programs to suit even the frailest of skeleton

- This involves high-intensity and impact training under specialised supervision, given that this type of exercise approach can have risks in those with already frail skeletons.

- This unique weight-lifting program is already showing impressive improvements in bone density for the participants.

- To understand what type of exercise program is best for bones, Professor Beck explains that there are four very important misconceptions that can sabotage a good bone-building exercise routine:

    1. Positive changes in bone strength and quality may not be obvious on BMD DEXA scans. That means that improving T-scores does not guarantee reduced fracture risk and conversely static T-scores in a woman who is exercising well does not mean she is failing to reduce fracture risk.

    2. Individuals with low bone density will show greater improvement in bone strength with exercise. In other words, the lower your bone density, the greater your improvement will be with targeted and supervised weight training. Clinical trials using subjects with normal bone density will be less likely to show improvement with a robust exercise routine.

    3. The importance and potential of the exercise component to reverse low bone density is grossly under-estimated as most of these trials exclude people with osteoporosis.

    4. The exercise trials in the past have not concentrated on increasing the weight load on muscles and bone—recent research shows this to be the key.

### KEEP YOUR EYE ON THE PRIZE

Like any tool to help us maintain wellbeing, you must keep your eye focused on the end game: for osteoporosis, the end game is reducing your risk of bone fractures as you age.

If you have established osteoporosis, embark on a targeted weights program only under the supervision of a trained expert who understands how to do this safely. This is often an exercise physiologist (a very under-utilised expert in the movement field) or a physiotherapist who is hands-on with you in the gym. This choice can be life-changing—strong, bigger muscles mean better bones, lower risk of falls and fractures, more confidence and a reduced risk of Type 2 diabetes.

If you have normal bone density and want to keep it that way as you move through the decades ahead, hit the gym with a trainer who can safely guide you on proper technique in weight training to support healthy bones.

### SLEEP, CIRCADIAN RHYTHM AND BONE HEALTH

Studies on shift workers, who have a potential added risk of low bone density gave researchers clues that sleep is a player in maintaining bone care. Like all biochemical processes that occur in your body, bone cells are programmed to a tight schedule of 'repair and replace' based on your circadian bio-clock. Bone building and repair occurs overnight, peaking around 4 am.

#### SOLUTIONS

- Melatonin supplementation (1 to 3 mg daily) can improve hip bone density.
- Reconsider night shift as you move toward menopause. If continued night-shift work is non-negotiable for you, be proactive about the other lifestyle choices and strategies that support good bone health.

### HORMONAL BALANCE

Have your hormones assessed by women's health expert. If the risk/benefit consideration is supportive of HRT, a combination of bioidentical oestradiol and progesterone will slow the rate of bone loss after menopause. If oestrogen is not for you, consider bioidentical progesterone supplementation. See page 179 on bioidentical hormones.)

Testosterone is also a bone density player—this hormone provides energy, drive, libido and bone density support. It's important to engage with an experienced women's health doctor for this as more testosterone is not better! Side effects usually occur when the dose exceeds your unique sweet spot. (See page 673 for our Spotlight on Testosterone.)

Emerging research highlights melatonin as a safe, long-term option for supporting bone density. If you're aged over 55, it's available over the counter at pharmacies. Otherwise, you may need to provide medical references (see our Resource section on page 691) to convince your doctor to provide a script for this natural hormone. Globally, melatonin is often sold over the counter, and in the USA, it's classified as a dietary supplement, available freely in various forms and dosages.

## KEY TAKEAWAYS

- Begin early with preventive strategies like optimising vitamin D and other bone support nutrients, avoiding bone saboteurs.

- Exercise to supports good bone density into the menopause years.

- Have your bone density checked when approaching menopause to understand your baseline.

- Reconsider night shift as you move toward menopause. If continued night-shift work is non-negotiable for you, take extra care with bone-supporting lifestyle changes.

- Consider a dedicated bone support strength training based on the Onero protocol.

- Address suboptimal bone density (osteopenia) with herbal, hormonal, or other supportive measures.

- Regularly reassess and adapt your plan based on test results, lifestyle changes or medical needs.

- When hormones start to change and periods falter, know your baseline bone density and be proactive before a medical label of low bone density applies to you.

- If bone density is suboptimal for your age (osteopenia) then look at herbal or hormonal options as add-ons to your basic nutritional and lifestyle commitments to strong bones moving forward.

**TIP**

Be proactive! Start young.

# SPOTLIGHT ON
# Brain Care

### THE DIFFERENCE BETWEEN THE COGNITIVE DECLINE OF AGEING AND DEMENTIA

Cognitive decline with ageing is a normal process where memory, attention, and problem-solving may become slower but do not significantly interfere with daily life. Dementia, on the other hand, is a progressive condition caused by nerve cell damage, often driven by inflammation and oxidative stress. It involves severe memory loss, confusion and difficulties with reasoning, language, and other mental abilities, which disrupt daily living and independence. There are different forms of dementia, the most common are Alzheimer's and vascular dementia.

### DEMENTIA AND WOMEN'S COGNITIVE HEALTH

Dementia has taken the top spot as the leading cause of death for women in both Australia and the UK. Our New Zealand sisters are faring slightly better, with dementia ranked third, behind cancer and heart disease. However, the rising trend in dementia cases is worrying as in 2014, dementia wasn't even in New Zealand's top ten causes of death.

We can't stop ageing, but research shows that several key drivers of cognitive decline can be prevented with lifestyle changes:

- Type 2 diabetes, with high blood glucose a major risk for cognitive decline
- Cardiovascular disease—especially uncontrolled high blood pressure
- Micronutrient deficiencies—despite diets high in calories
- Lifestyle habits like excessive alcohol and low physical activity.

We can't stop ageing but we know through research that all the risk factors above can be mitigated by adhering to core wellness principles. This is essential if you have a family history of dementia or cognitive decline.

> **MEDICATIONS AND DEMENTIA RISK**
>
> Some medications—particularly those with strong sedative or anticholinergic effects—have been linked to an increased risk of cognitive decline and dementia. This is especially relevant during and after the menopause transition, when hormonal changes can already impact memory and mood.
>
> Medications to be aware of include:
> - Over-the-counter sleep aids such as doxylamine (Restavit, Dozile)
> - Benzodiazepines like diazepam (Valium) and temazepam
> - Seroquel (quetiapine), used for mood or sleep issues
> - Bladder medications such as oxybutynin (Ditropan) and tolterodine.
>
> While these may be necessary in certain circumstances, they shouldn't be used long-term without regular review. If you're taking any of these, speak with your doctor about safer alternatives, dosage reduction or tapering options where appropriate.

### PUBERTY

The surge in oestrogen and testosterone reshapes the prefrontal cortex (the brain's 'CEO') which is responsible for decision-making and emotional regulation. Girls in puberty often experience heightened emotions as the brain organises its neural connections through neuroplasticity. Meanwhile, the hippocampus, responsible for memory and learning, grows rapidly.

### THE FERTILE YEARS

Oestrogen takes on a neuroprotective role, helping the brain adapt and reorganise itself. This is often when women experience peak cognitive performance. Testosterone, which peaks in women in their late 20s, also supports energy, drive, and brain function. High oestrogen levels interact with serotonin and dopamine, promoting emotional wellbeing.

### PERIMENOPAUSE

As oestrogen levels fluctuate, women experience mood swings, difficulty concentrating and sleep disturbances. These hormonal changes affect mood and cognitive function.

### MENOPAUSE—THE BIG BRAIN RESET

Two key changes occur in the brain during menopause:

1. The brain changes how it sources fuel.
2. Lower oestrogen levels make brain cells more vulnerable to inflammation.

Before menopause, the brain relies primarily on glucose for energy. However, post-menopause, hormonal shifts—particularly the drop in oestrogen—make the brain less efficient at processing glucose. This can lead to an 'energy crisis', where the brain struggles to function as well as it used to. To compensate, it begins to use ketones (derived from fatty acids stored in the liver) for fuel. However, this shift can also lead to increased inflammation, further impacting brain health.

Despite this decline, lifelong habits like continuous learning, social engagement and trying new things can support brain health and reduce the risk of cognitive decline. Testosterone also plays a role, with levels often increasing around age 70, supporting memory, problem-solving, and cognitive function.

### BRAIN HEALTH IN THE AGE OF WISDOM

If you have already transitioned to the Age of Wisdom, our Wellness Action Plan for Supporting Brain Health on page 639 is even more important for you. Now is the time to look at your lifestyle choices and tighten the boundaries to enhance your ability to navigate this stage with energy, vigour and good cognitive health.

## PRODUCTS CLINICALLY PROVEN TO SUPPORT COGNITION

Pharmaceutical options for improving cognitive health are limited, however Souvenaid, a product clinically proven to slow dementia progression, has become a valuable tool for neurologists treating early dementia. It's available over the counter at pharmacies and includes a range of ingredients beneficial for brain health.

| COMPONENT | | AMOUNT IN SOUVENAID |
|---|---|---|
| DHA | = | 1200 mg |
| EPA | = | 300 mg |
| UMP | = | 625 mg |
| Choline | = | 400 mg |
| Phospholipids | = | 106 mg |
| Folic Acid | = | 400 µg |
| Vitamin B6 | = | 1 mg |
| Vitamin B12 | = | 3 µg |
| Vitamin C | = | 80 mg |
| Vitamin E | = | 40 mg |
| Selenium | = | 60 µg |

This product is a game-changer for those already experiencing some cognitive decline or have been diagnosed with early dementia. We encourage you to research it and discuss it with your doctor. The key takeaway is that all the ingredients found in Souvenaid are also present in a healthy, plant-based diet so eat well in your early years. Essentially, this product supplements any gaps and supports a brain that may be struggling.

> **TIP**
>
> Before rushing out to buy Souvenaid, if your brain is in good shape, we suggest revisiting Spotlight on Nourishment on page 393. The research backing our Core Food Principles is rooted in studies on dementia prevention and the outstanding health of those living in the Blue Zones. The best medicine for your brain is often found right on your plate when you invest in nourishing both your body and mind.

## WELLNESS ACTION PLAN
# SUPPORTING BRAIN HEALTH

Menopause brings significant hormonal changes, especially a decrease in oestrogen, which impacts how brain cells use fuel. With this shift, brain cells become less efficient at using glucose and may increasingly rely on ketones for energy. Here are some practical strategies to support this transition.

### SUPPORTING BRAIN HEALTH DURING MENOPAUSE

Studies at Johns Hopkins Research Unit show that adapting your diet to promote ketone production can help maintain brain health.

### DIETARY ADJUSTMENTS

- **Increase healthy fats**: Despite any concerns about mid-section fat, now is not the time to skimp on healthy fats.
  - Include sources like avocados, olive oil, nuts, seeds, and fatty fish in your meals.

- **Eliminate processed carbs and sugars**: After menopause, refined sugars are particularly harmful to brain health.

- **Enjoy grains and starchy vegetables**: Don't cut these out because your body still needs the nutrients they provide.

- **Focus on low-carb vegetables**: Prioritise leafy greens, broccoli and cauliflower to support brain health.

- **Moderate protein intake**: Include lean meats, fish, eggs and legumes in your diet without over-consuming protein, which can interfere with ketosis.

- **Intermittent fasting:** Enhances ketone production and improves brain function. Two common methods are:
  - **16/8 method**: Fast for 16 hours and eat during an 8-hour window each day.
  - **5:2 method**: Eat normally for five days and reduce calorie intake on two non-consecutive days.

> **TIP**
> A plant-based diet reduces the risk of getting dementia by 53%.

### STAY PHYSICALLY ACTIVE

Exercise plays a key role in supporting brain health and promoting ketone production. Aim for a combination of:

- **Aerobic exercise**: Activities like walking, running, cycling, and swimming improve brain function.

- **Strength training**: Resistance exercises and weightlifting help maintain muscle mass and metabolic health by using glucose without relying on insulin.

- **Flexibility and balance**: Practices like yoga and Tai Chi improve circulation and reinforce healthy nerve pathways.

### INCORPORATE BRAIN-BOOSTING SUPPLEMENTS

- **Omega-3 fatty acids**: Found in fish oil, these help to reduce inflammation and support brain health.

- **Curcumin**: The active compound in turmeric, a natural anti-inflammatory food for the brain, shown to have neuroprotective properties.

### STAY HYDRATED

Drinking plenty of filtered water is essential for optimal brain function.

### REDUCE EXPOSURE TO BLUE LIGHT AT NIGHT

Recent research has discovered a strong link between this and dementia risk—more studies are underway. (See Spotlight on Sleep for tips on page 351.)

## MANAGE STRESS AND SLEEP

Both can negatively impact brain health. Revisit Spotlight on Restorative Practices on page 372 and consider embracing the following:

- **Mindfulness and meditation**
- **Sleep hygiene**: See Spotlight on Sleep on page 351.

## REDUCE OR STOP ALCOHOL

- Alcohol is a neurotoxin—it can accelerate both cognitive decline and the oxidative stress of dementia. (See Spotlight on Alcohol on page 287.)

- Your vulnerability may also depend on the efficiency of your detoxification pathways. Improve these by reviewing our Spotlight on Liver Care on page 592.

## KEEP YOUR BRAIN ACTIVE

Engage in activities that challenge and stimulate cognitive function:

- **Puzzles and games**: Try crosswords, Sudoku, or brain-training apps.
- **Learning new skills**: Pick up a new hobby or learn a new language.
- **Social interaction**: Participate in meaningful conversations and social activities.
- **Creative problem-solving**: Engage your brain in different ways—write a book, for instance!

Finally, review our Spotlight on Serotonin (page 648) as studies show that serotonin is low in those with cognitive decline. Although it's not clear if this is a cause or result, it's worthwhile supporting this wonderful mood hormone.

By adopting these strategies, you can help your brain transition to using ketones for energy, and supporting cognitive health during and after menopause.

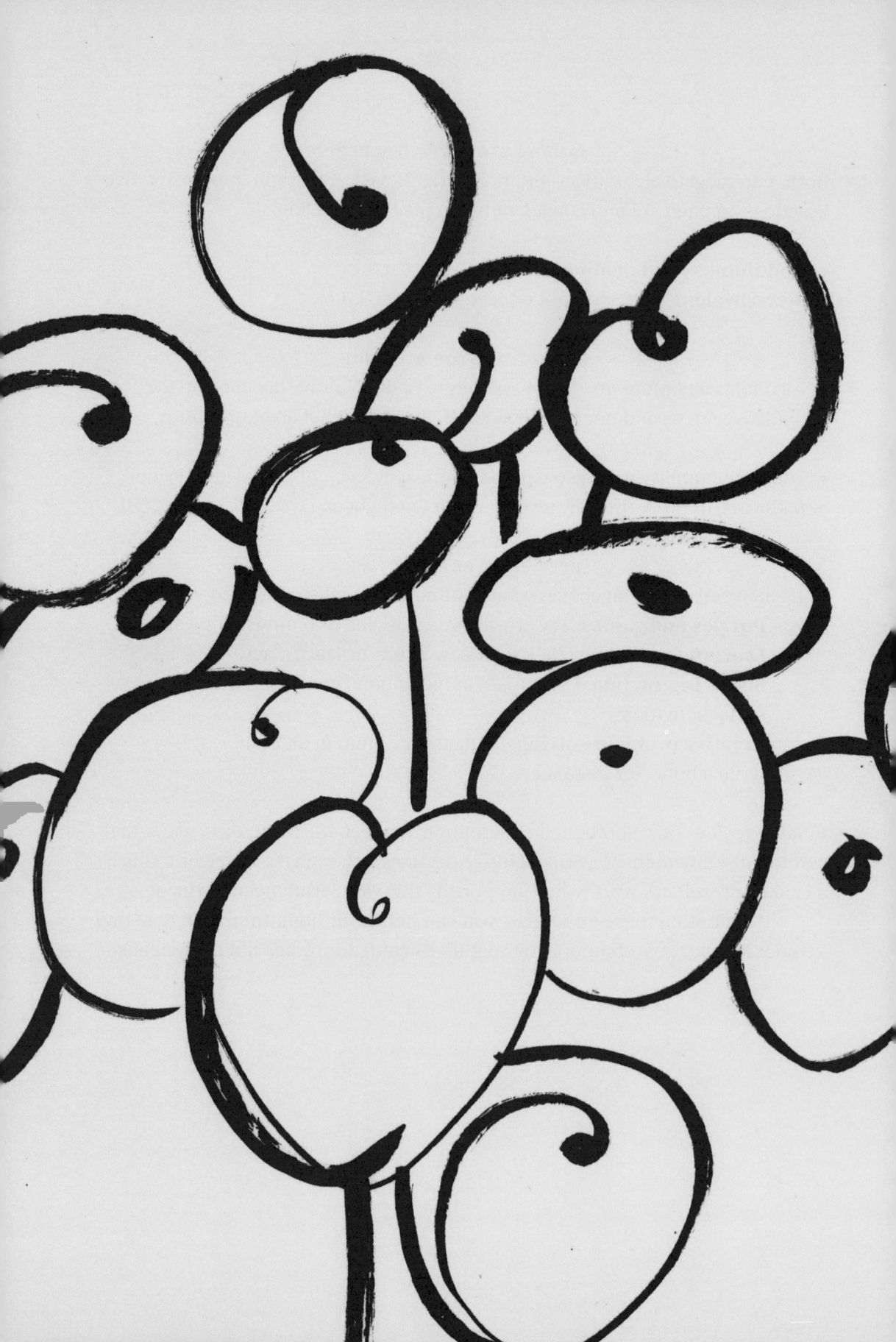

# 4.
# MEET YOUR HORMONAL SUPPORT TEAM

This section invites you to explore the vital network of supportive hormones that work in harmony with your primary fertility hormones to sustain balance and wellbeing. Often underestimated, these hormones are essential for achieving and maintaining hormonal harmony, supporting your health through every chapter of life.

**YOUR MOOD HORMONES PAGE 645**

**SPOTLIGHT ON:**

**SEROTONIN PAGE 648**
**DOPAMINE PAGE 658**
**GABA FOR RELAXATION PAGE 667**
**TESTOSTERONE PAGE 673**
**OXYTOCIN PAGE 683**

# Your Mood Hormones

Achieving an optimal balance of mood hormones can be a game-changer for your wellbeing. These include GABA, serotonin, dopamine, and oxytocin—the powerful team that helps you feel emotionally balanced, socially connected, and motivated. GABA and serotonin provide calm and emotional stability, while dopamine fuels your drive and reward system, Oxytocin, often called the 'bonding hormone', deepens your sense of connection with others, playing a key role in relationships and overall happiness.

By understanding how to nurture and balance these hormones, you can take control of your mood and emotional health. Once you've explored the introduction to each hormone, complete the Mood Hormone Risk Audit on the following page for a deeper self-assessment.

**THE INTERPLAY OF MOOD HORMONES AND YOUR CYCLE**
The balance between mood and fertility hormones is a delicate dance that influences our emotional wellbeing throughout life's stages. Serotonin and dopamine, for instance, share a see-saw relationship—when one is high, it often dampens the other. Finding the right equilibrium is key, particularly through puberty, when hormonal shifts can create mood swings, and in menopause, as oestrogen levels drop, impacting both serotonin and dopamine, contributing to mood shifts, anxiety and waning motivation.

But there's more to this hormonal symphony. GABA, a calming neurotransmitter, partners with progesterone to bring feelings of relaxation, help stabilise moods and supports relaxation for quality sleep, especially during times of stress or hormonal fluctuation. Melatonin, the sleep hormone, connects to serotonin in ways that affect sleep quality, indirectly impacting mood stability. Together, these hormones create a web of interactions that supports not only emotional balance but also readiness for each life stage, reminding us how profoundly our moods are connected to the rhythms of our bodies.

### THE DANCE OF MOOD HORMONES

These hormones work together to keep your emotions balanced. Nurturing serotonin, dopamine, and GABA requires nourishing your body with the right nutrients, regular exercise, restful sleep, and mindful stress management.

### MOOD HORMONE RISK AUDIT

Use this audit to assess your lifestyle habits that may be affecting your mood hormone balance. Keep a record of your answers and use them as a guide for improvement.

**CONSCIOUS EATING**
- I'm too busy to sit down at mealtime.
- I rush through meals without chewing thoroughly.
- I often skip meals.
- I drink water during meals.

**FOOD CHOICES**
- I am mostly vegetarian.
- I don't prioritise protein.
- I rarely add nuts or seeds to my meals.
- I eat processed sugar daily.
- I eat high-fat takeaway more than twice a week.

**GUT HEALTH**
- ○ I take antacid or heartburn medication.
- ○ I drink large glasses of water during meals.
- ○ I have taken antibiotics in the past two years.
- ○ I experience bloating or gut pain most days.
- ○ I've been diagnosed with inflammatory bowel disease.

**STRESS AND SLEEP**
- ○ I experience a lot of stress in my life.
- ○ I feel anxious or wired most days.
- ○ I struggle to get restful sleep.
- ○ I work night shifts.

### WHAT YOUR AUDIT MEANS

These responses highlight areas where lifestyle or nutritional choices might be sabotaging your mood hormone production. Our next section explores strategies for nourishing these mood messengers, helping you build happiness, stability and joy into your life.

## SPOTLIGHT ON
# Serotonin

Let's learn how to boost your happiness, naturally. Serotonin, often called the 'happy hormone,' is at the heart of your emotional balance, working alongside other mood hormones to bring happiness to life. This chemical messenger, or neurotransmitter, plays a critical role in transmitting signals between nerve cells, ensuring that essential communication flows smoothly throughout your brain and body.

Serotonin's magic happens when it binds to specific receptors on nerve cells. Once this connection is made, a cascade of actions occurs within the cells, influencing how you feel and function. For example, serotonin enhances happiness and reduces anxiety in the brain's emotional centres, while in the digestive system, it regulates bowel movements and hunger signals.

When serotonin levels are balanced, your body's communication network functions efficiently, promoting calmness, focus, and a sense of wellbeing. This hormone also plays a crucial role in sleep quality, as serotonin is converted into melatonin, your sleep hormone, helping you feel balanced during the day and well-rested at night.

However, when serotonin's pathways are disrupted—by stress, poor diet or other factors—communication gets messy. This can lead to mood swings, anxiety, depression, and poor sleep. A vicious cycle can develop; low serotonin affects your ability to sleep deeply and without, deep sleep, your body struggles to produce serotonin.

In short, serotonin helps keep your mind and body in sync, setting the emotional tone for your day. Here are some signs that you might have low serotonin levels:

- Persistent sadness, low mood, or depression.
- Increased anxiety and worry.
- Difficulty sleeping.
- Craving carbs and sugar.
- Digestive issues like nausea or bloating.
- Fatigue and low energy.
- Poor concentration and memory.
- Irritability and mood swings.
- Unexplained aches and pains.
- Loss of interest in hobbies.
- Withdrawal from social connections.

### UNDERSTANDING SEROTONIN

Whether you're dealing with mood swings, sleep problems, or gut health issues, understanding serotonin can be the key to improving your wellbeing. So, let's dive into how your body produces serotonin and the simple steps you can take to boost this crucial hormone.

### THE RECIPE FOR MAKING SEROTONIN

Serotonin production begins with what you eat. It's a three-step process that starts in your mouth, where nutrient-rich foods are broken down. The conversion of food into serotonin involves essential nutrients like zinc, vitamin B6, and probiotics, which help extract an amino acid called tryptophan—the backbone of serotonin.

But before we get into the recipe, let's touch on a common problem. Many of us are not chewing our food properly, which can undermine our body's ability to produce serotonin.

#### HOW TO CHEW YOUR FOOD

Conscious chewing is one of the simplest yet most overlooked habits in supporting serotonin production. How many times should you chew your food before swallowing? The answer—more than 30 times, or until it's completely mushy! Proper chewing breaks down food efficiently, allowing your stomach to do its job in extracting the nutrients you need for serotonin production.

## CREATING HAPPINESS: SEROTONIN PRODUCTION

Once your well-chewed food reaches your stomach, the real work begins. Your stomach, with its highly acidic environment, continues the digestion process that began in your mouth. This acidity, along with zinc, vitamin B6 and probiotics, helps extract tryptophan from your food. Tryptophan is the essential building block of serotonin, making it the first crucial step in boosting your mood naturally.

By focusing on nutrient-dense foods, supporting your gut health, and ensuring you're getting the right nutrients, you can help your body produce the serotonin it needs to keep you feeling calm, happy and emotionally balanced.

### STEP 1:
### SUPPORTING SEROTONIN PRODUCTION—
### THE ROLE OF AMINO ACIDS

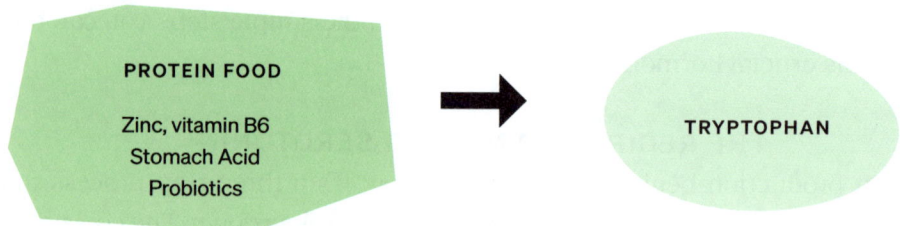

All protein-rich foods broken down in the stomach release amino acids, which go on to form different hormones. Tryptophan, the amino acid essential for serotonin production, is found in foods like white meat, dairy and tofu. However, simply eating these foods isn't enough—your body must properly digest and absorb these amino acids to effectively create serotonin.

#### SABOTEURS OF PROTEIN BREAKDOWN

To make sure your body gets the most out of these tryptophan-rich foods, it's important to avoid common factors that can sabotage protein digestion:

1  A beautifully acidic stomach

Your stomach needs to be acidic enough to break down protein and extract amino acids like tryptophan. Consider enhancing your stomach's acidity with a dash of apple cider vinegar or lemon juice before meals. These natural acids can aid in digestion and maximise nutrient absorption.

**2   Drinking water with meals**

Do you drink water with your meals? If so, you may unknowingly dilute the acidity of your stomach, reducing its ability to digest protein efficiently. For better digestion and serotonin production, it's best to drink water away from meals.

**3   Are you zinc deficient?**

Stomach acidity also plays a role in the absorption of essential minerals like zinc. Zinc partners with probiotics to help your body break down and absorb protein. Zinc deficiency can negatively impact serotonin production, so it's important to maintain healthy levels. Anti-ulcer drugs and similar medications can interfere with zinc absorption, making it harder for your body to produce serotonin.

For more tips on boosting zinc levels, check out our Spotlight on Vitamins and Minerals on page 472.

## STEP 2:
## IRON'S ROLE IN SEROTONIN PRODUCTION

Once the raw ingredients like zinc, calcium and tryptophan are prepared, iron steps into the process. Iron is crucial for delivering oxygen to cells and facilitating enzyme reactions that contribute to serotonin production. Without enough iron, serotonin synthesis can slow down, affecting your overall mood and energy levels.

By ensuring your body is getting the right nutrients—like tryptophan, zinc and iron—and avoiding digestion saboteurs, you can significantly improve your serotonin production and boost your mood naturally. Keep these simple tips in mind to maximise your body's serotonin-building potential!

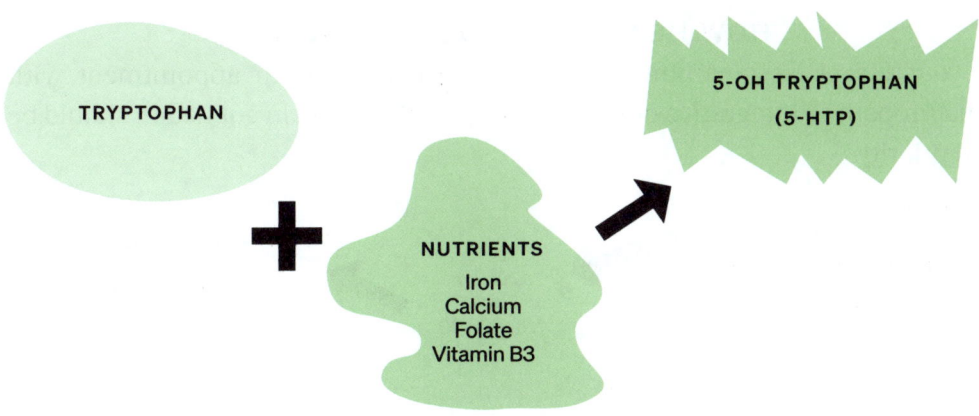

## SUPPORTING STEP 2
### COULD YOU BE LOW IN THE FOLLOWING NUTRIENTS?

- **Iron:** Low iron levels can affect oxygen delivery to your cells, slowing down enzyme reactions necessary for serotonin production. Symptoms of iron deficiency include fatigue, weakness, and pale skin.

- **Calcium:** Calcium plays a role in nerve function and is vital for neurotransmitter release. A deficiency in calcium can impair the communication between brain cells, affecting mood and serotonin levels.

- **Vitamin B3 (Niacin):** This vitamin is important for converting tryptophan into serotonin. A deficiency can lead to issues with serotonin synthesis, contributing to mood instability and low energy.

- **Folate (Vitamin B9):** Folate deficiency is particularly problematic for serotonin production, as folate is essential for neurotransmitter function. Some women are genetically predisposed to folate deficiency, making it harder for their bodies to process this nutrient. Additionally, women taking the oral contraceptive pill often experience reduced folate levels as a side effect.

To ensure your B-vitamin team is supporting your mental health and mood, see page 411 on how to boost all the essential B-vitamins for hormonal wellbeing. Keeping these nutrients in balance can help optimise serotonin production, improving mood, energy, and overall happiness.

## STEP 3:
### HOW HEALTHY IS YOUR GUT WALL?

If your bowel is screaming at you after every meal, an appointment with a naturopath or integrative doctor with a special interest in gut health should be top priority.

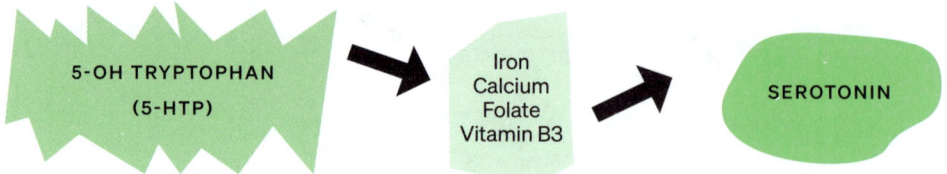

### GUT HEALTH FACTS

- 94% of serotonin is made in the bowel, your 'second brain'. The other 6% is made in the brain!
- Ask yourself the question, 'Is my gut health where it should be?'
- Is your main serotonin production factory (your gut) on fire?
- Gut support is one of the fundamental steps to support hormonal harmony at any age.
- If you have a medically diagnosed bowel disease, you will need to put extra effort into gut support (see page 424 on Gut Health).
- Antibiotics will alter the balance of healthy bacteria in your gut. This adds to the problem of low numbers of probiotic families that may already exist.
  - Include pre- and probiotic foods such as kimchi, kefir, yoghurt and sauerkraut when you are taking antibiotics.
  - Recent gut research suggests adding a probiotic may not be the best solution but check in with you naturopath for individual advice.

### SLEEP HEALTH FACT

The gut cells work the nightshift, tirelessly transforming 5-HTP into the final masterpiece of happiness—your serotonin. Serotonin production ramps up in restorative deep sleep. Good quality sleep ensures the production factory is working efficiently, and broken sleep can quickly domino into low serotonin 'blues'.

### PROCESSED SUGAR AND SEROTONIN

Eating high-sugar foods spikes insulin, which can affect the availability of amino acids like tryptophan. Insulin can block the movement of tryptophan across the blood-brain barrier—think of this like an impenetrable wall with door access permits issued only to essential brain personnel only—insulin blocks the door designed to allow amino acids into the brain. This is how sugar hits serotonin pathways, exacerbating those low moods.

## IMPORTANT POINTS FOR YOU TO REMEMBER

- A high dietary sugar load is poison to serotonin.

- Processed sugars disrupt the balance of your gut microbiome, leading to microscopic gut wall inflammation. Since the majority of serotonin is produced in the gut, this has a direct effect on the production factory

- A high-sugar diet is a missed opportunity to eat nutrient-dense food that has an essential role to play in human health.

- A high-sugar diet is deficient in vitamins B6, B12 and magnesium, at the very least.

Several studies highlight the critical role of iron, zinc, and magnesium in brain function, neurotransmitter regulation and overall mental health. Your amazing body can only do so much if the raw ingredients to keep you in top mental and physical condition are not in your body's pantry.

    Check your scores:
- Iron deficiency is officially experienced by 15% of premenopausal women
- Zinc deficiency is common to 20% of all women
- Magnesium deficiency occurs in up to 60% of all women

Now that we've explored the intricacies of serotonin production and its essential role in our wellbeing, it's time to turn knowledge into action. Follow the Wellness Action Plan to support and boost your serotonin naturally.

## WELLNESS ACTION PLAN
# SEROTONIN

The following wellness strategies will start to gently nudge your natural serotonin support networks in the right direction.

### MENTAL AND EMOTIONAL SUPPORT

- Talking to friends or family when we feel low can be one of the best therapies to help maintain serotonin levels.

- Counselling services can also assist you in implementing this plan if you feel stuck in a low serotonin state.

- A list of counselling support services is available in our Resource Section on page 691.

- If you have been diagnosed with depression or are currently on antidepressants, check in with your doctor. They can monitor your mood and symptoms while you work through your Wellness Action Plan.

- Always follow your doctor's advice and consult them if medication is needed to help your nervous system recalibrate.

## SUPPORT THE FUNDAMENTAL NEEDS OF SEROTONIN PRODUCTION PATHWAYS

- **Good gut health:** See Core Food Principle number 5 on page 424.
- **Nourishment:** Consume the raw ingredients. Making serotonin is like baking a cake; you need all the ingredients, or it won't be that same cake!
  - Tryptophan foods: Chicken, turkey, sardines, eggs, yoghurt, tofu, chickpeas, lentils.
  - Cofactor foods: Zinc, B-vitamins, iron, calcium, magnesium, vitamin C.

- **Prioritise quality sleep:** See Spotlight on Sleep page 351.
- **Regular exercise and movement:** Actively boosts serotonin, and other feel-good hormones!
- **Start a meditation practice:** Proven in research to raise serotonin levels. (See Spotlight on Restorative Practices on page 372.)

### STOP ALL NERVOUS SYSTEM DISRUPTORS OF SEROTONIN

- Sugar (see Core Food Principle Number 8 on page 430)
- Caffeine
- Alcohol
- Stress depletes serotonin faster (see page 314 for Stress Resilience)

### SUPPORT HYDRATION

Drink at least 2 litres of clean filtered water each day—dehydration directly impact serotonin levels.

### LIFESTYLE OPTIONS

Pick the ones that sing to you. The more you choose, the happier you will become!

- Practice gratitude by reflecting on positive experiences.
- Keep a gratitude diary: Read your entries to reinforce positive feelings about the people and things that you value.
- Stay connected: Social interactions boost serotonin.
- Spend time outdoors in nature: Morning sunlight helps to release bubbles of serotonin to boost happiness for the day.
- Herbal teas like Tulsi can gently support serotonin pathways by boosting the production of the enzymes you use for converting your food into happiness! (See page 349 for more on Tulsi.)

## HERBAL OPTIONS

If you feel like your serotonin may need a little boost, these herbs may be a perfect fit for you. Be guided by your health practitioner on good quality brands and doses.

- Herbs like turmeric, valerian, lavender, chamomile and passionflower are often used in herbal preparations to support symptoms of depression. Seek out an experienced naturopath who can individualise a herbal tonic for you. If you are on medication, these can still be useful but they can have a sedative effect, so are best taken in the evening. Your naturopath will guide you here. Herbal teas with these ingredients are safe to use even if you are on antidepressant medication.

- Herbs like rhodiola and St John's Wort work like mini antidepressants. This means that they must not be taken with medication—it's like doubling up on your dose for the day. If you feel like your serotonin may need a little boost, these herbs may be a perfect fit for you.

> **TIP**
>
> Studies on St John's Wort suggest it can effectively improve symptoms of mild to moderate anxiety and depression, showing results comparable to antidepressant medications but often with fewer side effects.

Maintaining buoyant levels of serotonin is all about balance. By integrating regular exercise, a nutrient-rich diet, stress management techniques, quality sleep, and perhaps some herbal support, you will not only nurture your nervous system but also enhance your overall wellbeing, helping you feel happier, energetic and more stress resilient.

# SPOTLIGHT ON
# Dopamine

## DOPAMINE: THE 'FEEL-GOOD' NEUROTRANSMITTER

Dopamine is often celebrated as the 'feel-good' neurotransmitter—a chemical messenger responsible for reward, motivation and overall wellbeing. Think of it as the conductor of your emotions and drive, orchestrating everything from joy to focus and guiding you toward activities that bring pleasure and satisfaction. Beyond mood, dopamine affects focus, memory and motor control.

When dopamine levels are balanced, you feel motivated, focused, and ready to take on challenges with enthusiasm. It's the excitement from a job well done or the contentment after achieving a goal. Dopamine also keeps you alert, helping you learn and remember new information.

However, dopamine is easily disrupted by diet, lifestyle, stress, and gut health. Low dopamine can lead to feelings of apathy, fatigue and even depression. You might seek risky behaviours for that dopamine 'hit', and it can even drive addictive behaviours like drug use and gambling. In short, when dopamine is low, that zest for life fades, leaving you feeling unmotivated and sluggish.

Understanding dopamine, how it's produced in the body, and how to keep it balanced is essential for mental sharpness, emotional balance and staying fully engaged in life.

## SIGNS OF LOW DOPAMINE

**BEHAVIOURAL SYMPTOMS:**
- Cravings for sugar, stimulants or unhealthy foods.
- Increased susceptibility to addiction (for example, drugs, alcohol, gambling).
- Difficulty concentrating or focusing.
- Procrastination or inability to complete tasks.
- Withdrawal from social interactions.

**EMOTIONAL SYMPTOMS:**
- Irritability or mood swings.
- Lack of motivation or drive.
- Inability to experience pleasure or joy.
- Increased feelings of apathy.
- Low self-esteem or feelings of worthlessness.
- Reduced libido (sex drive).
- Persistent low mood.

**PHYSICAL SYMPTOMS:**
- Fatigue or low energy.
- Poor coordination or motor control.
- Muscle stiffness or tremors.
- Restless legs syndrome.
- Sleep disturbances (insomnia or excessive sleepiness).
- Unexplained aches and pains.
- Weight gain or difficulty losing weight.

**COGNITIVE SYMPTOMS:**
- Memory problems or forgetfulness.
- Reduced ability to plan or organise tasks.
- Slow thought processes.
- Difficulty learning new things.

There's overlap between low dopamine and low serotonin symptoms. If serotonin-related issues like digestion problems (nausea or bloating) dominate, think serotonin. If sugar cravings, irritability and procrastination stand out, dopamine might be the issue. Supporting both neurotransmitters is key for optimal mental health.

## DOPAMINE AND HORMONES: FLUCTUATIONS THROUGHOUT LIFE

Dopamine's relationship with hormones shifts throughout a woman's life. Oestrogen boosts dopamine activity, supporting mood, focus and motivation. In contrast, progesterone dampens dopamine, contributing to low mood and decreased motivation, especially in perimenopause.

### PUBERTY

Dopamine peaks: Oestrogen surges during puberty, enhancing dopamine activity. This increase leads to the heightened emotions, risk-taking and mood swings typical of adolescence. Dopamine activity fluctuates as oestrogen rises and falls during the menstrual cycle.

### THE FERTILE YEARS

Dopamine stabilises during the Fertile Years, thanks to more predictable hormone cycles. Oestrogen peaks in the first half of the cycle, boosting dopamine, while progesterone's rise in the second half causes a slight dip. If baseline dopamine is healthy, this fluctuation goes unnoticed. But if it's low, you may experience mood dips, low motivation, and cravings—particularly for sweets.

### PERIMENOPAUSE—THE DOPAMINE ROLLERCOASTER

Perimenopause brings hormonal fluctuations that disrupt dopamine production. As oestrogen becomes inconsistent, so does dopamine activity, often resulting in low motivation, fatigue, and that 'I just can't be bothered' feeling. These symptoms tend to overlap with the emotional rollercoaster that is perimenopause.

### MENOPAUSE

As oestrogen levels drop, the dopamine system doesn't work as efficiently. This can contribute to brain fog, mood swings, and diminished focus—common complaints during menopause. These dopamine fluctuations can even mimic mild depression or heightened anxiety, making this phase a real challenge for both emotional and cognitive wellbeing.

### THE AGE OF WISDOM—STABILISE AND ADAPT!

As oestrogen fluctuations settle, dopamine stabilises but at lower levels. While extreme highs and lows are less frequent, motivation and pleasure may still feel diminished. However, many women find new sources of joy and motivation in social connections, intellectual pursuits and meaningful life experiences.

**BOOSTING DOPAMINE NATURALLY**

Understanding dopamine fluctuations can help you take control of your mood and motivation. Through dietary choices, exercise, stress management, and bio-hacks, you can maintain balanced dopamine levels and stay mentally sharp through each phase of life.

On the following pages you will find our science-backed strategies to naturally boost dopamine and thrive through all stages of your hormonal journey.

**CASE STUDY | DR KAREN**

# Sue

### Navigating the dopamine drought

Sue had always been the go-getter in her circle of friends. She juggled work, family, and her social life with ease, finding joy in the simplest of accomplishments—whether it was nailing a work presentation or just whipping up an Easter outfit for her kids' school event. But recently, something had shifted. Sue couldn't quite put her finger on it, but the spark that usually drove her had dimmed.

At first, she brushed it off as 'just one of those days'. But as the weeks rolled on, that 'off day' feeling became more persistent. Every morning felt like dragging herself through quicksand, and things that once excited her now felt like chores. She'd sit at her desk at work, staring blankly at her computer, knowing she had a to-do list but lacking any drive to tackle it. Even activities she once loved—yoga, dinner with friends, and binge-watching her favourite show—felt … meh.

It wasn't that Sue was sad exactly; she wasn't down in the dumps or crying at TV commercials. It was more like a dullness had crept in. Her energy had evaporated, and with it, her motivation to do much of anything. Her family noticed too. 'Mum, are you okay?', her teenage daughter asked one evening. 'You seem kind of … flat.' And flat was exactly how she felt.

One day, during a routine check-up, Sue mentioned her low energy and lack of drive to me, half-expecting to be told to get more sleep. I asked her a few questions (my serotonin and dopamine checklist) and then explained something Sue hadn't considered. It wasn't just stress or being tired—it could be her dopamine levels taking a dip. I explained how dopamine, the 'feel-good' chemical, is responsible for motivation, pleasure, and drive. When it's low, everything can feel like a slog. It was like a lightbulb went off in Sue's head. She wasn't lazy or unmotivated; her dopamine was just on holidays.

As Sue learned more, she realised she'd been ignoring some classic low dopamine signs like that overwhelming need for a sugar hit mid-afternoon. Yep, her brain's cheeky way of begging for a quick dopamine boost. And that lack of joy from things she usually loved? Another hallmark of low dopamine levels.

Sue's journey wasn't about being down or depressed; it was about realising that her brain chemistry was shifting. And as she stepped into her late 40s, with hormones dancing around unpredictably, she now understood that dopamine was a piece of the puzzle she needed to start focusing on.

With this newfound knowledge, Sue began making small changes. She swapped out her afternoon sugar hit for a walk in the fresh air, giving her brain a natural dopamine boost—that habit was hard to break, but she put some motivational Post-it notes around the kitchen as a reminder.

Sue tweaked her diet to include foods that support dopamine production (see our Wellness Action Plan on page 665 for more details). She started practising mindfulness to help her brain reset. Slowly but surely, the spark returned, and Sue found herself, if not sprinting, at least strolling with purpose again.

## WHAT LOW DOPAMINE CAN FEEL LIKE

Low dopamine doesn't always look like sadness or depression; sometimes, it's just that 'blah' feeling that creeps in and sticks around. Sue's story reminds us that recognising the signs and taking small steps can make all the difference in getting back to feeling like yourself again.

## HOW YOU MAKE DOPAMINE

The right food:
- Protein-rich foods like chicken, dairy, soy products, and certain nuts and seeds are key sources of tyrosine, the amino acid needed to produce dopamine.
- Your body can create tyrosine in the gut from other proteins (unlike tryptophan, which must come directly from your diet).

Like the 'mood hormone' serotonin, dopamine also starts its journey in your diet. This time, raw ingredients move to the brain for further transformation in a three-step process.

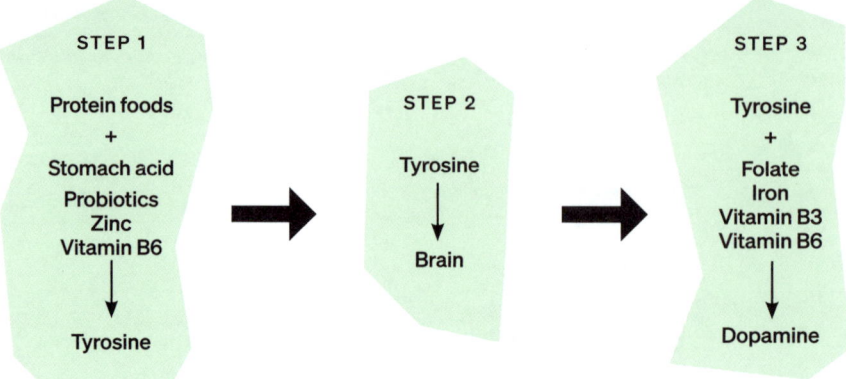

### TIP FOR VEGETARIANS:

Combine these plant-based food to feed your mind. These food duos contain all 9 essential amino acids:

- Hummus (chickpeas) and pita bread
- Peanut butter and whole wheat bread
- Beans and rice

## WELLNESS ACTION PLAN
# DOPAMINE

### NOURISHMENT—SOURCE THESE RAW INGREDIENTS
- **Tyrosine-rich foods**: Beef, pork, chicken, fish, eggs, dairy, soy, nuts, seeds, avocados, bananas.
- **Cofactor foods:** Magnesium, zinc, iron, vitamins B6 and C, and folate.

### SUPPORT HYDRATION
Drink at least 2 litres of water daily to maintain dopamine levels.

### QUALITY SLEEP
Ensure 7 to 9 hours of sleep each night to support dopamine production.

**EXERCISE**
- **Regular exercise** boosts dopamine receptors in the brain. Try:
  - Aerobic exercise: Running, cycling, swimming.
  - Strength training: Lifting weights and resistance exercises.
  - High-intensity interval training (HIIT) for a dopamine surge.

- **Team sports:** Combining physical exertion and social interaction enhances dopamine production.

**OUTDOOR ACTIVITIES**
Morning sunlight and spending time in nature boost dopamine.

### LIFESTYLE HACKS

- **Stay connected:** Social interactions naturally increase dopamine.
- **Herbal teas:** Tulsi, ginseng, and ginkgo biloba teas gently support dopamine production.

### HERBAL SUPPLEMENTS

- **Ginseng:** Enhances mental clarity and supports dopamine.
- ***Ginkgo biloba***: Improves brain blood flow and dopamine.
- ***Mucuna pruriens***: A natural source of L-DOPA, a direct dopamine precursor.

### GUT HEALTH AND DOPAMINE

The gut-brain connection, via the vagus nerve, plays a crucial role in dopamine production and signalling, which impacts mood and cognitive function. (For more on gut health, see Core Food Principle Number 5 on page 424.)

### REDUCE CHRONIC STRESS

Chronic stress and high cortisol levels interfere with dopamine production and its messaging within the brain. (For more, see Spotlight on Psychological Stress page 290.)

### PRESCRIPTION MEDICATIONS

Bupropion (Wellbutrin or Zyban) is a medication that works on dopamine and norepinephrine pathways. Unlike many antidepressants that target serotonin, bupropion helps boost dopamine, enhancing mood and energy. It's often used for smoking cessation but is also prescribed off-label for depression in Australia, New Zealand, and the UK.

### FURTHER READING

For a deeper dive into dopamine, consider reading *The Dopamine Brain* by Dr Anastasia Hronis, clinical psychologist and founder of the Australian Institute for Human Wellness.

**SPOTLIGHT ON**
# GABA for Relaxation

Gamma-aminobutyric acid (GABA) is often called the brain's natural sedative. This calming neurotransmitter is your Blue Zone superpower, helping to maintain calm and balance within your nervous system (for more on zones see page 295). Think of GABA as a gentle guardian, soothing neurons and preventing overstimulation, allowing you to relax and unwind.

GABA is essential for reducing stress, promoting restful sleep, and fostering a sense of inner peace. When your GABA levels are optimal, you feel serene and composed, able to handle life's challenges with ease—this is the true essence of the Blue Zone. But when GABA levels are low, anxiety, restlessness, and difficulty sleeping can creep in.

In this chapter, we'll dive into the science of GABA, explore its profound effects on mental and emotional wellbeing, and offer practical strategies to naturally enhance its levels. By nurturing this crucial neurotransmitter, you can achieve a more balanced, tranquil mind and increase resilience to stress.

Unlike serotonin and dopamine, where raw ingredient supply can be a problem, GABA's production process is simpler. GABA is made from the abundant amino acid glutamine, which is easily sourced from food or converted from other amino acids in the body. From glutamine, it quickly becomes glutamate, needing only water and an enzyme called glutaminase. One more step converts glutamate into GABA, which is stored in tiny pods at the ends of specially designed nerve cells known as GABAergic neurons, scattered throughout the brain.

From these neurons, GABA plays a vital role in balancing stimulation and inhibition within the nervous system. This balance contributes to three key aspects of wellness:

1   **Regulating anxiety**: GABA is your natural anxiety-reducer, calming an overstimulated mind.

2   **Promoting sleep**: As a sedative, GABA helps you relax and drift into restful sleep.

3   **Maintaining muscle tone**: GABA ensures your muscles have the right amount of tone and control for smooth physical movement.

GABA's release follows your body's circadian rhythm, with levels peaking between 2 and 4 am to promote deep sleep and dropping to their lowest point 12 hours later supporting you to be alert and productive into your afternoon.

By understanding how GABA works and supporting its natural production, you can foster a more relaxed, resilient state of being.

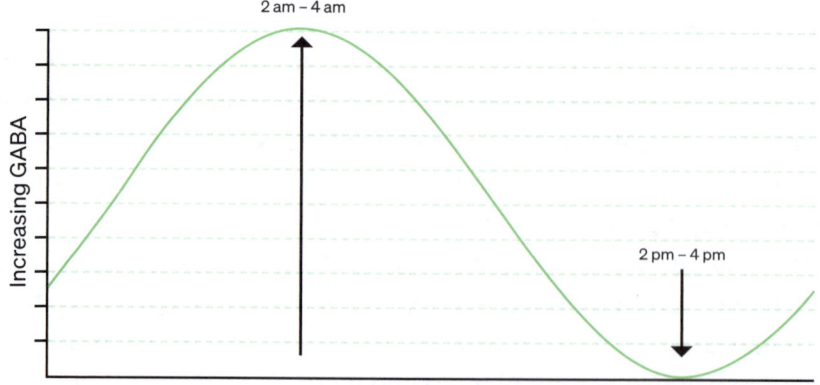

**THE GABA CONTROL CENTRE OF YOUR NERVOUS SYSTEM**

Your body is equipped with a perfect balancing system to control how much stimulation or soothing your brain and nervous system need. GABA, through its flexible conversion from glutamate and back, helps regulate your nervous system, allowing you to de-stress and relax as needed.

Unlike some other mood hormones, GABA levels need to be flexible. At times, such as in the evening when you're winding down for sleep, higher levels of GABA are perfect. During the day, a moderate level of GABA helps with concentration and productivity. Without enough GABA, your nervous system can go into overdrive, leaving you in a state of fight-or-flight, especially if adrenaline takes over. Think of GABA as the 'calm controller'—without it, your brain can turn into a chaotic hub of overstimulation.

### SYMPTOMS OF TOO MUCH GABA

When GABA is too high, it can overly dampen your nervous system, resulting in:

- Drowsiness or sleepiness
- Muscle weakness
- Excessive calmness
- Impaired coordination and balance
- Slowed thinking and reaction times
- Difficulty concentrating
- Sedation or feeling unusually relaxed.

### SYMPTOMS OF TOO LITTLE GABA

When GABA levels are too low, your nervous system fires up, leading to:

- Anxiety or panic attacks
- Insomnia
- Restlessness
- Irritability
- Muscle tension or cramps
- Difficulty relaxing
- Increased sensitivity to stress.

### GABA AND ALCOHOL

GABA and alcohol have a complicated relationship. Alcohol mimics GABA, disrupting its natural balance almost immediately after consumption. This leads to a temporary calming effect, but as the alcohol is metabolised, it causes a rebound effect—often resulting in anxiety, restlessness, and disrupted sleep. Prolonged alcohol use changes the sensitivity of GABA receptors, making it harder to achieve the same level of relaxation without more alcohol. Over time, this can lead to tolerance, withdrawal symptoms, and even seizures as the nervous system becomes unregulated without GABA's influence.

### GABA AND ADRENALINE—BALANCE IS EVERYTHING

Balancing both GABA and adrenaline is crucial for your overall wellbeing. While GABA promotes calmness, adrenaline prepares your body for action. Ideally, adrenaline should be triggered only in times of real danger, but in today's world, it's often activated unnecessarily, leading to heightened stress and anxiety.

### GABA AND SEROTONIN—THE PERFECT PARTNERSHIP

GABA and serotonin are closely linked in their roles within your nervous system. GABA helps you relax, while serotonin works to regulate mood and lower anxiety. Serotonin can even stimulate the release of GABA, reinforcing a calm, balanced state. Together, these neurotransmitters are vital for maintaining mental health and emotional stability.

By understanding GABA's role in your nervous system and how it interacts with other mood hormones, you can take proactive steps to support relaxation, reduce stress, and promote mental and physical wellbeing.

### GABA'S ROLE IN PMS AND PMDD

Recent research shows that disruptions in GABA signalling may contribute to PMS and PMDD symptoms. For more information on managing these conditions, refer to the Wellness Action Plan for PMS on page 80 and Resources for PMDD support on page 691.

### THE LIFE CYCLE OF GABA

After calming the nervous system, GABA breaks down into succinate, a vital compound for cellular energy production in the Krebs cycle, keeping your mitochondria—your body's powerhouses—running smoothly.

> **(NOT SO) FUN FACT**
>
> The drug Valium, once known as 'mother's little helper' in the 1950s and 1960s, was named after the GABA-supporting herb Valerian. Intended to help women manage their nervous systems while juggling domestic responsibilities, it was marketed as a quick fix for GABA depletion caused by boredom and stress. Unfortunately, Valium is highly addictive, leading to a generation of women numbed by GABA overstimulation, which limited their ability to reach their full potential.

## WELLNESS ACTION PLAN
# GABA

**Nourish your body** with GABA-boosting Foods: A balanced diet with GABA-friendly nutrients can help elevate GABA levels. Try including:

- Fermented foods: Kimchi, sauerkraut, yoghurt, kefir.
- Green tea: Contains L-theanine, which enhances GABA production.
- Magnesium-rich foods: Spinach, pumpkin seeds, almonds, dark chocolate.
- Whole grains: Brown rice, oats, barley.
- Nuts and seeds: Sunflower seeds, walnuts, peanuts.
- Bananas and oranges: These fruits help with GABA synthesis.

**Optimise your gut health:** Good gut health supports neurotransmitter production, including GABA:
- Eat a variety of fibre-rich foods.
- Include probiotics from fermented foods or supplements.
- Limit processed foods and excess sugar, which can disturb gut flora.

**Get quality sleep**—GABA plays a key role in sleep regulation, so aim for 7 to 9 hours of rest:
- Stick to a regular sleep schedule.
- Create a calming sleep environment.
- Avoid screen time before bed.
- Skip caffeine and heavy meals close to bedtime.

Manage stress effectively: Chronic stress can reduce GABA levels. To counter this:
- Exercise regularly (walking, swimming, etc).
- Practise mindfulness and meditation (see page 382 for techniques).
- Spend time outdoors in nature.
- Engage in relaxation practices: To boost GABA, incorporate relaxation techniques into your routine
    - Yoga: Promotes GABA production through mindful movement.
    - Acupuncture: Has been shown to increase GABA levels.
    - Engage in calming activities like listening to music, painting, or journaling.

**Consider herbal supplements:** Certain herbs and nutrients naturally enhance GABA levels.
- Valerian root: Known for its calming effects.
- Passionflower: Reduces anxiety and promotes relaxation.
- Withania (ashwagandha): Supports stress management and GABA levels.
- Magnesium: An essential cofactor for GABA function.

**Limit nervous system disruptors:** Avoid substances that interfere with GABA. Reduce or remove:
- Caffeine: Can reduce GABA's calming effects.
- Alcohol: Disrupts GABA function and negatively impacts sleep.
- Nicotine: Lowers GABA and raises anxiety levels.

**Lifestyle options**: Incorporate lifestyle habits that naturally boost GABA.
- Gratitude practice: Reflect on positive experiences or keep a journal.
- Stay connected: Meaningful social interactions enhance wellbeing.
- Sunlight and fresh air: Boost mood and support GABA levels.

> **TIP**
>
> Diaphragmatic breathing stimulates the vagus nerve causing the synapsis in your brain to release GABA. This means you can self-medicate with GABA by using this essential breathing technique. Help support your GABA levels and promote calmness, relaxation, and overall wellbeing.

### SPOTLIGHT ON
# Testosterone

**ENHANCING FEMALE STRENGTH AND VITALITY**

Testosterone, often dubbed the 'libido hormone', remains your ally from puberty well into the Age of Wisdom. It might be best known as a 'male hormone', but it's just as vital for women. In women, testosterone is produced in the ovaries, adrenal glands, and other areas like fatty tissue. Though present in smaller amounts than in men, it plays a crucial role in maintaining overall health, particularly during reproductive years and beyond.

### WHAT TESTOSTERONE DOES IN WOMEN:

- Supports muscle and bone health: Helps maintain muscle mass and bone density, which is crucial for strength and resilience.
- Drives libido: Plays a key role in sexual desire and arousal.
- Boosts energy and mood: Contributes to a sense of vitality and emotional wellbeing.
- Aids in hormone balance: Acts as a precursor, converting into oestrogen when needed by the body.
- Promotes cognitive function: Supports memory, focus, and overall mental sharpness.

## HEALTHY TESTOSTERONE THROUGH YOUR LIFE

Unlike oestrogen and progesterone, which fluctuate monthly and decline as you age, testosterone peaks in your 20s and then gradually declines into your 60s. Before menopause the ovaries produce it, handing over production to the adrenals as they retire. At that point, it levels out, quietly supporting your hormonal health in the background. But then—something surprising happens!

Around age 70, testosterone levels start to slowly rise again, eventually levelling out at amounts similar to when you were 30. It's even measurable in 90-year-old women, sometimes matching the levels seen in their stressed-out grandchildren (because yes, stress can diminish testosterone levels in all women and men).

This fascinating shift in testosterone suggests that even in later years, your body still values its role in keeping you strong and balanced.

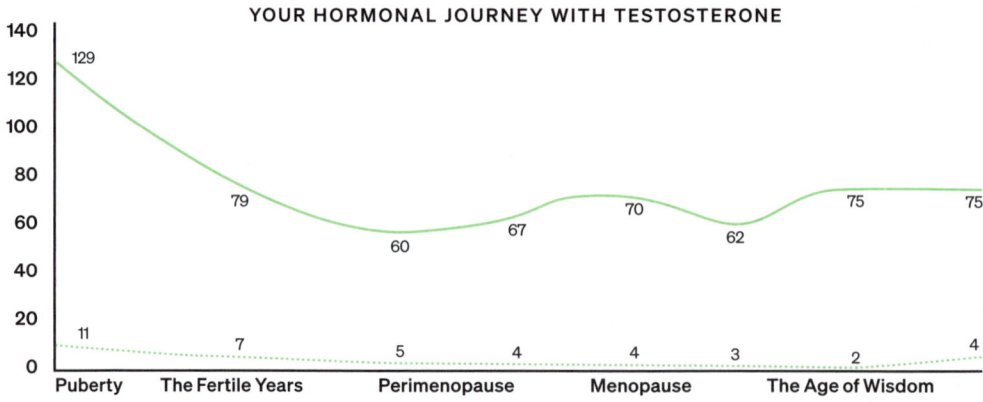

The solid line represents the highest potential for testosterone levels through the decades. The dotted line is the cut-off for the lowest levels. The ideal level is around the middle of the two lines, while aiming towards the higher.

## TESTOSTERONE FLUCTUATIONS ACROSS THE HORMONAL STAGES

### PUBERTY

Testosterone helps build muscle mass and strength. It stimulates bone growth, repairs muscle fibres, and boosts red blood cell production. Testosterone also plays a role in skin oiliness and, for some girls, contributes to unwanted hair growth and acne.

### THE FERTILE YEARS

In the Fertile Years, testosterone continues to be vital. It helps grow egg follicles in the ovaries, supports oestrogen production, and influences mood, cognitive function, energy levels and libido. Women with low testosterone during this phase might experience symptoms like:

- Low libido
- Fatigue
- Difficulty maintaining muscle mass
- Low mood and reduced motivation.

### PERIMENOPAUSE

Testosterone remains important during perimenopause. It helps maintain muscle mass and bone strength, supports brain function, and stabilises mood and libido. However, stress often causes testosterone levels to dip, leading to symptoms such as:

- Mood swings and irritability
- Weaker muscles
- Fatigue
- Low libido
- Increased belly fat.

### MENOPAUSE

As oestrogen declines in menopause, testosterone becomes more significant, helping to maintain energy, muscle tone, bone density, and mood stability. It also supports heart health by reducing inflammation and promoting blood vessel health. Symptoms of low testosterone in menopause include:

- Forgetfulness
- Fatigue
- Loss of libido
- Mood swings
- Muscle weakness
- Increased belly fat.

**AGE OF WISDOM**

Even into the later years, testosterone continues to support muscle mass, energy, cognitive function, and a balanced immune response. It remains crucial for bone health and libido. However, chronic illness or stress can still impact testosterone levels, leading to:

- Fragility and muscle loss
- Reduced energy
- Forgetfulness and difficulty focusing
- Loss of libido
- Increased aches and pains.

**THE HORMONAL COST OF STRESS**

Chronic stress can deplete testosterone, with effects varying depending on which stage of life you're in and how stress impacts your oestrogen and progesterone levels.

**HOW YOUR TESTOSTERONE INTERACTS WITH OTHER HORMONES**

Beyond its direct effect, testosterone acts as a buffer throughout the ebbs and flows of your other fertility hormones. It helps build and maintain muscle and bone strength, and can even be converted into oestrogen when your body needs it. Like all hormones, your body requires just the right balance—not too much and not too little.

**IS TESTOSTERONE REPLACEMENT THERAPY A GOOD CHOICE FOR ME?**

Women low in testosterone are the ones who benefit the most from supplementation and are less likely to experience side effects. It can often take time to get the dose 'just right'. Working with an integrative doctor with experience with bioidentical hormones is the key to long term success.

As with other medical interventions, you need to consider both the benefits and the risks. While testosterone can be beneficial, balance is key—more is not always better.

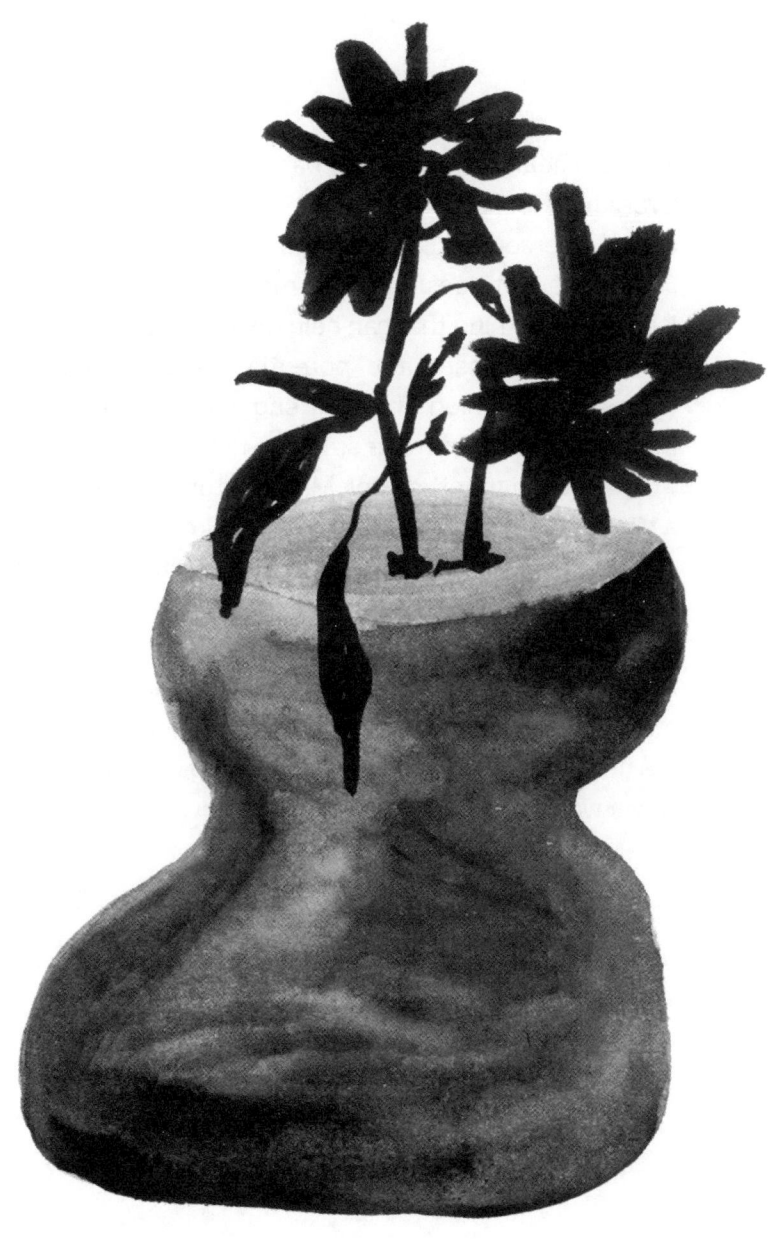

**CASE STUDY | DR KAREN**

# Maree

## More of a good thing: libido

Maree, a healthy 74-year-old patient, came to see me for her final cervical smear. Everything looked perfect, and I asked my usual question about vaginal comfort during intercourse. She responded with a laugh, saying, 'Comfort is fine, but my libido is zero. It doesn't bother me, but my husband is constantly asking for sex. Is there something that can help my sex drive?'

We discussed the potential benefits of a small dose of transdermal testosterone, which she was eager to try. Maree left with a prescription for bioidentical testosterone cream.

Several months later, Maree returned to my office for travel advice before a trip to Fiji. At the end of the visit, I asked, 'How's your libido going?'

With a grin, she replied, 'Oh, the testosterone was amazing—I've never felt so horny in my life!'

Knowing her previous script had no repeats, I offered another prescription. Maree, still smiling, said, 'Good grief, no! After a week of intense sex, I ended up chasing my husband around the kitchen for a second session that day. He told me he couldn't keep up, that I was going to kill him, and begged to go back to the way it was before. We're both happy now!'

Maree left my office with us both giggling like teenagers.

## TOO MUCH TESTOSTERONE AT ANY AGE

The following may be indications your body has too much testosterone:
- Increased appetite and weight gain
- Skin breakouts reminiscent of puberty
- Unwanted facial and body hair growth
- A deeper voice
- Irritability and sudden rage
- An overactive sex drive.

## USING BIOIDENTICAL TESTOSTERONE AND DHEA

Bioidentical testosterone replacement can be tricky to manage, but many women experience fantastic results and are willing to work with their doctor to find the right dose. If side effects like weight gain and hair growth persist, switching to a gentler male hormone, DHEA, may be a better option.

DHEA is easier to manage long-term in capsule form, with typical doses ranging from 10 to 25 mg daily. If side effects remain stubborn, a transition to 7-keto DHEA may offer a smoother option. Always consult your doctor for guidance on dosage and adjustments.

## TESTOSTERONE'S VERY INTIMATE RELATIONSHIP WITH OESTROGEN

Oestrogen plays a role in regulating the production of testosterone. When oestrogen levels are low, the brain releases hormones that stimulate the ovaries to produce more testosterone. Testosterone can then be recycled in other pathways that lead to oestrogen. This can make it unsuitable as a choice for women with oestrogen-sensitive breast cancer. On the flip side, high levels of oestrogen can suppress testosterone production sometimes contributing to a roller-coaster of oestrogen highs and lows—women with PCOS will sometimes experience this.

Testosterone replacement at menopause has been well-researched by endocrine specialists from the Melbourne-based Jean Hailes Foundation for Women's Health. It is a safe and useful option for hormone support through to the Age of Wisdom.

## WELLNESS ACTION PLAN
# TESTOSTERONE SUPPORT

Integrating natural strategies, proven herbal remedies, and bioidentical hormone options to optimise testosterone and boost libido.

### NOURISH TESTOSTERONE PRODUCTION WITH THESE FOODS

- **Healthy fats**: Support hormone production with avocado, olive oil, fatty fish, and coconut oil.
- **Zinc and magnesium**: Include zinc-rich foods like pumpkin seeds, oysters, and lean meats, and magnesium-rich options like spinach and almonds to support testosterone synthesis.
- **Protein balance**: Choose lean proteins (eggs, chicken, legumes) to maintain muscle tone and support hormones.
- **Adaptogenic herbs**: Incorporate withania (ashwagandha) or maca root to boost natural testosterone by reducing stress-induced hormone imbalance.

### HERBS TO BOOST TESTOSTERONE AND LIBIDO

- *Tribulus terrestris*: Traditionally used to enhance libido and support testosterone levels, it may help improve sexual function.
- **Fenugreek**: Known for its testosterone-boosting effects, it can also improve energy and libido.
- **Maca root**: Often referred to as 'Peruvian ginseng,' maca supports libido and energy while balancing hormones.
- **Shatavari (*Asparagus racemosus*)**: A traditional Ayurvedic herb that supports hormonal balance and enhances libido in women.

## CONSIDER BIOIDENTICAL HORMONE THERAPY (BHT)

- **Testosterone cream or gel**: Low-dose topical applications can effectively improve libido, energy and mood. Work with a healthcare provider to create a customised formula based on individual needs.

- **DHEA**: High stress depletes DHEA, a vital precursor for testosterone production. Unlike direct testosterone supplementation, DHEA self-regulates its conversion, reducing the risk of pushing testosterone levels above optimal. Ask your healthcare provider to test your DHEA levels. If suitable, DHEA can be prescribed as capsules, creams or troches (sublingual lozenges) to support balanced testosterone levels.

- **Monitoring**: Regular testing ensures that levels are optimised and side effects (for example, acne or excessive hair growth) are avoided.

## STRENGTHEN WITH TARGETED MOVEMENT

- **Resistance training**: Builds muscle and stimulates testosterone production.
- **High-intensity interval training (HIIT)**: Short bursts of intense activity naturally enhance testosterone.
- **Restorative practices**: Yoga or Pilates can help reduce stress and maintain hormonal balance.

## PRIORITISE REST AND RECOVERY

- **Sleep**: Deep, restorative sleep (7 to 9 hours) is essential for testosterone production.
- **Circadian rhythms**: Support hormonal cycles with sunlight exposure during the day and limited screen time at night.

## MANAGE STRESS AND OPTIMISE CORTISOL

- **Stress management**: Chronic stress raises cortisol, suppressing testosterone. Practise mindfulness, meditation, or gentle exercise.
- **Adaptogens**: Herbs like rhodiola, holy basil, and withania (ashwagandha) help balance cortisol and indirectly support testosterone.

## DETOX AND REDUCE ENDOCRINE DISRUPTORS

- **Toxin avoidance**: Eliminate exposure to BPA, phthalates, and other hormone disruptors by using glass containers and organic personal care products.
- **Liver support**: Enhance detox pathways with cruciferous vegetables (broccoli, cauliflower, kale) and herbs like milk thistle.

## SUPPLEMENTATION

- **Vitamin D**: Crucial for testosterone production. Maintain optimal levels (100–150 nmol/L).
- **Omega-3 fatty acids**: Found in fatty fish or supplements, these support cell membranes and hormone function.
- **B-vitamins**: Support hormonal pathways and energy, particularly B6 and B12.

## HERBS TO ENHANCE LIBIDO

- **Damiana (*Turnera diffusa*)**: A traditional aphrodisiac known to support sexual health and libido.
- ***Ginkgo biloba***: Improves circulation, which may enhance sexual function.
- **Saffron:** Shown in studies to improve sexual desire and satisfaction.

## MONITOR AND SEEK EXPERT GUIDANCE

- **Hormonal testing**: Regularly check testosterone and other hormone levels to ensure balance.
- **Personalised care**: Work with a healthcare provider for tailored advice on herbs, supplementation, and BHT.

By combining lifestyle adjustments, herbal remedies and options like bioidentical hormone therapy, you can effectively support healthy testosterone levels, enhance libido, and improve overall vitality for life.

# SPOTLIGHT ON
# Oxytocin

Oxytocin, often called the 'love hormone' or 'bonding hormone,' is a multitasking molecule crucial to your overall wellbeing. This ancient hormone has played a key role in shaping human evolution by fostering social connections and emotional bonds, allowing humans to form cohesive communities for survival. Oxytocin surges when we connect with others—whether through a hug, shared laughter, or even a simple conversation—strengthening our relationships and boosting emotional resilience.

## PUBERTY

During puberty, oxytocin acts as a chemical messenger in the brain. It helps manage stress, fights inflammation and serves as an antioxidant, offering protection when life gets tough. Oxytocin influences your nervous and immune systems, and it's deeply connected to the feel-good moments that come from social interactions and bonding experiences.

> **EARLY LIFE STRESS AND OXYTOCIN PATHWAYS**
>
> Prolonged early-life or childhood stress can have lasting effects on oxytocin pathways. If childhood trauma is part of your story, it's especially important to focus on nurturing your oxytocin pathways. See the Wellness Action Plan on page 687 for ways to boost oxytocin naturally.

## THE FERTILE YEARS

Oxytocin also contributes to overall mental and emotional health throughout all stages of life. This graph shows oxytocin levels during your menstrual cycle.

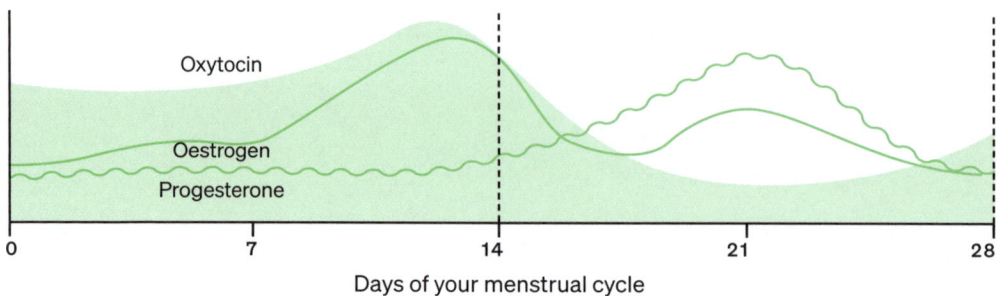

## OXYTOCIN'S ROLE IN CHILDBIRTH AND BEYOND

Oxytocin helps with emotional bonding—it's a superstar during childbirth as well. This hormone supports effective contractions during labour, and it even acts as a natural pain reliever by suppressing pain signals in the spinal cord. Immediately after birth, a final surge of oxytocin reduces postpartum bleeding, which can be lifesaving for the mother.

Once breastfeeding begins, powerful pulses of oxytocin promote the 'let-down' reflex, helping milk flow more easily, which reduces the baby's effort during feeding.

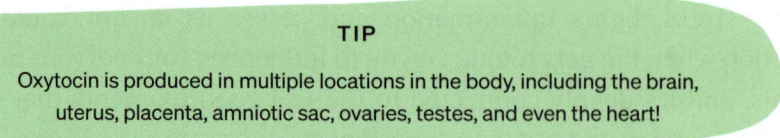

**TIP**

Oxytocin is produced in multiple locations in the body, including the brain, uterus, placenta, amniotic sac, ovaries, testes, and even the heart!

## OXYTOCIN BEYOND PREGNANCY AND BREASTFEEDING

Oxytocin's benefits extend far beyond childbirth and nursing. It also plays important roles in:

- Insulin production: Supports healthy insulin levels.
- Kidney function: Helps balance salt and water levels in the body.
- Empathy: Aids in the development of emotional understanding.
- Language skills: Enhances practical language abilities in women.
- Bone health: Works with oestrogen to maintain strong bones.
- Mood stabilisation: Acts as a mood-balancing hormone.
- Energy regulation: Helps reduce appetite and support healthy body weight.

### SIGNS OF LOW OXYTOCIN

When oxytocin levels are low, it can lead to:
- Increased period pains.
- Higher vulnerability to anxiety and depressive disorders.
- Reduced empathy and difficulty forming deep relationships.
- A tendency to gain weight.
- Greater risk of postnatal depression and difficulty breastfeeding.

### SYNTHETIC OXYTOCIN AND POSTNATAL HEALTH

It's important to keep an eye on the mental health of mums after delivery, especially if synthetic oxytocin (Syntocinon) was used during labour or postpartum to help with contractions or bleeding. This treatment is vital for safety but can sometimes increase the risk of postnatal mood changes like depression or anxiety. Mums who have elective caesarean deliveries may also miss the natural surges of oxytocin during labour, which can affect their mood.

If you or someone you care for is a new mum, encourage her to prioritise emotional support, seek help early for any mood changes, and discuss concerns with her healthcare provider. Emotional support is essential during this time.

### OXYTOCIN IN MENOPAUSE

As we age, oxytocin production naturally slows, yet like many other hormones, its levels never drop to zero. Oxytocin continues to play a vital role in supporting emotional wellbeing, physical health and social connections throughout menopause and beyond.

### THE AGE OF WISDOM

Oxytocin is a key player in promoting longevity and vitality as part of the Age of Wisdom phase. This is how oxytocin continues to benefit women during this life stage:

- **Reduces cardiovascular risk:** Oxytocin lowers stress levels, helping to protect your heart by improving coronary artery health.
- **Regulates insulin production:** Reduces the risk of Type 2 diabetes.
- **Supports bone health:** Oxytocin, in partnership with oestrogen, plays a role in maintaining strong bones.
- **Reduces risk of urinary incontinence:** It supports the health of the pelvic floor muscles and the urethral lining, reducing symptoms of urinary incontinence.

- **Fosters healthy social connections:** Strong social bonds are enhanced by oxytocin, which boosts emotional resilience and wellbeing.

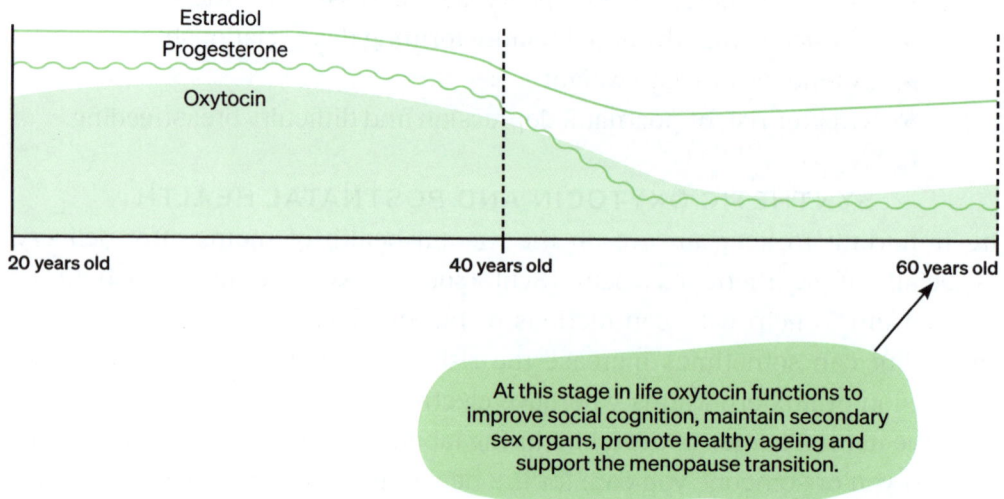

At this stage in life oxytocin functions to improve social cognition, maintain secondary sex organs, promote healthy ageing and support the menopause transition.

## VAGINAL OXYTOCIN

Vaginal oxytocin preparations can be particularly effective for managing symptoms of 'urogenital ageing', such as urinary incontinence and vaginal discomfort during intercourse. Research shows that oxytocin improves the health of the urethra's lining and boosts vaginal comfort with minimal side effects compared to vaginal oestrogen preparations. This is especially beneficial for women who have side effects from oestrogen or who are at higher risk of breast cancer.

### TIP
Contact your local compounding pharmacy for advice on sourcing integrative doctors who can prescribe vaginal oxytocin.

**WELLNESS ACTION PLAN**
# OXYTOCIN

- Hugs: A six-second hug can boost oxytocin levels for several hours, promoting emotional wellbeing.

- Laughter: Sharing a good laugh with friends or family is a great way to naturally increase oxytocin.

- Music and singing: Listening to music or singing in a group, like with friends or family, stimulates oxytocin production.

- Magnesium: Optimise your magnesium levels, as this mineral acts as a cofactor for oxytocin receptors, helping them function properly.

- Eye contact: Engaging in eye contact during conversations can naturally raise oxytocin levels, fostering deeper connections.

- Cold therapy: Exposure to cold, such as cold showers or ice baths, increases oxytocin levels, along with other benefits for wellbeing. If cold therapy isn't for you, try a warm bath to relax and boost oxytocin.

**TIP**

Cholesterol Caution: Cholesterol supports oxytocin receptor binding, so be aware that cholesterol-lowering statin drugs may impact oxytocin communication with cells.

**DID YOU KNOW?**

- Kissing for longevity: Men who kiss their loved ones goodbye live, on average, two years longer. This strategy works for women too, as it boosts oxytocin levels.

- Hugging pets: Hugging your pet raises oxytocin for both you and your furry friend, promoting bonding and wellbeing for both!

By weaving these simple bio-hacks into your daily life, you'll naturally boost your oxytocin, deepen your social connections, and improve your health. Try incorporating some of these practices and enjoy the benefits of this powerful hormone.

## It's time to feel the love!

## Recommended reading

**Women's hormonal health and wellness**

*How to Be Well: A Handbook for Women* by Dr Karen Coates and Sharon Kolkka

*The Dopamine Brain* by Dr Anastasia Hronis

*What Your Doctor May Not Tell You About Menopause* by Dr John R Lee MD

*Natural Fertility* by Francesca Naish

*What Am I Supposed to Eat?* by Dr Libby Weaver

**Women's wisdom and emotional wellbeing**

*The Red Tent* (fiction) by Anita Diamant

*Women Who Run with the Wolves* by Clarissa Pinkola Estés

*Inward* by Yung Pueblo

**Hormones and your brain**

*The XX Brain* by Dr Lisa Mosconi

*Brainstorm: The Power and Purpose of the Teenage Brain* by Dr Daniel J Siegel

**Mindfulness and meditation**

*Learn to Meditate* by Dr David Fontana

Writings and teachings by Pema Chödrön, Thich Nhat Hanh, Dr Daniel J Siegel and Jon Kabat-Zinn

## Medical references

Scan the QR code to find a list of sources the authors referred to while researching and writing this book.

# Resources

### Accredited naturopaths, TCM and Ayurvedic practitioners

Australia

**NHAA**
nhaa.org.au

**ATMS**
atms.com.au

New Zealand

**NZAMH**
nzamh.org.nz

**NMHNZ**
naturopath.org.nz

**NHPNZ**
nhpnz.org

United Kingdom

**CNHC**
cnhc.org.uk

**British Acupuncture Council**
acupuncture.org.uk

**General Naturopathic Council**
gncouncil.co.uk

### Alcohol support services

Australia

**Alcoholics Anonymous**
aa.org.au

**Al-Anon Family Groups**
al-anon.org.au

**Hello Sunday Morning**
hellosundaymorning.org

**SMART Recovery Australia**
smartrecoveryaustralia.com.au

New Zealand

**Alcoholics Anonymous NZ**
aa.org.nz

**Al-Anon NZ**
al-anon.org.nz

**Living Sober**
livingsober.org.nz

**CADS Auckland**
cads.org.nz

United Kingdom

**Alcoholics Anonymous UK**
alcoholics-anonymous.org.uk

**Al-Anon Family Groups UK**
al-anonuk.org.uk

**SMART Recovery UK**
smartrecovery.org.uk

### Apps for health and mindfulness

Brain and focus

*Lumosity*
lumosity.com

*Waking Up*
wakingup.com

Menstrual and fertility tracking

*Flo*
flo.health

*MyNFM*—Natural Fertility Management
naturalfertility.com

Mindfulness and calm

*Headspace*
headspace.com

*Calm*
calm.com

### Compounding pharmacies

Australia

**ACPharm**
acpharm.com.au

New Zealand

**CompoundLabs**
compoundlabs.co.nz

**Optimus Healthcare**
optimushealth.co.nz

**Waimauku Pharmacy**
waimaukupharmacy.co.nz

United Kingdom

**Roseway Labs**
rosewaylabs.com

**Specialist Pharmacy**
specialist-pharmacy.com

**Compounding Chemist**
cchemist.com

RESOURCES

## Bone Health and Physio

**The Bone Clinic and the Onero Principle**
theboneclinic.com.au

**Australian Physiotherapy Association**
australian.physio

## Crisis support services

### Australia

**Lifeline**
13 11 14—lifeline.org.au

**Beyond Blue**
1300 22 4636—beyondblue.org.au

### New Zealand

**1737**—call or text

**Lifeline NZ**
0800 543 354

**Suicide Crisis Helpline**
0508 828 865 (0508 TAUTOKO)

**Youthline**
0800 376 633 or text 234—youthline.co.nz

### United Kingdom

**NHS 111 (mental health option)**

**Samaritans**
116 123—samaritans.org

**SANEline**
0300 304 7000—sane.org.uk

## Domestic violence services

### Australia

**1800RESPECT**
1800 737 732, 1800respect.org.au

### New Zealand

**Women's Refuge Crisisline**
0800 733 843, womensrefuge.org.nz

### United Kingdom

**National Domestic Abuse Helpline**
0808 2000 247, nationaldahelpline.org.uk

## Gender clinics and transgender support

### Australia

**Royal Children's Hospital Gender Service (Melbourne)**
rch.org.au

**The Identity Clinic (Sydney)**
theidentityclinic.com.au

### New Zealand

**Gender Minorities Aotearoa**
genderminorities.com

**Auckland DHB**
adhb.health.nz

### United Kingdom

**Tavistock and Portman NHS Gender Clinic**
tavistockandportman.nhs.uk

**GenderCare**
gendercare.co.uk

**Gender Plus**
genderplus.co.uk

## Genetic testing for health and wellness

**BRCA Gene Testing (Breast/Ovarian Cancer)**—Speak with your doctor about genetic counselling and testing options.

## Health and wellbeing genes (e.g. COMT, detox pathways)

### Australia

**Fitgenes**
fitgenes.com.au

### New Zealand

**Fitgenes NZ**
fitgenes.com.au

**The Apothecary**
the-apothecary.co.nz

### United Kingdom

**United Kingdom
Body Fabulous**—mybodyfabulous.co.uk

## Integrative medicine practitioners

### Global

**Institute for Functional Medicine (IFM)**
ifm.org

### Australia

**ACNEM**
acnem.org

**ACPharm**
acpharm.com.au

### New Zealand

**ACNEM**
acnem.org

### United Kingdom

**MTHFR Support UK**
mthfr-genetics.co.uk

## Natural skin and body care

Australian skincare brands

**Eco Tan—certified organic tanning, skincare and body care:**
ecotan.com.au

**Phyt's—certified organic French skincare**
phyts.com.au

**Subtle Energies—aromatherapy and ayurvedic skincare**
subtleenergies.com.au

**ACPharm—vitamin and mineral-based
skincare and tinted sunscreens**
acpharm.com.au

Scent and pheromones

**The Athena Institute—women's pheromone fragrance**
athenainstitute.com

## Menopause and hormonal health

Education and clinics

**Australian Menopause Centre**
menopausecentre.com.au

PMDD resources

Australia

**Professor Jayashri Kulkarni (MAPrc)—PMDD explainer video**
youtu.be/AXHR4mOuYcs

**Dr Len Kliman**
drlenkliman.com.au/articles/premenstrual-dysphoric-disorderpmdd/

New Zealand

**Family Health Diary**
familyhealthdiary.co.nz/pmdd/

United Kingdom

**Hormone Health**
hormonehealth.co.uk/treatments/premenstrual-dysphoric-disorder-pmdd

**Marion Gluck Clinic**
mariongluckclinic.com

Endometriosis

**RATE Tool (RANZCOG)**
ranzcog.edu.au

## Self-referral pathology testing

Australia

**iMedical**
imedical.com.au

**QML Pathology**
qml.com.au

New Zealand

**MyTests by Awanui**
mytests.co.nz

**i-screen NZ**
i-screen.co.nz

United Kingdom

**Nuffield Health—
Pathology Direct**
nuffieldhealth.com/pathology-direct

**Private Blood Tests UK**
privatebloodtests.co.uk

## Sleep health

**Dr Matt Walker**
sleepfoundation.org

# Index

## #
4-7-8 breathing 385
5:2 or 16/8 fasting 640
5-HTP 187, 651, 652, 653

## A
acceptance 330
acne 46-8, 343
acupuncture 83, 106, 115, 174, 336, 672
acute stress response 337-8
adaptogens 143, 190, 201, 336, 345, 349, 680, 681
adenomyosis 403, 518-19
adrenal disruptors 478, 481-2
adrenal exhaustion 335, 343, 497
adrenal glands 239, 294, 334-41
adrenal support 115, 201, 347-8
adrenaline 102, 187, 196, 275, 335, 336-41
  stress and 187, 200, 275, 276, 291, 310, 335
  wellness action plan 339-41
aerobic glycolysis 367
Age of Wisdom 25, 166, 236-65
  exercise plan 247-9
  hormone levels 240-2
  medical checklist 251-2
  spiritual connection and growth 254-65
  wellness action plan 243-6
alcohol 176, 239, 272, 282, 287-9, 345, 528
  bladder health 532
  bone health 629
  breast cancer and 287, 288, 587
  breast health 287, 570, 573, 577
  dementia and 641
  fatty liver disease 596, 597
  fertility and 106, 114
  GABA production and 669, 672
  liver and 280, 287, 288, 359
  menopause 166, 176, 182, 197, 225, 288, 359
  oxidative stress 282, 287
  perimenopause 158, 159, 288, 359
  PMS and 81
  postnatal recovery and 108
  sleep and 176, 359, 363, 364, 365
  standard drink definitions 288
  stress hormones and 176, 301
  sugar and 435
aldosterone 336
alpha linolenic acid (ALA) 416, 419-20, 568
Alzheimer's disease 352, 370, 401, 635
amygdala 49, 102, 311-13, 317
anaemia 70, 109, 133, 139, 202, 412, 454, 460
androgens 336, 558
anti-inflammatory foods 82, 107, 246, 271, 346
  breast health 574
  endometriosis management 543
  menopause 177, 192, 226, 271
  ovarian health 528
  stress management 271, 349
antioxidants 82, 93, 248, 282-5, 408-10
  breast health 287, 570, 573, 575
  cervical health 516
  menopause 186, 190, 193, 194, 226, 271
  ovarian health 528
  stress relief 282-5, 349
apple cider vinegar 426, 507, 567, 650
arthritis 221, 247, 417, 491
artificial additives 398, 437-40
ashwagandha *see* withania
assisted reproduction 23, 105-9, 368
autoimmune disorders 109, 270, 276, 602
Ayurveda 41, 43, 79, 131, 335, 336

## B
B-vitamins *see* vitamin B
Beck, Belinda 628, 631
berberine 568
beta-caryophyllene 350
Biobran/Ribraxx 577, 590
bioidentical hormones *see* hormone replacement therapy
biotin 194
bisphosphonates 623-4
black cohosh 174, 177, 230, 630
bladder 126, 157, 182-4, 530-3
bloating 33, 45, 82, 157, 125-8, 224, 595
blood pressure 200, 201, 220, 244, 463
blood sugar 81, 176, 200, 205, 251, 347, 398, 528
blood tests 111, 139, 140
blue light 355-6, 368, 640
Blue Zone (calm) 295, 296, 299-305, 373
  activating 304-5, 311, 346, 373-80
Blue Zones (longevity) 95, 96, 238-9, 393
body fat 31, 151, 203-5, 239, 245
body image boosters 217
bone health/density 245, 612-34
  alcohol and 629
  bisphosphonates 623-4
  calcium 229, 231, 233, 462, 468-71, 612
  denosumab 624
  early menopause 229, 231, 233, 615
  exercise for 209, 628, 631-3
  herbal support 315-16
  HRT and 626, 629, 633
  melatonin 205-6, 369, 629, 633
  menopause 161, 178, 194, 205, 209, 210, 470, 627
  nutrition 619, 622
  osteopenia 613, 615
  osteoporosis 206, 271, 291, 369, 613-18
  oestrogen and 34, 69, 160, 229, 245, 619
  oxytocin and 685
  perimenopause 126
  progesterone and 619, 626
  sleep and 628, 633
  testing 613-15, 621
  testosterone 629, 633, 673
  vitamin D 229, 231, 233, 246, 445-7, 614, 621, 622, 627
  wellness action plan 627-34
boric acid pessaries 509, 510
BPA 113, 440, 479-80, 536, 560-1
brain 635-41
  Age of Wisdom 25, 247-8, 637
  amygdala 49, 102, 311-13, 317
  dementia *see* dementia
  fog 151, 158, 169, 188-91, 232, 291, 345, 588
  improving function 188-91 639-41
  meditation benefits 387-8
  melatonin and 370
  menopause 152, 158, 188-91, 279, 637, 639-41
  nutrition for 188-90, 401, 639-40
  oestrogen, role of 34, 35, 69, 156
  orgasms improving function 221
  oxidative stress and 277, 279
  perimenopause 126, 133, 140, 143, 636
  pharmaceuticals supporting 638
  puberty 29, 30, 49-50, 636
  reshaping 310
  resting brain state 301
  rewiring 313, 320, 321-5
  wellness action plan 639-41
breast cancer 230-1, 578-91
  alcohol and 287, 288, 587
  antioxidants protecting against 284
  black cohosh and 177, 230
  BPA and 560
  cortisol and stress 281
  Depo-Provera and risk of 117
  exercise/movement 588-9
  hormone-receptor positive 230-1
  HRT and 172, 230-1, 571
  melatonin and 367-8, 577
  nutrition 586-8
  olive oil and 421
  omega-3s 586
  oxidative stress and 277, 279, 286
  phytoestrogens reducing risk 404
  screening for 171, 571-2, 578
  self-care 584-5
  stress and 242, 581
  Tamoxifen 587-8

## INDEX

breasts 569-91
  alcohol and 287, 570, 573, 577
  antioxidants protecting 284
  bra 207
  cortisol and stress 281
  dense 572
  fertile years 64, 78, 570
  fibrocystic 126, 572
  herbal support 573
  menopause 157, 171, 207-8, 224, 570
  microbiome 574
  oestrogen, role of 35, 69, 207
  oxidative stress 571
  perimenopause 124-6, 136, 570
  puberty 22, 28, 35, 42, 569
  screening 171, 571-2
  self-examination 208
  synthetic hormones and 571
  tenderness 42, 45, 64, 78, 124-6, 224
  vitamin D and 445
  wellness action plan 575-7
breathing/breathwork 261, 297, 340, 381-5
  Blue Zone, activating 374, 377, 378
  fertile years 74, 89, 91, 93, 104, 115
  menopause 186, 187, 201, 227
  perimenopause 134
butter 422

## C

C-Reactive Protein (CRP) test 251, 252
caffeine 82, 108, 110, 114, 182, 197, 225, 433
  adrenal health and 341, 345
  bladder health 532
  bone health 628
  breast health 577
  GABA production and 672
  sleep and 357-8, 363
  tips for reducing intake 358
calcium 194, 229, 231, 233, 462, 468-71
  bone health 612, 614, 627
  serotonin and 651, 652, 656
cancer 77, 238
  alcohol and 287, 288
  artificial additives and 438
  breast *see* breast cancer
  cervical 511-16
  HRT and 168, 177, 228
  iron deficiency 453
  olive oil and 420
  ovarian 277, 280, 284, 524, 526
  phytoestrogens reducing risk 404
  skin 193
  stress and 242, 291
*Candida see* vaginal *Candida*
carbohydrates 56, 113, 205, 400-3, 559, 639
cardiovascular exercise *see* exercise/movement
cardiovascular health 60, 79, 238, 244, 251, 280

alcohol and 287, 288
lifestyle factors 238, 271, 272
magnesium 464
menopause 154, 172, 200, 202, 203, 209, 233
nutrition 245, 395, 417, 420
orgasms and 220
oxytocin and 685
Carman, Dr Judy 428-9
cartilage protection 192, 195
catalase 280
catastrophising 324, 325
catecholamines 335, 336
cell housekeeping 280-1
cervical cancer 511-16
cervical caps 117
cervical smear tests 111, 250, 251, 512
cervix 511-16
chamomile 82
Chaste Tree 37, 44, 45, 573
chemical menopause 216, 227
cholesterol 244-5, 445
choline 576, 577, 638
chronotypes 353, 365
circadian rhythm 99, 134, 175, 186, 205, 299, 343, 354-5, 367, 681
clean foods 85, 112, 397, 405-7
COAL state of mind 326, 329-30
coconut oil 180, 217, 250, 397, 416, 422-3, 508
cognitive behavioural therapy 83, 133, 187, 317-24, 364, 386
cognitive function *see* brain
collagen 192, 193, 194, 207, 284
COMT enzyme 86, 93, 169, 224, 275
conception 94-115
  egg and cell health 278-9
  IVF 105-9, 368
  wellness action plan 111-15
contraception 23, 69, 71, 116-18
contraceptives 48, 83, 116-18
  the Pill 23, 37, 41, 48, 71, 76, 83, 538
cooling strategies 161, 175, 198
copper 473, 476-7, 515
core strength 31
cortisol 299, 336, 342-50
  bone health 628
  breasts and 281
  low levels 110
  management 68, 88, 170, 187, 343-6, 383
  over-exercising and 68, 101, 144, 283, 345
  oxidative stress and 281, 282
  PCOS and 553-4
  rhythm 169
  sleep and 169, 176, 345-7, 355
  stress and 102, 137, 205, 275, 276, 282, 291, 311
  wellness action plan 347-8
Cramp Bark 45, 72, 74
creative practices 258, 305, 306, 378-9

creator mindset 327-8
critical planning 324
cruciferous vegetables 86, 226, 284, 400, 522, 570, 573, 577, 528, 598
curcumin 284, 573, 640
curiosity 329
Cutler, Dr Winnifred 218
cyclic breathing 383-4
CYP1B1 169, 224

## D

dehydration 182, 190, 194, 201
dementia 138, 238, 248, 635-41
  brain health *see* brain
  HRT and 172, 173
  risk of 164, 172, 635-41
  stress and 291
denosumab 624
depression 156, 163, 185-7, 232, 240
  postnatal 107, 109, 163
  premenstrual 43
detox apps 484
detox pathways 145, 483, 522
DHEA 278, 286, 335, 336, 348, 681
diabetes 111, 238, 245, 685
  Type 2 203, 245, 251, 269, 401, 431, 434, 565
diaphragmatic breathing 385, 391, 672
diaphragms 116-17
diet *see* nourishment
DIM (diindolylmethane) 137, 522, 543, 573
dizziness 42, 126, 157, 197, 200-2
DNA methylation 272
domestic violence 293
Dong quai 158, 178, 544
dopamine 240, 335, 336, 645, 653-66
  boosting 185-9, 661-6
  gut health and 425, 666
  low, symptoms of 658-9, 662-4
  menopause 164, 169, 189, 223, 661
  nutrition 185, 189, 664, 665
  sugars disrupting 398
DUTCH test 168-9, 171, 348, 608
dyspareunia 213

## E

early menopause 216, 227-34
egg freezing 94, 230, 231
electrolyte imbalance 197
embracing emotions 322-3
empowering language 319
emulsifiers 86, 439
endocrine-disrupting chemicals (EDCs) 31, 405, 478-84, 527
endometrial ablation 83
endometrial hyperplasia 171
endometriosis 23, 75, 107, 126, 534-45
  folate and 403
  hysterectomy 153

oophorectomy 228
oxidative stress and 286, 291, 536
progesterone receptor resistance 537
wellness action plan 542–5
endorphins 220, 221
epigenetics 269–76, 431, 535, 602
equanimity 311–12, 321, 324, 327
eugenol 349
eustress 292, 293, 295
evening primrose oil 45, 82, 178
exercise/movement 58–61, 485–97
  adrenaline, controlling 339–41
  Age of Wisdom 246, 247–9, 488, 495
  balanced 60, 283, 486–97
  bone health 628, 631–3
  brain health 640
  breast cancer 588–9
  breast health 576
  cardiovascular 60, 61, 89, 210–12, 246, 488, 494
  cortisol management 348
  destress toolkit 304
  dopamine boost 186, 189, 665
  endometriosis management 542
  endurance training 490
  fertile years 87–93, 488, 494
  flexibility 60, 61, 212, 213, 488, 493
  GABA support 144
  hormone balance 87–93
  intensity 489
  menopause 170, 179, 186, 189, 198, 201, 204, 208–12, 488, 495
  mood boosting 186
  over-exercising 68, 101, 114, 283, 488, 497, 619
  PCOS management 559–60
  perimenopause 134, 137, 144, 271, 488, 494
  preconception 114
  puberty 45, 58–61, 488, 494
  restorative 376
  serotonin boost 656
  stability 60, 61, 211, 212, 488, 493
  strength 59, 61, 88–91, 208–12, 246, 488, 490–5
  testosterone support 681
  yin and yang 486–91

## F

facial hair 192
fast 800 diet 566
fasting, intermittent 191, 640
fats 56, 81, 188, 191, 245
  healthy see healthy fats/oils
fatty liver disease 596
fenugreek 568, 680
fermented foods 86, 186, 248, 397, 424–6, 567, 671
fertile years 23, 63–118, 270
  conception see conception
  menstrual cycle see menstrual cycle
  wellness action plan 85–93

fertility 23, 94–104
  Blue Zones 95, 96, 393
  disruption 101–4
  early menopause and 231, 232
  egg and cell health 278–9
  endometriosis and 537, 538
  melatonin and 367, 368
  oxidative stress and 278–9
fibre 56, 86, 205, 226, 345, 399, 402, 521, 575
fibroids, uterine 126, 517–20
fish/seafood 56, 57, 80, 81, 89, 344
  big fish and pregnancy 113
  farming 417
  omega-3 56, 81, 186, 189, 192, 205, 414, 417
  sleep support 362
  thyroid support 610
  vitamin D 448
  wild seafood 113, 483
fish oil supplements 416–17
flaxseeds 284
float therapy 375
fluctuating hormones 22, 23, 24, 30
  menopause 153, 154, 174, 196, 200, 223
  perimenopause 124, 136, 140, 142, 146, 279
fluid retention 81, 82, 125, 157, 595
focus see memory and focus
folate 186, 190, 287, 371, 403, 411–15
  breast health 576
  cervical health 515
  dopamine and 664, 665
  PCOS management 556, 563
  serotonin and 652
folic acid 403, 515, 638
follicle-stimulating hormone (FSH) 71, 99, 103, 368
food see nourishment
food labels 440
forest bathing (Shinrin-Yoku) 374
'forever chemicals' 145, 481–2
free radicals 100, 193, 274–82
  see also oxidative stress

## G

GABA 82, 141–4, 185, 195, 223, 645, 667–72
  calming effect 185, 196, 645, 668
  nutrition for 82, 185, 671
  serotonin and 646, 670
  sleep support 362, 668
gabapentin 179, 230
gamma-aminobutyric acid see GABA
gender identity 54
genetically modified (GMO) foods 398, 428–9
geothermal bathing 375
Giedd, Jay 49
GliSODin 285
glucocorticoid receptors (GRs) 342–3

glutathione 280, 284
glycation end products (AGEs) 280
glyphosate reduction 406, 585
goal setting 146, 189, 237, 314, 322
gratitude 263, 265, 315, 316, 319, 332, 378, 672
Graves disease 602
growth mindset 315
gut health 80, 86, 113, 226, 397, 402, 424–6
  artificial additives and 438
  dopamine and 425, 666
  endometriosis management 544
  GABA production 671
  insulin resistance and 567
  iron intake and 451, 459
  magnesium intake and 466
  mood hormones and 647
  serotonin and 425, 650–2, 656
  vitamin supplements and 444
gymnema sylvestre 568

## H

hair loss 126, 157, 192, 233
healthy fats/oils 56, 86, 106, 397, 416–23
  alpha linolenic acid (ALA) 416, 419–20
  brain health 639
  maintaining fat distribution 205
  menopause 188, 201
  omega-3 see omega-3 fatty acids
  omega-6 246, 416, 418–23
  perimenopause 144, 271
  testosterone support 680
  thyroid support 610
  uterine health 521
heart health see cardiovascular health
herbal tea 182, 201, 305, 361, 377, 527, 544
  Tulsi 201, 341, 348, 349–50, 610, 666
high-intensity interval training (HIIT) 492
Highly Sensitive CRP (HsCRP) test 252
histone modification 272
homeostasis 310–11
hormonal balance/imbalance
  Age of Wisdom 240–2
  alcohol and 287
  bone health and 633
  breast health and 571
  DUTCH test 168–9, 171, 348, 608
  epigenetics and lifestyle choices 270–1
  exercise plan 87–92, 134
  healthy fats for 205, 416
  iron, role of 449
  lifestyle and herbal remedies 41, 43–5, 143
  menstrual cycle 23, 31, 64, 79
  orgasms and 220

PCOS 536, 537, 558
Pill for 37, 41, 71, 76, 83
puberty 23, 31, 270, 278
sleep and 351, 352, 364
stress and 79, 83, 242, 270, 291
sulforaphane and 401
vitamin D and 445
Hormonal Health Pillars 43, 223, 267–497
hormonal patches 117
hormonal stages 22–5
hormonal testing 31, 38
hormone replacement therapy (HRT) 162–4, 172–3
  benefits and risks 164, 172–3
  bioidentical hormones 139, 179, 225
  bone health 626, 629, 633
  breast cancer and 172, 230–1, 571
  early menopause 233
  hot flushes, for 179
  menopause 25, 151, 162–4, 168, 172–3, 192
  mood balancing 187
  oestrogen replacement 162–4, 179, 228
  oral form 173, 226
  perimenopause 119, 139–41, 143
  progesterone 139–41, 143, 168, 199, 228, 610
  safety 162, 172, 173
  sublingual delivery 173
  testosterone 179, 676, 679, 681
  thyroid support 610
  timing 172
  transdermal delivery 173, 225, 226
horny goat weed 217
hot flushes 24, 174–9
  cortisol and 344
  early menopause 232
  herbal support 174, 177, 230–1
  HRT for 179
  lifestyle choices to reduce 179, 271
  menopause 159, 163–6, 174–9, 363
  palpitations and 197, 198
  perimenopause 24, 124, 126, 271, 363
  pharmaceutics for 179, 230
  stress and 291
HPA axis dysfunction 107, 110
HRT *see* hormone replacement therapy
human papilloma virus (HPV) 511–15
hyaluronic acid (HA) 194–5
hydrating foods 175, 186, 190, 201
hydration 182, 194, 197, 201, 208, 366
hyperthyroidism 600, 601
hypothyroidism 600, 607
hysterectomy 140, 153, 164, 227

# I

immune system 68, 109, 112, 252, 537
  adrenals supporting 335, 336, 338
  alcohol and 287
  cortisol and 342–6
  endometriosis and 536, 543
  iron, role of 449
  oxidative stress and 277–8, 280
  sleep and 352
  stress and 292, 299, 311, 321
in vitro fertilisation (IVF) 105–9, 368
incontinence *see* bladder
infertility 101–4
inflammation 245, 246, 251, 270, 277, 345
  CRP test 251, 252
  infertility and 101
  reducing *see* anti-inflammatory foods
inflammatory bowel diseases 425, 438, 439, 459, 619
insulin 251, 280, 286, 398, 424, 685
insulin resistance 107, 204, 245, 286, 401, 564–8
  fatty liver disease and 596
  liver health and 598
  PCOS and 559, 562, 564
  wellness action plan 566–8
insulin sensitivity 170, 200, 203, 558
intermittent fasting 191, 640
intrauterine devices (IUDs) 117, 171
iodine 187, 458, 576, 577, 609
iron 449–61
  anaemia 70, 109, 133, 139, 202, 412, 454, 460
  audit 451
  B-vitamins and 412
  brain function 654
  causes of low 458
  deficiency 70, 133, 202, 348, 412, 413, 449–55, 652
  dopamine and 664, 665
  excessive 457
  Ferinject 460
  fertile years 89, 100, 109, 270, 461
  food sources 45, 460
  optimum level 283
  oxidative stress reduction 283–4
  perimenopause 133, 134, 139, 461
  puberty 45, 461
  serotonin and 651, 652, 656
  sleep and 363
  tests 455–6
  thyroid support 609
  wellness action plan 459
isoflavones 175, 178, 570, 588

# J

jet lag 364
joints 192, 195, 221, 246, 247
  exercise for 59, 60, 247, 491
  pain or stiffness 126, 157, 192, 195, 246
journaling 258, 261, 322, 379, 606, 611

# K

ketones 188, 191
kidneys 111, 112, 114, 139, 251, 288
kissing and longevity 688
KNDy neurons 175, 177, 179

# L

L-theanine 144
*Lactobacillus* 504, 505, 507, 557, 563
Lazar, Dr Sara 387
leafy greens 133, 186, 284, 400
leaky gut 425, 439
Lee, Dr John 242
legumes 133, 171, 248, 399
libido 24, 84, 103, 116, 216–18, 352
  loss of 125, 126, 157, 213, 214–18
  testosterone and 673, 675, 678, 682
lifestyle choices 15, 55, 173, 204, 223
  epigenetics and 269, 270–1
  fertility and 96, 112, 142
linalool 350
liver 112–14, 139, 176, 286, 592–8
  alcohol and 280, 287, 288, 359
  breast health and 573
  clean 113, 137, 176
  detoxifying 280, 286, 522, 528, 592–4
  enzymes 594–5
  fatty liver disease 596
  testosterone support 682
  wellness action plan 597–8
longevity 238–9, 688
love 330, 332, 683
luteal progesterone 83
luteinising hormone (LH) 71, 99, 103, 132, 368

# M

maca root 178, 680
magnesium 462–8
  adrenal health 340, 344, 345, 348
  blood pressure regulation 201, 244, 463
  bone health 245, 614, 627
  brain function 186, 189, 654
  calcium and 462, 465, 468, 614
  deficiency checklist 465
  endometriosis management 544
  fertile years 86, 464
  food sources 45, 246–8, 466, 469
  GABA production 671, 672
  insulin resistance and 566
  intravenous 468

melatonin and 371
  menopause 185, 186, 189, 197, 201, 226, 465
  oil 467
  oxytocin and 687
  PCOS management 555, 556, 563
  perimenopause 137, 144, 464
  potassium and 468
  pre-eclampsia 463
  serotonin and 248, 654, 656
  sleep and 363
  stress relief 305
  testosterone support 680
  thyroid support 610
  toxicity 467
  transdermal 466
magnolia bark 177
manganese 100, 280, 283, 610, 627
manganese superoxide dismutase (MnSOD) 280
massage 115, 208, 307, 375, 467
'me time' 74, 89, 108, 167, 302
meat, grass-fed, free-range 397, 427
medically-induced menopause 227-34
meditation 134, 258, 386-92
  adrenal health 336, 344
  Blue Zone activation 377-8
  breast health 576
  endometriosis management 542
  fertile years 89, 91, 93, 114
  how to meditate 389-92
  menopause 179, 187, 189, 201, 227, 235
  serotonin boost 656
  sleep and 364
  stress reduction 304, 305, 306, 308
Mediterranean diet 395, 417, 421, 566
melatonin 170, 205-6, 367-71
  Age of Wisdom 240, 369
  blue/red light and 355, 356, 368
  body weight and 206, 369
  bone health 205-6, 369, 629, 633
  breast cancer support 367-8, 577
  fertile years 367, 368
  food sources 170, 368, 369, 371
  menopause 170, 205-6, 367, 369
  moon decreasing 99
  oxidative stress and 286, 370
  perimenopause 369
  pistachio nuts 362
  puberty 368
  serotonin and 355, 371, 645
  sleep and 169-71, 205-6, 347, 355, 362, 363, 365, 366
  sugar and 359
  supplementation 170, 369
  topical 193
memory and focus see also brain
  early menopause 232
  improving 188-91
  lapses 126, 138, 157, 188-91
  meditation benefits 387-8
  oestrogen, role of 34, 35, 69
  testosterone, role of 673

menarche 35
menopausal hormone therapy (MHT) see hormone replacement therapy (HRT)
menopause 24-5, 149-235
  action plan 225-7
  early/premature 216, 227-34
  exercise plan 209-13
  herbal support 161, 164
  HRT see hormone replacement therapy (HRT)
  induced 216, 227-34
  nutrition 170-1, 175-6, 185-6, 204, 205, 271
  oestrogen deficiency 24, 156, 158-61, 213, 279
  oxidative stress 279
  sexual health 180-1, 213-21
  symptoms 156-8
  wellness action plan 174-9
menstrual cycle 22, 23, 31-45, 67-83, 87
  balanced cycle 42, 66, 74
  celebrating end of 237-8
  cortisol and 344, 346
  erratic periods 24, 36, 38, 125, 147, 159, 165, 525
  fertile years 67-83, 97
  follicular phase 40, 70-1, 89
  hormonal imbalance 31, 37, 43, 64, 70-1
  iron deficiency 452, 458
  natural fertility and contraception 69, 71, 97
  night-time flooding 129, 138
  normal cycle 38-9, 42, 74
  overall health, reflecting 66
  oxidative stress and irregularity 279
  perimenopause 124-9, 138, 143
  PMS see premenstrual syndrome
  puberty 22, 28-45, 51
  red flags 43, 70-1, 77
  thyroid, role of 600, 602
  tracking 31, 33, 37, 69, 97
milk thistle 573
mindfulness see also meditation
  Blue Zone activation 377-8
  cortisol management 344-6
  creative practices 378-9
  embracing emotions 322-3
  health benefits 387-8
  meditation 387-92
  menopause 179, 187, 189, 201, 217
  perimenopause 134, 142, 144
  stress reduction 93, 298, 304, 306, 321, 387
  stress resilience 315, 320, 332
mindfulness-based cognitive therapy (MBCT) 386
mindfulness-based stress reduction (MBSR) 386
mineralocorticoid receptors (MRs) 342
monounsaturated fats 416, 420-1

mood hormones 645-7
  see also dopamine; GABA; oxytocin; serotonin
mood swings and irritability
  Age of Wisdom 240
  cortisol and 343, 344, 346
  early menopause 232
  HRT alleviating 164
  lifestyle choices to reduce 271
  meditation benefits 387-8
  menopause 156, 157, 159, 174, 185-7, 224
  nutritional support 185-6, 248
  oxidative stress and 279
  perimenopause 124, 125, 126, 127, 138, 139, 271
  premenstrual 44, 45, 64, 78
  processed sugars and 398
  progesterone, role of 35, 36, 69
  puberty 22, 31, 36, 39, 278, 343
moon 97, 99, 128, 262, 333, 364
Mosconi, Dr Lisa 248
movement see exercise/movement
multivitamins 443-4
music 378-9, 687
myo-inositol 557, 562, 567

# N

N-acetyl cysteine (NAC) 597
Naish, Francesca 97
natural contraception 69, 71, 116, 118
natural fertility 95-100
nature, connecting with 186, 260-3, 374
naturopathy checklist 252
negative thoughts 297, 314, 317-20
nervous system 293-303
  parasympathetic 294, 295, 383
  sympathetic 294
neuroplasticity 313
nicotine 359, 433, 672
night sweats 126, 151, 157, 158, 164, 232, 344, 363
noradrenaline 275, 335-8
nourishment 393-442
  acne management 48
  adrenal support 344-8
  Age of Wisdom 248, 272
  allergies and intolerances 438
  artificial additives 398, 437-40
  balanced diet 55-7, 201, 204, 217, 235, 377
  Blue Zones 393
  bone health 619, 622
  brain health 188-90, 639-40
  breast cancer 586-8
  breast health 575-7
  clean foods 85, 112, 397, 405-7
  Core Food Principles 396-442
  cortisol regulation 344-8
  destress toolkit 304
  epigenetics and lifestyle choices 270-2
  fertile years 85-6, 89-92

fresh, local, seasonal foods 85, 397, 408-15
GABA support 144
genetically modified goods 398, 428-9
grass-fed, free-range meat 397, 427
ideal food pyramid 395
low-inflammatory foods 85
Mediterranean diet 395, 417, 421, 566
melatonin sources 170, 368, 369, 371
menopause 170-1, 175-6, 185-6, 204, 205, 271
mood hormone balance 185-6
organic foods 397, 405-7, 483, 544
oxidative stress reduction 283
PCOS management 556-9
perimenopause 133, 134, 144, 271
plant-based 393-5, 397, 399-404
PMS management 80-1
postnatal recovery 108
preconception 112-14
preservatives and colourings 398, 437-40
puberty 22, 37, 48, 55-6, 270, 344
real food 55
restorative 376
serotonin and 185, 649-54
sleep support 170, 362, 371
testosterone support 680
thyroid support 610
whole foods 393-5, 397, 399-404, 483

## O

ocimumosides 349
oestradiol 168, 183, 224
oestriol cream 181, 183, 193, 217, 508, 509, 533
oestrobolome 226, 424
oestrogen
  Age of Wisdom, ideal level 240
  brain function 34, 35, 69, 156
  deficiency 24, 25, 156, 158-61, 233
  dominance 75-6, 103, 124, 135-47, 402, 424, 473, 478, 517-23
  environmental 224
  fertile years 23, 69-76, 79, 82-93, 278
  menopause, decline in 156, 158-61, 196, 207, 213, 279
  menstrual cycle 31, 34-9, 69-76, 87
  metabolism 168, 224
  oxidative stress and 278-9, 286
  perimenopause phases 124-47, 279
  puberty 22, 31, 34-9, 278
  replacement therapy 162-4, 179, 228
  role of 34, 35, 69, 156, 207
  sensitivity 224, 225
  stress hormones and 291
  testosterone and 679
Okinawa Blue Zone 95, 96, 393
olive oil 56, 81, 180, 188, 245, 397, 416, 418, 420, 423

omega-3 fatty acids 245, 416-23, 521
  antioxidants 284
  brain health 189, 248, 640
  breast cancer and 586
  breast health 570, 572, 575, 577
  chemotherapy and 586
  cortisol management 344, 346
  endometriosis management 543
  food sources 248, 397, 417-18
  insulin resistance and 568
  menopause 183, 186, 189-93, 205
  PCOS management 563
  PMS reduction 81
  puberty 45, 56
  testosterone support 682
  thyroid support 610
omega-6 fatty acids 246, 416, 418-19
oophorectomy 227, 228
openness 329
organic foods 397, 405-7, 483, 544, 585
orgasms 182, 219-21
osteonecrosis 623, 624
osteopenia 613, 615
osteoporosis 206, 271, 291, 369, 613-18
ovarian cancer 284, 524, 526
  endometriosis and risk of 538
  oxidative stress and 277, 280, 284, 524, 527
  testing and screening 526
ovarian cysts 526, 529
  PCOS *see* polycystic ovary syndrome
ovaries 72, 524-9
  antioxidants protecting 284
  conception *see* conception
  egg and cell health 278-9
  melatonin protecting 367
  oxidative stress and 280, 284, 524, 527
  rejuvenation 106
  retiring 122, 124, 126, 127, 227
over-exercising 68, 101, 114, 144, 283, 488, 497
  bone health and 619-20
  cortisol and 68, 101, 144, 283, 345
  fertility and 101
ovulation 36, 38-40, 71-2, 97-100
oxidative stress 273-86
  alcohol and 282, 287
  antioxidants *see* antioxidants
  breast health and 571
  causes 274-5
  eggs susceptible to 100
  hormones and 278-80
  infertility 101
  melatonin and 370
  oestrogen and 278-9, 286
  ovaries and 277, 280, 284, 524, 527
  over-exercising 101
  reducing 282-6, 399
oxytocin 220, 240, 645, 683-8
  wellness action plan 686-8

## P

palpitations 126, 157, 196-9
panic attacks 339-41
parasympathetic nervous system 114, 294, 295, 337
  activating 339, 372, 373, 383
passionflower 143, 177, 341, 361, 657, 672
PCOS *see* polycystic ovary syndrome
pelvic floor exercises 182, 221, 247, 532
pelvic wellness 501-10
perimenopause 24, 119-47, 271
  nutrition 133, 134, 144, 271
  oestrogen decline 124, 151
  ovaries retiring 122, 124, 126, 127
  phases, overview 123-7
  pregnancy during 141, 142
perimenopause phase one 124-35
  herbal support 132-3
  lifestyle support 134
  mood swings and irritability 127
  progesterone decline 124-35, 279
  sleep 127, 129, 134, 363
  support team 131
  symptoms 125, 127-8
  wellness action plan 132-5
perimenopause phase two 124-6, 135-47
  herbal support 143
  monitoring and support 146
  oestrogen dominance 124, 135-47, 279
  progesterone replacement therapy 139-41, 143
  symptoms 125-6, 136-7
  wellness action plan 137, 139, 143-7
perimenopause phase three 124, 126, 147, 150-7
  menopause transition *see* menopause
period tracking 31, 33, 37, 69, 71, 97
periods *see* menstrual cycle
personal growth 331
PFAS 145, 398, 441-2, 481-2
pheromones 116, 217-18
phospholipids 82, 638
phytoestrogens 86, 161, 175, 226, 230, 242, 248, 399, 404, 424
  breast cancer and 587
  breast health 574, 576
  ovarian health 527
  uterine health 521
Pilates 59, 60, 88-92, 144, 210, 247, 491, 493
pituitary glands 22
plant-based diet 393-5, 397, 399-404
PMDD *see* premenstrual dysphoric disorder
PMS *see* premenstrual syndrome
polycystic ovary syndrome (PCOS) 23, 75, 286, 546-63
  cortisol and 553-4
  epigenetics and lifestyle 270, 431, 551
  fatty liver disease and 596

melatonin and 368
nutrition 552, 556-9
stress and 291, 553
symptom checklist 550-1
wellness action plan 556-63
polyunsaturated fats (PUFAs) 416-20
pomegranate 171, 284, 404
positive affirmations 317
positive thoughts 315
post-menopause *see* Age of Wisdom
postnatal recovery 107-9, 163, 685
postnatal thyroiditis 603, 607
posture 208
potassium 197, 336, 468
prebiotics 56, 425, 426, 503, 505, 653
preconception health 23, 111-15
pre-eclampsia 463
pregnancy 71, 94-115
   B-vitamins 403, 412
   calcium 470, 471
   folate and 403, 412
   iron deficiency 453, 459, 461
   melatonin and 368
   oestrogen, role of 34, 69
   oxytocin, role of 684-5
   perimenopause, during 141, 142
   postnatal recovery 107-9, 163
   postnatal thyroiditis 603, 607
   progesterone, role of 35, 36, 69
   stress management 102
   unintended/unexpected 95, 142, 163, 316
   vaginal health 504-5
premenstrual dysphoric disorder (PMDD) 75, 76 153
   GABA and 670
   wellness action plan 80-3
premenstrual syndrome (PMS) 39, 75-83
   cortisol and 344, 346
   GABA and 670
   PMS-like symptoms in puberty 36, 39
   stress and 75, 79, 291
   symptoms 42, 45, 64, 77-9
   wellness action plan 80-3
probiotics 80, 183, 226, 397, 425, 503, 650, 653
processed foods, avoiding 57, 81, 114, 283
progesterone
   Age of Wisdom, ideal level 240
   balancing with oestrogen 226, 228
   bone health 619, 629
   early menopause, 228, 233
   endometriosis management 537, 543
   fertile years 23, 64, 67-75, 79, 82-93
   luteal progesterone 83
   menopause, lower level 24, 156, 158, 196, 200
   menstrual cycle 31, 34-9, 69-74, 87
   oxidative stress and 278-9

perimenopause, decline in 24, 124, 125, 127-35
puberty 22, 31, 34-9
replacement *see* hormone replacement therapy
role of 35, 69, 99, 175
sleep and 360, 362-3
stress hormones and 291
supplementation 228-9
vaginal health 507, 510
progesterone-supporting foods 86
progressive muscle relaxation 340
Promensil 177-8, 231
Prometrium 168, 169, 610
protein 56, 57, 90, 113, 186, 189, 205, 345, 346, 614, 680
proton pump inhibitors (PPIs) 617, 618
psychological stress *see* stress
puberty 22, 27-62, 270
   cortisol management 343-4
   emotional wellbeing 51-3
   nutrition 22, 37, 48, 55-6, 270, 344
   oxidative stress 278
   periods *see* menstrual cycle
   PMS-like symptoms in 36, 39
   talking to girls about 29, 52-3
   wellness action plan 55-7
Purple Zone 292, 295, 296, 298-301, 304-5, 373

## Q

Qigong 89, 91, 376, 391, 486, 491, 493, 497

## R

rainbow diet 56
reactive oxygen species (ROS) 100, 277, 423
red clover 177-8, 231, 622, 630, 631
red light 355-6, 361, 368
Red Zone 294-7, 301, 311, 320
relaxing environment 377
rescue mindset 326, 327
restless legs 363, 450, 659
restorative practice 372-92
rewiring your brain 313, 320, 321-5
rewriting your story 309-13, 325-8
rhodiola 190, 336, 345, 348, 544, 657, 681
rites of passage 51, 52, 255-6
ROS *see* reactive oxygen species
rosehip oil 193, 370
rosmarinic acid 349

## S

sacred journey 259-65
saturated fats 81, 416, 421-2
schisandra 170, 544
selective serotonin reuptake inhibitors

(SSRIs) 179
selenium 100, 280, 283, 477, 514, 528, 563, 575, 610, 638
self-care 93, 94, 98, 108, 167, 286, 302, 306-8, 332, 375
self-revolution 309-13, 325-8
serotonin 164, 169, 185, 223, 248, 645, 648-57
   brain health and 641
   exercise to boost 186
   GABA and 646, 670
   gut health and 425, 650-2, 656
   herbal support 657
   HRT supporting 187
   melatonin and 355, 371, 645
   nutrition 185, 248, 649-54, 656
   production 649-53
   red light/sunlight and 355
   wellness action plan 655-7
serum ferritin test 456, 457
serum iron test 455, 456-7
sex drive *see* libido
sexual health 180-1, 213-21, 232
sexually transmitted infections 511-14
shift work 364-6, 368
Siegel, Daniel 50, 317
silica 194
skin 46-8, 192-4, 233, 279, 370, 371
sleep 351-66
   adrenal support 343-6
   alcohol and 176, 359, 363, 364, 365
   bedtime routine 134, 170, 175, 186, 305, 360-1
   blue/red light and 355-6, 361, 368, 640
   bone health and 628, 633
   chronotypes 353, 365
   cortisol and 169, 176, 345-7, 355
   deprivation 351, 352
   disturbances 24, 126, 127, 157, 174, 191, 232, 357, 364
   fertile years 93, 104, 108
   foods supporting 170, 362, 371
   GABA production 671
   herbal mix for 132, 137, 170, 362
   HRT benefits 164
   melatonin 99, 169-71, 205-6, 347, 355, 362, 363, 365
   menopause 157-9, 169, 170, 174, 187, 191, 201, 205, 363
   mood hormones and 647
   oestrogen, role of 34, 35
   orgasms improving 221
   perimenopause 126, 127, 132, 134, 137, 143, 363
   power naps 308
   preconception 115
   progesterone and 143, 169, 360, 362-3
   promoters 134, 170, 175, 360-3
   puberty 22, 35, 37, 55, 270, 344
   quality sleep, factors for 354-66
   saboteurs 357-60, 363, 364

serotonin and 653
shift work and 364-6
stress and lack of 198, 205, 364
support 187
temperature control 175, 356-7, 361
testosterone support 681
sleep apnoea 352, 360
sleep-wake pattern 353
smoking 272, 283, 359, 672
soy products 171, 178, 404, 420, 630
spiritual connection and growth 254-65
St John's wort 45, 82, 143, 164, 169, 171, 187, 657
St Mary's thistle 158, 522, 597
Stapper, Dr Maarten 429
steroid hormones 336
storytelling 257
strength training 59, 488, 490-2
   Age of Wisdom 246, 488, 495
   brain health 640
   early menopause 229, 231, 233
   fertile years 88-91, 488, 494
   menopause 194, 208, 208-12, 488, 495
   perimenopause 144, 145, 488
   puberty 59, 61, 488, 494
Strep vaginitis 506, 509
stress 273-333
   acute 292, 337-8
   adrenalin and 187, 196, 200, 275, 276, 291, 310, 335
   blood pressure and 244
   Blue Zone see Blue Zone (calm)
   breast health and 576
   cholesterol levels and 245
   chronic 292, 311, 343, 666
   cortisol and 102, 137, 205, 275, 282, 342-3
   destress toolkit 304-5
   development of baby, affecting 102
   distress 292
   epigenetic impact 93, 270-2, 274, 276
   eustress 292, 293
   GABA production and 672
   hormonal imbalance and 79, 83, 242, 291
   infertility and 101, 102
   IVF causing 105
   management 93, 102, 114, 133, 137, 187, 197, 235, 271, 286, 314-33
   menopause 165, 166, 179, 205
   mood hormones and 647
   orgasms reducing 221
   oxidative see oxidative stress
   palpitations 196, 197
   perimenopause 130, 133, 137, 271
   PMS and 75, 79, 291
   preconception 114-15
   psychological 275, 282, 290-333
   puberty 37, 39, 43, 270
   Purple Zone 292, 295, 296, 298-301, 304-5, 373
   real vs imagined 293
   Red Zone 294-7, 301, 311, 320, 337
   self-care to reduce 302, 306-8
   sleep and 198, 205, 364
   testosterone and 681
   Tulsi for stress relief 349-50
   types of 274-5, 292
stress hormones see also adrenaline; cortisol
   adrenal glands 335-8
   alcohol and 176, 301
   cholesterol and 245
   fertility and 101, 102, 114
   menstrual cycle and 74, 79, 88, 93
   over-exercising and 68, 101, 114, 144, 283
stress resilience 314-33
   COAL state of mind 326, 329-30
   cognitive behavioural therapy 317-20
   cortisol management 343-5
   mindfulness 187, 298, 304, 306, 321
   PCOS management 560
   personal growth 331
   rewiring your brain 313, 320, 321-5
   rewriting your story 309-13, 325-8
sugar (processed) 81, 92, 398, 430-6
   addiction to 431, 432, 436
   adrenal health and 341, 344
   alcohol and 435
   breast cancer and 586
   insulin resistance and 567
   menopause 176, 197, 200, 205, 271
   serotonin and 653, 654
   sleep and 359
sulforaphane 86, 226, 284, 285, 401, 516, 543, 577
   breast cancer 589
   liver support 598
sunlight 355-6, 672
sunscreen 47, 193, 283, 448, 536

## T

T3 (triiodothyronine) 599, 600, 604
   reverse T3 605
T4 (thyroxine) 599, 600, 604, 605
Tai Chi 345, 486, 493, 640
Tamoxifen 587-8
tampon toxins 480
temperature
   control 161, 175, 198
   hot flushes see hot flushes
   ovulation 97, 98
   pregnancy, avoiding overheating 115
   sleep environment 175, 356-7, 361
testosterone 87, 88, 240, 673-82
   bone health 629, 633, 673
   brain health 637, 637
   facial hair 192
   healthy levels 674
   libido and 673, 675, 678
   menopause 213, 674, 675-6
   nutrition 680
   oestrogen and 679
   orgasms and 220
   PCOS and 554
   perimenopause 142, 674, 675
   replacement therapy 179, 676, 679, 681
   stress and 676
   wellness action plan 680-2
thelarche 35
therapeutic bandwidth 222-3
thermostat neurons see KNDy neurons
thrush 504, 506, 509-10
thyroid 599-611
   bone health and 619
   fertile years 69, 602-3, 607
   Hashimoto's thyroiditis 279
   hormones 599, 600, 604, 605
   menopause 187, 202, 603
   oxidative stress and 277, 279
   perimenopause 279, 603, 604-5, 608
   postnatal thyroiditis 603, 607
   progesterone and 599, 601-4, 610
   puberty 35, 602, 606
   testing 609
   vitamin D and 446
   wellness action plan 609-11
thyroid-binding globulin (TBG) 602, 604
thyroid stimulating hormone (TSH) 600, 604, 606-9
topical hormones 193
total iron-binding capacity (TIBC) test 456, 457
toxic stress 292, 293, 294
toxin exposure 93, 101, 270, 271, 274, 478-84, 536
   reducing 93, 483-4, 522, 544, 560, 682
toxoplasmosis in cats 112
Traditional Chinese Medicine 41, 43, 79, 115, 131, 335, 336, 348, 362, 543
transferritin saturation test 456, 457
tryosine 664, 665
tryptophan 186, 650-3, 656
Tulsi tea 201, 341, 348, 349-50, 361, 610, 666
turmeric 248, 284, 346, 522, 573, 597, 640, 657

## U

urethral bulking agents 184
urinary alkalinisers 182, 532
urinary tract infections 126, 182, 183
ursolic acid 350
uterine fibroids 126, 517-20
uterus 517-23

## V

vaginal *Candida* (thrush) 504, 506, 509–10
vaginal dryness 126, 156, 180, 213, 217, 232, 249–50, 505, 508
vaginal health 111, 156, 180–1, 217, 249, 503–10
vaginal microbiome 180, 183, 249, 503–7
vaginal mucus 71, 97, 99, 249
vaginal odour 503–4
vaginal oestrogen cream 181, 183, 217, 250, 508, 533
vaginal oxytocin 686
vaginal pessaries 509, 510, 533
vaginal rings 117, 183, 533
vaginitis 502, 506
vaginosis 502, 506, 509–10
vagus nerve stimulation 340, 362
valerian 202, 362, 657, 670, 672
venlafaxine 230
Veoza (Fezolinetant) 179, 230
victim mindset 325, 326–7
vitamin A 284, 409, 422, 432, 515
vitamin B 80, 108, 410–15
   B1 (thiamine) 80, 185, 410, 411, 414, 415
   B2 (riboflavin) 410, 411, 414, 415, 516
   B3 (niacin) 370, 411, 413, 414, 415, 652
   B5 345, 414, 415
   B6 45, 80–2, 186, 371, 410–15, 638
   B7 414, 415
   B9 *see* folate
   B12 111, 185, 186, 371, 411–15, 432, 577, 638
   cortisol management 344, 345, 348
   deficiency checklist 413
   dopamine and 664, 665
   food sources 248, 399, 414–15, 426
   menopause 185, 186, 226, 412
   serotonin and 651, 652, 656
   testosterone support 682
   thyroid support 610
vitamin C 133, 193, 284, 370, 409, 528
   adrenal health 344, 345, 348
   brain health 638
   breast health 575
   cervical health 515
   iron absorption 459, 461
vitamin D 160, 161, 194, 445–8
   adrenal health 346
   bone health 229, 231, 233, 246, 445–7, 614, 621, 622, 627
   boosting naturally 448
   breast health 570, 575, 577
   cervical health 515
   endometriosis management 543
   food sources 422, 447–8
   insulin resistance and 567
   liver metabolising 593
   PCOS management 555, 556, 557, 562, 563
   receptors (VDRs) 445
   sleep and 363
   testing 111, 139, 627
   testosterone support 682
   thyroid support 609, 610
   wellness action plan 447
vitamin E 193, 208, 284, 422, 515, 528, 563, 575, 638
vitamin K 190, 422, 426, 614, 627
vitamin supplements 443–8
*Vitex agnus-castus see* Chaste Tree
VO2 max 209, 210, 212
vulva 501–2

## W

Walker, Dr Matt 351, 363
walking 491–2
walking meditation 390–1
water
   being near 374
   contaminants 441, 482
   filtered 398, 441–2, 482, 483
   foods rich in 175, 186, 190, 201
   rinsing food 406
   serotonin and drinking 651, 656
Wave Brilliance Chair 533
weight gain 126, 158, 203–6, 245, 271, 279, 369
weight training 59, 89, 229, 231, 233, 247
   *see also* strength training
   bone health 614, 622
what are hormones 21
whole foods 393–5, 397, 399–404
whole grains 171, 402, 404, 414
withania 68, 130, 132, 143, 170, 187, 190, 201
   adrenal support 336, 345, 348
   breast health 573
   GABA production 672
   ovarian health 528
   PCOS management 562
   sleep support 362
   testosterone support 680, 681
   thyroid support 610
women's lore 255–7
writing 258, 261, 379

## X

xenoestrogens 75, 145, 224, 225, 478–80

## Y

yoga 60, 145, 247, 258, 376, 491, 492
   adrenal health 336, 344, 346
   brain health 640
   fertile years 83, 89–92, 104
   GABA production 672
   menopause 179, 187, 209, 235
   restorative 376, 492

## Z

zinc 472–7
   bone health 627
   brain function 654
   cervical health 515
   deficiency 270, 343, 475, 651
   dopamine and 664, 665
   food sources 82, 185, 344, 346, 348, 475–6
   PCOS management 555, 556, 563
   serotonin and 650, 651, 656
   testosterone support 680
   thyroid support 609, 610
ziziphus 132, 137, 362
Zones *see* Blue Zone; Purple Zone; Red Zone

## Acknowledgments

With deep gratitude, we again thank Julie Gibbs for her unwavering encouragement and belief in our ability to bring another book to life. To the team at Simon & Schuster—thank you for believing in our vision once again and supporting the publication of our second book. We are especially grateful to our editors: Charmaine Yabsley, who worked with us on the first drafts, and Katrina O'Brien whose thorough final editing of this very big and comprehensive book helped bring clarity and consistency. Our sincere appreciation also goes to the brilliant final proofread by Puddingburn who combed through every detail. Evi O—we love your work, your creative flair once again brought our words to life. Your page designs are simple and beautiful, and make our words much easier to absorb.

To all the women whose real-life experiences are reflected in the case studies in these pages; your names have been changed but your hormonal challenges remain true. And to every woman who shared a personal story so others might benefit from your journey, we honour your courage and generosity.

**HORMONAL HARMONY: A WOMAN'S GUIDE TO PUBERTY, FERTILITY, MENOPAUSE AND BEYOND**

First published in Australia in 2025 by
Simon & Schuster (Australia) Pty Limited
Level 4, 32 York St, Sydney NSW 2000

A JULIE GIBBS BOOK
for
SIMON & SCHUSTER
New York · Amsterdam/Antwerp · London · Toronto · Sydney · New Delhi

10 9 8 7 6 5 4 3 2 1

New York Amsterdam/Antwerp London Toronto Sydney New Delhi
Visit our website at www.simonandschuster.com.au

© Dr Karen Coates and Sharon Kolkka 2025

All rights reserved. No part of this publication may be reproduced, stored in a retrieval system, or transmitted in any form or by any means, electronic, mechanical, photocopying, recording or otherwise, without prior permission of the publisher.

A catalogue record for this book is available from the National Library of Australia

ISBN: 9781761426728

Publisher: Julie Gibbs
Structural editor: Charmaine Yabsley
Copy editor: Katrina O'Brien
Cover and internal design: Evi O. Studio
Printed and bound in China by RR Donnelley

MIX
Paper | Supporting responsible forestry
FSC® C144853

The paper this book is printed on is certified against the Forest Stewardship Council® Standards. RR Donnelley (Guangdong) Printing Solutions Company Limited holds chain of custody certification NC-COC-032126. FSC® promotes environmentally responsible, socially beneficial and economically viable management of the world's forests.